Wáng Zhízhōng's 王執中

# 針灸資生經

# The Classic of Supporting Life with Acupuncture and Moxibustion

*Zhēn Jiǔ Zī Shēng Jīng*

Volumes IV - VII

Dr. Yue Lu, L.Ac., Dipl.Ac.

Lorraine Wilcox L.Ac., Ph.D.

The Chinese Medicine Database
www.cm-db.com
*Portland, Oregon*

# The Classic of Supporting Life with Acupuncture and Moxibustion

# 針灸資生經

## *Zhēn Jiǔ Zī Shēng Jīng*

Volume IV - VII

Yue Lu

Lorraine Wilcox



1017 SW Morrison #306
Portland, OR 97205 USA

COMP designation original Chinese work and English translation

Cover Design by Jonathan Schell L.Ac.
Library of Congress Cataloging-in-Publication Data:

Zhízhōng, Wáng, fl. 1140-1207
[The Classic of Supporting Life with Acupuncture and Moxibustion. English]
Zhen Jiu Zi Sheng Jing = The Classic of Supporting Life with Acupuncture and Moxibus tion/ translation Yue Lu, edit Lorraine Wilcox
p. cm.
Includes Index.
ISBN 978-0-9799552-9-7 (alk. paper)
Medicine, Chinese I. Lu, Yue. II. Title: The Classic of Supporting Life with Acupuncture and Moxibustion
III. Title: Vol. IV - VII



International Standard Book Number (ISBN): 978-0-9799552-9-7
Printed in the United States of America

# Contents

## Appendices



## Indices

# Foreword

## *The Life-Promoting Classic of Acupuncture and Moxibustion*

The *Sòng* Dynasty (960-1279) was a time when China was finally able to shake off the political upheaval of the Five Dynasties and forge ahead to rediscover the sophistication and glory last seen in the *Táng* Dynasty. Wood block printing had already been invented, and a publishing boom ensued to complement the explosion in the newly found confidence of a flourishing, cultured society. There was new hope in the air, science, philosophy, literature, art and medicine advanced with renewed vigour and purpose. It was into this world that Wáng Zhízhōng was born. A humble tutor, he made a living by teaching in schools at provincial level in Húnán 湖南 and Húběi 湖北 provinces. Due to a combination of ill health and an inquisitive nature, he developed a keen and life long interest in medicine, that led to him setting up practise to treat patients himself, gaining inspiration and insights from the classical texts available to him at the time such as the *Bronze Statue Illustrated Classic of Acupuncture Points, Prescriptions Worth a Thousand Pieces of Gold* and the *Sage-like Prescriptions of the Tài Píng Era* to name a few.

During his studies of these exalted works, he discovered certain errors that inspired him to embark upon compiling his own magnum opus, the *Life-Promoting Classic of Acupuncture and Moxibustion,* today considered amongst a dozen or so of the most important and influential of classical texts on acupuncture & moxibustion. To do this he did not confine himself solely to studying scholarly works however, but pursued his own investigations by questioning many doctors of his age, and testing his knowledge by applying what he learned in actual clinical practice. In the process he cleared up many inconsistencies in point identification, and established standardised ways of locating points on the body as well as fixing more accurately proportional measurements (including the middle joint of the middle finger cùn measurement). He included illustrations of channels along with detailed instructions on how to locate, needle and apply moxibustion to each point. Subsequently those amended guiding notes were incorporated in to the *Míng* and *Qīng* Dynasty bronze man models that formed the basis of the point locations that we use today.

Another fascinating aspect of his work that made it so well thought of and studied by later generation is its insightful and detailed case histories. These were not only derived from his own experiences (including interestingly details of his as well as members of his own family's ill health), but also from the historical sources he studied. He crystallised a wealth of clinical experience along with hundreds of appropriate acupuncture point combinations into an accessible and well-structured treatise. In it he instructs us how to treat the broadest range of diseases, covering the widest spectrum of specialities from gynaecology and gastroenterology, to dermatology and urinary disorders.

Not only did he include the tried and tested formulae that had been passed down through the ages, as was the standard approach in classical writings, but he also put forward and commented upon numerous original and innovative combinations that he developed in the course of his own practice or heard of during his studies.

In some instances he urges the reader to rely on the miraculous efficacy of prescriptions that he himself has successfully used, whilst in others, where he freely admits to only having heard of the value of a particular combination, he encourages the need to verify effectiveness by personal experience. Many of these combinations have proved their worth and are still studied and used today.

Although the *Life-Promoting Classic of Acupuncture and Moxibustion* is a product of one man's tireless efforts, dedication and scholarship, and gives us a fascinating window into the art of acupuncture and moxibustion of the *Sòng* Dynasty, it is much more than just an historical record worthy of study for the snap shot it gives us of those ancient times. This quintessentially classical work forms a significant part of a jigsaw of medical delights that create a rich backdrop of all that we apply and practice in the modern era of Chinese medicine.

The legacy of Wáng Zhízhōng and his work the *Life-Promoting Classic of Acupuncture and Moxibustion* is without question secure. Now we must be grateful to Dr. Yue Lu for her masterful translation and for making this book available to the emerging Chinese medicine community that would not otherwise have access to this foundational masterpiece. With such a celebrated classic now available for all non-Chinese readers to scrutinise, acupuncture is truly on the path to coming of age in the West.

Mazin Al-Khafaji,

Brighton, UK 2014

# Introduction to
# *Zhēn Jiǔ Zī Shēng Jīng* 《針灸資生經》

*Zhēn Jiǔ Zī Shēng Jīng* 《針灸資生經》Life-Promoting Classic of Acupuncture and Moxbustion was written by Wáng Zhízhōng 王執中 during the *Sòng* Dynasty, approximately between 1180-1195. It has seven volumes.

The author, Wáng Zhízhōng (c. 1140-1207) was from Ruì'ān 瑞安, (modern-day Wēnzhōu 温州 in Zhèjiāng 浙江 province), but he was posted as a low ranking officer in Húnán 湖南 and Húběi 湖北 where he taught in schools at the provincial level. Because he was often ill, Wáng treated himself and so began gathering medical information. In his research, he focused on the classics of acupuncture-moxibustion but collected prescriptions from the practices of the common people (including acupuncture, moxibustion, dietary, and miscellaneous treatments). He also visited local doctors and herb stores. Wáng was obviously very well-educated; in his book, he frequently cited historical cases, philosophical texts, or ancient poetry. Wáng practiced medicine himself, testing whatever he learned. He recorded what he found to be effective.

The title of the book - 'Life-Promoting' (*Zī Shēng* 資生) is a reference to people's reliance on stomach qì for life. In Volume 3, Wáng wrote, "人仰胃氣為主 。是人資胃氣以生矣 。People rely on stomach qì as the governing principle; this means people should *promote* stomach qì in order to *live*."

Volume 1 describes the location and acupuncture techniques for 365 points. The information about the points is mainly quoted from *The Bronze Statue Illustrated Classic of Acupuncture Points* and from Volumes 99 and 100 of *Sage-like Prescriptions of Tài Píng Era.*

Earlier sources often disagreed on the location of certain points. In Volume 1, Wáng compared the location from different sources and tried to verify the proper position of these points. He especially investigated the location of abdominal points and the distance of their channels from the midline. This had great influence in later generations.

Volume 2 discusses various issues, including contraindications for acupuncture, the distance between points, proportional measurement (using same-body cùn), similarities and differences in the names of points, how to locate points, and moxibustion (the number and size of cones, how to treat moxa sores, etc.). It is a general introduction to acupuncture-moxibustion. Although Wáng frequently used passages from earlier texts, most of the text of Volume 2 is Wáng's own opinion. He presented some new ideas by researching information from many different books and combining this with his own experience.

Volumes 3 through 7 provide point indications and point prescriptions arranged according to categories of disorder. Those volumes cite the many earlier texts including *Sage-like Prescriptions of Tài Píng Era, Prescriptions Worth a Thousand Piece of Gold* and *Supplement to Prescriptions Worth a Thousand Piece of Gold*, and *The Bronze Statue*. As in the earlier volumes, Wáng compared similar passages from these books, noting and differences.

Throughout the book, Wáng is quite concerned with comparing words and phrases from various sources, trying to parse out which is correct. This was not only an issue for Wáng, but it is also an issue in translation. Because Wáng used so many different sources, both ancient and contemporary, terminology was inconsistent. Various sources may have used different terms for the same thing (point names, symptoms, diseases, and so forth) or the same term for different things. Wáng wrote many paragraphs musing over this and it was also an issue for the translator. Footnotes have been added to clarify, when possible.

Wáng included many case studies in the later volumes. Some are historical, some from people he knew or had treated, and many were about himself or his mother. Through these cases, we see glimpses of what treatment actually looked like during the *Sòng* Dynasty. We also get to know a little of Wáng Zhízhōng's personality, which is especially evident in the cases. These case studies and 'secret' formulas that were recorded made *Zī Shēng Jīng* popular in later generations.

Although acupuncture and moxibustion are both in the title of the book, it is obvious that Wáng gave as much or more respect to moxibustion as to acupuncture. He also often described herbal treatment in his own comments or in the case studies.

*Zī Shēng Jīng* influenced authors for hundreds of years, even up to the present. Here are some of the contributions that are still used today:

- Wáng gave references for all his sources and also made it obvious when he himself was commenting. This was quite unusual at the time.
- Wáng promoted proportional measurement, especially the use of the middle joint of the middle finger as one cùn.
- Wáng organized indications and point formulas according to category of disorder, so the book was easy to use in the clinic.
- Wáng corrected the location of many points, especially those on the abdomen. Many later books followed his point locations, including Huá Shí's *Sì Jīng Fā Huī* 滑壽《十四經發揮》, Gāo Wǔ's *Zhēn Jiǔ Jù Yīng* 高武《針灸聚英》, Xú Fèng's *Zhēn Jiǔ Dà Quán* 徐鳳《針灸人全》, and Yang Jizhou's *Zhen Jiu Dà Chéng* 楊繼洲《針灸大成》.

- Wáng discussed various types of contraindications. At that time, it was popular to calculate certain days when acupuncture was prohibited. Wáng was not opposed to this in principle, but felt that in urgent cases, the prohibitions could be ignored. Besides this, some points had contraindications, for example moxibustion might be forbidden on a particular point. But if moxibustion seemed to be indicated, especially in an urgent case, the contraindication need not be followed. See Xīn Shù 心俞 (UB 15) and Tiān Yǒu 天牖 (SJ 16) in Volume 1.

- In Volume 2, Wáng discussed *ā shì* points or treatment of the affected area. Sūn Sīmiǎo 孫思邈 had mentioned *ā shì* points earlier, but Wáng contributed to the theory, and added specific examples in the volumes on treatment. He suggested pressing Fèi Shù 肺俞 (UB 13) for wheezing and asthma, Dàn Zhōng 膻中 (Rèn 17) for cough, Tiān Shū 天樞 (UB 25) for intestinal abscess, Dài Mài 帶脈 (GB 26) for abnormal vaginal discharge, and so forth. If these points were found to be sore, they would be effective.

Overall, having a translation *Zhēn Jiǔ Zī Shēng Jīng* is a great contribution to the community of English-speaking practitioners of Chinese medicine.

## Acknowledgements

I would like to express my appreciation to Lorraine Wilcox. I thank her for encouraging my work. Her comments and suggestions on the translation have been priceless. Without her help, this book would not have been possible.

I would also like to thank Jerome Jiang for his help during the translation. His knowledge of ancient literature is impressive.

A special thanks also goes to Jonathan Schell for introducing this ancient Chinese acupuncture classic to the English-speaking world.

Finally, I would like to express appreciation to my family. Your support is what has sustained me thus far and given me incentive to work towards my goal.

# Publisher's Note

A few things about this book:

1) Notes in the lateral margin. These are the Chinese characters for the section headings which Wáng included in the text, for example: ( 見尸厥 ) which means (see the section on deathlike reversal). In the lateral margin, you will see the Chinese character for 尸厥 and underneath it, a number. This is the page number for this section. We hope that by including these, it makes the book more usable, and let's the reader quickly check Wáng's reference. For the sake of brevity, if the reference appears twice on a single page, it is only displayed once in the lateral margin, in the order with which it appears in the Chinese text on that page.

2) On a page by page basis, when characters were repeated, such as with point names, we have chosen not to repeat them in the second instance. Thus, under the Chinese passage, in the English translation, if Pū Cān 僕參 (UB 61) is mentioned, then on the second reference on the same page, it will appear as Pū Cān (UB 61). This is the same with book titles, so if on the first instance it reads (*Qiān* 《千》), then on the second instance for that page it will read (*Qiān*). These are not mistakes, only an effort to save space. It was apparent from the outset that this was going to be a very large, and very dense book, therefore we instigated methods from the beginning to try to keep the size of the book manageable.

3) We have chosen to break this book into two volumes, even though in its original state it would have comprised a single book of seven volumes. For this material we decided it was better to have two 400+ page books, then it would to be have one 1,000 page book. The book you hold in your hands, has the full Table of Contents, as well as a master index for both books. The index as you will note spans a massive 137 pages. To some, this may seem excessive, but to the clinician-scholar, ease of access to the information you want, is everything. The index is large, because it not only covers numerous indications and patterns of Chinese medicine (some of which have never been translated before), but also serves as a gloss for the student and researcher of Chinese medicine. We have included the foreword and introduction in both books, in the off case that someone only purchases one of the two volume set. The page numbers of the two books are sequential from the end of chapter 3, to the beginning of chapter 4 of the next book. At the end of this book, the page numbers of the appendix and index begin at page A-1. Thus, these sections are not part of the final page numbering of the content of the two volumes.

Jonathan Schell L.Ac.
Publisher
August 8th, 2015

*Zhēn Jiǔ Zī Shēng Jīng*

# 《針灸資生經·第一》

# 4.01
## *Xīn Tòng*
## 心痛
## Heart pain

凡心實者，則心中暴痛，虛則心煩惕然不能動，失智，內關主之（《千》）。凡卒心痛，汗出，刺大敦出血立已。心俞、膻中、通谷、巨闕、太倉、神府、郄門、曲澤、大陵主心痛。期門、長強、天突、俠白、中衝主心痛短氣。尺澤主心痛膨膨然，心煩亂悶，少氣不足息。然谷主心如懸，少氣不足以息。

In repletion of the heart, there is violent pain of the heart; in vacuity, there is vexation of the heart, fear with inability to move, and dementia; Nèi Guān 內關 (PC 6) governs it (*Qiān*《千》).

For sudden heart pain and sweating, bleeding Dà Dūn 大敦 (LV 1) immediately cures the disease.

Xīn Shù 心俞 (UB 15), Dàn Zhōng 膻中 (Rèn 17), Tōng Gǔ 通谷 (KI 20 or UB 66), Jù Quē 巨闕 (Rèn 14), Tài Cāng 太倉 (Rèn 12), Shén Fǔ 神府 (Rèn 15), Xī Mén 郄門 (PC 4), Qū Zé 曲澤 (PC 3), and Dà Líng 大陵 (PC 7) govern heart pain.

Qī Mén 期門 (LV 14), Cháng Qiáng 長強 (Dū 1), Tiān Tū 天突 (Rèn 22), Xiá Bái 俠白 (LU 4), and Zhōng Chōng 中衝 (PC 9) govern heart pain and shortness of breath.

Chǐ Zé 尺澤 (LU 5) governs heart pain with a feeling of inflation, vexation of the heart and oppression, qì shortage, and inability to breath.

Rán Gǔ 然谷 (KI 2) governs a feeling as if the heart is suspended, qì shortage, and inability to breathe.

心悶痛，上氣牽引小腸：灸巨闕二七壯。腎俞、復溜、大陵、雲門主心痛如懸。間使主心懸如飢。支溝、太溪、然谷主心痛如錐刺，甚者手足寒至節者死。行間主心痛，色蒼蒼然如死灰狀，終日不得太息（《銅》）。鳩尾主心寒脹滿不得食，息賁唾血，厥心痛，善噦，心疝太息。中管主心痛，難俯仰（《甲》云：身寒心疝衝胃，死不知人）。

Heart pain and oppression, and pulling qì ascent that radiates to the small intestine: Apply two times seven cones of moxibustion on Jù Quē 巨闕 (Rèn 14).

臍 466 腹痛 441

Shèn Shù 腎俞 (UB 23), Fù Liū 復溜 (KI 7), Dà Líng 大陵 (PC 7), and Yún Mén 雲門 (LU 2) govern heart pain when the heart feels like it has been suspended.

Jiān Shǐ 間使 (PC 5) governs a feeling as if the heart is suspended and as if famished.[1]

Zhī Gōu 支溝 (SJ 6), Tài Xī 太溪 (KI 3), and Rán Gǔ 然谷 (KI 2) govern heart pain that feels like being punctured by an awl; in a severe case, the patient will die when his hands and feet become cold up to the joints.

Xíng Jiān 行間 (LV 2) governs heart pain, pale complexion that looks like a dying ember, and inability to sigh all day long (*Tóng* 《銅》 agrees).

Jiū Wěi 鳩尾 (Rèn 15) governs coldness, distention and fullness of the heart, inability to eat, rushing respiration and spitting of blood, reversal heart pain, frequent hiccups, heart *shàn*-mounting, and sighing.

Zhōng Guǎn 中管 (Rèn 12) governs heart pain and difficulty bending forward and backward (*Jiǎ* 《甲》 says: generalized cold, heart *shàn*-mounting surging upward into the stomach, and unconsciousness).

臨泣主胸痹心痛，不得反側（《甲》云：不得息，痛無常處）。腹結（見臍）、行間（見腹痛）主痛搶心。通里主卒痛煩心，心中懊憹，數欠頻伸，心下悸悲（《千》與《銅》同）。靈道主心痛，悲恐相引，瘛瘲。

Lín Qì 臨泣 (GB 41) governs chest *bì*-impediment with heart pain, and inability to turn to the sides (*Jiǎ* says: inability to breathe and pain without a fixed location).

Fù Jié 腹結 (SP 14) (see the section on the umbilical [pain]) and Xíng Jiān 行間 (LV 2) (see the section on abdominal pain) govern pain prodding the heart.

Tōng Lǐ 通里 (Rèn 11) governs sudden pain, vexation and anguish in the heart, frequent yawning and stretching, palpitations, and sorrow below the heart (*Qiān* 《千》 and *Tóng* agree).

Líng Dào 靈道 (HT 4) governs heart pain, sorrow and fear affecting each other, and tugging and slackening.

1. Zhāng Jièbīn 張介賓 commented on this in the *Categorized Classic*: "When the heart and kidneys do not communicate, essence and spirit separate and scatter. Thus the heart is suspended. When there is yīn vacuity, the interior is hungry, so it is constantly as if it were famished."

胸痹 476
心滿 445
胸脅 449

建里主心痛上搶心，不欲食（《明》云：心痛身腫）。章門主心痛而嘔。太泉主心痛肺脹，胃氣上逆。鳩尾主心寒脹滿，不得食。大都、太白主暴泄心痛，腹脹，心痛尤甚。上管主心痛，有三蟲，多涎，不得反側。不容、期門主心切痛，喜噫酸。

Jiàn Lǐ 建里 (Rèn 11) governs heart pain prodding upward into the heart with no desire to eat (*Míng*《明》says: heart pain and generalized swelling).

Zhāng Mén 章門 (LV 13) governs heart pain and vomiting.

Tài Quán 太泉 (LU 9) governs heart pain, lung distention, and counterflow ascent of stomach qì.

Jiū Wěi 鳩尾 (Rèn 15) governs coldness, distention, and fullness of the heart, and inability to eat.

Dà Dōu 大都 (SP 2) and Tài Bái 太白 (SP 3) govern violent diarrhea, heart pain, and abdominal distention, but especially serious heart pain.

Shàng Guǎn 上管 (Rèn 13) governs heart pain, the three worm diseases,[2] copious drool, and inability to turn to the sides.

Bù Róng 不容 (ST 19) and Qī Mén 期門 (LV 14) govern cutting pain of the heart and frequent belching of sour fluids.

少衝主心痛而寒。商丘主心下有寒痛。胸痹心痛：天井、臨泣主之；或灸膻中百壯（見胸痹）。膻中、天井主胸心痛。心腹諸病，心痛：灸太倉、肝俞（見心滿）。心腹胸滿痞痛：灸肝俞（見胸脅脹）。中管治心痛（《銅》見心滿）。

Shào Chōng 少衝 (HT 8) governs heart pain and coldness.

Shāng Qiū 商丘 (SP 5) governs coldness and pain below the heart.

Chest *bì*-impediment with heart pain: Tiān Jǐng 天井 (SJ 10) and Lín Qì 臨泣 (GB 41) can govern it; or apply a hundred cones of moxibustion on Dàn Zhōng 膻中 (Rèn 17) (see the section on chest *bì*-impediment pain).

Dàn Zhōng (Rèn 17) and Tiān Jǐng (SJ 10) govern pain of the chest and heart.

Diseases of the heart and abdomen, as well as heart pain: Apply moxibustion on Tài Cāng 太倉 (Rèn 12) and Gān Shù 肝俞 (UB 18) (see the section on fullness [and distention] of the heart).

2. The three worm diseases indicate infection with *cháng chóng* 長蟲 [long worms - ascaris lumbricoides], *chì chóng* 赤蟲 [red worms - fascidopsiasis] and *náo chóng* 蟯蟲 [called pinworms in the US and threadworms in the UK - enterobius].

Fullness, glomus, and pain of the heart, abdomen, and chest: Apply moxibustion on Gān Shù 肝俞 (UB 18) (see the section on distention of the chest and rib-sides).

痃癖 433
月事 735

Zhōng Guǎn 中管 (Rèn 12) treats heart pain (see the section on fullness [and distention] of the heart) in *Tóng*《銅》).

建里療心痛(《明》見上氣)。膈俞治心痛周痹(見痃癖)。足臨泣治心痛周痹，痛無常處(見月事)。魚際療心痹(《明》見氣逆)。

Jiàn Lǐ 建里 (Rèn 11) cures heart pain (see the section on qì ascent in *Míng*《明》).

Gé Shù 膈俞 (UB 17) treats heart pain and generalized *bì*-impediment (see the section on strings and aggregations).

Zú Lín Qì 足臨泣 (GB 41) treats heart pain and generalized *bì*-impediment, the pain is without a fixed location (see the section on menstruation).

Yú Jì 魚際 (LU 10) cures heart *bì*-impediment (see the section on qì counterflow in *Míng*).

荊婦舊侍親疾，累日不食，因得心脾疼。發則攻心腹，後心痛亦應之，至不可忍，則與兒女別。以藥飲之，疼反甚；若灸則遍身不勝灸矣。不免令兒女各以火針微刺之，不拘心腹，須臾痛定，即欲起矣，神哉。

[Author's notes:] Once there was a lady from Jīng [Prefecture] who took care of her sick parents. The daughter had not been able to eat for a couple of days, and suffered pain of the heart and spleen. When the pain occurred, it attacked her heart and abdomen, and also responded with pain behind the heart; this became unbearable. [The daughter thought she was dying] so she bid farewell to her children. Her pain worsened after drinking herbs; and her body could not bear moxibustion either. So I asked her children to puncture her gently with a fire needle, without restrictions for the heart or abdomen [areas]. The pain stopped after a while and she wanted to get up. It was a miracle.

治心腹冷痛，玉抱肚法：針砂四兩，炒似煙出；入白礬半兩，硇砂、粉霜各半錢，新水拌勻，微濕，以皮紙貼安懷中。候熱發，置臍中，氣海、石門、關元穴，大補本元。或置其他冷處，汗出立瘥(予自用驗)。此藥燥則不熱，再以新水拌，再熱。可用十餘次。如藥力盡，卻曝乾，再入礬等，依舊熱。舍弟叔浩傳一方：只用針砂、泥礬，功效亦同，豈以硇砂、粉霜價不廉而不用耶。

To treat cold pain of the heart and abdomen, *yù bào dù* 玉抱肚 (jade holding the abdomen) method can be used: stir-fry 4 *liǎng* of *zhēn shā* 針砂 [needle filings - acus pulvis] until they seem to be smoking; then add 0.5 *liǎng* of *bái fán* 白礬 [alum - alumen], and 0.5 *qián* each of *gāng shā* 硇砂 [sal ammoniac - ammonium chloride][3] and refined calomel; blend with fresh water till it is slightly moist. Then stick it on bark paper and put on the chest. Wait until it becomes hot, then apply it on the center of the umbilicus, as well as on Qì Hǎi 氣海 (Rèn 6), Shí Mén 石門 (Rèn 5), and Guān Yuán 關元 (Rèn 4). It will strongly supplement the root and origin. Or apply it to other cold sites; it will cure the disease immediately once there is sweating. (I used this on myself and it was effective). This medicine will not be hot when it dries out; but it will become hot again when mixed with fresh water once more. This method can be repeated more than ten times. When the medicinal strength is gone, dry it in the sun and add *fán* [alum], etc; it will get hot again. My younger brother Shūhào gave me a formula that only uses *zhēn shā* [needle filings - acus pulvis] and *ní fán* 泥礬, but has same effects. How can we not use *lǔ shā* 硵砂 [sal ammoniac - ammonium chloride] and refined calomel, just because they are expensive?

予舊患心痹，發則疼不可忍。急用瓦片置炭火中，燒令通紅，取出投米醋中，漉出，以紙三二重裹之，置疼處，稍止，冷即再易。耆舊所傳也，後閱《千金方》，有云：凡心腹冷痛，熬鹽一半熨。或熬蠶砂、燒磚石蒸熨，取其里溫暖止；或蒸土亦大佳。始知予家所用，蓋出《千金方》也。它日心疼甚，急灸中管數壯，覺小腹兩邊有冷氣自下而上，至灸處即散，此灸之功也。《本事方》載王思和論心忪，非心忪也。胃之大絡，名曰建里，絡胸膈及兩乳間，虛而有痰則動，更須臾發一陣熱，是其證也。審若是，又當灸建里矣。但不若中管為要穴云。

[Author's notes:] I suffered heart *bì*-impediment before. The pain was unbearable when it occurred. I put a tile into a charcoal fire and let it burn until it became completely red. Then I took it out and threw it into vinegar. Then, I wrapped it with two or three layers of the paper and applied it on the painful area. The pain decreased. The tile is changed when it becomes cold. This was passed down from old. Later, I read in *Qiān Jīn Fāng* 《千金方》 where it says: For all cold pain of the heart and abdomen, partially dry-fry salt and iron the patient with it. Or dry-fry *cán shā* 蠶砂 [silkworm droppings - bombycis faeces] or roast a brick, then steam or iron the patient. The pain will stop after warming with them. Or steaming earth [in a hot pack] is also very good. I didn't realize the method I used before is from *Qiān Jīn Fāng*.

I suffered severe heart pain the other day. I applied several cones of moxibustion on Zhōng Guǎn 中管 (Rèn 12), then I felt cold qì surging upward from the sides of my smaller abdomen, and scattering when it arrived at the moxibustion site. This is the effect of moxibustion.

3. *Gāng shā* 硇砂 should be *lǔ shā* 硵砂 according to *Shì Zhāi Bǎi Yī Xuǎn Fāng* 《是齋百一選方》 (One in a Hundred Formulas Selected by Shì Zhāi) by Wáng Qíu 王璆 whose penname was Shì Zhāi, published in 1196.

[*Pǔ Jì*] *Běn Shì Fāng*《本事方》recorded the discussion about heart palpitations by Wáng Sīhé 王思和, but that was not really heart palpitations. The great network vessel of the stomach is named Jiàn Lǐ 建里 (Rèn 11).[4] It connects the chest, diaphragm, and both breasts. In vacuity, there is phlegm which then stirs; and there are bouts of heat occurring later. These are the symptoms [mentioned by Wáng Sīhé]. If the case looks like this, we should apply moxibustion on Jiàn Lǐ (Rèn 11). But this is not as important as Zhōng Guǎn 中管 (Rèn 12).

霍亂 267
咳逆 417
煩心 335
月事 735
上氣 420
腹痛 441
腸鳴 263

靈道治心痛，悲恐相引，瘈瘲肘攣，暴喑不能言。俠白治心痛，乾嘔煩滿。極泉治心痛乾嘔。太淵治心痛唾血，振寒咽乾，狂言口僻。陰郄（見霍亂）、中衝治心痛煩滿，舌強。厥陰俞（見咳逆）、神門（見煩心）、臨泣治心痛（見月事）。

Líng Dào 靈道 (HT 4) treats heart pain with sorrow and fear affecting each other, tugging and slackening, hypertonicity of the elbows, sudden loss of voice and inability to speak.

Xiá Bái 俠白 (LU 4) treats heart pain, dry vomiting, vexation and fullness.

Jí Quán 極泉 (HT 1) treats heart pain and dry vomiting.

Tài Yuān 太淵 (LU 9) treats heart pain, spitting of blood, quivering with cold, dry throat, manic raving, and deviation of the mouth.

Yīn Xī 陰郄 (HT 6) (see the section on cholera [sudden turmoil disease]) and Zhōng Chōng 中衝 (PC 9) treat heart pain, vexation and fullness, and stiffness of the tongue.

Jué Yīn Shù 厥陰俞 (UB 14) (see the section on coughing counterflow), Shén Mén 神門 (HT 7) (see the section on vexation of the heart), and Lín Qì 臨泣 (GB 41) treat heart pain (see the section on menstruation).

齦交治面赤心煩痛。天井治心胸痛（見上氣）。下管治心痛不可忍。外陵治心如懸下痛（見腹痛）。大陵、上管治心痛不可忍（《明》云不可臥）。章門治喘息心痛（見腸鳴）。涌泉、建里治心下痛，不欲食（許云：心疼是有涎，宜針建里）。幽門治女子心痛，逆氣善吐，食不下。期門治產餘疾，食不下，胸脅滿，心切痛，善噫。

Yín Jiāo 齦交 (Dū 28) treats red face, vexation, and pain of the heart.

Tiān Jǐng 天井 (SJ 10) treats pain of the heart and chest (see the section on qì ascent).

Xià Guǎn 下管 (Rèn 10) treats unbearable heart pain.

4. *Sù Wèn*《素問》Chapter 18 says: The great network vessel of the stomach is named Xū Lǐ 虛里, not Jiàn Lǐ 建里 (Rèn 11).

唾血 402 Wài Líng 外陵 (ST 26) treats a feeling like the heart is suspended and pain below the heart (see 腹痛 441 the section on abdominal pain).

痰飲 399 Dà Líng 大陵 (PC 7) and Shàng Guǎn 上管 (Rèn 13) treat unbearable heart pain (*Míng*《明》says: inability to lie down).

Zhāng Mén 章門 (LV 13) treats panting breath and heart pain (see the section on rumbling intestines).

Yǒng Quán 涌泉 (KI 1) and Jiàn Lǐ 建里 (Rèn 11) treat pain below the heart and no desire to eat (Xǔ[5] said: When there is heart pain with drooling, it is appropriate to needle Jiàn Lǐ (Rèn 11)).

Yōu Mén 幽門 (KI 21) treats heart pain in women, qì counterflow with frequent vomiting, and difficulty getting food down.

Qī Mén 期門 (LV 14) treats diseases after childbirth, difficulty getting food down, fullness of the chest and rib-sides, cutting pain of the heart, and frequent belching.

巨闕療凡心痛有數種：冷痛、蛔蟲心痛、蠱毒、霍亂不識人(《明》)。《銅》云：治蛔蟲心痛，蠱毒。中管治心匿不能食，反胃，霍亂心痛。曲澤(見唾血)、督俞(見腹痛)、膈俞(見痰飲)療心痛。

Jù Quē 巨闕 (Rèn 14) cures several types of heart pain: cold pain, heart pain caused by roundworms, *gǔ*-toxins, sudden turmoil [cholera], and loss of consciousness (*Míng*). *Tóng*《銅》says: It treats heart pain caused by roundworms and *gǔ*-toxins.

Zhōng Guǎn 中管 (Rèn 12) cures heart *nì*,[6] inability to eat, stomach reflux, sudden turmoil [cholera], and heart pain.

Qū Zé 曲澤 (PC 3) (see the section on spitting of blood), Dū Shù 督俞 (UB 16) (see the section on abdominal pain), and Gé Shù 膈俞 (UB 17) (see the section on phlegm-rheum) cure heart pain.

涌泉療心痛不嗜食。少衝療卒心痛。心俞療寒熱心痛，背相引痛，胸滿悶，咳嗽不得息，煩心多涎。巨闕療心痛不可忍，嘔血煩心(《下》)。張仲文療卒心痛不可忍，吐冷酸水，及元藏氣：灸足大指、次指內橫文中各一壯，炷如小麥，立愈。

5. Xǔ 許 refers to Xǔ Shūwēi 許叔微, the author of *Pǔ Jì Běn Shì Fāng*《普濟本事方》(Skillful Formulas for Universal Salvation). See the book appendix.

6. The meaning of this symptom is unclear. *Xīn nì* 心匿 could be a typographical error for *xīn nì* 心䘌, which is a disease with heart pain, fullness, and vexation, as well as cold limbs and hands. It is caused by qì vacuity of the viscera and a warm attack of the intestines.

Yǒng Quán 涌泉 (KI 1) cures heart pain with no desire to eat.

Shào Chōng 少衝 (HT 9) cures sudden heart pain.

Xīn Shù 心俞 (UB 15) cures pain, cold or hot heart pain, pain radiating to the back, fullness and oppression of the chest, cough and inability to breathe, vexation of the heart, and copious drool.

Jù Quē 巨闕 (Rèn 14) cures unbearable heart pain, vomiting of blood, and vexation of the heart (*Xià*《下》). Zhāng Zhòngwén treated sudden unbearable heart pain and vomiting of cold sour water, as well as *yuán zàng qì* 元藏氣[7]: apply one cone of moxibustion on the transverse crease inside the big toe and second toe. The cones should be the size of a grain of wheat. This will cure the disease immediately.

心懊憹憹，微痛煩逆：灸心俞百壯（《千》）。心痛如錐刀刺，氣結：灸膈俞七壯。心痛冷氣上：灸龍頷百壯，在鳩尾頭上行一寸半，不可刺。心痛惡氣上脅急痛：灸通谷五十壯，在乳下二寸。心痛暴絞，急絕欲死：灸神府百壯，在鳩尾正心，有忌。

Heart anguish, mild pain, vexation, and counterflow: Apply a hundred cones of moxibustion on Xīn Shù (UB 15) (*Qiān*《千》).

Heart pain that feels like the piercing of an awl, qì binding: Apply seven cones of moxibustion on Gé Shù 膈俞 (UB 17).

Heart pain and ascent of cold qì: Apply a hundred cones of moxibustion on Lóng Hàn 龍頷 (Dragon's Chin) which is located 1.5 cùn above the tip of the xyphoid. Acupuncture is not allowed.

Heart pain and evil qì ascending to the rib-sides with acute pain: Apply fifty cones of moxibustion on Tōng Gǔ 通谷 (KI 20), which is located 2 cùn below the nipple.

Heart pain with a violent gripping feeling, quickly expiring, and about to die: Apply a hundred cones of moxibustion on Shén Fǔ 神府 (Rèn 15), right in the center of the xiphoid. There are contraindications.

心痛暴惡風：灸巨闕百壯。心痛堅煩氣結：灸太倉百壯。心痛：灸臂腕橫文三七壯，又灸兩虎口白肉際七壯（《千》）。腎心痛：先取京骨、崑崙，發針不已，取然谷。胃心痛：取大都、太白。脾心痛：取然谷、太溪。肝心痛：取行間、太衝。肺心痛：取魚際、太淵。

7. *Yuán zàng qì* 元藏氣: This phrase literally says *original storage qì* or *original visceral qì*. It is possible that 元 is a typographical error for *wǔ* 五 (five), in which case it would mean *qì of the five viscera*. In any case, the exact meaning of this phrase is unknown.

驚 323 Heart pain with sudden aversion to wind: Apply a hundred cones of moxibustion on Jù Quē 巨闕 (Rèn 14).

Heart pain, hardness, vexation, and qì binding: Apply a hundred cones of moxibustion on Tài Cāng 太倉 (Rèn 12).

Heart pain: Apply three times seven cones of moxibustion on the transverse crease between the arm and wrist; seven cones of moxibustion can also be applied on the border of the white flesh at the two tiger mouths (*Qiān*《千》).

Kidney and heart pain: needle Jīng Gǔ 京骨 (UB 64) and Kūn Lún 崑崙 (UB 60) first; if not effective, then select Rán Gǔ 然谷 (KI 2).

Stomach and heart pain: select Dà Dū 大都 (SP 2) and Tài Bái 太白 (SP 3).

Spleen and heart pain: select Rán Gǔ (KI 2) and Tài Xī 太溪 (KI 3).

Liver and heart pain: select Xíng Jiān 行間 (LV 2) and Tài Chōng 太衝 (LV 3).

Lung and heart pain: select Yú Jì 魚際 (LU 10) and Tài Yuān 太淵 (LU 9).

心痛不可按，煩心：巨闕主之。心痛有三蟲，多涎，不得反側：上管主之。心痛身寒，難以俯仰，心疝衝冒，死不知人，中管主之。心痛如針錐刺，然谷及太溪主之。心腹中卒痛：石門主之。行間、陰郄主心痛（見驚）。

Heart pain that cannot be pressed, with vexation of the heart: Jù Quē (Rèn 14) governs it.

Heart pain with the three worms, copious drooling, and inability to turn to the sides: Shàng Guǎn 上管 (Rèn 13) governs it.

Heart pain with generalized cold, difficulty bending forward and backward, heart *shàn*-mounting surging upward, and unconsciousness: Zhōng Guǎn 中管 (Rèn 12) governs it.

Heart pain that feels like the piercing of an awl: Rán Gǔ (KI 2) and Tài Xī (KI 3) govern it.

Sudden pain of the heart and abdomen: Shí Mén 石門 (Rèn 5) governs it.

Xíng Jiān (LV 2) and Yīn Xī 陰郄 (HT 6) govern heart pain (see the section on [heart] fright [and fear]).

間使治卒心痛，多驚，喑不得語，咽中如鯁（《銅》）。曲澤治心痛善驚。郄門治心痛衄血，嘔噦，驚恐畏人，神氣不足。天泉治心病，胸脅支滿咳逆，膺背胛臂內廉痛。太溪治久瘧咳逆，心痛如錐刺，手足寒至節，喘息者死。

Jiān Shǐ 間使 (PC 5) treats sudden heart pain, frequent fright, loss of voice with inability to speak, and feeling like a fishbone is stuck in the throat (*Tóng*《銅》).

Qū Zé 曲澤 (PC 3) treats heart pain with susceptibility to fright.

Xī Mén 郄門 (PC 4) treats heart pain and nosebleeds, vomiting and retching, fright and fear of people, and insufficiency of spirit qì.

Tiān Quán 天泉 (PC 2) treats heart disease, propping fullness of the chest and rib-sides, coughing counterflow, and pain of the chest, back, scapula and medial aspect of the arm.

Tài Xī 太溪 (KI 3) treats enduring malaria, coughing counterflow, heart pain that feels like the piercing of an awl, and cold hands and feet up to the joints. People who are panting may die.

心痛有九種，乃心脾疼，而非真心痛。真心痛則朝發夕死，夕發朝死，如《難經疏》所載是已。然此疾亦有所自。《產論》嘗謂產後心痛，若誤以為有所傷療之，則虛極而心絡寒甚，傳心之正經，則變為真心痛。此一說也。巫臣以夏姬之故，怨子反曰：余必使汝疲於奔命以死。子反於是一歲七奔命，遂遇心疾而卒。則又因用心而成疾矣，然則如之何。平居當養其心，使之和平，疾自不作。其次，則當服鎮心丹之類，以補養之可也，若疾將作而針灸，抑亦可以為次矣。

[Author's notes:] There are nine types of heart pain; [one is] heart and spleen pain, but this is not true heart pain. True heart pain arises in the morning and the patient dies in the evening; or arises in the evening and the patient dies in the morning. This is just like what was written in *Nàn Jīng Shū*《難經疏》. This disease also has its causes. Once *Chǎn Lùn*《產論》(Discussion on Obestetry) said: As for heart pain after childbirth, if it is mistakenly taken as damage [from childbirth] and treated, the patient will become severely vacuous and the heart networks will be extremely cold. When the cold transfers to the heart's primary channel, it becomes true heart pain. This is one theory. Because of Concubine Xià, Wū Chén complained about Zǐ Fǎn saying[8]: I must let you die of tiredness from constantly running around. Zǐ Fǎn had to run around seven times a year, and so he died from heart disease. The disease also could have been caused by using the heart-mind too much [excessive mental work]. Then what could be done? People should nourish their heart in daily life, making it calm and peaceful. Then the disease will not emerge. Secondly, people can take formulas like *Zhèn Xīn Dān* 鎮心丹 (Settle the Heart Elixir) to supplement and nourish themselves. Applying acupuncture when the disease is about to emerge is also fine.

8. From the time of the *Zhōu* (周) Dynasty (1046–770 BCE) until the *Hàn* (漢) Dynasty (206 BCE–220 CE), a varying number of vassal states existed in Ancient China. These ranged in size from small city states to vassals which controlled large swathes of territory. One of these vassal states went on to conquer China and unite the country under the first emperor, Qín Shǐhuáng 秦始皇. Wū Chén 巫臣 was a senior official in the state of Chǔ 楚 during that period. Zǐ Fǎn 子反 was the younger brother of the ruler of the Chǔ 楚. Conbubine Xià 夏 was a princess of the Zhèng 鄭 state.

狂
345
邪癲
343

# 4.02
## Xīn Huǎng Hū (Yú Jiàn Fèi Zhòng Fēng)
## 心恍惚（餘見肺中風）

## Heart abstraction[9]
(for the remainder, see wind stroke in the lungs)

心俞、天井、神道（《明》上、下同）治悲愁恍惚（《千》見悲愁）。狂驚恍惚：灸足陽明。狂癲恍惚：灸腦戶等。狂言恍惚：灸天樞（並見狂）。卒中邪魅恍惚（見邪癲），左手關後尺中陰實者，腎實也。

Xīn Shù 心俞 (UB 15), Tiān Jǐng 天井 (SJ 10), Shén Dào 神道 (Dū 11) (*Míng Shàng*《明上》and *Xià*《下》agree) govern sorrow, anxiety and abstraction (see the section on sorrow and anxiety in *Qiān*《千》).

Mania, fright, and abstraction: Apply moxibustion on Foot Yángmíng [Chōng Yáng 衝陽 (ST 42)].

Mania, withdrawal and abstraction: Apply moxibustion on Nǎo Hù 腦戶 (Dū 17), and so forth.

Manic raving and abstraction: Apply moxibustion on Tiān Shū 天樞 (ST 25) (for all, see the section on mania).

Sudden strike by evils and demons, abstraction (see the discussion of evil withdrawal), and yīn repletion in the *chǐ* position which is posterior to the *guān* position on the left hand: This is kidney repletion.

若恍惚健忘，目視睆睆，耳聾悵悵善鳴：刺足少陰治陰。巨闕治恍惚不知人（《銅》見痰）。百會療少心力，忘前失後，心神恍惚（《明下》）。陰都療心恍惚（《千》）。

Abstraction and forgetfulness, blurred vision, deafness with susceptibility to tinnitus: puncture foot shàoyīn (Tài Xī 太溪 (KI 3)) to treat yīn.

9. Heart abstraction is usually caused by internal damage from the seven emotions or profuse sweating which injuries heart qì; the patient loses the ability to concentrate and is easily startled.

心痛 312
傷寒 661
憂疝 331
心煩 335
疝 220
狂 345

Jù Quē 巨闕 (Rèn 14) treats abstraction and unconsciousness (see the section on phlegm in *Tóng* 《銅》).

Bǎi Huì 百會 (Dū 20) cures shortage of heart strength, forgetfulness, and abstraction of heart spirit (*Míng Xià* 《明下》).

Yīn Dū 陰都 (KI 19) cures heart abstraction (*Qiān* 《千》).

## 4.03
## *Xīn Jīng Kǒng*
## 心驚恐
## Heart fright and fear

曲澤治心痛善驚（《銅》）。靈道治悲恐（見心痛）。下廉治暴驚。魚際治心痹悲恐。少衝治悲恐善驚（見傷寒）。上管治心風驚悸（《明》同，作心忪）。少府治悲恐畏人（見憂疝）。神門（見心煩）、蠡溝（見疝）、巨闕治驚悸少氣（見狂）。

Qū Zé 曲澤 (PC 3) treats heart pain with susceptibility to fright (*Tóng*).

Líng Dào 靈道 (HT 4) treats susceptibility to fear (see the section on heart pain).

Xià Lián 下廉 (LI 8 or ST 39) treats sudden fright.

Yú Jì 魚際 (LU 10) treats heart *bì*-impediment, sorrow, and fear.

Shào Chōng 少衝 (HT 9) treats sorrow, fear, and susceptibility to fright (see the section on cold damage).

Shàng Guǎn 上管 (Rèn 13) treats heart wind and fright palpitations (*Míng* 《明》 agrees but says heart palpitations).

Shào Fǔ 少府 (HT 8) treats sorrow, fear, and fear of people (see the sections on anxiety and *shàn*-mounting).

Shén Mén 神門 (HT 7) (see the section on vexation of the heart), Lí Gōu 蠡溝 (LV 5) (see the section on prominent *shàn*-mounting), and Jù Quē (Rèn 14) treat fright palpitations and qì shortage (see the section on mania).

心痛 312
傷寒 690
風勞 371
瘧 301
淋 222
風癇 366
頭痛 643
風痹 377
狂 345
目眩 575
水腫 459

梁丘治大驚乳痛。陰郄、間使（見心痛）、二間、厲兌治多驚。《明下》云：間使療驚悸（見傷寒無汗）、五里治驚恐（見風勞）。京骨（見瘧）、大鐘（見淋）、太陵治喜驚恐。百會（見風癇）、神道（見頭痛）、天井（見風痹）、液門（見狂）治驚悸。

Liáng Qiū 梁丘 (ST 34) treats great fright and pain of the breasts.

Yīn Xī 陰郄 (HT 6), Jiān Shǐ 間使 (PC 5) (see the section on heart pain), Èr Jiān 二間 (LI 2), and Lì Duì 厲兌 (ST 45) treat frequent fright. *Míng Xià*《明下》says: Jiān Shǐ (PC 5) cures fright palpitations (see the section on cold damage with absence of sweating). Wǔ Lǐ 五里 (LI 13 or LV 10) treats fright and fear (see the section on wind taxation).

Jīng Gǔ 京骨 (UB 64) (see the section on malaria), Dà Zhōng 大鐘 (KI 4) (see the section on dribbling), and Dà Líng 大陵 (PC 7) treat frequent fright and fear.

Bǎi Huì 百會 (Dū 20) (see the section on wind epilepsy), Shén Dào 神道 (Dū 11) (see the section on headache), Tiān Jǐng 天井 (SJ 10) (see the section on wind *bì*-impediment), and Yè Mén 液門 (SJ 2) (see the section on mania) treat fright palpitations.

通谷（見目眩）、章門治善恐（見水腫）。天衝治癲疾，風痙，牙腫，善驚恐。支正治風，虛驚恐狂惕。《明下》云：療驚恐悲愁。郄門治驚恐畏人（見心痛）。神庭治驚悸不得安寢。腦空治腦風頭痛，目瞑心悸。三間、合谷、厲兌主吐舌，戾頸喜驚（《千》）。

Tōng Gǔ 通谷 (UB 66 or KI 20) (see the section on dizzy vision) and Zhāng Mén 章門 (LV 13) treat susceptibility to fear (see the section on edema).

Tiān Chōng 天衝 (GB 9) treats epilepsy diseases, wind tetany, swelling of the teeth, and susceptibility to fright and fear.

Zhī Zhèng 支正 (SI 7) treats wind, vacuity fright and fear, and mania and fear. *Míng Xià* says: It governs fright, fear, sorrow, and anxiety.

Xī Mén 郄門 (PC 4) treats fright and fear, and fear of people (see the section on heart pain).

Shén Tíng 神庭 (Dū 24) treats fright palpitations and inability to sleep peacefully.

Nǎo Kōng 腦空 (GB 19) treats brain wind, headache, dimness of vision, and heart palpitations.

Sān Jiān 三間 (LI 3), Hé Gǔ 合谷 (LI 4), and Lì Duì (ST 45) govern protrusion of the tongue, perverse neck [torticollis or wryneck], and frequent fright (*Qiān*《千》).

曲澤、大陵主心下澹澹喜驚（《甲》作內關）。通里主心下悸。《明下》云：療悲恐畏人。然谷（《銅》同）、陽陵泉（《明》同）主心下惕恐，如人將捕之。大鐘、郄門主驚恐畏人，神氣不足。氣海、陰交、大巨主驚不得臥。大巨主善驚。厲兌主多臥好驚（《明》同）。

Qū Zé 曲澤 (PC 3) and Dà Líng 大陵 (PC 7) govern a rolling sensation below the heart and frequent fright (*Jiǎ*《甲》says Nèi Guān 內關 (PC 6)).

Tōng Lǐ 通里 (HT 5) governs palpitations below the heart. *Míng Xià*《明下》says: It cures sorrow and fear of people.

Rán Gǔ 然谷 (KI 2) (*Tóng*《銅》agrees) and Yáng Líng Quán 陽陵泉 (GB 34) (*Míng*《明》agrees) govern apprehension and fear below the heart as if about to be arrested.

Dà Zhōng 大鐘 (KI 4) and Xī Mén 郄門 (PC 4) govern fright, fear of people, and insufficient spirit qì.

Qì Hǎi 氣海 (Rèn 6), Yīn Jiāo 陰交 (Rèn 7), and Dà Jù 大巨 (ST 27) govern fright and inability to sleep.

Dà Jù (ST 27) governs susceptibility to fear.

Lì Duì 厲兌 (ST 45) governs somnolence and frequent fear (*Míng* agrees).

液門主喜驚妄言面赤。少府主數噫，恐悸，氣不足。神門主數噫，恐悸不足。巨闕主驚悸少氣。陰蹻主臥驚視如見鬼。解溪主瘛瘲而驚。少衝主太息煩滿，少氣悲驚。行間主心痛數驚，心悲不樂。手少陰、陰郄主氣驚心痛。少衝療悲恐畏人，善驚。神庭療驚不安寢（《明》見癲癇）。

Yè Mén 液門 (SJ 2) governs frequent fright, frenetic speech, and red face.

Shào Fǔ 少府 (HT 8) governs frequent belching, fear with palpitations, and insufficient qì.

Shén Mén 神門 (HT 7) governs frequent belching and fear with palpitations due to insufficiency.

Jù Quē 巨闕 (Rèn 14) governs fright palpitations and qì shortage.

Yīn Qiāo 陰蹻 (KI 6 or KI 8) governs fright, appearing as if one is seeing a ghost during sleep.

Jiě Xī 解溪 (ST 41) governs tugging and slackening as well as fright.

Shào Chōng 少衝 (HT 9) governs sighing, vexation and fullness, qì shortage, sorrow, and fright.

Xíng Jiān 行間 (LV 2) governs heart pain, frequent fright, and sorrowful heart.

足寒 513
瘛瘲 354
月事 735
心煩 335
悲 331
臥 338
上氣 420
驚癇 363

Shǒu Shào Yīn 手少陰, Yīn Xī 陰郄 (HT 6),[10] governs qì fright and heart pain.

Shào Chōng 少衝 (HT 9) cures sorrow, fear of people, and susceptibility to fright.

Shén Tíng 神庭 (Dū 24) cures fright and inability to sleep peacefully (see the section on withdrawal and epilepsy in *Míng*《明》).

曲澤療喜驚。梁丘（見足寒）療大驚。瘈脈療小兒驚恐（見瘛瘲）。陰蹻療婦人驚悲不樂（見月事），又療大風，臥驚視如見星。風府療多悲恐驚悸（《下》）。鳩尾療心驚悸，神氣耗散。兒睡中驚，目不合：灸屈肘橫文中上三分，各一壯。兒睡中驚掣：灸足大指次指端，去爪甲如韭葉，各一壯。然谷主兒善驚（《千》）。

Qū Zé 曲澤 (PC 3) cures frequent fright.

Liáng Qiū 梁丘 (ST 34) (see the discussion of cold legs) cures great fright.

Chì Mài 瘈脈 (SJ 18) cures fright and fear in children (see the section on tugging and slackening).

Yīn Qiāo 陰蹻 (KI 6 or KI 8) cures fright and sorrow in women (see the section on menstruation). It also cures great wind [leprosy], fright, and appearing as if one is seeing stars during sleep.

Fēng Fǔ 風府 (Dū 16) cures frequent sorrow, fear, and fright palpitations (*Xià*《下》).

Jiū Wěi 鳩尾 (Rèn 15) cures fright palpitations in the heart and dissipated spirit qì.

Awakening from fright during sleep in children and inability to close the eyes: Apply one cone of moxibustion each on the site 3 fēn above the midpoint of the transverse crease of elbow.

Pulling movements from fright during the sleep in children: Apply one cone of moxibustion each on the tip of the second toe, a leek leaf's distance from the corner of the nail.

Rán Gǔ 然谷 (KI 2) governs susceptibility to fright in children (*Qiān*《千》).

驚怖心忪少力：灸大橫五十壯。上管療驚悸（《明》見心煩）。天井療驚悸（《明下》見悲）。厲兌療善驚（見臥）。彧中等主悸坐不安席（《千》見上氣）。長強主小兒驚恐失精（見驚癇）。

Fright and fear, heart palpitations, and lack of strength: Apply fifty cones of moxibustion on Dà Héng 大橫 (SP 15).

10. Shǒu Shàoyīn 手少陰 and Yīn Xī 陰郄 (HT 6) are both names for HT 6.

Shàng Guǎn 上管 (Rèn 13) cures fright palpitations (see the section on vexation of the heart in *Míng* 《 明 》).

Tiān Jǐng 天井 (SJ 10) cures fright palpitations (see the section on sorrow in *Míng Xià* 《 明下 》).

Lì Duì 厲兌 (ST 45) cures susceptibility to fright (see the section on somnolence).

Yù Zhōng 彧中 (KI 26), and so forth govern palpitations and inability to sit on the mat calmly (see the section on qì ascent in *Qiān* 《 千 》).

Cháng Qiáng 長強 (Dū 1) governs fright, fear, and loss of essence [possibly 'semen'] in children (see the section on fright epilepsy).

癲狂 345
四肢 528
中風 379
傷寒 690
癲癇 357
脊 555
氣逆 420
目翳 584
瘛瘲 354

# 4.04

## *Xīn Xǐ Xiào (Nù Mà)*

# 心喜笑（怒罵）

## Susceptibility to laughter

**(Angry cursing)**

神門、陽谷主笑若狂（《千》）。勞宮、大陵主喜笑不止（見癲狂）。列缺主喜笑，（見四肢厥）。勞宮治悲笑（《銅》見中風）。大陵治喜笑不休（見傷寒無汗）。陽溪治狂言喜笑見鬼。水溝（見癲癇，《銅》同），失笑無時節（《明》）。復溜（見脊），勞宮治善怒（《銅》見中風）。

Shén Mén 神門 (HT 7) and Yáng Gǔ 陽谷 (SI 5) govern laughter as if manic (*Qiān*《千》).

Láo Gōng 勞宮 (PC 8) and Dà Líng 大陵 (PC 7) govern incessant laughter (see the section on withdrawal and mania).

Liè Quē 列缺 (LU 7) governs susceptibility to laughter (see the section on limb reversal).

Láo Gōng (PC 8) treats sorrow and laughter (see the section on wind stroke in *Tóng*《銅》).

Dà Líng (PC 7) treats incessant laughter (see the section on cold damage with absence of sweating).

Yáng Xī 陽溪 (LI 5) treats manic raving, susceptibility to laughter as if seeing a ghost.

Shuǐ Gōu 水溝 (Dū 26) (see the section on withdrawal and epilepsy; *Tóng* agrees) treats spontaneous uncontrollable laughter (*Míng*《明》).

Fù Liū 復溜 (KI 7) (see the section on the spine) and Láo Gōng (PC 8) treat susceptibility to anger (see the section on wind stroke).

魚際療心痹悲怒（《明》見氣逆）。肝俞療多怒（《下》見目翳）。身柱主怒欲殺人（《千》見瘛瘲，《明》、《銅》同）。狂風罵撾斫人，名熱陽風：灸口兩吻邊燕口處赤白際，各一壯；又陰囊縫三十壯（《千》）。

Yú Jì 魚際 (LU 10) cures heart *bì*-impediment, sorrow, and anger (see the section on qì counter flow in *Míng*).

Gān Shù 肝俞 (UB 18) cures susceptibility to anger (see the section on eye screens in *Xià*《下》).

Shēn Zhù 身柱 (Dū 12) governs anger with desire to kill people (see the section on tugging and slackening in *Qiān*《千》; *Míng*《明》and *Tóng*《銅》agree).

Manic wind, cursing, striking and attacking people. This is called hot yáng wind [*rè yáng fēng* 熱陽風]: Apply one cone of moxibustion each on both corners of the mouth and on the border of the red and white flesh near Yàn Kǒu 燕口 [swallow mouth, non-channel];[11] thirty cones of moxibustion can also be applied on the seams of the scrotum (*Qiān*).

癇 357
風癇 366
頭痛 643
胸痛 469
勞瘵 188

## 4.05

## *Xīn Qì (Jiàn Wàng, Wú Xīn Lì, Shī Zhì)*

# 心氣（健忘　無心力　失志）

## Heart qì

**(Forgetfulness, absence of heart strength, loss of mind)**

心俞療心氣亂（《明》見癇）。百會（《下》同）治無心力，忘前失後（見風癇）。百會治中風心煩，驚悸健忘（《銅》）。神道（見頭痛）、幽門（見胸痛）、列缺、膏肓俞治健忘（見勞瘵）。百會、天府、曲池、列缺主惡風邪氣，泣出喜忘（《千》）。

Xīn Shù 心俞 (UB 15) cures disordered heart qì (see the section on withdrawal and epilepsy in *Míng*).

Bǎi Huì 百會 (Dū 20) (*Xià* agrees) cures weakness of the heart and forgetfulness (see the section on wind epilepsy).

Bǎi Huì (Dū 20) treats wind stroke, vexation of the heart, fright palpitations, and forgetfulness (*Tóng*).

Shén Dào 神道 (Dū 11) (see the section on headaches), Yōu Mén 幽門 (KI 21) (see the section on chest pain), Liè Quē 列缺 (LU 7), and Gāo Huāng Shù 膏肓俞 (UB 43) treat forgetfulness (see the section on consumption).

11. Yàn Kǒu 燕口 [swallow's mouth] is the name of a point. It is located at the corner of the mouth, on the border of dark and light skin, near Dì Cāng 地倉 (ST 4). It has the appearance of the mouth of the swallow, hence its name.

恍惚 322
驚 323
風癇 366
癲癇 354
心煩 335
尸厥 531
心痛 312
癲 360
驚癇 363
口啞 594

Bǎi Huì 百會 (Dū 20), Tiān Fǔ 天府 (LU 3), Qū Chí 曲池 (LI 11), and Liè Quē 列缺 (LU 7) govern evil wind and qì, tearing, and frequent forgetfulness (*Qiān*《 千 》).

健忘：刺足少陰（ 見恍惚 ）。心忪少力：灸大横五十（ 見驚 ）。百會（ 見風癇 ）、巨闕（ 見驚癇 ）療無心力（ 《 明 》 ）。上管療心中悶（ 明見心煩 ）。委陽（ 見尸厥 ）治失志（ 《 銅 》 ）。秦承祖云：中衝療神氣不足失志（ 《 明下 》 ）。內關主失志（ 《 千 》見心痛 ）。通谷主心中憒憒（ 見癲 ）。鳩尾療心中氣悶，不喜聞人語（ 《 明 》見驚癇 ）。心俞療小兒心氣不足，不語（ 見口啞 ）。

Forgetfulness: Puncture Zú Shàoyīn 足少陰 (KI 3) (see the section on abstraction).

Heart palpitations and shortage of strength: Apply fifty cones of moxibustion on Dà Héng 大横 (SP 15) (see the section on fright).

Bǎi Huì 百會 (Dū 20) (see the section on wind epilepsy) and Jù Quē 巨闕 (Rèn 14) (see the section on fright epilepsy) cure weakness of the heart (*Míng*《 明 》).

Shàng Guǎn 上管 (Rèn 13) cures oppression of the chest (see the section on vexation of the heart in *Míng*).

Wěi Yáng 委陽 (UB 39) (see the section on deathlike reversal) treats loss of the will (*Tóng*《 銅 》).

Qín Chéngzǔ said: Zhōng Chōng 中衝 (PC 9) cures insufficiency of spirit qì and loss of the will (*Míng Xià*《 明下 》).

Nèi Guān 內關 (PC 6) governs loss of the will (see the section on heart pain in *Qiān*).

Tōng Gǔ 通谷 (UB 66 or KI 20) governs fretting of the heart (see the section on withdrawal).

Jiū Wěi 鳩尾 (Rèn 15) cures oppression of the heart and dislike of hearing people talk (see the section on fright epilepsy in *Míng*).

Xīn Shù 心俞 (UB 15) cures pediatric insufficiency of heart qì and loss of speech (see the section on muteness).

予舊患心氣，凡思慮過多，心下怔忪，或至自悲感慨，必灸百會。則以百會有治無心力、忘前失後證故也（兼服鎮心丹）。

[Author's notes:] I suffered from heart qì in the past. If I worried too much, I would get fright palpitations below the heart, or sorrow, or I would sigh with emotions. I needed to apply moxibustion on Bǎi Huì 百會 (Dū 20). This is because Bǎi Huì (Dū 20) can treat absence of heart strength and forgetfulness (at the same time, take *Zhèn Xīn Dān* 鎮心丹 (Settle the Heart Elixir)).

# 4.06

## *Xīn Yōu Bēi (Kū Qì, Yú Jiàn Diān Xié)*

腸鳴 263
心痛 312
頭痛 643
咽乾 628
傷寒 661

## 心憂悲（哭泣　餘見癲邪）

## Anxiety and Sorrow of the Heart

**(see the section on crying; for the rest, see the section on withdrawal evils)**

漏谷主心悲（《千》見腸鳴）。商丘（見腸鳴）治心悲（《銅》）。靈道治悲恐（見心痛）。神道治恍惚悲愁（見頭痛）。天井、心俞（《明下》同）。神道主悲愁恍惚，悲傷不樂。

Lòu Gǔ 漏谷 (SP 7) governs sorrowful heart (see the section on rumbling intestines in *Qiān*《千》).

Shāng Qiū 商丘 (SP 5) (see the section on rumbling intestines) treats sorrowful heart (*Tóng*《銅》).

Líng Dào 靈道 (HT 4) treats sorrow and fear (see the section on heart pain).

Shén Dào 神道 (Dū 11) treats abstraction, sorrow, and anxiety (see the section on headaches).

Tiān Jǐng 天井 (SJ 10), Xīn Shù 心俞 (UB 15) (*Míng Xià*《明下》agrees), and Shén Dào (Dū 11) govern sorrow, anxiety, abstraction, sadness, and unhappiness.

天井主大風默默不知所痛，悲傷不樂。《明下》云：療驚悸悲傷。大橫治大風逆氣，多寒善悲（《銅》）。照海（見咽乾）治善悲不樂。日月治太息善悲，小腹熱欲走，多唾，言語不正，四肢不收（《明下》）。少衝治悲恐善驚（見傷寒）。

Tiān Jǐng (SJ 10) governs great wind (leprosy) and quietness, inability to feel pain, sorrow and unhappiness. *Míng Xià* says: It cures fright palpitations and sorrow.

Dà Héng 大橫 (SP 15) treats great wind (leprosy) and counterflow qì, pronounced cold, and susceptibility to sorrow (*Tóng*).

Zhào Hǎi 照海 (KI 6) (see the section on dry throat) treats frequent sorrow and unhappiness.

中風 379
癲癇 354
心煩 335
癲 360
傷寒 690
口噤 605
癲狂 345
心痛 312
驚 323

Rì Yuè 日月 (GB 24) treats sighing and susceptibility to sorrow, heat in the abdomen and desire to walk, copious spittle, abnormal speech, and loss of use of the limbs (*Míng Xià* agrees).

Shào Chōng 少衝 (HT 9) treats sorrow, fear, and susceptibility to fright (see cold damage).

少府治煩滿少氣，悲恐畏人，掌熱（《明下》同），股腋攣急，胸痛，手卷不伸。支正療驚恐悲愁（《明下》）。勞宮治悲笑（《銅》見中風）。心俞（見癲癇）、神門（見心煩）、解溪（見癲）、大陵（見傷寒無汗）治喜悲泣。

Shào Fǔ 少府 (HT 8) treats vexation and fullness, qì shortage, sorrow and fear of people, hot palms (*Míng Xià*《明下》agrees), hypertonicity of the thighs[12] and axilla, chest pain, and curled hands that are unable to stretch.

Zhī Zhèng 支正 (SI 7) cures fright, fear, sorrow, and anxiety (*Míng Xià*).

Láo Gōng 勞宮 (PC 8) treats sorrow and laughter (see the section on wind stroke in *Tóng*《銅》).

Xīn Shù 心俞 (UB 15) (see the section on withdrawal and epilepsy), Shén Mén 神門 (HT 7) (see the section on vexation of the heart), Jiě Xī 解溪 (ST 41) (see the section on withdrawal), and Dà Líng 大陵 (PC 7) (see the section on cold damage with absence of sweating) treat frequent sorrow and crying.

小兒夜啼，上燈啼，雞鳴止者：灸中指甲後一分，中衝穴一壯。新生兒不吮奶，多啼（見口噤）：先灸承漿七壯，次灸頰車各七壯，炷如雀屎。間使主善悲（《千》見癲狂）。通里（見心痛）主悸悲。行間（見驚）主心悲。勞宮等主心悲（見癲狂）。

Night crying in children; the crying starts when the lamp is lit (evening) and ends when the cock crows: Apply one cone each on the site 1 fēn posterior to the nail of the middle finger, which is Zhōng Chōng 中衝 (PC 9).

Newborns who do not suckle, crying a lot (see the section on clenched jaw): First apply seven cones of moxibustion on Chéng Jiāng 承漿 (Rèn 24), then seven cones of moxibustion each on Jiá Chē 頰車 (ST 6). The cones are the size of sparrow droppings.

Jiān Shǐ 間使 (PC 5) governs susceptibility to sorrow (see the section on withdrawal and mania).

Tōng Lǐ 通里 (HT 5) (see the section on heart pain) governs palpitations and sorrow.

12. This should say *zhóu yè* 肘腋 (elbow and axilla), based on *Tóng Rén Tú Jīng*《銅人圖經》.

Xíng Jiān 行間 (LV 2) (see the section on fright) governs sorrowful heart. 健忘 329

Láo Gōng 勞宮 (PC 8) and so forth governs sorrowful heart (see the section on withdrawal and mania). 驚 323

上氣 420

瘌 354

百會等主泣出（ 見健忘 ）。陰蹻療婦人驚悲（ 《 明 》見驚 ）。憂主心：灸絕骨（ 見上氣 ）。百會療小兒驚啼（ 見癇 ），又療多哭 。水溝治乍哭（ 《 銅 》見癲癇 ）。

Bǎi Huì 百會 (Dū 20) and so forth govern tearing (see the section on forgetfulness).

Yīn Qiāo 陰蹻 (KI 6 or KI 8) cures fright and sorrow in women (see the section on fright in *Míng* 《 明 》).

Anxiety governing the heart: Apply moxibustion on Jué Gǔ 絕骨 (GB 39) (see the section on qì ascent).

Bǎi Huì 百會 (Dū 20) cures fright-crying in children (see the section on withdrawal and epilepsy); it also cures incessant crying.

Shuǐ Gōu 水溝 (Dū 26) treats sudden bouts of crying (see the section on withdrawal and epilepsy in *Tóng* 《 銅 》).

執中母氏久病，忽泣涕不可禁，知是心病也，灸百會而愈。執中凡遇憂愁淒愴，亦必灸此。有此疾者，不可不之信也。

[Wang] Zhízhōng's mother had been sick for a long time, when she suddenly began crying uncontrollably. I knew this was heart disease. I applied moxibustion on Bǎi Huì (Dū 20) and cured the disease. I, Zhízhōng, always apply moxibustion on this [point] when I encounter anxiety, worry and sorrow. Believe it for someone who has this kind of disease.

心痛 312
腸鳴 263
悲愁 331
口喎 591

# 4.07
## *Tàn Xī (Tài Xī)*
# 嘆息（太息）

## Sighing
**(Great respiration [sighing])**

少衝主太息煩滿，少氣悲驚（《千》）。行間主不得太息（見心痛）。凡好太息，不嗜食，多寒熱汗出，病至則喜嘔，嘔已乃衰，即取公孫及井俞。實則腸中切痛，厥，頭面腫起，煩心狂，多飲不嗜臥；虛則鼓脹，腹中氣滿熱痛，不嗜食，霍亂：公孫主之。商丘（見腸鳴）、日月治太息善悲（《銅》見悲愁）。行間治太息（見口喎）。丘墟療胸脅痛，善太息，胸滿膨膨（《明下》）。

Shào Chōng 少衝 (HT 9) governs sighing, vexation and fullness, qì shortage, sorrow, and fright (*Qiān*《千》).

Xíng Jiān 行間 (LV 2) governs inability to sigh (see the section on heart pain).

Susceptibility to sighing, no desire to eat, frequent [sensations of] cold and heat, sweating, frequent retching at the onset of the disease, but the symptoms wane after retching: select Gōng Sūn 公孫 (SP 4) and the *jǐng*-well point.

In repletion, cutting pain of the intestines, reversal, swelling of the head and face, vexation of the heart, mania, drinking a lot, and no desire to sleep; in vacuity, drum distention, qì fullness and hot pain of the abdomen, no desire to eat, and sudden turmoil [cholera]: Use Gōng Sūn (SP 4) to govern it.

Shāng Qiū 商丘 (SP 5) (see the section on rumbling intestines) and Rì Yuè 日月 (GB 24) treat sighing and frequent sorrow (see the section on sorrow and anxiety in *Tóng*《銅》).

Xíng Jiān (LV 2) treats sighing (see the section on deviated mouth).

Qiū Xū 丘墟 (GB 40) cures pain of the chest and rib-sides, frequent sighing, and chest fullness with a feeling of inflation (*Míng Xià*《明下》).

# 4.08

## *Xīn Fán Mèn (Xīn Bì, Dǎn Fēng Rè, Yú Jiàn Xīn Qì)*

## 心煩悶（心痹　膽風熱　餘見心氣）

### Vexation of the heart and oppression

**(Heart *bì*-impediment, gallbladder wind-heat, for the rest, see the section on heart qì)**

瘧
301
胸痛
469
善噫
281
狂言
345
癲
360
頭痛
643
風
379

神門治瘧，心煩甚，欲得飲冷，惡寒則欲處溫中，咽乾不嗜食，心痛數噫，恐悸，少氣不足，手臂寒，喘逆身熱，狂悲哭，嘔血遺溺（《銅》）。上管治心中熱煩。陰都（見瘧）、巨闕治心中煩滿。玉堂治煩心（見胸痛）。魚際、少商（見善噫）、公孫（見狂言）、解溪（見癲）、至陰（見頭痛）、完骨治頭痛煩心。

Shén Mén 神門 (HT 7) treats malaria, severe vexation of the heart, desire for cold drinks; aversion to cold with desire to stay in warm places; dry throat, no desire to eat; heart pain, frequent belching, fear with palpitations, qì shortage, cold arms, panting counterflow, generalized heat, mania, sorrow and crying, vomiting blood, and enuresis (*Tóng*《銅》).

Shàng Guǎn 上管 (Rèn 13) treats heat and vexation of the heart.

Yīn Dū 陰都 (KI 19) (see the section on malaria) and Jù Quē 巨闕 (Rèn 14) treat vexation and fullness of the heart.

Yù Táng 玉堂 (Rèn 18) treats vexation of the heart (see the section on chest pain).

Yú Jì 魚際 (LU 10), Shào Shāng 少商 (LU 11) (see the section on frequent belching), Gōng Sūn 公孫 (SP 4) (see the section on manic raving), Jiě Xī 解溪 (ST 41) (see the section on withdrawal), Zhì Yīn 至陰 (UB 67) (see the section on headaches), and Wán Gǔ 完骨 (GB 12) treat headaches and vexation of the heart.

陽溪治熱病煩心。百會（見風）、強間、承光治煩心（見頭痛）。曲差治心中煩滿，汗不出。完骨主風頭耳後痛，煩心（《千》）。關衝主舌卷口乾，心煩悶。幽門治心煩悶（見胸痛）。

Yáng Xī 陽溪 (LI 5) treats heat disease and vexation of the heart.

嘆息 334
脅痛 476
心痛 312
癲狂 345
風癇 366
賁豚 430

Bǎi Huì 百會 (Dū 20) (see the section on wind), Qiang Jian 強間 (Dū 18), and Chéng Guāng 承光 (UB 6) treat vexation of the heart (see the section on headaches).

Qū Chā 曲差 (UB 4) treats vexation and fullness of the heart and absence of sweating.

Wán Gǔ 完骨 (GB 12) governs wind, pain of the head and behind the ears, and vexation of the heart (*Qiān* 《千》).

Guān Chōng 關衝 (SJ 1) governs curled tongue, dry mouth, and vexation and oppression of the heart.

Yōu Mén 幽門 (KI 21) treats vexation and oppression of the heart (see the section on chest pain).

少衝療煩心上氣(《明》)。紫宮療胸脅支滿，痹痛骨疼，食不下，嘔逆，上氣煩心。玉堂療胸滿，不得喘息，膺痛骨疼，嘔逆上氣煩心。公孫主煩心(《千》見嘆息)。尺澤、少澤主心煩(見脅痛)。凡心虛則心煩：內關主之(見心痛)。通里主煩心(《千》見心痛)。

Shào Chōng 少衝 (HT 9) cures vexation of the heart and qì ascent (*Míng* 《明》).

Zǐ Gōng 紫宮 (Rèn 19) cures propping fullness of the chest and rib-sides, *bì*-impediment pain, bone pain, difficulty getting food down, retching counterflow, qì ascent, and vexation of the heart.

Yù Táng 玉堂 (Rèn 18) cures chest fullness, inability to pant, pain of the chest, bone pain, retching counterflow and qì ascent, and vexation of the heart.

Gōng Sūn 公孫 (SP 4) governs vexation of the heart (see sighing in *Qiān*).

Chǐ Zé 尺澤 (LU 5) and Shào Zé 少澤 (SI 1) govern vexation of the heart (see the section on pain of the rib-sides).

Vexation of the heart occurring after heart vacuity (see the section on heart pain): Nèi Guān 內關 (PC 6) can govern it.

Tōng Lǐ 通里 (HT 5) governs vexation of the heart (see the section on heart pain in *Qiān*).

巨闕、心俞療煩心(《明》見心痛)。太乙治心煩(《銅》見癲狂)。上管療心風驚悸(《銅》同)，不能食，心中悶發噦。百會療心熱悶，心煩(見風癇)。巨闕療心中煩悶(見風癇)。中脘療心悶(見賁豚)。

Jù Quē 巨闕 (Rèn 14) and Xīn Shù 心俞 (UB 15) cure vexation of the heart (see the section on heart pain in *Míng*).

上氣 420
頸項 636
心痛 312
風癇 366
中風 379
月事 735
痃癖 433

Tài Yī 太乙 (ST 23) treats vexation of the heart (see the section on withdrawal and mania in *Tóng* 《銅》).

Shàng Guǎn 上管 (Rèn 13) cures heart wind, fright palpitations (*Tóng* agrees), inability to eat, oppression of the heart, and hiccups.

Bǎi Huì 百會 (Dū 20) cures oppression and heat in the heart, and vexation of the heart (see the section on wind epilepsy).

Jù Quē 巨闕 (Rèn 14) cures vexation and oppression in the heart (see the section on wind epilepsy).

Zhōng Wǎn 中脘 (Rèn 12) cures oppression of the heart (see the section on running-piglet qì).

紫宮等主心煩（見上氣）。曲澤療心痛出血，則心下澹澹喜驚，身熱煩心，口乾，逆氣唾血，肘瘛瘲，喜搖頭，清汗出不過肩（《明》）。曲差療心煩（《明》見頸項）。心悶痛：灸巨闕二七壯（《千》見心痛）。百會治心熱悶（見風癇）。

Zǐ Gōng 紫宮 (Rèn 19) and so forth govern vexation of the heart (see the section on qì ascent).

Qū Zé 曲澤 (PC 3) cures heart pain and bleeding, a rolling sensation below the heart, susceptibility to fright, generalized heat, vexation of the heart, dry mouth, counterflow qì, spitting of blood, tugging and slackening of the elbows, frequently shaking of the head, and perspiration of clear sweat that does not go beyond the shoulders (*Míng* 《明》).

Qū Chā 曲差 (UB 4) cures vexation of the heart (see the section on the neck and nape in *Míng*).

Heart pain and oppression: Apply two times seven of moxibustion on Jù Quē (Rèn 14) (see heart pain in *Qiān* 《千》).

Bǎi Huì (Dū 20) treats heat and oppression of the heart (see the section on wind epilepsy).

絕骨治風心煩（並見中風）。魚際療心痹（《銅》見上氣）。臨泣（月事）、膈俞治心痛周痹（《銅》見痃癖）。

Jué Gǔ 絕骨 (GB 39) treats wind and vexation of the heart (for all, see the section on wind stroke).

Yú Jì 魚際 (LU 10) cures heart *bì*-impediment (see the section on qì ascent in *Míng*).

Lín Qì 臨泣 (GB 41) (menstruation) and Gé Shù 膈俞 (UB 17) treat heart pain and generalized *bì*-impediment (see strings and aggregations in *Tóng*).

肺氣 412
頭痛 643
癎 357
小腹 209
食不 291
勞 188

## 4.09
## *Dǎn Xū (Dǎn Rè)*
# 膽虛（膽熱）
## Gallbladder vacuity
**(Gallbladder heat)**

中府治膽熱嘔逆上氣（《銅》見肺氣）。膽虛：灸三陰交各二十壯。

Zhōng Fǔ 中府 (LU 1) treats gallbladder heat, vomiting counterflow, and qì ascent (see the section on lung qì in *Tóng*《銅》).

Gallbladder vacuity: Apply twenty cones of moxibustion on Sān Yīn Jiāo 三陰交 (SP 6).

## 4.10
## *Shì Wò*
# 嗜臥
## Somnolence

囟會（見頭痛，《銅》同）、百會（見癎）療多睡（《明》）。陰蹻（見小腹痛）、膈俞（見食不下）療嗜臥。腎俞療好獨臥（見勞）。二間（《下》同）、三間療多臥喜睡。

Xìn Huì 囟會 (Dū 22) (see the section on headaches; *Tóng* agrees) and Bǎi Huì 百會 (Dū 20) (see the section on withdrawal and epilepsy) cure sleepiness [somnolence] (*Míng*《明》).

Yīn Qiāo 陰蹻 (KI 6 or KI 8) (see the section on pain of the smaller abdomen) and Gé Shù 膈俞 (UB 17) (see the section on difficulty getting food down) cure somnolence.

Shèn Shù 腎俞 (UB 23) cures liking only to sleep (see the section on taxation).

Èr Jiān 二間 (LI 2) (*Xià*《下》agrees) and Sān Jiān 三間 (LI 3) cure somnolence.

厲兌療多睡善驚(《千》同)。脾俞療四肢煩熱，嗜臥怠惰，四肢不欲動(《下》)。三陽絡療嗜臥，身不欲動。五里(見風勞)、太溪(見傷寒無汗)、大鐘、照海(並見淋)、二間治嗜臥(《銅》)。膈俞主傷寒嗜臥(《千》)。三陽絡治嗜臥，身體不欲動。厲兌、大敦治喜寐(見小腹痛)。天井主嗜臥(《千》見四肢厥)。

風勞 371
傷寒 690
淋 222
小腹 209
四肢 528

Lì Duì 厲兌 (ST 45) cures sleepiness and susceptibility to fright (*Qiān*《千》agrees).

Pí Shù 脾俞 (UB 20) cures vexation heat in the four limbs, somnolence with fatigue, and no desire to move the limbs (*Xià*).

Sān Yáng Luò 三陽絡 (SJ 8) cures somnolence and no desire to move the body.

Wǔ Lǐ 五里 (LI 13 or LV 10) (see the section on wind taxation), Tài Xī 太溪 (KI 3) (see the section on cold damage and absence of sweating), Dà Zhōng 大鐘 (KI 4), Zhào Hǎi 照海 (KI 6) (for all, see the section on dribbling), and Èr Jiān 二間 (LI 2) treat somnolence (*Tóng*《銅》).

Gé Shù 膈俞 (UB 17) governs cold damage and somnolence (*Qiān*).

Sān Yáng Luò (SJ 8) treats somnolence with no desire to move the body.

Lì Duì (ST 45) and Dà Dūn 大敦 (LV 1) treats fondness for sleep (see the section on pain of the smaller abdomen).

Tiān Jǐng 天井 (SJ 10) governs somnolence (see the section on limb reversal in *Qiān*).

《千金》云：食多身瘦，名曰食晦：先取脾俞，後取季脅。又云：凡身重不得，食無味，喜臥，皆針胃管太倉，服建中湯平胃丸。今人嗜臥，與夫食罷則脾困欲臥，縱不能針，豈可不灸。予與人灸中管膏肓，遂皆不困，故既言之。

[Author's notes:] *Qiān Jīn*《千金》says: Thin body despite large food intake is called *shí huì* 食晦. Treat it with Pí Shù 脾俞 (UB 20) first, then Jì Xié 季脅 (LV 13). It also is said: For generalized heaviness, inability to taste food, and fondness for sleep [somnolence], needle Wèi Guǎn 胃管 (Rèn 13) and Tài Cāng 太倉 (Rèn 12); take *Jiàn Zhōng Tāng* 建中湯 (Center Fortifying Decoction) and *Píng Wèi Wán* 平胃丸 (Stomach Calming Pill). Nowadays, people have somnolence; or they suffer an encumbered spleen after eating, resulting in desire to sleep. If acupuncture is unavailable, moxibustion should be tried. When I apply moxibustion on Zhōng Guǎn 中管 (Rèn 12) and Gāo Huāng 膏肓 (UB 43), [the spleen] is no longer encumbered [and people do not feel sleepy anymore]. So I talk about it here.

上氣 420
腸鳴 263
霍亂 267
胸痹 476
腹脹 449
中惡 379
水腫 459
癲癇 357
肺 412
足麻 509
勞 188
瘧瘕 354

# 4.11
## *Bù Wò*
## 不臥
## Insomnia

神庭治驚悸不得安寢（《銅》）。氣衝（見上氣）、章門治不得臥（見腸鳴）。期門治大喘不得臥（見霍亂）。太淵治咳嗽，煩怒不得臥（見胸痹）。白環俞治腰脊冷痛，不得久臥（《明》云：不識眠睡）。隱白（見腹脹）、天府（見中惡）、陰陵泉（見水腫）治不得臥。

Shén Tíng 神庭 (Dū 24) treats palpitations and inability to sleep peacefully (*Tóng*《銅》).

Qì Chōng 氣衝 (ST 30) (see the section on qì ascent) and Zhāng Mén 章門 (LV 13) treat inability to lie down (see the section on rumbling intestines).

Qī Mén 期門 (LV 14) treats severe panting and inability to lie down [sleep] (see the section on cholera [sudden turmoil disorder]).

Tài Yuān 太淵 (LU 9) treats cough, vexation, anger, and inability to lie down [sleep] (see the section on chest *bì*-impediment [pain]).

Bái Huán Shù 白環俞 (UB 30) treats cold pain of the spine and low back with inability to lie down [sleep] for long (*Míng*《明》says: cannot sleep).

Yǐn Bái 隱白 (SP 1) (see the section on abdominal fullness), Tiān Fǔ 天府 (LU 3) (see the discussion of malignity stroke), and Yīn Líng Quán 陰陵泉 (SP 9) (see the section on edema) treat inability to lie down [sleep].

神庭療風癇驚悸，不得安寢（《明》見癲癇）。太淵、肺俞（見肺）、上管（見霍亂）、條口（見足麻）、隱白（見腹脹）療不可臥。譩譆（見勞）、環跳，岐伯云：療臥伸縮回轉不得。大椎療臥不安（《下》見瘧瘕）。

Shén Tíng (Dū 24) cures wind epilepsy, fright palpitations, and inability to sleep peacefully (see the section on withdrawal and epilepsy in *Míng*).

Tài Yuān 太淵 (LU 9), Fèi Shù 肺俞 (UB 13) (see the section on lung [qì]), Shàng Guǎn 上管 (Rèn 13) (see the section on sudden turmoil [cholera]), Tiáo Kǒu 條口 (ST 38) (see the section on numbness of the legs), and Yǐn Bái 隱白 (SP 1) (see the section on abdominal fullness) cure inability to sleep.

嘆息 334 癲狂 345

Yī Xī 譩譆 (UB 45) (see the section on taxation) and Huán Tiào 環跳 (GB 30): Qí Bó said they cure inability to stretch, contract, and turn around while sleeping.

Dà Zhuī 大椎 (Dū 14) cures unquiet sleep (see the section on tugging and slackening in *Xià*《下》).

氣海、陰交、大巨主驚不得臥（《千》）。公孫主不嗜臥（見嘆息）。攢竹等主不得臥（見癲狂）。

Qì Hǎi 氣海 (Rèn 6), Yīn Jiāo 陰交 (Rèn 7), and Dà Jù 大巨 (ST 27) govern fright and inability to lie down [sleep] (*Qiān*《千》).

Gōng Sūn 公孫 (SP 4) governs no desire to sleep (see the section on sighing).

Zǎn Zhú 攢竹 (UB 2) and so forth govern inability to lie down [sleep] (see the section on withdrawal and epilepsy).

人不得臥，亦有因心氣使然，宜服俞山人鎮心丹。此丹以酸棗仁微炒過，則令人得睡故也（《指迷》云：若頭痛筋攣，驚不嗜臥，謂之腎厥頭痛。宜灸關元百壯，服玉真丸。）

[Author's notes:] The reason for inability to lie down [insomnia] can also be heart qì. It is appropriate to take *Zhèn Xīn Dān* 鎮心丹 (Settle the Heart Elixir) from Yú Shān Rén 俞山人. This pill has *suān zǎo rén* 酸棗仁 (Spiny Jujube Semen) that is stir-fried a little, so it can make people fall asleep (*Zhǐ Mí*《指迷》says: Headaches, hypertonicity of the sinews, fright and inability to lie down [insomnia]; this is called kidney reversal headache. It is appropriate to apply a hundred cones of moxibustion on Bǎi Huì 百會 (Dū 20) and take *Yù Zhēn Wán* 玉真丸 (True Jade Pill).

# 4.12
## *Mèng Yǎn (Zá Mèng)*
## 夢魘（雜夢）
## Oppressive ghost dreams [nightmares]
**(And miscellaneous dreams)**

商丘治魘夢（《銅》）。《千》云：主喜魘夢。天牖療夜夢顛倒，面青黃無顏色（《明》）。右手關後尺中陰絕者，無腎脈也。若足逆冷，上搶胸痛，夢入水，見鬼，善魘寐，黑色物來掩人上：刺足太陽治陽（《千》）。

Shāng Qiū 商丘 (SP 5) treats oppressive ghost dreams (*Tóng*《銅》). *Qiān*《千》says: It governs susceptibility to oppressive ghost dreams.

Tiān Yǒu 天牖 (SJ 16) cures dreams in deranged sequence, with green-blue or yellow facial complexion and abnormal color (*Míng*《明》).

[If there is] yīn expiry in the right *chǐ* position, which is posterior to the *guān* position: there is no kidney pulse. Reversal cold of the feet, pain prodding upward into the chest, dreams of entering the water and seeing ghosts, susceptibility to oppressive ghost dreams of black things coming and covering people: Puncture foot Tài Yáng 足太陽 [UB 60] to treat yáng (*Qiān*).

凡魘死，不得著燈火照，亦不得近前急喚，多殺人，但痛咬其足跟及足拇指。邊並多唾其面即活。又灸足大指聚毛中三七壯（《集效》）。魘不覺：兩足大指聚毛中三十壯（《千翼》）。

When someone dies from oppressive ghost dreams, it is not appropriate to light a lamp, or come close and wake him. That would kill him. Just give a painful bite to his heel and big toe, and spit a lot on his face;[13] this will revive him. Three times seven cones of moxibustion can also be applied to the tuft of hair on the big toe (*Jí Xiào*《集效》).

Oppressive ghost dreams and inability to wake up: Apply thirty cones of moxibustion on the tuft of hair on both big toes (*Qiān Yì*《千翼》).

13. In ancient China it was said that ghosts were afraid of spittle.

有婦人夜多魘，蓋因少年侍親疾用心所致也。後服定志丸，遂不常魘。灸固不可廢，藥亦不可不服也。



[Author's notes:] A lady suffered frequent oppressive ghost dreams at night. This might be because she took care of her sick parents when she was young and used her heart too much. After she took *Dìng Zhì Wán* 定志丸 (Will Stabilizing Pill), the oppressive ghost dreams decreased. Though we cannot abandon moxibustion, we also need to take medication.

# 4.13
## *Diān Xié (Guǐ Xié)*
## 癲邪（鬼邪）
## Withdrawal evils
**(Ghost evils)**

〇扁鵲針邪病十三穴見《千金》

* Thirteen points which are used by Biǎn Què to treat evil-disease, see *Qiān Jīn*《千金》

黃帝灸神邪鬼魅（《明下》見狂言）。岐伯療鬼神邪：灸間使。攢竹療神邪鬼魅（見狂）。秦承祖灸狐魅神邪，及癲狂病，醫治不瘥者：並兩手大指，用軟絲繩急縛，灸三壯。艾炷著四處，半在甲上，半在肉上。四處盡燒，一處不燒，其疾不愈，神效。小兒胎癇、奶癇、驚癇，依此灸一壯，炷如麥。

The Yellow Emperor applied moxibustion to treat [diseases caused by] evils and ghosts (see the section on manic raving in *Míng Xià*《明下》). Qí Bó treated [diseases caused by] evils and ghosts by applying moxibustion on Jiān Shǐ 間使 (PC 5).

Zǎn Zhú 攢竹 (UB 2) cures [diseases caused by] evils and ghosts (see the section on mania).

Qín Chéngzǔ applied moxibustion to treat diseases that could not be cured by other doctors: fox spirits,[14] spirit evils, and mania-withdrawal. He tightly tied both thumbs together with a soft silk string and applied three cones of moxibustion by putting each moxa cone on four sites [simultaneously]: half on the nail, the other half on the flesh. It is burned on the four sites together. The disease

14. In Chinese folk tales, fox spirits often bewitched people.

狂言 345

will not be cured if one of the four sites is not burned. This has divine effects. Based on this method, apply one cone of moxibustion to treat fetal epilepsy, milk epilepsy, and fright epilepsy in children. Use a grain-of-wheat size cone.

陽溪、僕參、溫溜治狂言見鬼（見狂言）。狂邪鬼語：灸天窗九壯，或伏兔百壯（《千》）。悲泣鬼語：灸天府五十。悲泣邪語，鬼忙歌哭：灸慈門五十。卒中邪魅，恍惚振噤：灸鼻下人中，及兩手足大指爪甲本節。令艾丸半在爪上，半在肉上，各七壯，不止，十四壯，炷如雀屎。

Yáng Xī 陽溪 (LI 5), Pū Cān 僕參 (UB 61), and Wēn Liū 溫溜 (LI 7) treat manic raving as if seeing the ghosts (see the section on manic raving).

Manic evils and ghost speech: Apply nine cones of moxibustion on Tiān Chuāng 天窗 (SI 16); or burn a hundred cones of moxibustion on Fú Tù 伏兔 (ST 32) (*Qiān*《千》).

Sorrowful crying and ghost speech: Apply fifty cones of moxibustion on Tiān Fǔ 天府 (LU 3).

Sorrowful crying and evil talking, the ghost is busy singing and crying: Apply fifty cones of moxibustion on Cí Mén 慈門 (unknown).[15]

Sudden strike by evils and demons, abstraction, shivering and clenched jaws: Apply moxibustion on Rén Zhōng 人中 (Dū 26) below the nose, and [the site between] the nails and the base joints of both thumbs and big toes. Let half of the moxa cones stay on the nails, and the other half on the flesh. Burn seven cones of moxibustion; if the disease does not stop, burn fourteen cones. The cones are the size of a sparrow's droppings.

風邪：灸間使隨年壯；又承漿七壯；又心俞七壯；又三里七壯。鬼魅：灸入發一寸百壯；又灸間使、手心各五十壯。狐魅：合手大指，縛指，灸合間三七壯，當狐鳴即瘥。風府主邪病，臥瞑瞑不自知。囟上主邪病鬼癲。尺澤主邪病，四肢腫痛。諸雜候，狂癇哭泣：灸手逆注三十（扁鵲針邪病十三穴，見《千金》）。

Wind evils: Apply the same number of cones of moxibustion as the age of the patient on Jiān Shǐ 間使 (PC 5); and seven cones of moxibustion on Chéng Jiāng 承漿 (Rèn 24), Xīn Shù 心俞 (UB 15) and Sān Lǐ 三里 (ST 36).

Ghosts demons: Apply a hundred cones of moxibustion on the site 1 cùn within the hairline; and fifty cones of moxibustion on Jiān Shǐ (PC 5) and in the center of the palm.

Fox demons: Tie the thumbs together, apply three times seven cones of moxibustion on the space between [the thumbs]. The disease will be cured when the fox howls.

15. Cí Mén 慈門: The identification of this point is uncertain. Cí Gōng 慈宮 is a name for SP 12.

Fēng Fǔ 風府 (Dū 16) governs evil diseases with sleepiness and unconsciousness.

Xìn Shàng 囟上 (Dū 22) governs evil diseases and ghost withdrawal.

Chǐ Zé 尺澤 (LU 5) governs evil diseases, and swelling and pain of the four limbs.

All miscellaneous symptoms, mania, epilepsy, and crying: Apply thirty cones of moxibustion on Shǒu Nì Zhù 手逆注 (LI 7).

(For the thirteen points which were used by Biǎn Què for evil diseases, see *Qiān Jīn* 《千金》).

## 4.14
## *Diān Kuáng (Kuáng Zǒu, Kuáng Yán)*
## 癲狂（狂走　狂言）
## Withdrawal and mania
**(Manic walking, manic raving)**

溫溜、液門、京骨主狂僕(《千》)。神門、陽谷主笑若狂。勞宮、大陵主風熱善怒，心中悲喜，思慕歔欷，喜笑不休。飛揚、太乙、滑肉門主癲狂，吐舌。溫溜、僕參主癲疾，吐舌鼓頷，狂言見鬼。長強主癲發如狂，面皮敦敦者不治。《明下》云：療癲狂。風府(《銅》云：治狂走，目注視)。肺俞主狂走欲自殺。

Wēn Liū 溫溜 (LI 7), Yè Mén 液門 (SJ 2), and Jīng Gǔ 京骨 (UB 64) govern manic collapse (*Qiān* 《千》).

Shén Mén 神門 (HT 7) and Yáng Gǔ 陽谷 (SI 5) govern laughter as if manic.

Láo Gōng 勞宮 (PC 8) and Dà Líng 大陵 (PC 7) govern wind heat, susceptibility to anger, sorrow and joy in the heart, thinking of someone and sighing, and incessant laughter.

Fēi Yáng 飛揚 (UB 58), Tài Yǐ 太乙 (ST 23), and Huá Ròu Mén 滑肉門 (ST 24) govern withdrawal, mania and protrusion of the tongue.

Wēn Liū (LI 7) and Pū Cān 僕參 (UB 61) govern madness, protrusion of the tongue, chattering of the jaws, and manic raving as if seeing ghosts.

瘛瘲 354 Cháng Qiáng 長強 (Dū 1) governs the onset of the untreatable madness as if manic with thick
膝攣 536 facial [skin]. *Míng Xià*《 明下 》says: It cures withdrawal and mania.

Fēng Fǔ 風府 (Dū 16) (*Tóng*《 銅 》 says: It treats manic walking and visual hallucinations).

Fèi Shù 肺俞 (UB 13) governs manic walking and desire to commit suicide.

筋縮、曲骨、陰谷、行間主驚癇狂走癲疾。絡卻、聽會、身柱主狂走瘛瘲，恍惚不樂。攢竹、小海、後頂、強間主癲發瘛瘲，狂走不得臥。衝陽、豐隆主狂妄行，登高而歌，棄衣而走。天柱、臨泣主狂易，多言不休，目上反。支正、魚際、合谷、少海、曲池、腕骨主狂言。

Jīn Suō 筋縮 (Dū 8), Qū Gǔ 曲骨 (Rèn 2), Yīn Gǔ 陰谷 (KI 10), and Xíng Jiān 行間 (LV 2) govern fright epilepsy, manic walking, withdrawal and mania.

Luò Què 絡卻 (UB 8), Tīng Huì 聽會 (GB 2), and Shēn Zhù 身柱 (Dū 12) govern manic walking, tugging and slackening, abstraction and unhappiness.

Zǎn Zhú 攢竹 (UB 2), Xiǎo Hǎi 小海 (SI 8), Hòu Dǐng 後頂 (Dū 19), and Qiáng Jiān 強間 (Dū 18) govern withdrawal, tugging and slackening, manic walking, and inability to lie down [sleep].

Chōng Yáng 衝陽 (ST 42) and Fēng Lóng 豐隆 (ST 40) govern manic behavior, climbing to high places and singing, taking the clothes off and walking.

Tiān Zhù 天柱 (UB 10) and Lín Qì 臨泣 (GB 15) govern susceptibility to mania, incessant talking, and upturned eyes.

Zhī Zhèng 支正 (SI 7), Yú Jì 魚際 (LI 10), Hé Gǔ 合谷 (LI 4), Shào Hǎi 少海 (HT 3), Qū Chí 曲池 (LI 11), and Wàn Gǔ 腕骨 (SI 4) govern manic raving.

下廉、丘墟主狂言非常。巨闕、築賓主狂易，妄言怒罵。陽溪、陽谷主吐舌戾頸妄言。間使主驚狂善悲，面赤目黃，瘖不言（並《千》）。筋縮（《下》同）療驚癇，狂走癲疾，脊急強，目轉上垂（《明》）。陽谷、身柱（見瘛瘲）、腦空、京骨（見膝攣）療癲疾強走。

Xià Lián 下廉 (LI 8 or ST 39) and Qiū Xū 丘墟 (GB 40) govern unusual manic raving.

Jù Quē 巨闕 (Rèn 14) and Zhù Bīn 筑賓 (KI 9) govern susceptibility to mania, manic raving and angry cursing.

Yáng Xī 陽溪 (LI 5) and Yáng Gǔ 陽谷 (SI 5) govern protrusion of the tongue, perverse neck [torticollis or wryneck], and manic raving.

驚癇 363
鬼邪 343
熱病 661
心憂 331
目眩 575

Jiān Shǐ 間使 (PC 5) governs fright, mania and tenancy to sorrow, red face, yellowing of the eyes, muteness and inability to speak (all in *Qiān*《千》).

Jīn Suō 筋縮 (Dū 8) (*Xià*《下》agrees) cures fright epilepsy, manic walking, withdrawal and mania, acute stiffness of the spine, spinning of the eyes, and drooping upper [eyelids] (*Míng*《明》).

Yáng Gǔ 陽谷 (SI 5), Shēn Zhù 身柱 (Dū 12) (see the section on tugging and slackening), Nǎo Kōng 腦空 (GB 19), and Jīng Gǔ 京骨 (UB 64) (see the section on hypertonicity of knees) cure madness and stiff walking.

風府療狂走欲自殺，目反妄視（《下》同）。束骨療癲狂（見驚癇）。攢竹，但是尸厥癲邪，神狂鬼魅，皆療之。秦承祖灸神邪癲狂（見鬼邪）。衝陽治久狂，登高而歌，棄衣而走（《銅》）。光明治卒狂（見熱病無汗）。

Fēng Fǔ 風府 (Dū 16) cures manic walking, desire to commit suicide, upturned eyes, and visual hallucinations (*Xià* agrees).

Shù Gǔ 束骨 (UB 65) cures withdrawal and mania (see the section on fright epilepsy).

Zǎn Zhú 攢竹 (UB 2) cures all deathlike reversal, epilepsy evils, and spirit demons. Qín Chéngzǔ applied moxibustion on it to treat spirit evils, withdrawal and mania (see the discussion of ghost evils).

Chōng Yáng 衝陽 (ST 42) treats enduring mania, climbing to high places and singing, taking the clothes off and walking (*Tóng*《銅》).

Guāng Míng 光明 (GB 37) treats sudden mania (see the discussion of heat diseases without sweating).

間使治卒強，胸中澹澹，惡風寒，嘔吐，怵惕，寒中少氣，掌熱腋腫，肘攣。《明下》云：療卒狂驚悸。日月治小腹熱欲走（見心憂悲）。絲竹空治發狂吐涎沫（見目眩）。太乙治癲疾狂走，心煩吐舌（《銅》）。陽谷治癲疾狂走。

Jiān Shǐ (PC 5) treats sudden rigidity, a rolling sensation in the chest, aversion to wind-cold, vomiting, apprehensiveness, cold strike and qì shortage, heat in the palms, axillary swelling, and hypertonicity of the elbows. *Míng Xià*《明下》says: It cures sudden mania, fright and palpitations.

Rì Yuè 日月 (GB 24) treats heat in the smaller abdomen with desire to walk (see the section on anxiety and sorrow of the heart).

Sī Zhú Kōng 絲竹空 (SJ 23) treats mania with vomiting of drool and foam (see the section on dizzy vision).

勞瘵 188
驚恐 323
傷寒 690

Tài Yǐ 太乙 (ST 23) treats withdrawal and mania, manic walking, vexation of the heart, and protrusion of the tongue (*Tóng*《銅》).

Yáng Gǔ 陽谷 (SI 5) treats withdrawal and manic walking.

心俞治心中風，狂走發癇，語悲泣，心胸悶亂煩滿，汗不出，結積，寒熱嘔吐，不下食，咳唾血（《明》同）。腕骨治狂惕。巨闕治發狂不識人，驚悸少氣。曲泉、膏肓俞治發狂（見勞瘵）。神門治身熱狂悲哭。陽交治寒厥驚狂。少海治目眩發狂，嘔吐涎沫，項不得顧。

Xīn Shù 心俞 (UB 15) treats heart wind-strike, manic walking, epilepsy, sorrowful speech, oppression and derangement of the heart, vexation and fullness, absence of sweating, binding accumulations, [sensations of] cold and heat, vomiting, inability to get food down, cough, and spitting of blood (*Míng*《明》agrees).

Wàn Gǔ 腕骨 (SI 4) treats mania and fear.

Jù Quē 巨闕 (Rèn 14) treats mania, loss of consciousness, fright palpitations, and qì shortage.

Qū Quán 曲泉 (LV 8) and Gāo Huāng Shù 膏肓俞 (UB 43) treat mania (see the section on consumption).

Shén Mén 神門 (HT 7) treats generalized heat, mania, sorrow and weeping.

Yáng Jiāo 陽交 (GB 35) treats cold reversal, fright and mania.

Shào Hǎi 少海 (HT 3) treats dizzy vision, mania, vomiting of drool and foam, and inability to turn the neck.

支正治風虛狂惕（見驚恐）。大陵治狂言不樂（見傷寒無汗）。陽谷治妄言，左右顧，瘛瘲目眩。陽溪治狂言，喜笑見鬼（《銅》）。僕參治癲癇，狂言見鬼。偏歷治癲疾多言（《下》同）。溫溜治癲疾吐涎，狂言見鬼。《明下》云：癲癇吐舌，鼓頷狂言。

Zhī Zhèng 支正 (SI 7) treats wind vacuity, mania, and fear (see the section on [heart] fright and fear).

Dà Líng 大陵 (PC 7) treats manic raving and unhappiness (see the section on cold damage with absence of sweating).

Yáng Gǔ (SI 5) treats manic raving, turning the head to the left and right, tugging and slackening, and dizzy vision.

驚 323
心痛 312
癲癇 357
驚癇 363

Yáng Xī 陽溪 (LI 5) treats manic raving and susceptibility to laughter as if seeing a ghost (*Tóng*《銅》).

Pū Cān 僕參 (UB 61) treats withdrawal and epilepsy, manic raving, and seeing ghosts.

Piān Lì 偏歷 (LI 6) treats withdrawal and mania as well as continual talking (*Xià*《下》agrees).

Wēn Liū 溫溜 (LI 7) treats madness, vomiting of drool, and manic raving as if seeing a ghost. *Míng Xià*《明下》says: withdrawal and epilepsy, protrusion of the tongue, chattering of jaws, and manic raving.

下廉治狂言（見驚）。築賓治癲疾狂言。《明下》云：小兒癲病吐舌。公孫治卒面腫，煩心狂言。太淵治狂言（《明下》同），口僻（見心痛）。液門治驚悸妄言。陽谷療吐舌戾頸妄言，不得左右顧，瘛瘲，頭眩目痛（《明》）。筋縮療癇病多言（《下》）。鳩尾療癲癇狂歌，不擇言。

Xià Lián 下廉 (ST 39) treats manic raving (see the discussion of fright).

Zhù Bīn 筑賓 (KI 9) treats madness and manic raving. *Míng Xià* says: withdrawal disease in children and protrusion of the tongue.

Gōng Sūn 公孫 (SP 4) treats sudden facial swelling, vexation of the heart, and manic raving.

Tài Yuān 太淵 (LU 9) treats manic raving (*Míng Xià* agrees) and deviation of the mouth (see the section on heart pain).

Yè Mén 液門 (SJ 2) treats fright, palpitations, and manic raving.

Yáng Gǔ 陽谷 (SI 5) cures protrusion of the tongue, perverse neck [torticollis or wryneck], manic raving, inability to turn the neck to the left or right, tugging and slackening, dizzy head, and eye pain (*Míng*《明》).

Jīn Suō 筋縮 (Dū 8) cures epilepsy and continual talking (*Xià*).

Jiū Wěi 鳩尾 (Rèn 15) cures withdrawal and epilepsy, manic singing, and speaking without choosing the right words.

黃帝療鬼邪魅，及癲狂，語不擇尊卑：灸上唇里面中央肉弦上一壯，炷如小麥；又用鋼刀決斷更佳。《銅》云：水溝治語不識尊卑（見癲癇）。液門主妄言（《千》見驚癇）。狂言恍惚：灸天樞百壯。狂邪發無常，披頭大喚，欲殺人，不避水火，及狂言妄語：灸間使三十壯（亦灸驚恐歌哭）。

The Yellow Emperor's treatment for ghosts and evil demons, withdrawal and mania, speaking without regard for social rank or age: Apply one cone of moxibustion on the string-like flesh on the center of the inside of the upper lip, using a grain-of-wheat size cone. It is even better to cut it with a knife. *Tóng*《銅》says: Shuĭ Gōu 水溝 (Dū 26) treats speaking without regard for the social rank or age (see the section on withdrawal and epilepsy).

Yè Mén 液門 (SJ 2) governs manic raving (see the section on fright epilepsy in *Qiān*《千》).

Manic raving and abstraction: Apply a hundred cones on Tiān Shū 天樞 (ST 25).

Mania occurring without consistency, hair hanging down, shouting loudly, desire to kill people, no regard for water and fire, and manic raving: Apply thirty cones of moxibustion on Jiān Shĭ 間使 (PC 5) (also apply moxibustion for fright, fear, and [uncontrollable] singing and crying).

狂癲鬼語：灸足太陽四十壯。狂癲驚走風恍惚，嗔喜罵笑，歌哭鬼語：悉灸腦戶、風池、手陽明、太陽、太陰、足陽明、陽蹻、少陽、太陰、陰蹻、足跟，皆隨年壯。狂走刺人，或欲自死，罵詈不息，稱神鬼語：灸口吻頭赤白際一壯；又兩肘內屈中五壯；又背胛中間三壯；報灸之。

Mania-withdrawal and ghost speech: Apply forty cones of moxibustion on Foot Tàiyáng 足太陽 (UB 60).

Mania and withdrawal, fright walking, wind, abstraction, anger, laughing and cursing, singing and crying, and ghost speech: Apply moxibustion on all of the following: Năo Hù 腦戶 (Dū 17), Fēng Chí 風池 (GB 20), Shŏu Yángmíng 手陽明 (unknown), Tàiyáng 太陽 (unknown), Tàiyīn 太陰 (unknown), Zú Yángmíng 足陽明 (ST 42), Yáng Qiāo 陽蹻 (UB 62), Shàoyáng 少陽 (unknown), Tàiyīn 太陰 (SP 6), Yīn Qiāo 陽蹻 (KI 6 or KI 8) and the heel. Burn the same number of the cones as the age of the patient.[16]

Manic walking and stabbing people, or desire to commit suicide, incessant chiding and cursing, speaking of spirits and ghosts: Apply one cone of moxibustion on the border of red and white flesh at the corners of the mouth; or burn five cones of moxibustion on the center of inner aspect of both elbows while they are flexed; or burn three cones of moxibustion on the center of the scapula. Apply moxibustion in sessions.

倉公法神效。卒狂言鬼語，以甑帶急合縛兩手大指，便灸左右脅下對屈肋頭。兩處火俱起，各七壯。須臾，鬼自道姓名乞去，徐徐問之，乃解其手。卒狂鬼語，針其足大拇指爪甲下，入少許即止。人中主邪病語不止，及諸雜候。凡人中惡，先掐鼻下是也。

16. The identification of many of these points is uncertain. It is possible that these refer to channels instead of points.

中風 379
癲邪 343

The methods of Master Cāng are divinely effective. Sudden manic raving and ghost talk: quickly tie both thumbs together with a cattail belt,[17] then apply moxibustion on the corresponding end of the curved ribs under the left and right rib-sides; burn the seven cones of moxibustion simultaneously on both sides. After a while, the ghost will say his name and ask to leave. Slowly and gently ask this of him, and then release his hands.

Sudden mania and ghost talk: Needle below the nail of the big toe. It will stop a little while after insertion.

Rén Zhōng 人中 (Dū 26) governs evil disease, incessant talking, and all other miscellaneous symptoms.

Dig in the nails under the nose whenever someone has malignity strike.

邪鬼妄語：灸懸命十四壯，穴在口唇里中央弦，用鋼刀決斷佳。治肺中風狂言（見中風）。狂邪鬼語：灸天窗、伏兔。悲泣鬼語：灸天府、慈門（並見癲邪）。

Ranting about evils and ghosts: Apply forty cones of moxibustion on Xuán Mìng 懸命. The point is located on string-like flesh in the center of the inside of the upper lip. It is even better to cut it with knife. This treats wind attacking the lungs and manic raving (see the section on wind stroke).

Manic evils and ghost talk: Apply moxibustion on Tiān Chuāng 天窗 (SI 16) and Fú Tù 伏兔 (ST 32).

Sorrow, weeping and ghost talk: Apply moxibustion on Tiān Fǔ 天府 (LU 3) and Cí Mén 慈門 (unknown) (for all, see the section on withdrawal evils).

有士人妄語異常，且欲打人，病數月矣。予意其是心疾，為灸百會。百會治心疾故也。又疑是鬼邪，用秦承祖灸鬼邪法：並兩手大拇指，用軟帛繩急縛定，當肉甲相接處灸七壯，四處皆著火而後愈（灸法見癲邪門）。更有二貴人子，亦有此患，有醫僧亦為灸此穴愈。

[Author's notes:] There was scholar who, for several months, ranted in an unusual way and wanted to beat people. I thought it was heart disease, so I applied moxibustion on Bǎi Huì 百會 (Dū 20). Bǎi Huì can treat heart disease. I also suspected it was ghost evils, so I followed the moxibustion method of Qín Chéngzǔ for treating ghost evils: I put both thumbs together, and tied them with soft silk string; then I applied seven cones of moxibustion on the junction of the flesh and the nail, burning all four corners. He was cured afterwards (see the moxibustion method in the section on withdrawal evils). Two sons of an honourable person also suffered this disease, so a monk-doctor applied moxibustion on this point, and also cured the disease.

17. According to ancient medicinal texts, cattail belts can unblock qì.

上氣
420

狂走掣瘲：灸玉枕上三寸；一法，項後一寸百壯（《千》）。狂走癲疾：灸項後二寸十二壯。狂走驚癇：灸河口五十壯，在腕後陷中動脈是。此與陽明同也。狂走癲疾：灸大幽百壯。

Manic walking, pulling and slackening: Apply moxibustion on the site 3 cùn above Yù Zhěn 玉枕 (UB 9); another method is to apply a hundred cones on the site 1 cùn above the nape (*Qiān*《千》).

Manic walking and withdrawal disease: Apply twelve cones of moxibustion on the site 2 cùn above the nape.

Manic walking and fright epilepsy: Apply fifty cones of moxibustion on Hé Kǒu 河口 which is located on pulsating vessel in the depression proximal to the wrist. It is the same as Yáng Míng 陽明 (LI 5).

Manic walking and withdrawal disease: Apply a hundred cones of moxibustion on Dà Yōu 大幽 (unknown).

狂走癲癇：灸季肋端三十。狂走喜怒悲泣：灸巨覺（一作巨攪），隨年壯。在背上甲內側，反手所不及者，骨芒穴上捻之痛者是。狂走驚恍惚：灸足陽明三十壯。狂走易罵：灸八會隨年壯，在陽明下五分。

Manic walking, withdrawal and epilepsy: Apply thirty cones of moxibustion on the end of the free ribs.

Manic walking, joy, anger, sorrow and weeping: Apply the same number of the cones as the age of the patient on Jù Jiào 巨覺[18] (another says Jù Jiǎo 巨攪). It is located on the back, on the medial aspect of the scapula where it cannot be reached by turning the hand backward; this is the Gú Máng 骨芒 point (unknown) and it is painful when twisted with the fingers.

Manic walking, fright and abstraction: Apply thirty cones of moxibustion on Foot Yángmíng 足陽明 (ST 42).

Manic walking and tendency to curse: Apply the same number of the cones as the age of the patient on Bā Huì 八會 which is located 5 fēn below Yángmíng 陽明 (ST 42).

筋縮（《銅》同）等主狂走。三里主邪病大喚罵走遠。狂走癲厥如死人：灸足大指三毛中九壯（《翼》云灸大敦）。狂走易氣等：灸絕骨（見上氣）。

Jīn Suō 筋縮 (Dū 8) (*Tóng*《銅》agrees) and so forth govern manic walking.

18. According to some texts, Jù Jiào 巨覺 may refer to Gāo Huāng Shù 膏肓俞 (UB 43).

Sān Lǐ 三里 (ST 36) governs evil diseases, shouting and cursing loudly, as well as running far.

Manic walking, withdrawal and deathlike reversal: Apply nine cones of moxibustion to the three hairs [the region proximal to the base of the nail] on the big toe (*Yì* 《 翼 》 says to apply moxibustion on Dà Dūn 大敦 (LV 1)).

Manic walking, tendency toward anger, and so forth: Apply moxibustion on Jué Gǔ 絕骨 (GB 39) (see the section on qì ascent).

**鬼語狂走，當依法灸之。若傷寒鬼語癲狂，惟宜用四物湯加黃芪等分，七八錢重作一服，水一碗煎七分服。滓即用水一碗煎半碗連服。予屢用之神效，故附著於此。**

[Author's notes:] For ghost talk and manic walking, follow the methods [above] and apply moxibustion. For cold damage, with ghost talk, withdrawal and mania, it is appropriate to use equal portions of [each herb in] *Sì Wù Tāng* 四物湯 (Four Agents Decoction) plus *huáng qí* 黃芪 (Astragali Radix). Take 7 or 8 *qián* as one dose, cook it down to seventy percent of one bowl of water and drink it. Then cook the residue in one bowl of water to fifty percent and drink again. I use this method a lot and it gives divine effects, so I attach it here.

身腫
459
狂言
345
唾血
402

# 4.15
## *Diān Xián Chì Zòng (Xiǎo Ér Chì Zòng)*
## 癲癇瘛瘲（小兒瘛瘲）
## Withdrawal, epilepsy, tugging and slackening
**(Tugging and slackening in children)**

命門治瘛瘲里急，腰腹相引痛（《銅》）。大杼治瘛瘲，氣實脅滿。屋翳治瘛瘲不仁（見身腫）。陽谷（見狂言，《明》同）治瘛瘲。曲澤療肘瘛瘲（《明》見唾血）。少澤療瘛瘲。承筋主瘛瘲腳酸（《千》）。曲池、少澤主瘛瘲，癲疾。

Mìng Mén 命門 (Dū 4) treats tugging and slackening with abdominal tension, and pulling pain of low back and abdomen (*Tóng*《銅》).

Dà Zhù 大杼 (UB 11) treats tugging and slackening, qì excess, and fullness of the rib-sides.

Wū Yì 屋翳 (ST 15) treats tugging and slackening and numbness (see the section on generalized swelling).

Yáng Gŭ 陽谷 (SI 5) (see the section on manic raving; *Míng*《明》agrees) treat tugging and slackening.

Qū Zé 曲澤 (PC 3) cures tugging and slackening in the elbows (see the section on spitting of blood in *Míng*).

Shào Zé 少澤 (SI 1) cures tugging and slackening.

Chéng Jīn 承筋 (UB 56) governs tugging and slackening and sore legs (*Qiān*《千》).

Qū Chí 曲池 (LI 11) and Shào Zé (SI 1) govern tugging and slackening and withdrawal diseases.

身柱主癲疾瘛瘲，怒欲殺人，身熱狂走，譫言見鬼（《明》上、下同）。商丘主癇瘲。攢竹、小海、後頂、強間主癇發瘛瘲狂走。崑崙主癇瘛，口閉不開。陽溪、天井主驚瘲。解溪主瘛瘲而驚。上關主瘛瘲沫出，寒熱痓引骨痛。

Shēn Zhù 身柱 (Dū 12) governs withdrawal disease, tugging and slackening, anger with desire to kill people, generalized heat, manic walking, and dream talking as if seeing a ghost (upper and lower *Míng* 《 明 》 agree).

Shāng Qiū 商丘 (SP 5) governs epilepsy and slackening.

Zǎn Zhú 攢竹 (UB 2), Xiǎo Hǎi 小海 (SI 8), Hòu Dǐng 後頂 (Dū 19), and Qiáng Jiān 強間 (Dū 18) govern onset of epilepsy, tugging and slackening, and manic walking.

Kūn Lún 崑崙 (UB 60) governs epilepsy, slackening, and clenched jaws.

Yáng Xī 陽溪 (LI 5) and Tiān Jǐng 天井 (SJ 10) govern fright and tugging.

Jiě Xī 解溪 (ST 41) governs tugging and slackening and fright.

Shàng Guān 上關 (GB 3) governs tugging and slackening, spitting of foam, and cold-heat tetany with pain radiating to the bones.

巨闕 、照海主瘛瘲引臍腹，短氣 。命門主瘛瘲里急，腰腹相引痛（ 《 銅人 》 、《 明 》同 ）。腦戶 、聽會 、聽宮 、風府 、翳風主骨酸眩狂，瘛瘲口噤，喉鳴沫出，喑不能言 。

Jù Quē 巨闕 (Rèn 14) and Zhào Hǎi 照海 (KI 6) govern tugging and slackening that radiates to the umbilicus and abdomen, and shortness of breath.

Mìng Mén 命門 (Dū 4) governs tugging and slackening, abdominal tension, and pulling pain of low back and abdomen (*Tóng Rén* 《 銅人 》 and *Míng* agree).

Nǎo Hù 腦戶 (Dū 17), Tīng Huì 聽會 (GB 2), Tīng Gōng 聽宮 (SI 19), Fēng Fǔ 風府 (Dū 16) and Yì Fēng 翳風 (SJ 17) govern aching bones, dizziness, mania, tugging and slackening, clenched jaws, throat rales, spitting of foam, and loss of voice.

五處 、身柱 、委中 、委陽 、崑崙主脊強反折，瘛瘲，癲疾頭痛 。絡卻 、聽會 、身柱主狂走瘛瘲，恍惚不樂（ 並《 千 》 ）。啞門治寒熱風痓，背強反折，瘛瘲癲疾頭重（ 《 銅 》 ）。五處治頭風目眩，瘛瘲，目戴上不識人 。巨髎治瘛瘲，口喎（ 《 明 》同 ）。上關治瘛瘲口沫出，目眩，牙車不開，口噤 。

Wǔ Chù 五處 (UB 5), Shēn Zhù 身柱 (Dū 12), Wěi Zhōng 委中 (UB 40), Wěi Yáng 委陽 (UB 39), and Kūn Lún 崑崙 (UB 60) govern arched-back rigidity, tugging and slackening, withdrawal diseases, and headaches.

風痹 377 小腹 209 驚癇 363

Luò Què 絡卻 (UB 8), Tīng Huì 聽會 (GB 2), and Shēn Zhù 身柱 (Dū 12) govern manic walking, tugging and slackening, abstraction and unhappiness (for all, see *Qiān*《千》).

Yǎ Mén 啞門 (Dū 15) treats [sensations of] cold and heat, wind tetany, arched-back rigidity, tugging and slackening, withdrawal diseases, and heaviness of the head (*Tóng*《銅》).

Wǔ Chù (UB 5) treats head wind, dizzy vision, tugging and slackening, upturned eyes, and loss of consciousness.

Jù Liáo 巨髎 (ST 3) treats tugging and slackening with deviation of the mouth (*Míng*《明》agrees).

Shàng Guān 上關 (GB 3) treats tugging and slackening, spitting of foam, dizzy vision, and clenched jaws.

少澤治臂痛瘛瘲，咳嗽，頸項急，不可顧。跗陽（見風痹）、天井治瘛瘲（《千》見風痹）。腕骨治驚風瘛瘲，五指掣。帶脈治婦人里急瘛瘲（見小腹痛）。大椎療癲病瘛瘲，身熱目昡，項急，臥不安（《明下》）。

Shào Zé 少澤 (SI 1) treats arm pain, tugging and slackening, cough, stiff neck and nape, and inability to turn the neck.

Fū Yáng 跗陽 (UB 59) (see the section on wind *bì*-impediment) and Tiān Jǐng 天井 (SJ 10) treat tugging and slackening (for all, see the section on wind *bì*-impediment in *Qiān*).

Wàn Gǔ 腕骨 (SI 4) treats fright wind, tugging and slackening, and pulling of the five fingers.

Dài Mài 帶脈 (GB 26) treats abdominal tension in women and tugging and slackening (see the section on pain of the smaller abdomen).

Dà Zhuī 大椎 (Dū 14) cures withdrawal diseases, tugging and slackening, generalized heat, dizzy vision, tension of the nape, and unquiet sleep (*Míng Xià*《明下》).

顱囟治小兒發癇瘛瘲，嘔吐涎沫，驚恐失精，瞻視不明（《銅》）。瘈脈治小兒驚癇瘛瘲，嘔吐泄痢無時，驚恐眵瞢，目睛不明（《明》同）。前頂治小兒驚癇風癇瘛瘲（見驚癇）。崑崙治小兒發癇瘛瘲。

Lú Xìn 顱囟 (SJ 19) treats pediatric epilepsy with tugging and slackening, vomiting of drool and foam, fright and fear, seminal loss,[19] and indistinct vision (*Tóng*).

19. *Shī jīng* 失精 (seminal loss) is corrected from *shī jiá* 失頰 (loss of jaw) based on *Tóng Rén Tú Jīng*《銅人圖經》.

Chì Mài 瘈脈 (SJ 18) treats pediatric fright epilepsy with tugging and slackening, vomiting, incessant diarrhea, fright and fear, copious eye discharge, and diminished vision (*Míng* 《明》 agrees).

Qián Dǐng 前頂 (Dū 21) treats pediatric fright epilepsy wind epilepsy, and tugging and slackening (see the section on fright epilepsy).

Kūn Lún 崑崙 (UB 60) treats pediatric onset of epilepsy and tugging and slackening.

## 4.16
## *Diān Xián (Xián Fù, Yú Lùn Jiàn Fēng Xián)*
# 癲癇（癇附　餘論見風癇）
## Withdrawal and epilepsy
**(Epilepsy is attached; for further discussion, see the section on wind epilepsy)**

天柱主卒暴癇眩（《千》）。攢竹、小海、後頂、強間主癇發瘛瘲狂走。商丘主癇瘛。絲竹空、通谷主風癇癲疾，涎沫狂煩。金門、僕參主癲疾馬癇（《千》）。天井、小海主癲疾，羊癇吐舌，羊鳴戾頸。

Tiān Zhù 天柱 (UB 10) governs sudden and violent epilepsy and dizziness (*Qiān* 《千》).

Zǎn Zhú 攢竹 (UB 2), Xiǎo Hǎi 小海 (SI 8), Hòu Dǐng 後頂 (Dū 19), and Qiáng Jiān 強間 (Dū 18) govern onset of epilepsy, tugging and slackening, and manic walking.

Shāng Qiū 商丘 (SP 5) governs epilepsy and tugging.

Sī Zhú Kōng 絲竹空 (SJ 23) and Tōng Gǔ 通谷 (UB 66 or KI 20) govern wind epilepsy, withdrawal diseases, [spitting of] drool and foam, mania, and vexation.

Jīn Mén 金門 (UB 63) and Pū Cān 僕參 (UB 61) govern withdrawal diseases and horse epilepsy (*Qiān*).

Tiān Jǐng 天井 (SJ 10) and Xiǎo Hǎi 小海 (SI 8) govern withdrawal diseases, goat epilepsy with protrusion of the tongue and sounds like the bleating of a goat, and perverse neck [torticollis or wryneck].

懸釐、束骨主癲疾互引，善驚羊鳴。筋縮、曲骨、陰谷、行間主驚癇狂走癲疾。列缺主熱癇驚而有所見。水溝治失笑無時，癲癇，語不識尊卑（《下狂走 345 經》同），乍喜乍哭，牙關不開（《銅》）。心俞治發癇悲泣（見狂走）。
狂言 345 筋縮治驚癇，狂走癲疾，脊急強，目轉上垂。

尸厥 531 Xuán Lí 懸釐 (GB 6) and Shù Gǔ 束骨 (UB 65) govern withdrawal diseases affecting each other, susceptibility to fright, and sounds like the bleating of a goat.

Jīn Suō 筋縮 (Dū 8), Qū Gǔ 曲骨 (Rèn 2), Yīn Gǔ 陰谷 (KI 10), and Xíng Jiān 行間 (LV 2) govern fright epilepsy, manic walking, and withdrawal diseases.

Liè Quē 列缺 (LU 7) governs heat epilepsy and fright as if seeing something.

Shuǐ Gōu 水溝 (Dū 26) treats uncontrollable laughter, withdrawal and epilepsy, speaking without regard to a person's proper rank (*Xià Jīng*《下經》agrees), bouts of laughter and crying, and clenched jaws (*Tóng*《銅》).

Xīn Shù 心俞 (UB 15) treats the onset of epilepsy and sorrowful weeping (see the section on manic walking).

Jīn Suō (Dū 8) treats fright epilepsy, manic walking, withdrawal diseases, acute stiffness of the spine, upturned eyes, and drooping.[20]

僕參（見狂言）、金門（見尸厥）治癲癇。脊中治風癇癲邪。神門治大小人五癇。金門治小兒發癇，張口搖頭，身反折。脊俞療風癇癲邪（《明》）。神庭療腫氣風癇，癲風不識人，羊鳴，角弓反張，披髮而上歌下哭，多學人語，驚悸不安寢。

Pū Cān 僕參 (UB 61) (see the section on manic raving) and Jīn Mén 金門 (UB 63) (see the section on deathlike reversal) treat withdrawal and epilepsy.

Jǐ Zhōng 脊中 (Dū 6) treats wind epilepsy and withdrawal evils.

Shén Mén 神門 (HT 7) treats the five epilepsies[21] in adults and children.

Jīn Mén 金門 (UB 63) treats onset of epilepsy in children, open mouth, shaking of the head, and arched-back rigidity.

Jǐ Shù 脊俞 (Dū 6) cures wind epilepsy and withdrawal evils (*Míng*《明》).

Shén Tíng 神庭 (Dū 24) cures qì swelling and wind epilepsy, withdrawal and loss of consciousness, [sounds like] the bleating of a goat, arched-back rigidity, disheveled the hair, ascending to high

20. What is meant by *drooping* is unclear.

21. Different references have variations in the list of the five epilepsies. According to this text (later in this section), they are horse epilepsy, goat epilepsy, chicken epilepsy, pig epilepsy, and ox epilepsy.

places and singing, descending to lower places and crying, frequently copying people's speech, fright palpitations, and unquiet sleep.

肺俞、僕參（ 見尸厥 ）療癲癇。少海療癲癇吐舌，沫出羊鳴。狂癲風癇吐舌：灸胃管百壯，不針。倉公法：狂癇不識人，癲病眩亂：灸百會九壯。

Fèi Shù 肺俞 (UB 13) and Pū Cān 僕參 (UB 61) (see the section on deathlike reversal) cure withdrawal and epilepsy.

Shào Hǎi 少海 (HT 3) cures withdrawal and epilepsy with protrusion of the tongue, spitting of foam and sounds like the bleating of a goat.

Manic withdrawal and wind epilepsy with protrusion of the tongue: Apply a hundred of cones of moxibustion on Wèi Guǎn 胃管 (Rèn 12 or Rèn 13) but no acupuncture.

Master Cāng's method for manic epilepsy, loss of consciousness, withdrawal, dizziness, and confusion: Apply nine cones of moxibustion on Bǎi Huì 百會 (Dū 20).

《難經疏》云：狂病之候，不愛眠臥，不肯飲食，自言賢智，歌樂行走。此是陽氣盛之所為。故經言：重陽者狂。今世以此為癲病，謬矣。癲病發即僵僕倒地，故有癲蹶之言。陰氣大盛，故不得行立而倒也。今世以為癇病者，誤也。其剖析癲狂之病，曉然如此，而人終不信，豈亦傳習之誤，難以改歟（重陰者癲）。

[Author's notes:] *Nàn Jīng Shū* 難經疏 says: Symptoms of mania include: Dislike for sleep, no desire to eat and drink, calling oneself a sage, and [uncontrollable] walking and singing. These are caused by excess yáng qì. So the Classic says: Double yáng becomes mania. Nowadays, people think this is withdrawal disease, but that is wrong. When withdrawal disease attacks, [people] collapse suddenly on the ground, so it is called withdrawal stumbling.

When yīn qì is too excuberant, people cannot stand or walk, so they fall. Nowadays, people think this is epilepsy, but that is not correct. It is very clear after analyzing withdrawal and mania diseases, but people still do not believe it. This is a mistake in teaching and learning, and is difficult to correct (double yīn becomes withdrawal).

凡發狂則欲走，或自高貴稱神聖，皆須備諸火灸之，乃得永瘥。悲泣呻吟，此則為邪，非狂也，自依邪方法治（《千》）。

Whenever mania erupts, there is a desire to walk, or believing oneself to be nobility and calling oneself a divine sage; fire must be prepared for moxibustion so the disease will be cured forever.

癲癇 357 Sorrow, weeping and groaning are from evil and are not mania, so in that case treat the evil (*Qiān*《千》).

# 4.17

## *Diān Jí (Yú Lùn Jiàn Fēng Xián)*

## 癲疾（餘論見風癇）

## Withdrawal diseases

**(for further discussion, see wind epilepsy)**

解溪治癲疾，煩心悲泣（《銅》）。啞門治癲疾頭重。完骨治癲疾，頭面浮腫，齒齲。天衝治頭痛，癲疾，風痙，牙齦腫，善驚。筋縮治癲疾脊強（見癲癇）。申脈、後溪、前谷治癲疾。滑肉門治癲疾嘔逆吐舌。兌端（《明下》同）、本神治癲疾吐沫。

Jiě Xī 解溪 (ST 41) treats withdrawal disease, vexation of the heart, sorrow and weeping (*Tóng*《銅》).

Yǎ Mén 啞門 (Dū 15) treats withdrawal disease with heaviness of the head.

Wán Gǔ 完骨 (GB 12) treats withdrawal disease, puffy swelling of the head and face, and tooth decay.

Tiān Chōng 天衝 (GB 9) treats headaches, withdrawal disease, wind tetany, gum swelling, and susceptibility to fright.

Jīn Suō 筋縮 (Dū 8) treats withdrawal disease and stiffness of the spine (see the section on withdrawal and epilepsy).

Shēn Mài 申脈 (UB 62), Hòu Xī 後溪 (SI 3), and Qián Gǔ 前谷 (SI 2) treat withdrawal disease.

Huá Ròu Mén 滑肉門 (ST 24) treats withdrawal disease, retching counterflow, and protrusion of the tongue.

Duì Duān 兌端 (Dū 27) (*Míng Xià*《明下》agrees) and Běn Shén 本神 (GB 13) treat withdrawal disease and spitting of foam.

飛揚治癲疾寒痛。承山、崑崙療寒熱癲疾。尺澤療癲病不可向，手臂不得上頭（《下》）。解溪、陽蹻主癲疾（《千》）。神庭、上星、百會、聽會、聽宮、偏歷、攢竹、本神、築賓、陽溪、後頂、強間、腦戶、絡卻、玉枕主癲疾嘔。

Fēi Yáng 飛揚 (UB 58) treats withdrawal disease with cold pain.

Chéng Shān 承山 (UB 57) and Kūn Lún 崑崙 (UB 60) cure cold and heat withdrawal disease.

Chǐ Zé 尺澤 (LU 5) cures withdrawal disease; and inability to face [the hands] with inability of the arms to reach the head (*Xià*《下》).

Jiě Xī 解溪 (ST 41) and Yáng Qiāo 陽蹻 (UB 62) govern withdrawal disease (*Qiān*《千》).

Shén Tíng 神庭 (Dū 24), Shàng Xīng 上星 (Dū 23), Bǎi Huì 百會 (Dū 20),Tīng Huì 聽會 (GB 2), Tīng Gōng 聽宮 (SI 19), Piān Lì 偏歷 (LI 6), Zǎn Zhú 攢竹 (UB 2), Běn Shén 本神 (GB 13), Zhù Bīn 筑賓 (KI 9), Yáng Xī 陽溪 (LI 5), Hòu Dǐng 後頂 (Dū 19), Qiáng Jiān 強間 (Dū 18), Nǎo Hù 腦戶 (Dū 17), Luò Què 絡卻 (UB 8), and Yù Zhěn 玉枕 (UB 9) govern withdrawal disease and vomiting.

兌端、齦交、承漿、大迎、絲竹空、囟會、天柱、商丘主癲疾嘔沫，寒熱痙互引。承漿、大迎主寒熱淒厥鼓頷，癲痙口噤。臑會、申脈主癲疾腠氣。尺澤、然谷主癲疾手臂不得上頭。偏歷主癲疾，多言，耳鳴口僻。

Duì Duān 兌端 (Dū 27), Yín Jiāo 齦交 (Dū 28), Chéng Jiāng 承漿 (Rèn 24), Dà Yíng 大迎 (ST 5), Sī Zhú Kōng 絲竹空 (SJ 23), Xìn Huì 囟會 (Dū 22), Tiān Zhù 天柱 (UB 10), and Shāng Qiū 商丘 (SP 5) govern withdrawal disease, vomiting of foam, and cold and heat tetany pulling each other.

Chéng Jiāng 承漿 (Rèn 24) and Dà Yíng 大迎 (ST 5) govern cold and heat reversal, chattering jaws, withdrawal tetany, and clenched jaws.

Nào Huì 臑會 (SJ 13) and Shēn Mài 申脈 (UB 62) govern withdrawal disease and interstitial qì.[22]

Chǐ Zé (LU 5) and Rán Gǔ 然谷 (KI 2) govern withdrawal disease and inability of the arms to reach the head.

Piān Lì (LI 6) governs withdrawal disease, continual talking, tinnitus, and deviation of the mouth.

22. *Còu qì* 腠氣 (interstitial qì): The meaning is unclear.

瘛瘲 354
癲癇 357
驚癇 363

腦空、束骨主癲疾，大瘦頭痛。懸釐、束骨主癲疾互引，善驚羊鳴。天衝主頭痛癲疾，互引數驚。通谷主心中憒憒數，數欠，癲，心下悸恐，咽中澹澹。風池、聽會、復溜主寒熱癲僕。完骨主癲疾僵。曲池等主癲疾（見瘛瘲）。狂癲：灸胃管（見癲癇）；或灸巨陽（見驚癇）。

Nǎo Kōng 腦空 (GB 19) and Shù Gǔ 束骨 (UB 65) govern withdrawal disease, marked emaciation, and headache.

Xuán Lí 懸釐 (GB 6) and Shù Gǔ (UB 65) govern withdrawal diseases affecting each other, susceptibility to fright, and sounds like the bleating of a goat.

Tiān Chōng 天衝 (GB 9) governs headaches, withdrawal diseases affecting each other, and frequent fright.

Tōng Gǔ 通谷 (UB 66) governs fretting of the heart, frequent yawning, withdrawal, palpitations and fear below the heart, and a rolling sensation in the throat.

Fēng Chí 風池 (GB 20), Tīng Huì 聽會 (GB 2) and Fù Liū 復溜 (KI 7) govern [sensations of] cold and heat, withdrawal disease, and falling.

Wán Gǔ 完骨 (GB 12) governs withdrawal disease and stiffness.

Qū Chí 曲池 (LI 11) and so forth govern withdrawal disease (see the section on tugging and slackening).

Mania-withdrawal: Apply moxibustion on Wèi Guǎn 胃管 (Rèn 12 or Rèn 13) (see the section on withdrawal and epilepsy) or Jù Yáng 巨陽 (UB 63) (see the section on fright epilepsy).

有人患癇疾，發則僵僕在地，久之方蘇。予意其用心所致，為灸百會。又疑是痰厥致僵僕，為灸中管，其疾稍減，未除根也。後閲《脈訣》後通真子有“愛養小兒，謹護風池”之說。人來覓灸癇疾，必為之按風池穴，皆應手酸疼，使灸之而愈（小兒癇，恐亦可灸此。）

[Author's notes:] Someone suffered epilepsy, collapsing on the floor when it erupted and taking a long time to wake up. I thought it was caused by overuse of the heart, so I applied moxibustion on Bǎi Huì 百會 (Dū 20). I also suspected the sudden collapse was due to phlegm reversal, so I applied moxibustion on Zhōng Guǎn 中管 (Rèn 12). The disease got better, but the root was not gone. Later, after I read *Mài Jué*《脈訣》, I knew [Cuī] Zhēngzǐ had the theory of "loving and nurturing children by carefully protecting Fēng Chí (GB 20)." When people come and asked for moxibustion treatment for epilepsy, I always press Fēng Chí (GB 20) and pain is the response to pressure. After applying moxibustion on it, the disease is cured. (It is appropriate to apply moxibustion on this point for epilepsy in children).

# 4.18

## *Jīng Xián (Xiǎo Ér Jīng Xián, Jí Jīng Fēng, Màn Jīng Fēng)*

## 驚癇（小兒驚癇　急驚風　慢驚風）

### Fright epilepsy[23]

**(Fright epilepsy in children, acute fright wind, and chronic fright wind)**

囟會治驚癇，戴目上不識人（《銅》）。巨骨療驚癇破心，吐血（《明》）。鳩尾療心驚癇發，狀如鳥鳴，破心吐血，心中氣悶，不喜聞人語，心痛腹脹。少衝療驚癇，吐舌沫出。束骨療驚癇癲狂，身寒熱，頭痛目眩（《下》）。筋縮療驚癇狂走，癇病多言，脊強，兩目轉上及目瞪。

Xìn Huì 囟會 (Dū 22) treats fright epilepsy, upcast[24] eyes, and loss of consciousness (*Tóng*《銅》).

Jù Gǔ 巨骨 (LI 16) cures fright epilepsy breaking the heart open and vomiting blood (*Míng*《明》).

Jiū Wěi 鳩尾 (Rèn 15) cures heart fright and onset of epilepsy, [making sounds like] birds chirping, breaking the heart open and vomiting blood, qì oppression of the heart, dislike of hearing people talking, heart pain, and abdominal distention.

Shào Chōng 少衝 (HT 9) cures fright epilepsy, protrusion of the tongue, and spitting of foam.

Shù Gǔ 束骨 (UB 65) cures fright epilepsy, withdrawal and mania, generalized [sensations of] cold and heat, headaches, and dizzy vision (*Xià*《下》).

Jīn Suō 筋縮 (Dū 8) cures fright epilepsy and manic walking, epilepsy with continual talking, stiffness of the spine, upturned eyes, and staring eyes.

23. Generally, epilepsy is divided into eight categories: wind epilepsy, fright epilepsy, phlegm epilepsy, food epilepsy, heat epilepsy, stagnation epilepsy, vacuity epilepsy, and worm epilepsy.

24. *Jǐng Yuè Quán Shū* Volume 45《景岳全書·卷之四十五》(Jǐng Yuè's Complete Compendium) by Zhāng Jǐngyuè 張景岳, published in 1624, states: The symptom of upcast eyes occurs after suppuration of pox, or after severe sweating and diarrhea. It is usually characterized by upturned eyes with the white of eyes (sclera) showing.

小兒
354 瘈脉、長強主小兒驚癇瘛瘲，嘔吐泄注，驚恐失精，瞻視不明（《千》）。
風 囟會、前頂、本神、天柱主小兒驚癇。臨泣主兒癇反視。囟會主兒癇喘不得
379 息。前頂治小兒驚癇（《明下》同），風癇瘛瘲，發即先時鼻多清涕，頂腫
（《銅》）。

Chì Mài 瘈脈 (SJ 18) and Cháng Qiáng 長強 (Dū 1) govern fright epilepsy in children, tugging and slackening, vomiting and outpour diarrhea, fright, fear, seminal loss, and indistinct vision (*Qiān*《千》).

Xìn Huì 囟會 (Dū 22), Qián Dǐng 前頂 (Dū 21), Běn Shén 本神 (GB 13), and Tiān Zhù 天柱 (UB 10) govern fright epilepsy in children.

Lín Qì 臨泣 (GB 15) governs epilepsy in children and rolled back eyes.

Xìn Huì (Dū 22) governs epilepsy in children, panting, and inability to breathe.

Qián Dǐng (Dū 21) treats fright epilepsy in children (*Míng Xià*《明下》agrees), wind epilepsy, tugging and slackening, with copious clear snivel [nasal mucus], and swollen vertex during attacks (*Tóng*《銅》).

瘈脉、神道、顱囟治兒發癇瘛瘲（並見小兒瘛瘲）。長強、身柱療小兒驚癇。小兒但是風病：灸率谷（見風）。小兒先驚怖啼叫，後乃發驚癇：灸頂上旋毛中三壯，及耳後青絡脈。小兒驚癇：灸鬼錄穴一壯，在上唇內中央弦上，用鋼刀決斷更佳。小兒急驚風：灸前頂三壯；若不愈，須灸兩眉頭及人中穴。

Chì Mài (SJ 18), Shén Dào 神道 (Du 11), and Lú Xìn 顱囟 (SJ 19) treat epilepsy in children and tugging and slackening (see also the section on tugging and slackening in children).

Cháng Qiáng (Dū 1) and Shēn Zhù 身柱 (Dū 12) cure fright epilepsy in children.

Wind diseases in children: Apply moxibustion on Shuài Gǔ 率谷 (GB 8) (see the section on wind [stroke]).

First crying due to fright and fear in children, then fright epilepsy erupts: Apply three cones of moxibustion on the twirled hair [cowlick] at the vertex and on the green vessels behind the ear.

Fright epilepsy in children: Apply one cone of moxibustion on Guǐ Lù 鬼錄. It is located on the string-like flesh inside the upper lip in the center, or it is even better to cut it with a knife.

Acute fright wind in children: Apply three cones of moxibustion on Qián Dǐng (Dū 21). If it is not cured, also apply moxibustion on the two eyebrows and on Rén Zhōng 人中 (Dū 26).

秦承祖灸小兒驚癇等（ 見鬼邪 ），小兒緩驚風：灸尺澤各一壯 。狂邪驚癇病：灸承命三十壯，在內踝後上行三寸動脈上，亦灸驚狂走 。狂癲風驚，厥逆心煩：灸巨陽五十壯 。行間（ 見癲狂 ）主驚癇（ 《 千 》 ）。腕骨治驚風（ 《 銅 》見瘛瘲 ）。筋縮療驚癇（ 《 明 》見癲狂 ）。

鬼邪 343
癲狂 345
瘛瘲 354

Qín Chéngzǔ treated pediatric fright epilepsy, chronic fright wind, and so forth with moxibustion (see the discussion of ghost evils): Apply one cone of moxibustion on Chǐ Zé 尺澤 (LU 5).

Mania evils and fright epilepsy: Apply thirty cones of moxibustion on Chéng Mìng 承命 which is located on the pulsating vessel, 3 cùn above the medial malleolus; it is also good for fright and manic walking.

Mania, withdrawal, fright wind, reverse counterflow and vexation of the heart: Apply fifty cones of moxibustion on Jù Yáng 巨陽 (UB 60).

Xíng Jiān 行間 (LV 2) (see the section on withdrawal and mania) governs fright epilepsy (*Qiān* 《 千 》).

Wàn Gǔ 腕骨 (SI 4) treats fright wind (see the section on tugging and slackening in *Tóng* 《 銅 》).

Jīn Suō 筋縮 (Dū 8) cures fright epilepsy (see the section on withdrawal-mania in *Míng* 《 明 》).

急、慢驚風，非風也。古人謂之陰陽癇，猶傷寒之有陰陽證也。陽癇如陽證，當治以涼藥；陰癇如陰證，當治以溫藥。庸醫不知此例，以風藥治之，風藥多涼，或是慢驚，未有不罹其害者。戒之戒之。若灸驚風，惟灸慢驚、慢脾風為穩當云。

[Author's notes:] Acute or chronic fright wind is not really wind. Ancient people called it yīn and yáng epilepsy, like the yīn and yáng patterns of cold damage. Yáng epilepsy seems like a yáng pattern, so it should be treated with cooling herbs; yīn epilepsy seems like a yīn pattern, so it should be treated with warming herbs. Ordinary doctors do not know this rule, so they use herbs to treat wind. Wind herbs are usually cooling, [so if they are used to treat] chronic fright wind, the patient will be harmed. Beware of this. When applying moxibustion for fright wind, it is safer to use moxibustion for chronic fright wind or chronic spleen wind.

癲癇
357
目眩
575

# 4.19
## *Fēng Xián (Wǔ Xián)*
# 風癇（五癇）
## Wind epilepsy
**(The five epilepsies)**

神庭療癲風不識人，羊鳴（《明》見癲癇）。百會療風癇，青風心風，角弓反張，羊鳴，多哭，言語不擇，發時即死，吐沫心熱悶，頭風，多睡心煩，驚悸無心力，忘前失後，食無味，頭重，飲酒面赤鼻塞。《明下》云：療登高而歌，棄衣而走，角弓反張，羊癇吐舌。

Shén Tíng 神庭 (Dū 24) cures epilepsy, loss of consciousness, and making sounds like the bleating of a goat (see the section on withdrawal and epilepsy in *Míng*《明》).

Bǎi Huì 百會 (Dū 20) cures wind epilepsy, green-blue wind,[25] heart wind, arched-back rigidity, goat sounds, incessant crying, speaking without choosing the words, dying when the disease erupts, spitting of foam, heat and oppression of the heart, head wind, sleepiness and vexation of the heart, fright palpitations, weakness of the heart, forgetfulness, inability to taste food, heaviness of the head, and red face with nasal congestion after drinking alcohol. *Míng Xià*《明下》says: It cures climbing to high places and singing, taking the clothes off and walking, arched-back rigidity, epilepsy, and protrusion of the tongue.

百會治風癇，中風，角弓反張，或多哭，言語不擇，發即無時，盛即吐沫，心煩驚悸（《銅》）。神庭、絲竹空（見目眩）治風癇，目戴上不識人。巨闕療心中煩悶，熱風風癇，浪言或作鳥聲，不能食，無心力。會宗治肌膚痛，耳聾，風癇。

Bǎi Huì (Dū 20) treats wind epilepsy, wind stroke, and arched-back rigidity, or incessant crying and speaking without choosing the words. The disease could erupt at anytime, with spitting of foam when it reaches its peak, vexation of the heart, and fright palpitations (*Tóng*《銅》).

Shén Tíng (Dū 24) and Sī Zhú Kōng 絲竹空 (SJ 23) (see the section on dizzy vision) treat wind epilepsy, upcast eyes and loss of consciousness.

25. This could refer to wind in the spring-time. It is also the name of a disease that resembles glaucoma in Western medicine. However in this context, it should be related to epilepsy.

Jù Quē 巨闕 (Rèn 14) cures vexation and oppression in the heart, hot wind, wind epilepsy, manic raving or making sounds like the chirping of a bird, inability to eat, and weakness of the heart.

癲 357

頭風 640

Huì Zōng 會宗 (SJ 7) treats pain of the skin and flesh, deafness, and wind epilepsy.

脊中（見癲）、涌泉治風癇。前頂療風癇（《明》）。上管療風癇熱痛，可瀉而後補。脊俞療風癇癲邪。眉衝療目五般癇，頭痛鼻塞。涌泉、神聰（見頭風）、強間（岐伯云）療風癇。天井療癇病，羊鳴吐舌。

Jǐ Zhōng 脊中 (Dū 6) (see the section on withdrawal [and epilepsy]) and Yǒng Quán 涌泉 (KI 1) treat wind epilepsy.

Qián Dǐng 前頂 (Dū 21) cures wind epilepsy (*Míng*《明》).

Shàng Guǎn 上管 (Rèn 13) cures wind epilepsy and hot pain. It is appropriate to drain first, then supplement.

Jǐ Shù 脊俞 (Dū 6) cures wind epilepsy and withdrawal evils.

Méi Chōng 眉衝 (UB 3) cures the eyes, the five types of epilepsy, headaches, and nasal congestion.

Yǒng Quán 涌泉 (KI 1), Shén Cōng 神聰 (non-channel)[26] (see the section on head wind) and Qiáng Jiān 強間 (Dū 18): (Qí Bó said) they cure wind epilepsy.

Tiān Jǐng 天井 (SJ 10) cures epilepsy, making sounds like the bleating of a goat, and protrusion of the tongue.

癇病，小兒惡疾也。呼吸之間，不及求師，致困者不少（《下》）。小兒食癇者，先寒熱灑淅乃發：灸鳩尾上五分三壯。小兒風癇者，先屈手指如數物，乃發也：灸鼻柱上髮際宛中三壯。

Pediatric epilepsy is a malign disease. [Its onset is] as fast as the breath, there's not enough time to ask for help. So there are lots of children stranded in danger (*Xià*《下》).

Food epilepsy in children, first erupts with [sensations of] cold and heat, as if after being soaked in the rain: Apply three cones of moxibustion on the site 5 fēn above the Jiū Wěi 鳩尾 (Rèn 15).

Wind epilepsy in children that first erupts with bent fingers as if counting something: Apply three cones of moxibustion in the depression within the hairline above the nose pillar [the stem of the nose].

26. This refers to Sì Shén Cōng 四神聰, the four points surrounding Bǎi Huì 百會 (Dū 20).

小兒豬癇病，如尸厥，吐沫：灸巨闕三壯。小兒雞癇，善驚反折，手掣自搖：灸手少陰五壯，在掌後去腕半寸陷中。小兒羊癇，目瞪吐舌羊鳴：灸九椎下節間三壯。小兒牛癇，目直視腹脹，乃發：灸鳩尾三壯。小兒馬癇，張口搖頭，身反折，馬鳴：灸僕參各三壯。

Pig epilepsy in children, similar to deathlike reversal, with spitting of foam: Apply three cones of moxibustion on Jù Quē 巨闕 (Rèn 14).

Chicken epilepsy in children, with susceptibility to fright, arched-back rigidity, pulling and spontaneous shaking of the hands: Apply five cones of moxibustion on Shǒu Shàoyīn 手少陰 (HT 6) which is located in the depression 0.5 cùn proximal to the wrist, on the palmar aspect.

Goat epilepsy in children, with staring eyes, protrusion of the tongue and [sounds like] the bleating of a goat: Apply three cones of moxibustion on the site below the ninth vertebra.

Ox epilepsy in children, erupting with forward-staring eyes and abdominal distention: Apply three cones of moxibustion on Jiū Wěi 鳩尾 (Rèn 15).

Horse epilepsy in children, with mouth opened, shaking of the head, as well as arched-back rigidity, and [sounds like] the neighing of a horse: Apply three cones of moxibustion on Pū Cān 僕參 (UB 61).

馬癇，張口搖頭馬鳴，欲反折：灸項風府、臍中三壯（《千》：燒馬蹄末服良）。牛癇，目正直視腹脹：灸鳩尾骨及大椎，各三壯（燒牛蹄末服良）。羊癇，喜揚目吐舌：灸大椎上三壯。豬癇，喜吐沫：灸完骨兩旁各一寸，七壯。犬癇，手屈拳攣：灸兩手心、足太陽、肋戶，各一壯。雞癇，搖頭反折，喜驚自搖：灸足諸陽各三壯。

Horse epilepsy, with mouth opened, head shaking, [sounds like] the neighing of a horse, as well as arched-back rigidity: Apply three cones of moxibustion on Fēng Fǔ 風府 (Dū 16) and Qí Zhōng 臍中 (Rèn 8) (*Qiān*《千》says: It is good to cook powdered horse's hoof and drink it).

Ox epilepsy, with forward-staring eyes and abdominal distention: Apply three cones of moxibustion on Jiū Wěi (Rèn 15) and Dà Zhuī 大椎 (Dū 14) (it is good to cook powdered ox's hoof and drink it).

Goat epilepsy, tends to raise the eyes and stick out the tongue: Apply three cones of moxibustion on Dà Zhuī (Dū 14).

Pig epilepsy, tends to spit foam: Apply seven cones of moxibustion on the site that is 1 cùn lateral to Wán Gǔ 完骨 (GB 12).

Dog epilepsy, with fingers bent as well as hypertonicity of the fists: Apply one cone of moxibustion on the centers of the palms, Foot Tàiyáng 足太陽 (UB 60) and Lèi Hù 肋戶 (Rib Door).

Chicken epilepsy, with head shaking, arched-back rigidity, frequent fright and spontaneous shaking: Apply three cones of moxibustion on all the Foot Yáng [Channels].

驚癇
363
癲癇
357

神庭、脊俞療風癇（見驚癇）。前頂治小兒驚癇風癇（《銅》見癲癇）。小兒髮逆上，啼笑，面暗、色不變，是癇候，或鼻口青時小驚；或目閉青時小驚；或身熱頭常汗出；或身熱吐哯而喘；或身熱目時直視；或臥惕惕而驚，手足振搖；或臥夢笑，手足動搖；或意氣下而妄怒；或咽乳不利；或目瞳子卒大黑於常；或喜欠、目上視；或身熱小便難；或身熱目視不精；或吐痢不止，厥痛時起；或弄舌搖頭。諸候二十條，皆癇之初也。見其候，便爪其陽脈所應灸，爪之皆重手，令兒驟啼，及足絕脈，亦依方與湯。

Shén Tíng 神庭 (Dū 24) and Jǐ Shù 脊俞 (Dū 6) cure wind epilepsy (see the section on fright epilepsy).

Qián Dǐng 前頂 (Dū 21) treats fright epilepsy and wind epilepsy in children (see the section on withdrawal and epilepsy in *Tóng*《銅》).

Hair sticking up in children, with crying and laughing, dark facial complexion but no change in color. These are signs of epilepsy. There is minor fright when the nose and mouth turn blue-green, or there is minor fright when the eyes close and turn blue-green; or generalized heat and sweating on the head; or generalized heat and vomiting as well as panting; or generalized heat, with eyes frequently staring straight ahead; or fear when sleeping with shaking hands and feet; or sleeping and dreaming of laughter with hands and feet shaking; or descent of reflection-qì with frenetic anger; or inhibited swallowing of milk; or the pupils are suddenly larger and darker than usual; or frequent yawning and upward staring eyes; or generalized heat and difficult urination; or generalized heat and diminished vision; or incessant vomiting and dysentery with intermittent reversal pain; or hyperactive tongue and shaking head. All twenty symptoms indicate the initial stage of the epilepsy. When these symptoms are seen, pinch the yáng vessels and apply moxibustion on the sites that responded. Pinch with heavy hands [heavily]; and make the child suddenly cry; if the foot vessels expire, also give the decoctions based on the formula books.

直視瞳子動，腹滿轉鳴下血，身熱口噤不得乳，反張脊強，汗出發熱，為臥不悟，手足掣瘲，喜驚。凡八條，癇之劇者也。如有此，非復湯爪所能救，當時而灸之。

Staring forward with pupils moving; abdominal distention and rumbling with bloody stool; generalized heat, clenched jaws, and inability to get milk; arched-back rigidity; sweating with fever; sleep without awakening; pulling and slackening of the hands and feet; and susceptibility to fright. All eight symptoms indicate severe epilepsy. If someone has these, he cannot be saved by decoctions or pinching; he should get frequent moxibustion.

徐嗣曰：風眩之病，起於心氣不足，胸上蓄熱實，痰熱相感而動風，風心相亂則悶瞀，故謂之風眩瞀。大人曰癲，小兒為癇。此方為治，萬無不愈。困急時但度灸穴，使大針針之，無不瘥者。初得針竟便灸最良。余業之以來三十餘年，所救活者，數千百人，病此而死，不逢嗣故也。（續命湯主眩發頓悶無知，口沫出，四體角弓，目反上，口噤不得言：竹瀝一升二合，生地黃汁一升，龍齒末、生薑、防風、麻黃去節，各四兩；防己、附子炮，各三兩；石膏十兩，桂二兩。合十味，水一斗煮取三升，分三服。有氣加附子一兩，紫蘇五合，橘皮半兩）。其論風眩癲癇甚有理，故並其方附於此（更有賁豚湯，詳見《千金》）。

[Author's notes:] Xú Sì[bó][27] said: Wind dizziness is caused by insufficient heart qì and repletion of accumulated heat in the chest. Mutual contraction of phlegm and heat stir up the wind and mutual derangement of the heart and wind lead to oppression; so this is called wind dizziness oppression. It is called withdrawal in adults and epilepsy in children. Using this formula to treat will cure all of it. In urgent situations, just locate the moxibustion points, and then needle with big needles. That will also cure the disease. It is best to apply moxibustion right after needling. I have saved several thousand people during the more than thirty years I have been in this career. People who die of this disease do so because they did not come across [the methods of] Xú Sì[bó]. (*Xù Mìng Tāng* 續命湯 (Life-Prolonging Decoction) governs the onset of dizziness, oppression, loss of consciousness, foaming at the mouth, arched-back rigidity, upward staring eyes, clenched jaws, and inability to speak. It consists of one *shēng* and two *gě*[28] of *zhú lì* 竹瀝 (Bamboo Succus); one *shēng* of *shēng dì huáng* 生地黃 (Fresh Rehmanniae); four *liǎng* each of *lóng chǐ* 龍齒 (Dentis Fossilia) powder, *shēng jiāng* 生薑 (Ginger), *fáng fēng* 防風 (Saposhnikovia Radix) and *má huáng* 麻黃(Ephedra Herba) (remove the nodes); three *liǎng* each of *fáng jǐ* 防己 (Stephaniae Tetrandrae Radix) and *fù zǐ* 附子 (Aconite) (blast fried); ten *liǎng* of *shí gāo* 石膏 (Gypsum Crudum); and two *liǎng* of *guì zhī* 桂枝 (Cinnamon Ramulus). Boil all ten herbs in one *dǒu*[29] of water, cooked down to three *shēng*, divide into three portions and drink it. If there is qì, add one *liǎng* of *fù zǐ* (Aconite), five *gě* of *zǐ sū* 紫蘇 (Perilla Folium), and half a *liǎng* of *jú pí* 橘皮 (Citri Reticulatae Pericarpium). This discussion of wind dizziness and epilepsy is reasonable. So I attach it and the formula here (there also is *Bēn Téng Tāng* 奔豚湯 (Running-piglet Decoction), for details, see *Qiān Jīn*《千金》).

但小兒癇非心氣不足爾。《千金》有風、食、驚癇三種。《本事》有陰、陽癇、慢脾風三證（慢脾即食癇。宜醒脾丸、人參散）。右方有三癇丸，治小兒百二十種驚癇（荊芥穗二兩，礬一兩，半生半枯，為

27. Xú Sìbó 徐嗣伯 was a famous doctor during the *Nán Qí* 南齊 (Southern Qí) (479-502 AD) and *Nán Běi* 南北 (Southern and Northern) Dynasties.

28. *Gě* 合: A unit of measurement equal to 1/10 of a *shēng* 升 (a unit of dry measurement for grain; one *shēng* equaled about 664 milliliters during the *Sòng* (宋) Dynasty).

29. *Dǒu* 斗: A unit of dry measure for grain. One *dǒu* equals 10 *shēng*.

末，面糊丸，黍米大，朱砂衣，薑湯下二十丸）。吾謂慢驚用來復丹，急驚三癇丸，食癇醒脾丸可也。

But in children, epilepsy is not caused by insufficient heart qì. *Qiān Jīn*《 千金 》has three types of epilepsy: wind, food and fright epilepsy. *Běn Shì* 《 本事 》has three patterns: yīn and yáng epilepsy, as well as chronic spleen wind (chronic spleen [wind] is food epilepsy. It is appropriate to use *Xǐng Pí Wán* 醒脾丸 (Spleen-Arousing Pill) and *Rén Shēn Sǎn* 人參散 (Ginseng Powder). The formula below is *Sān Xián Wán* 三癇丸 (Three Epilepsies Pill); it treats over a hundred and twenty types of pediatric fright epilepsy: two liǎng of *jīng jìe suì* 荊芥穗 (Schizonepetae Flos), and one liǎng of [*bái*] *fán* 白礬 (Alumen, half unprocessed and half dried). Grind the above into a powder, make pills the size of millet using flour paste, and coat them with *zhū shā* 朱砂 (Cinnabaris). Take twenty pills with ginger juice). I say that *Lái Fù Dān* 來復丹 (Return Again Elixir) is used to treat chronic fright [wind]; *Sān Xián Wán* is used to treat acute fright [wind]; while *Xǐng Pí Wán* is used for food epilepsy.

## 4.20
## *Fēng Láo (Yú Jiàn Láo)*
# 風勞（餘見勞）

## Wind taxation
**(for further discussion, see taxation)**

大杼治風勞，氣咳嗽（《明》有氣急字），胸中鬱鬱，身熱目眩（《銅》）。大椎治風勞食氣。風門治風勞，嘔逆上氣，胸背痛，喘氣，臥（《明》作短）不安。膀胱俞治風勞，腰脊痛。

Dà Zhù 大杼 (UB 11) treats wind taxation, qì cough (*Míng*《 明 》has rapid breathing), chest oppression, generalized heat, and dizzy vision (*Tóng*《 銅 》).

Dà Zhuī 大椎 (Dū 14) treats wind taxation and consumption of qì.

Fēng Mén 風門 (UB 12) treats wind taxation, retching counterflow, qì ascent, pain of the chest and back, panting, and unquiet sleep (*Míng* says short sleep).

Páng Guāng Shù 膀胱俞 (UB 28) treats wind taxation and pain of the low back and spine.

附分治風勞，臂肘不仁。五里治風勞驚恐吐血，肘臂痛，嗜臥，四肢不得動。曲泉治風勞，失精，身體極痛，泄水下利膿血，陰腫胻痛。關元俞、膀胱俞療風勞，腰痛(《明》)。伏兔療風勞，痹逆狂邪，膝冷手節攣縮，身癮疹，腹脹，少氣。頭重，風勞：腦戶五壯，針三分補之(《千翼》)。

Fù Fēn 附分 (UB 41) treats wind taxation and numbness of the arms and elbows.

Wǔ Lǐ 五里 (LI 13 or LV 10) treats wind taxation, fright and fear, vomiting of blood, elbow and arm pain, somnonlence, and inability to move the four limbs.

Qū Quán 曲泉 (LV 8) treats wind taxation, seminal loss, extreme pain of the body; diarrhea with water, pus, and blood; genital swelling, and leg pain.

Guān Yuán Shù 關元俞 (UB 26) and Páng Guāng Shù 膀胱俞 (UB 28) cure wind taxation and lower back pain (*Míng*《明》).

Fú Tù 伏兔 (ST 32) cures wind taxation, *bì*-impediment and counterflow, manic evils, cold knees, hypertonicity of the finger joints, dormant papules, abdominal distention, and qì shortage.

Heaviness of the head and wind taxation: Apply five cones of moxibustion on Nǎo Hù 腦戶 (Dū 17); needle 3 fēn deep and supplement it (*Qiān Yì*《千翼》).

灸風勞，發背癰疽：用麻繩一條蠟過；從手中指第二節，量至心坎骨截斷(須直伸臂)，折過，自前項下取中，纏至後心相對令齊，閉口量兩吻闊狹，以此為則，對灸七壯。(澧州井司法馬司法云神效)。

To apply moxibustion for wind taxation, flat and welling-abscesses with sores on the back: Wax a piece of linen string; measure from the second joint of the middle finger to the xyphoid process (stretch out the arm), cut and then fold it. Wrap the string around the front of the neck with the mid-point on the midline, and then let the string hang down in back to the posterior aspect of the heart. Make the [two ends of the string] even with each other. Measure the width between the two corners of the mouth when mouth is closed and take this measurement as the standard; apply seven cones of moxibustion correspondingly.[30] (Law Officiers Jǐng and Mǎ of the Lǐ Province both said that it is divinely effective.)

30. While this passage does not explicitly say it, based on similar sets of directions elsewhere, the string that is measured to the width of the mouth is then centered on the site on the spine found before. The string is spread horizontally and the moxibustion point is located on both sides, more or less on the inner bladder channel.

月事 735
中風 379
絕子 721

# 4.21
## *Fēng Jìng (Jiǎo Gōng Fǎn Zhāng)*
# 風痓（角弓反張）

## Wind tetany
**(Arched-back rigidity)**

顱囟治風痓（《銅》）。大迎治風痓口噤，牙疼頬腫，惡寒，舌強不能言。啞門治寒熱風痓，脊強反折，瘛瘲。天衝治癲疾風痓，牙齦腫，善驚。脾俞、膀胱俞主熱痓引骨痛（《千》）。上關主瘛瘲，沫出，寒熱痓引骨痛。

Lú Xìn 顱囟 (SJ 19) treats wind tetany (*Tóng*《銅》).

Dà Yíng 大迎 (ST 5) treats wind tetany, clenched jaws, toothache, swelling of the cheeks, aversion to cold, stiffness of the tongue and inability to speak.

Yǎ Mén 啞門 (Dū 15) treats [sensations of] cold and heat, wind tetany, arched-back rigidity, and tugging and slackening.

Tiān Chōng 天衝 (GB 9) treats madness, wind tetany, swollen gums, and frequent fright.

Pí Shù 脾俞 (UB 20) and Páng Guāng Shù 膀胱俞 (UB 28) govern heat tetany that induces bone pain (*Qiān*《千》).

Shàng Guān 上關 (GB 3) governs tugging and slackening, spitting of foam, cold and heat tetany that induces bone pain.

腎俞、中膂俞、長強主寒熱痓反折。肝俞主筋寒熱痓，筋急手相引。魚際主痓上氣，失喑不言。腰俞主反折（見月事）。小兒身強角弓反張：灸鼻上入髮際三分三壯，次大椎下節間三壯（《明下》）。百會治角弓反張（《銅》見中風）。上窌（見絕子）、腰俞主脊強反折（《千》）。

Shèn Shù 腎俞 (UB 23), Zhōng Lǚ Shù 中膂俞 (UB 29), and Cháng Qiáng 長強 (Dū 1) govern cold and heat tetany with arched-back rigidity.

Gān Shù 肝俞 (UB 18) governs cold sinews, heat tetany, and tension of the sinews with pulling of the hands.

Yú Jì 魚際 (LU 10) governs tetany, qì ascent, loss of voice, and inability to speak.

Yāo Shù 腰俞 (Dū 2) governs arched-back rigidity (see the section on menstruation).

Pediatric hypertonicity of the body and arched-back rigidity: Apply three cones of moxibustion on the site 3 fēn within the hairline above the nose; next apply moxibustion the joint space below Dà Zhuī 大椎 [the seventh cervical vertebra][31](*Míng Xià*《明下》).

Bǎi Huì 百會 (Dū 20) treats arched-back rigidity (see the section on wind stroke in *Tóng*《銅》).

Shàng Liáo 上窌 (UB 31) (see the section on infertility) and Yāo Shù (Dū 2) govern arched-back rigidity (*Qiān*《千》).

《産論》云：痙者口噤不開，背強而直，如發癇狀，搖頭馬鳴，身反折。宜速灌小續命湯，是也（此見二十論）。又云：産後中風，如角弓狀，無治法（見十八章）。後人惟用荊芥穗末酒服二錢七，立效。若是則灸未必如藥之速見效也。

[Author's notes:] *Chǎn Lùn*《産論》says: Tetany [has the symptoms of] clenched jaws, rigidity of the back as if it is the onset of epilepsy, shaking head, neighing like a horse, and arched-back rigidity. It is appropriate to give *Xiǎo Xù Mìng Tāng* 小續命湯 (Minor Life-Prolonging Decoction) immediately (for this, see the 20th discussion). It also says: There is no treatment for postpartum wind stroke with arched-back rigidity (see the 18th chapter). Later generations take two *qián* of *jīng jiè suì* 荊芥穗 (Schizonepetae Flos) powder with liquor. It takes effect right away, so the effects of moxibustion may not be as fast as this herbal-medicine.

31. Dà Zhuī 大椎 can refer to the seventh cervical vertebra or the point just below it (Dū 14). Here the text describes the location of Dū 14, but the term Dà Zhuī 大椎 refers to the vertebra.

# 4.22

## *Fēng Xuàn*

## *(Yú Jiàn Tóu Mù Xuàn, Yú Lùn Jiàn Fēng Xián)*

# 風眩（餘見頭目眩　餘論見風癇）

## Wind dizziness

**(for further discussion, see the sections on dizziness, and the head and eyes; for further discussion, see the discussion of wind epilepsy)**

頭風 640
目痛 568
偏頭 643
腰腳 542
項風 640
目眩 575

完骨療風眩，項痛，頭強寒熱（《明》）。當陽、臨泣療卒不識人，風眩鼻塞。後頂（見頭風）、玉枕（見目痛）、頷厭（見偏頭痛）療風眩（《千》）。陽谷主風眩，驚，手卷（《甲乙》手卷作手腕痛），泄風汗出，腰項急。承光治風眩頭痛，嘔吐心煩。

Wán Gǔ 完骨 (GB 12) cures wind dizziness and pain of the nape, hypertonicity of the head, and [sensations of] cold and heat (*Míng*《明》).

Dāng Yáng 當陽 (non-channel)[32] and Lín Qì 臨泣 (GB 15 or GB 41) cure sudden loss of consciousness, wind dizziness, and nasal congestion.

Hòu Dǐng 後頂 (Dū 19) (see the section on head wind), Yù Zhěn 玉枕 (UB 9) (see the section on eye pain), and Hàn Yàn 頷厭 (GB 4) (see the section on hemilateral headaches) cure wind dizziness (*Qiān*《千》).

Yáng Gǔ 陽谷 (SI 5) governs wind dizziness, fright, curled hands (*Jiǎ Yǐ*《甲乙》has wrist pain instead of curled hands), discharge of wind with sweating, and tension of the low back and nape.

Chéng Guāng 承光 (UB 6) treats wind dizziness, headache, vomiting, and vexation of the heart.

申脈治坐如在舟車中（見腰腳）。神庭、上星、囟會主風頭眩（《千》）。天牖等、前頂等主風眩（見項風）。攢竹療頭目風眩（見目眩）。

Shēn Mài 申脈 (UB 62) treats a sensation as if sitting in a boat or wagon (see the section on low back and leg [pain]).

32. Dāng Yáng 當陽 is located directly above the pupils, 1 cùn within the anterior hairline.

Shén Tíng 神庭 (Dū 24), Shàng Xīng 上星 (Dū 23), and Xìn Huì 囟會 (Dū 22) govern wind and dizzy head (*Qiān*《千》).

Tiān Yǒu 天牖 (SJ 16) and so forth, and Qián Dǐng 前頂 (Dū 21) and so forth govern wind dizziness (see the section on head wind).

Zǎn Zhú 攢竹 (UB 2) cures wind dizziness of the head and eyes (see the section on dizzy vision).

《千金方》載徐嗣之言曰：風眩之病，起於心氣不足，胸上蓄熱實，痰熱相感而動風，風心相亂則悶瞀，故謂之風眩瞀。大人曰癲，小兒為癇，則是風眩癲癇本一疾也。不知後人何為析而三之。予因分為三門，且從為之辭，以釋世醫之疑云。

[Author's notes:] *Qiān Jīn Fāng*《千金方》recorded what Xú Sì[bó] 徐嗣[伯] said: Wind-dizziness is caused by insufficient heart qì and repletion heat accumulation in the chest. Mutual contraction of phlegm and heat stir up wind and mutual derangement of the heart and wind lead to oppression; so it is called wind-dizziness oppression. It is called withdrawal in adults and epilepsy in children, so wind-dizziness, withdrawal, and epilepsy are one disease at the root. This was not understood by later generations so they broke it into three diseases. Because of this, I divided it into three categories, and explain the misgivings of generations of doctors.

# 4.23

## *Fēng Bì (Yú Jiàn Jiān Yú Xué)*

## 風痹（餘見肩髃穴）

### Wind *bì*-impediment

**(for further discussion, see the section on Jiān Yú 肩髃 (LI 15)).**

膝痛 539
腰脊 551
瘰歷 702
腳弱 524
身寒 682
腰痛 545
中風 379

天井治驚悸瘛瘲，風痹臂肘痛，捉物不得（《銅》）。肩貞治風痹手臂不舉，肩中熱痛。尺澤治風痹肘攣，手臂不舉。消濼治寒熱風痹，項痛肩背急（《明》云頭痛項背急）。膝關治風痹，膝內痛引髕，不可屈伸，喉咽痛。

Tiān Jǐng 天井 (SJ 10) treats fright palpitations, tugging and slackening, wind *bì*-impediment, arm and elbow pain, and inability to grasp things (*Tóng*《銅》).

Jiān Zhēn 肩貞 (SI 9) treats wind *bì*-impediment, inability to lift the arms, and hot pain of the shoulders.

Chǐ Zé 尺澤 (LU 5) treats wind *bì*-impediment, hypertonicity of the elbows, and inability to lift the arms.

Xiāo Luò 消濼 (SJ 12) treats cold, heat, and wind *bì*-impediment, nape pain, and tension of the back and shoulders (*Míng*《明》 says: headaches and tension of the back and nape).

Xī Guān 膝關 (LV 7) treats wind *bì*-impediment, pain on inner aspect of the knees that radiates to the patella, inability to flex and stretch [the knees], and sore throat.

跗陽治痿厥風痹，頭重頔痛，髀樞股胻痛，瘛瘲，風痹不仁，時有寒熱，四肢不舉。陽輔（見膝痛）、陽關（並見膝痛）治風痹不仁。委中（見腰脊）治風痹。少海（見瘰歷）療風痹（《明》）。委中（見腳弱）、下廉療風濕痹（見身寒痹）。環跳治冷風濕痹（見腰痛），治卒病肉痹不知人（見中風）。

Fū Yáng 跗陽 (UB 59) treats wilting reversal, wind *bì*-impediment, heaviness of the head, pain of the cheeks; pain of the thigh pivot, thigh, and lower leg, tugging and slackening, wind *bì*-impediment and numbness, frequent [sensations of] cold and heat, and inability to lift the four limbs.

Yáng Fǔ 陽輔 (GB 38) (see the section on knee pain) and Yáng Guān 陽關 (GB 33) (for all, see the section on knee pain) treat wind *bì*-impediment and numbness.

Wěi Zhōng 委中 (UB 40) (see the section on [pain of] the low back and spine) treats wind *bì*-impediment.

Shào Hǎi 少海 (HT 3) (see the section on scrofula) cures wind *bì*-impediment (*Míng*《明》).

Wěi Zhōng (UB 40) (see the section on weak legs) and Xià Lián 下廉 (ST 39) cure wind-damp *bì*-impediment (see the section on cold *bì*-impediment of the body).

Huán Tiào 環跳 (GB 30) treats cold, wind, and damp *bì*-impediment (see the section on lower back pain), sudden onset of flesh *bì*-impediment, and unconsciousness (see the section on wind stroke).

岐伯曰：中風大法有四：四曰風痹。巢氏曰：風寒濕三氣合而為痹，風多者為風痹。風痹之狀，肌膚盡痛，而復手足不隨也。醫者當以此求之，速與續命湯，依俞穴灸之云（詳見《千金》）。

[Author's notes:] Qí Bó said: There are four great laws of wind stroke; the forth is wind *bì*-impediment. Master Cháo said: wind, cold, and dampness combine together and become *bì*-impediment. If wind is predominant, it becomes wind *bì*-impediment. The symptoms of wind *bì*-impediment are: generalized pain of skin and flesh followed by hemiplegia of the extremities. Doctors should use this and seek [treatment]; immediately give *Xù Mìng Tāng* 續命湯 (Life-Prolonging Decoction), then apply moxibustion by selecting the proper points (*Qiān Jīn*《千金》).

# 4.24
## *Zhòng Fēng (Zhòng Fēng Hán Rè, Yú Lùn Jiàn Piān Fēng)*
# 中風（中風寒熱　餘論見偏風）

## Wind stroke
**(Struck by wind, cold, and heat; for further discussion, see the section on hemilateral wind)**

小兒但是風病，諸般醫治不瘥，灸率谷（《明下》）。黃帝療中風，眼戴上及不能語者：灸第二椎第五椎上，各十壯。齊下火，炷如半棗核大，立瘥。

Wind diseases in children when all other doctors cannot cure it: Apply moxibustion on Shuài Gǔ 率谷 (GB 8) (*Míng Xià*《明下》). The Yellow Emperor's treatment of wind stroke with upcast eyes and inability to speak: Apply ten cones of moxibustion each to the second and fifth vertebrae in one session. The moxa cones should be the size of half a date kernel. This will cure the disease immediately.

黃帝問岐伯曰：中風半身不遂，如何灸。答曰：凡人未中風一兩月前，或三五月前，非時足脛上忽酸重頑痹，良久方解。此將中風之候。急灸三里、絕骨四處三壯。後用蔥、薄荷、桃柳葉煎湯淋洗，驅逐風氣於瘡口出。灸瘡春較秋灸，秋較春灸，常令兩腳有瘡為妙。

Yellow Emperor asked Qí Bó: How is moxibustion applied for wind stroke with hemiplegia? Qí Bó answered: One or two months; or three or five months before someone suffers the wind stroke, there is frequent sudden onset of aching heaviness and persistent numbness in the lower leg; and it takes a long time [for the symptoms] to go away. These are the signs of wind stroke. Apply three cones of moxibustion immediately on the four sites of Sān Lǐ 三里 (ST 36) and Jué Gǔ 绝骨 (GB 39). Make a decoction of scallions, mint, peach and willow leaves to wash it, so the wind qì can be expelled through the opening of the moxa sores. When the moxa sores heal in the spring, apply moxibustion in the fall; when moxa sores heal in the fall, apply moxibustion in the spring;[33] it is excellent to have moxa sores on both legs.

33. This means apply a second treatment six months later.

凡人不信此法，飲食不節，酒色過度，忽中此風，言語謇澀，半身不遂。宜七處齊下火，各三壯，風在左灸右，右灸左。百會、耳前髮際、肩井、風市、三里、絕骨、曲池七穴，神效不能具錄。依法灸無不愈。

Ordinary people do not believe this method; they do not regulate their diet, they drink liquor and have sex excessively. Then they have a wind stroke, with sluggish speech and hemiplegia. It is appropriate to apply three cones of moxibustion to each of seven sites in one treatment. Apply moxibustion on the right side when wind strikes the left, and on the left side when wind strikes the right: Bǎi Huì 百會 (Dū 20), on the hairline anterior to the ear, Jiān Jǐng 肩井 (GB 21), Fēng Shì 風市 (GB 31), Sān Lǐ 三里 (ST 36), Jué Gǔ 絕骨 (GB 39) and Qū Chí 曲池 (LI 11). These seven points have divine effects which are too numerous to be recorded. When this method of moxibustion is followed, all will be cured.

灸風中腑：手足不隨，其狀覺手足或麻或痛，良久乃已。此將中腑之候。病左灸右，病右灸左。因循失灸廢者，灸瘡春較秋灸，秋較春灸，取盡風氣。（《集效》）

Moxibustion for wind striking the bowels, with paralysis of the extremities and other symptoms of long-lasting numbness or pain of the extremities. These are the signs of wind striking the bowels. Apply moxibustion on the right side for diseases of the left; apply moxibustion on the left side for diseases of the right. For those who are paralyzed because they followed [another method] and didn't receive moxibustion: When the moxa sores heal in the spring, apply moxibustion in the fall; when moxa sores heal in the fall, apply moxibustion in the spring.[34] This is how they can completely get rid of the wind qì (*Jí Xiào*《集效》).

百會、曲鬢、肩髃、曲池、風市、足三里、絕骨共十三穴，灸風中臟，氣塞涎上，不語。極危者，下火立效。其狀覺心中憒亂，神思不怡，或手足麻，此將中臟之候。不問風與氣，但依次自上及下，各灸五壯，日別灸隨年壯。凡遇春秋，常灸以泄風氣。素有風人，可保無虞。此能灸暴卒，百會、風池、大椎、肩井、曲池、間使、足三里共十二穴。

Bǎi Huì (Dū 20), Qū Bìn 曲鬢 (GB 7), Jiān Yú 肩髃 (LI 15), Qū Chí (LI 11), Fēng Shì (GB 31), Zú Sān Lǐ (ST 36) and Jué Gǔ (GB 39), a total of thirteen points [when you count both sides]. Apply moxibustion on them immediately for wind striking the viscera, with qì blockage, rising drool, and loss of speech. It will be effective right after moxibustion in very critical patients. The symptoms of oppression and derangement in the heart, unhappy thoughts, or numbness of the extremities are signs of wind striking the viscera. It is not necessary to ask if it is due to wind or qì; just apply five

34. As with the previous passage, this means apply two treatments, six months apart. This treatment will work preventively or if the wind stroke has already occurred and the patient is paralyzed.

cones of moxibustion on each [of the points] in turn from the top to the bottom. Every other day, burn the same number of cones as the age of the patient. Apply moxibustion regularly in the spring and fall in order to drain the wind qì. This will secure the peace [health] of those who are prone to the wind. Sudden death can also be treated by applying moxibustion on: Bǎi Huì 百會 (Dū 20), Fēng Chí 風池 (GB 20), Dà Zhuī 大椎 (Dū 14), Jiān Jǐng 肩井 (GB 21), Qū Chí 曲池 (LI 11), Jiān Shǐ 間使 (PC 5), Zú Sān Lǐ 足三里 (ST 36). This totals twelve points [when you count it bilaterally].

《集效方》云：治風莫如續命、防風、排風湯之類，此可扶助疾病。若救危急，必火艾為良。此論亦當。

[Author's notes:] *Jí Xiào Fāng*《集效方》says: To treat wind, nothing is better than using decoctions of the following types: *Xù Mìng* 續命 (Life-Prolonging [Decoction]), *Fáng Fēng* 防風 (Saposhnikovia [Decoction]), and *Pái Fēng* 排風 (Wind Expelling [Decoction]). These can help [treat] the disease. When rescuing critical and urgent [cases], it is good to apply moxibustion. This theory also is appropriate.

范子默自壬午五月間口眼喎斜，灸聽會等三穴即正。右手足麻無力，灸百會、髮際等七穴得愈。未年八月間，氣塞涎上，不能語，金虎丹加膩粉服至四丸半。氣不通，涎不下，藥從鼻出，魂魄飛揚，如墜江湖中，頃欲絕。灸百會風池等左右共十二穴。氣遂痛，吐幾一碗許，繼又下十餘行，伏枕半月餘遂平。爾後小覺意思少異於常，心中憒亂，即便灸百會風池等穴立效。

Fàn Zǐmò suffered deviation of the eyes and mouth since the fifth month of the Rén Wǔ 壬午 year.[35] After he received moxibustion on three points including Tīng Huì 聽會 (GB 2), he was back to normal. Numbness and weakness in his right extremities were also cured after receiving moxibustion on seven points including Bǎi Huì (Dū 20), Fà Jì 髮際 (Dū 24), and so forth. In the eighth month of the following year, he suffered qì blockage, rising drool, and inability to speak; he took four and a half pills of *Jīn Hǔ Dān* 金虎丹 (Golden Tiger Pill) plus *nì fěn* 膩粉 [calomel]. But qì was still blocked, drool could not descend, and the pills came out from his nose. His corporeal and ethereal souls were flying upward and he felt like he was drowning in a river or a lake; he was about to die. I applied moxibustion on the twelve points of Bǎi Huì (Dū 20), Fēng Chí (GB 20), and so forth. His qì unblocked, and he vomited almost a bowl [of drool]. This was followed by more than ten bouts of diarrhea. He recovered after laying in bed over half a month. Later on, whenever he felt his thoughts were a little bit different than normal, and experienced oppression

35. During the author's lifetime, 1162 was a Rén Wǔ 壬午 year. This may be the author's own case history since the book was published in 1165. It is also possible that this was another earlier doctor's case cited by the author. In that case, it would be 1102 or earlier, each possibility being earlier by sixty years.

and derangement in his heart; he would apply moxibustion on Bǎi Huì 百會 (Dū 20), Fēng Chí 風池 (GB 20), and so forth. It would be effective immediately.

《本事方》云：十二穴者，謂聽會、頰車、地倉、百會、肩髃、曲池、風市、足三里、絕骨、髮際、大椎、風池也。依而用之，立效。

[Pǔ Jì] Běn Shì Fāng《本事方》says: The twelve points are: Tīng Huì 聽會 (GB 2), Jiá Chē 頰車 (ST 6), Dì Cāng 地倉 (ST 4), Bǎi Huì (Dū 20), Jiān Yú 肩髃 (LI 15), Qū Chí 曲池 (LI 11), Fēng Shì 風市 (GB 31), Zú Sān Lǐ 足三里 (ST 36), Jué Gǔ 絕骨 (GB 39), Fà Jì 髮際 (Dū 24), Dà Zhuī 大椎 (Dū 14), and Fēng Chí (GB 20). Following this order when using them will be effective right away.

氣塞涎上，不能語，心中風候也。巢氏病源常論之。古方雖謂但得偃臥，悶絕汗出者，心中風之候，恐未盡也。范公灸得氣通，蓋灸百會之力。其吐幾一碗下十行者，豈服金虎丹加膩粉所致耶。（《必用方》戒人服金虎等丹。）

[Author's notes:] Qì blockage, rising drool, and inability to speak are symptoms of wind striking the heart. Master Cháo's *Bìng Yuán*《病源》[36] discusses it frequently. Ancient medical books say lying supine, extreme oppression, and sweating are symptoms of wind striking the heart, but this may not be complete. Master Fàn's qì unblocked after moxibustion [in the case presented above]; this is the effect of moxibustion on Bǎi Huì (Dū 20). Then he vomited almost a bowl of [drool] and had over ten bouts of diarrhea; this wouldn't be the effect of taking *Jīn Hǔ Dān* 金虎丹 (Golden Tiger Pill) plus *nì fěn* 膩粉 [calomel]. (*Bì Yòng Fāng* 必用方 warned people about taking *Jīn Hǔ Dān* (Golden Tiger Pill), and so forth.)

風池療大患風者，先補後瀉。少可患，以經取之（《明》）。肝俞療中風支滿，短氣不食，食不消，吐血，目不明，閉塞。陰蹻療偏枯不能行，大風暴不知人，臥驚視如見星。

Fēng Chí (GB 20) cures severe suffering from wind: supplement first then drain. For mild suffering, use the channel to treat it (*Míng*《明》).

Gān Shù 肝俞 (UB 18) cures wind stroke, propping fullness, shortness of breath, inability to eat, non-dispersion of food, vomiting blood, dim vision, and blockage.

36. *Bìng Yuán* 病源 indicates *Zhū Bìng Yuán Hóu Lùn* 諸病源候論 (The Origin and Indicators of Disease), by Cháo Yuánfāng 巢元方, published in 610.

Yīn Qiāo 阴蹻 (KI 8)[37] cures hemilateral withering, inability to walk, great wind [leprosy], sudden loss of consciousness, and fright vision as if seeing stars during sleep.

臨泣治卒中風不識人(《銅》)。解溪治風面浮腫，顏黑，厥氣上衝，腹脹，大便下重，瘈驚，膝股胻腫轉筋，目眩頭痛。勞宮治中風善怒，悲笑不休，手痹。內關治中風肘攣，實則心暴痛，虛則心煩惕惕。風頭耳後痛，煩心，足不收失履，口喎僻，頭項瘈痛，牙車急，完骨主之(《甲》)。

Lín Qì 臨泣 (GB 41) treats sudden onset of wind stroke with loss of consciousness (*Tóng*《銅》).

Jiě Xī 解溪 (ST 41) treats wind with puffy swelling of the face, dark complexion, reversal qì surging upward, abdominal distention, defection with rectal heaviness, tugging and fright, swelling and cramping of the knees, thighs and lower legs, dizzy vision, and headache.

Láo Gōng 勞宮 (PC 8) treats wind stroke, susceptibility to anger, incessant sorrow and laughter, and *bì*-impediment of the hands.

Nèi Guān 內關 (PC 6) treats wind stroke with hypertonicity of the elbows. There is violent heart pain in repletion; vexation of the heart and palpitations in vacuity.

For wind with headache and pain behind the ears, vexation of the heart, loss of use of the legs, inability to walk, deviation of the mouth, tugging and pain of head and nape, and tension of the tooth carriage [jaw]: use Wán Gǔ 完骨 (GB 12) to govern it (*Jiǎ*《甲》).

心俞治心中風，語悲泣(《銅》見狂走)。百會治風癇中風，角弓反張，或多哭，言語不擇，發即無時。盛即吐沫，心驚煩健忘(《銅》)。

Xīn Shù 心俞 (UB 15) treats wind stroke in the heart and sorrowful speech and weeping (see manic walking in *Tóng*).

Bǎi Huì 百會 (Dū 20) treats wind epilepsy and wind stroke, with arched-back rigidity, or frequent crying, and speaking without choosing the words with random onset. If exuberant [excessive], there is spitting of foam, fright, vexation, and forgetfulness (*Tóng*).

崑崙主狂易大風(《千》)。陰蹻主風暴不知人，偏枯不能行。照海主大風默默不知所痛，視如見星。天井主大風默默不知所痛，悲傷不樂。

37. Yīn Qiāo 阴蹻 could refer to Zhào Hǎi 照海 (KI 6) or Jiāo Xìn 交信 (KI 8) according to the discussion in Volume 1. But nearby in the text, Zhào Hǎi 照海 (KI 6) is referred to by name, so here it is likely to mean Jiāo Xìn 交信 (KI 8).

風癇 366 Kūn Lún 崑崙 (UB 60) governs mania and susceptibility to great wind (*Qiān*《千》).

中風 392 Yīn Qiāo 陰蹻 (KI 8) governs wind, sudden loss of consciousness, hemilateral withering, and inability to walk.

Zhào Hǎi 照海 (KI 6) governs great wind, silence,[38] inability to feel where it hurts, and seeing stars.

Tiān Jǐng 天井 (SJ 10) governs great wind, silence, inability to feel where it hurts, sorrow and unhappiness.

百會療青風心風（見風癇）。肩髃治偏風熱風（見中風不語）。

Bǎi Huì 百會 (Dū 20) cures green-blue wind and heart wind (see the section on wind epilepsy).

Jiān Yú 肩髃 (LI 15) treats hemilateral wind and hot wind (see the section on wind stroke and loss of speech).

岐伯曰：中風大法有四。一曰偏枯，二曰風痱，三曰風懿，四曰風痹。夫諸急卒病多是風，初得輕微，人所不悟，宜速與續命湯，依俞穴灸之。夫風者，百病之長。岐伯所言四者，說其最重也。

Qí Bó said: There are four laws of wind stroke: first is hemilateral withering; second is wind disablement;[39] the third is wind choking;[40] the forth is wind *bì*-impediment. All acute and sudden diseases are usually caused by wind. At the beginning when it is light, people usually do not realize it. Immediately give *Xù Mìng Tāng* 續命湯 (Life-Prolonging Decoction), then apply moxibustion according to the points. Wind is the chief of the hundred diseases. The four laws given by Qí Bó, are the most important.

凡風多從背五臟俞入。諸臟受病，肺病最急。肺主氣息，又冒諸臟故也。肺中風者，其人偃臥而胸滿，短氣冒悶，汗出者，肺風之證。

Wind usually enters the body through the back transport points of the five viscera. Among all diseases contracted by the viscera, lung disease is the most urgent. The lungs govern respiration, and also cover the other viscera. When wind strikes the lungs, people lie supine with chest fullness, shortness of breath, oppression, and sweating. These are the symptoms of lung wind.

38. Perhaps like catatonia.

39. *Fēng fèi* 風痱 (wind disablement) refers to symptoms of paralysis of the limbs without pain, inability to speak, and mental confusion.

40. *Fēng yí* 風懿 (wind choke) refers to symptoms of sudden loss of consciousness, stiff tongue, and a choking feeling in the throat caused by phlegm-fire.

視目下鼻上兩邊下行至口：色白者尚可治。急灸肺俞百壯，服續命湯，小兒減之。

Observe the area below the eyes and above the nose, down to the mouth on both sides: If the color is white, [lung disease] is treatable. Apply a hundred cones of moxibustion immediately on Fèi Shù 肺俞 (UB 13) and take *Xù Mìng Tāng* 續命湯 (Life-Prolonging Decoction); reduce the dosage for children.

若急黃者，此為肺已傷，化為血，不可復治。

If the color is very yellow, the lungs are damaged and [the heat disease] is transformed into blood; it is not treatable.

若為急風邪所中，便迷漠恍惚，妄言狂語，或少氣惙惙，不能復言。若不求師即治，宿昔而死。即覺，便灸肺俞及膈俞肝俞數十壯，急服續命湯可救。若涎唾出不收者，既灸，當立與湯也。

If [the lungs] were struck by violent wind evil, the patient has abstraction, manic raving; or qì shortage and loss of speech. If a master is not asked to treat the patient immediately, he will die in a short period. If the patient still lives, apply several tens of moxa cones on Fèi Shù (UB 13), Gé Shù 膈俞 (UB 17), and Gān Shù 肝俞 (UB 18); then take *Xù Mìng Tāng* (Life-Prolonging Decoction). It can save the patient. If there is incessant drool, give the decoction right after moxibustion.

諸陽受風，亦恍惚妄語，與肺病相似，然著緩可經久而死。

In wind contraction of all yáng [channels], there is also abstraction and manic raving; this is similar to lung disease, but the contraction is slower and people die after a long time.

肝中風者，其人但踞坐不得低頭，繞兩目連額上色微有青者，肝風之證。若唇色青面黃，尚可治。急灸肝俞百壯，服續命湯。

When wind strikes the liver, the patient can only crouch, unable to bow their head, with light green-blue color around both eyes and onto their forehead. These are symptoms of liver wind. It is treatable if the lips are green-blue and the facial color is yellow. Quickly apply a hundred cones of moxibustion on Gān Shù (UB 18) and take *Xù Mìng Tāng* (Life-Prolonging Decoction).

心中風者，其人但得偃臥，不得傾側，悶亂，冒絕汗出者。心風之證。若唇正赤，尚可治。急灸心俞百壯，服續命湯。

When wind strikes the heart, people can only lie supine, unable to lie on their sides, with oppression, vexation, and sweating that occurs when one is close to death. These are symptoms of heart wind. It is treatable when the mouth is red. Quickly apply a hundred cones of moxibustion on Xīn Shù 心俞 (UB 15) and take *Xù Mìng Tāng* 續命湯 (Life-Prolonging Decoction).

脾中風者，其人但踞坐而腹滿，身通黃。吐咸汁出者，尚可治。急灸脾俞百壯，服續命湯。

When wind strikes the spleen, the patient can only crouch with abdominal fullness and generalized yellowing. It is treatable if the patient vomits salty liquids. Quickly apply a hundred cones of moxibustion on Pí Shù 脾俞 (UB 20) and take *Xù Mìng Tāng* (Life-Prolonging Decoction).

腎中風者，其人踞坐而腰痛。視脅左右未有黃色如餅粢大者，尚可治。急灸腎俞百壯，服續命湯。

When wind strikes the kidneys, the patient has lower back pain after crouching. It is treatable if the patient does not have yellow patches the size of millet cakes on the left and right rib-sides. Quickly apply a hundred cones of moxibustion on Shèn Shù 腎俞 (UB 23) and take *Xù Mìng Tāng* (Life-Prolonging Decoction).

大腸中風者，臥而腸鳴不止。灸大腸俞百壯，可服續命湯。

When wind strikes the large intestine, the patient has incessant rumbling in the intestines while lying down. Apply a hundred cones of moxibustion on Dà Cháng Shù 大肠俞 (UB 25) and take *Xù Mìng Tāng* (Life-Prolonging Decoction).

鄉里有人忽覺心腹中熱甚，急投藥鋪說其狀。鋪家以為此中風之候，與治風藥而風不作。予中心藏之。

[Author's notes:] A person in town suddenly felt extreme heat in his heart and abdomen. He immediately went to the herb store and described his symptoms. The people in the store thought it was a symptom of wind stroke. They gave him herbs to treat wind and the wind did not break out. I stored this experience in my heart.

至夷陵，見一太守中夏忽患熱甚，不免以水灑地，設箪臥其上，令人扇之。次日，忽中風，數日而殂。人皆咎其臥水箪上而用扇也。

I arrived at Yí Líng and saw a prefect who suffered extreme heat in mid-summer [the month of the summer solstice]. He had splashed water on the ground, placed his bamboo mat there, and laid down on it; he also had people fan him. The next day, he suddenly suffered wind stoke and died several days later. People all blamed it on his lying on the wet bamboo mat and using fans.

暨到澧陽，見一老婦人夏中亦患熱，夜出臥廳上，次日中風。偶其子預合得小續命湯服，更召醫調理，數日愈。

I arrived at Lǐ Yáng and saw an old lady who also suffered from heat in mid-summer. She slept in the outer rooms one night, and suffered wind stroke next day. By chance her son got her to take *Xiǎo Xù Mìng Tāng* 小續命湯 (Minor Life-Prolonging Decoction) in time, and also asked doctors to care for her. She recovered several days later.

始知人之中風，心腹中多大熱而後作，而小續命湯不可不服也。

That was when I knew that wind stroke usually occurs after people suffer heat in the heart and abdomen, and they must take *Xiǎo Xù Mìng Tāng* (Minor Life-Prolonging Decoction).

王令患風，醫以青州白員子、排風湯、續命湯、四物湯、黃耆建中湯、朮附湯、嘉禾散各為一處，同和分數服，每服水一碗，棗三枚，生薑五片，同煎至七分，去滓溫服。

Wáng Lìng suffered from wind, so the doctors gave him equal portions of *Qīng Zhōu Bái Yuán Zǐ* 青州白員子 (White Pill from Qīng Zhōu), *Pái Fēng Tāng* 排風湯 (Wind Expelling Decoction), *Xù Mìng Tāng* 續命湯 (Life-Prolonging Decoction), *Sì Wù Tāng* 四物湯 (Four Agents Decoction), *Huáng Qí Jiàn Zhōng Tāng* 黃芪建中湯 (Astragalus Center-Fortifying Decoction), *Zhǔ Fù Tāng* 朮附湯 (White Atractylodes and Aconite Decoction), and *Jiā Hé Sǎn* 嘉禾散 (Good Millet Powder); mixed together and divided into several dosages. Each dose was cooked in one bowl of water with three dates and five slices of ginger. It was cooked down to seventy percent [of the volume], the dregs removed, and drank warm.

（自後與人服皆效。周戶傳三湯四散子。用四君子排風續命湯、嘉禾急風正氣勻氣散，一切風疾無不瘥。）

(I gave this to other people later. It was always effective. Zhōu's household has handed down *Sān Tāng Sì Sǎn Zǐ* 三湯四散子 (Three Decoction and Four Powder Pill). It contains *Sì Jūn Zǐ Tāng* 四君子[湯] (Four Gentlemen Decoction), *Pái Fēng* [*Tāng*] 排風 (Wind Expelling Decoction), *Xù Mìng Tāng* 續命湯 (Life-Prolonging Decoction) and *Jiā Hé Sǎn* 嘉禾散 (Good Millet Powder), *Jí Fēng Sǎn* 急風散 (Acute Wind Powder), *Zhèng Qì Sǎn* 正氣散 (Qì Righting Powder), and *Yún Qì Sǎn* 勻氣散 (Distribute Qì Evenly Powder). All wind diseases will be cured.)

肝風占候，其口不能言。灸鼻下人中，次灸大椎，次肝俞五十壯，餘處隨年壯。眼暗人灸之得明，二三百壯良。

A sign of liver wind stroke is inability to speak. Apply fifty cones of moxibustion on Rén Zhōng 人中 (Dū 26) which is located below the nose; followed by Dà Zhuī 大椎 (Dū 14); and Gān Shù 肝俞 (UB 18). Apply the same number of cones as the patient's age on the rest of the points. Moxibustion will brighten vision for people with dim vision; it is good to burn two or three hundred cones.

凡心風寒，灸心俞各五十壯。扁鵲曰：凡人心風，灸心俞兩邊各一寸二分，各五七壯。對心是肝俞二穴，主心風腹脹滿，食不消化，吐血酸痛，四肢羸露，不欲食飲，鼻血，目䀮䀮不明，肩頭脅下痛，小便急，灸二三百壯瘥，即止。

For wind-cold in the heart, apply fifty cones of moxibustion on Xīn Shù 心俞 (UB 15).

Biǎn Què said: For heart wind in people, apply five times seven cones of moxibustion to the site 1.2 cùn lateral to Xīn Shù (UB 15).

The bilateral point Gān Shù (UB 18) faces the heart. It governs heart wind, abdominal fullness, non-transformation of food, vomiting blood, aching pain, marked emaciation of the limbs, no desire to eat, nose bleed, blurred vision, pain of the shoulders and under the rib-sides and urgent urination. Apply two to three hundred cones of moxibustion and stop when [the symptoms are] cured.

扁鵲云：治卒中惡風，心悶煩毒欲死，急灸足大指下橫文隨年壯，立愈。若筋急不能行者：內踝筋急，灸內踝上四十壯；外踝筋急，灸外踝上三十壯，立愈。若眼戴精上插，灸目兩眥後二七壯。若不能語，灸第三椎上百壯。若不識人，灸季肋頭七壯。若眼反口噤，腹中切痛，灸陰囊下第一橫理十四壯，灸卒死亦良。

Biǎn Què said: To treat sudden strike of malign wind, with heart oppression, and vexation toxicity on the verge of dying; quickly apply moxibustion on the transverse crease on the bottom the big toe. Burn the same number of cones as the patient's age. This will cure the disease immediately.

For the tension of the sinews with inability to walk: When the tension is in the sinews of the medial malleolus, apply forty cones of moxibustion on medial malleolus; when the tension is in the sinews of the lateral malleolus, apply thirty cones of moxibustion on lateral malleolus. The disease will be cured right away.

For upcast eyes,[41] apply two times seven cones of moxibustion at the outer canthus.

For inability to speak, apply a hundred cones of moxibustion on the third vertebra.

For loss of consciousness, apply seven cones of moxibustion on the end of the free ribs.

For upturned eyes, clenched jaws, and cutting pain of the abdomen, apply fourteen cones of moxibustion on the first transverse crease behind the scrotum. This is also good for treating sudden death.

治大風卒風，緩急諸風卒發動，不自覺知，或心腹脹滿，或半身不隨，或口噤不言，涎唾自出，目閉耳聾，或舉身冷直，或煩悶恍惚，喜怒無節，或唇青口白，戴眼，角弓反張，始覺發動，即灸神庭七壯，次灸曲差，次上關，次下關，次頰車，次廉泉，次囟會，次百會，次本神，次天柱，次陶道，次風門，次心俞，次肝俞，次腎俞，次膀胱俞，次曲池，次肩髃，次支溝，次合谷，次間使，次陽陵泉，次陽輔，次崑崙，以上各七壯。

To treat great wind, sudden wind, acute or chronic wind, with sudden onset and unconsciousness; or distension and fullness of the heart and abdomen; or hemiplegia; or clenched jaws preventing speech, uncontrolled drooling and spitting, closed eyes and deafness; or generalized cold and stiffness; or vexation and oppression, abstraction, uncontrolled anger and joy; or pale green lips, upcast eyes, arched-back rigidity: If [these symptoms] have just started, apply seven cones of moxibustion on Shén Tíng 神庭 (Dū 24) first; then on the following points in order: Qū Chā 曲差 (UB 4), Shàng Guān 上關 (GB 3), Xià Guān 下關 (ST 7), Jiá Chē 頰車 (ST 6), Lián Quán 廉泉 (Rèn 23), Xìn Huì 囟會 (Dū 22), Bǎi Huì 百會 (Dū 20), Běn Shén 本神 (GB 13), Tiān Zhù 天柱 (UB 10), Táo Dào 陶道 (Dū 13), Fēng Mén 風門 (UB 12), Xīn Shù 心俞 (UB 15), Gān Shù 肝俞 (UB 18), Shèn Shù 腎俞 (UB 23), Páng Guāng Shù 膀胱俞 (UB 28), Qū Chí 曲池 (LI 11), Jiān Yú 肩髃 (LI 15), Zhī Gōu 支溝 (SJ 6), Hé Gǔ 合谷 (LI 4), Jiān Shǐ 間使 (PC 5), Yáng Líng Quán 陽陵泉 (GB 34), Yáng Fǔ 陽輔 (GB 38), and Kūn Lún 崑崙 (UB 60). Burn seven cones of moxibustion on each of the above points.

治風，灸上星二百壯；前頂二百四十壯；百會二百壯；腦戶、風府各三百壯。

41. *Jǐng Yuè Quán Shū* Volume 45 of《景岳全書·卷之四十五》(Jǐng Yuè's Complete Compendium) states: The symptom of upcast eyes occurs after suppuration of pox, or after severe sweating and diarrhea. It is usually characterized by upturned eyes, or the white of eyes (sclera) showing.

To treat wind, apply two hundred cones of moxibustion on Shàng Xīng 上星 (Dū 23), two hundred and forty cones of moxibustion on Qián Dǐng 前頂 (Dū 21), two hundred cones of moxibustion on Bǎi Huì 百會 (Dū 20), and three hundred cones of moxibustion each on Nǎo Hù 腦戶 (Dū 17) and Fēng Fǔ 風府 (Dū 16).

治大風，灸百會七百壯。治百種風，灸腦後項大椎平處，兩箱量二寸三分。須取病患指寸量兩箱各灸百壯，得瘥。治風耳鳴，從耳後量八分半裡許有孔，灸一切風，得瘥。狂者亦瘥，兩耳門前後各百壯。治卒病惡風欲死，不能語，及肉痹不知人，灸第五椎，名曰藏俞，百五十壯、三百壯便愈。大腸俞治風，腹中雷鳴，腸澼泄利，食不消化，小腹絞痛，腰脊疼強，或大小便難，不能飲食，灸百壯，三日一報。

To treat great wind, apply seven hundred cones of moxibustion on Bǎi Huì (Dū 20).

To treat the hundred types of wind, apply moxibustion on the posterior aspect of the head, 2.3 cùn lateral and level with Dà Zhuī 大椎 (Dū 14). Measure the distance with the patient's finger-cùn, and apply a hundred cones of moxibustion. The disease will be cured.

To treat wind with tinnitus, measure 8.5 fēn from the posterior aspect of the ear; there is a hollow on the medial side. All wind [diseases] will be cured after moxibustion is applied.

Mania also will be cured after a hundred cones of moxibustion are applied on the anterior and posterior aspect of both ear gates [tragus].

To treat sudden malign wind, about to die, unable to speak, with flesh *bi*-impediment and unconsciousness: Apply a hundred and fifty or three hundred cones of moxibustion on the fifth vertebra, which is named Zàng Shù 藏俞 (Dū 11). It will cure the disease.

Dà Cháng Shù 大腸俞 (UB 25) treats wind, with thunderous rumbling in the abdomen, intestinal afflux, diarrhea, non-transformation of food, gripping pain of the smaller abdomen, stiffness and pain of lower back and spine, or difficult urination and defecation with inability to eat. Apply a hundred cones of moxibustion and repeat every three days.

液門灸五十壯，主風。絕骨灸百壯，治風身重心煩，足脛疼。百會、天府、曲池、列缺主惡風邪氣，泣出喜忘。涌泉主風入腹中。商陽主耳中風生。臨泣主大風目痛(《甲》云：目外眥痛)。關衝主面黑濕風。解溪主風從頭至足，面目赤。

Apply fifty cones of moxibustion on Yè Mén 液門 (SJ 2) to govern wind.

Burn a hundred cones of moxibustion on Jué Gǔ 絕骨 (GB 39) to treat wind with generalized heaviness, vexation of the heart and leg pain.

Bǎi Huì 百會 (Dū 20), Tiān Fǔ 天府 (LU 3), Qū Chí 曲池 (LI 11), and Liè Quē 列缺 (LU 7) govern malign wind and evil qì, tearing, and forgetfulness.

Yǒng Quán 涌泉 (KI 1) governs wind entering the abdomen.

Shāng Yáng 商陽 (LI 1) governs wind engendered in the ears.

Lín Qì 臨泣 (GB 41) governs great wind with eye pain (*Jiǎ*《甲》says: pain at the outer canthus).

Guān Chōng 關衝 (SJ 1) governs dark facial complexion and wet wind.[42]

Jiě Xī 解溪 (ST 41) governs wind from head to feet with red eyes and face.

解益以醫風名。其進沉香半夏湯方云：夫人中風，心腎俱虛，百脈皆亂，氣散血凝。若使便服金銀、朱砂、腦麝涼藥，則手足不舉，經絡遂死。便服生附子，則益發虛熱，轉不能語，或下鮮血，故成廢疾。善治風者，當先主氣益心，去痰醒脾，然後療風，十愈八九。用炮附子一只，沉香等分、人參半兩、半夏二錢、南星一錢，各湯洗七次，為粗末（每服二大錢，水二盞，薑十片，煎至一盞，空心稍熱服，神效。其論治風有理。故附於此）。

[Author's notes:] Xiè Yì was famous for treating wind. He highly praised *Chén Xiāng Bàn Xià Tāng* 沉香半夏湯 (Aquilaria and Pinellia Decoction) for people suffering wind stroke, with vacuous heart and kidneys, chaos in the hundred vessels, scattered qì and congealed blood. If they were asked [by other doctors] to take cooling herbs like gold, silver, *zhū shā* 朱砂 (Cinnabar), [*lóng*] *nǎo* [龍]腦 (Borneol), and *shè* [*xiāng*] 麝[香] (Musk), their hands and feet became unable to raise up and their channels and network vessels would die. If they took raw *fù zǐ* 附子 (Aconite), they would have more vacuity heat, with inability to speak or fresh blood in the stool. Thus, disabling disease was formed. Those who are good at treating wind should first govern qì, supplement the heart, dispel phlegm, arouse the spleen, and then treat the wind. This will cure eighty or ninety percent. Use one piece of blast-fried *fù zǐ* (aconite), an equal amount of *chén xiāng* 沉香 (Aquilaria); half a *liǎng* (30g) of *rén shēn* 人參 (Ginseng), two *qián* (6g) of *bàn xià* 半夏 (Pinellia), and one *qián* (3g) of *nán xīng* 南星 (Arisaema). Wash it with hot water seven times and make a coarse powder. (Each time boil two *qián* in two bowls of water, with ten slices of ginger; boil it down to one bowl and drink it warm on an empty stomach. This is divinely effective. Xiè Yì's discussion of treating wind is reasonable, so it is appended here.)

液門主風寒熱（《千》）。內關主手中風熱。間使主頭身風熱。後溪主風身寒。俠溪主胸中寒如風狀。肺寒灸肺俞百壯。腎寒灸腎俞百壯。

42. Wet wind indicates the wind accompanied with rain or snow.

Yè Mén 液門 (SJ 2) governs wind, cold, and heat (*Qiān*《千》).

Nèi Guān 內關 (PC 6) governs wind heat in the hands.

Jiān Shǐ 間使 (PC 5) governs wind heat in the head and body.

Hòu Xī 後溪 (SI 3) governs wind with a cold body.

Xiá Xī 俠溪 (GB 43) governs cold in the chest as if wind [is striking].

Apply a hundred cones of moxibustion on Fèi Shù 肺俞 (UB 13) for cold in the lungs.

Burn a hundred cones of moxibustion on Shèn Shù 腎俞 (UB 23) for cold in the kidneys.

大橫治大風逆氣多寒(《銅》)。

Dà Héng 大橫 (SP 15) treats great wind, with qì counterflow in someone who is prone to cold (*Tóng*《銅》).

凡中風用續命湯、排風等湯;神精丹、茵芋酒;更加灸,必愈(《本事》)。

For wind stroke, use *Xù Mìng Tāng* 續命湯 (Life Prolonging Decoction), *Pái Fēng* [*Tāng*] 排風[湯] (Wind Expelling [Decoction), and so forth; also *Shén Jīng Dān* 神精丹 (Sharp Spirit Pill), *Yīn Yù* 茵芋 (Skimmia) liquor, plus moxibustion. The disease will certainly be cured (*Běn Shì*《本事》).

## 4.25
## *Zhòng Fēng Bù Yǔ*
### *(Zhòng Fēng Kǒu Jìn Fù, Yú Jiàn Kǒu Yǎ, Jǒu Yǎn Wāi)*

# 中風不語
## (中風口噤附　餘見口啞　口眼喎)

## Wind stroke with loss of speech
**(attached: wind stroke with clenched jaw;**
**see also the sections on muteness and deviation of the mouth and eyes)**

脾風占候，聲不出，或上下手，當灸手十指頭，次灸人中，次大椎，次兩耳門前脈，去耳門上下行一寸是，次兩大指節上下，各七壯。治脾風，灸脾俞脊兩邊各五十壯。凡人脾俞無定所，隨四季月應，病即灸藏俞是脾穴。此法甚妙。脾風者，總呼為八風。

The signs of wind striking the spleen are: loss of voice, or [uncontrollable] movement of the arms up and down. Apply moxibustion in the following order: the tips of the fingers, Rén Zhōng 人中 (Dū 26), Dà Zhuī 大椎 (Dū 14), the vessel approximately 1 cùn anterior to both ear gates [tragus], and above and below the thumb joints. Burn seven cones of moxibustion on each [site]. To treat spleen wind, apply fifty cones of moxibustion on Pí Shù 脾俞 (UB 20) on the both sides of the spine. There is no fixed place for the shù point of the spleen on people; the location corresponds to the four seasons and the month. When sick, apply moxibustion on the viscus-associated point. This is the point of the spleen. This method is excellent. Spleen wind is generally called *bā fēng* 八風 [the eight winds].[43]

猥腿風半身不遂失音不語者：灸百會，次本神，次承漿，次風府，次肩髃，次心俞，次手五冊，次手髓孔，次手少陽，次足五冊，次足髓孔，次足陽明，各五百壯。

*Wěi tuǐ fēng* 猥腿風 [flaccid leg wind][44] with hemiplegia and loss of speech: Apply moxibustion in the following order on Bǎi Huì 百會 (Dū 20), Běn Shén 本神 (GB 13), Chéng Jiāng 承漿 (Rèn 24), Fēng Fǔ 風府 (Dū 16), Jiān Yú 肩髃 (LI 15), Xīn Shù 心俞 (UB 15), Shǒu Wǔ Cè 手五冊,[45] Shǒu Suǐ Kǒng 手髓孔 (SI 4 or SI 5),[46] Shǒu Shào Yáng 手少陽,[47] Zú Wǔ Cè 足五冊,[48] Zú Suǐ Kǒng 足髓空,[49] and Zú Yáng Míng 足陽明 (ST 42).[50] Burn five hundred cones of moxibustion on each.

43. *Bā fēng* 八風 [eight winds] indicate wind coming from the eight directions according to *Líng Shū·Jiǔ Gōng Bā Fēng*《靈樞·九宮八風》(Magic Pivot 77, The Nine Palaces and the Eight Winds). Wind can cause disease when it comes from the opposite direction of the seasonal palace. Since spleen earth is located in the center, it has no direction of its own, but receives wind from all eight directions.

44. *Wěi tuǐ fēng* 猥腿風 [flaccid leg wind] is a disease with hemiplegia and loss of voice, according to *Qiān Jīn Yào Fāng*《千金要方》, Volume 8.

45. *Shǒu Wǔ Cè* 手五冊 is located on both sides of the transverse crease of the elbow, two points on each arm.

46. Shǒu Suǐ Kǒng 手髓孔 is located in the depression on the pointed bone proximal to the wrist according to *Qiān Jīn Yì Fāng*《千金翼方》(Appendix to Prescriptions Worth a Thousand Piece of Gold). This may refer to Wàn Gǔ 腕骨 (SI 4) or Yáng Gǔ 陽谷 (SI 5).

47. Shǒu Shào Yáng 手少陽: The location of this point is unknown.

48. Zú Wǔ Cè 足五冊 is located at the end of the transverse crease when the knee is flexed according to *Qiān Jīn Yì Fāng*《千金翼方》.

49. Zú Suǐ Kǒng 足髓空 is located one cùn posterior to the lateral malleolus according to *Qiān Jīn Yì Fāng* 千金翼方. It may refer to Kūn Lún 崑崙 (UB 60)

50. Zú Yáng Míng 足陽明 is another name for Chōng Yáng 衝陽 (ST 42).

中風
379
中風失音，不能言語，緩縱不隨：先灸天窗五十壯；息火，仍移灸百會五十壯畢；還灸天窗五十壯。若發先灸百會，則風氣不得泄，內攻五臟，喜閉伏，仍失音也。所以先灸天窗，次百會佳。一灸五十壯，悉泄火勢，復灸之。視病輕重，重者一處三百壯，大較。凡中風服藥益劇者，但是風穴，悉皆灸三壯，無不愈，神良。決定勿疑，不至心者，勿浪為灸。又灸風痱不能語，手足不遂（詳見《千金》）。治卒病欲死，不能語。治肺中風不能言（並見中風）。

Wind stroke with loss of voice, inability to speak, and hemiplegia: Apply fifty cones of moxibustion on Tiān Chuāng 天窗 (SI 16); after this is done, burn another fifty cones on Bǎi Huì 百會 (Dū 20); then another fifty cones on Tiān Chuāng (SI 16) again. If moxibustion is applied to Bǎi Huì (Dū 20) first, wind qì cannot be drained; it will attack the five viscera internally and tends to block and hide, causing loss of voice. So it is better to apply moxibustion to Tiān Chuāng (SI 16) first, and then Bǎi Huì (Dū 20). Burn fifty cones of moxibustion each time to discharge the fire completely, and repeat the moxibustion again.

Based on the severity of the disease, you can burn three hundred cones of moxibustion on one site for severe conditions; [the patient] will recover a lot.

For those wind stroke patients who get worse after taking herbs, apply three cones of moxibustion on all wind points. This will cure the disease and is very effective. Do not hesitate after making the decision; if you are unsure, do not apply moxibustion in vain.

Also apply moxibustion for wind disablement with inability to speak and paralysis of the limbs (for details see *Qiān Jīn*《千金》); [This method] can also treat sudden onset of disease when [the patient] is close to death and is unable to speak; and wind attacking the lungs with inability to speak (for all this, see the section on wind stroke).

巢氏云：脾脈絡胃夾咽，連舌本，散舌下。心之別脈，系舌本。心脾受風邪，故舌強不語（三陽之筋，並絡入頷頰，夾於口。諸陽為風寒所客，則筋急，故口噤不開）。

[Author's notes:] Master Cháo said: The spleen vessel nets with the stomach and lines the esophagus, links with the root of the tongue, and spreads over the lower surface of the tongue. The diverging vessel of the heart ties to the root of the tongue. When wind evils attack the heart and spleen, stiffness of the tongue and loss of speech occur (the sinews of the three yáng all net with the chin and cheeks and line the mouth. When wind-cold settles in all the yáng, tension of the sinews occurs and causes clenched jaws.)

卒中風，口噤不得：灸機關（《千金翼》名頰車）二穴。穴在耳下八分小近前，灸五壯即得語，又灸隨年壯。僻者逐僻左右灸（《千》）。

Sudden onset of wind stroke with clenched jaws: Apply moxibustion on the bilateral point Jī Guān 機關 (*Qiān Jīn Yì*《千金翼》named it Jiá Chē 頰車). The point is located eight fēn inferior to the ear and slightly anterior. The patient can speak after burning five cones of moxibustion, or applying the same number of cones as the age of the patient. Apply moxibustion on the left or right sides to expel deviation (*Qiān*《千》).

治卒中風口喎：筆筒長五寸，以一頭刺耳孔中，四畔以面密塞勿令泄氣；一頭內大豆一顆，並艾燒令燃，灸七壯瘥。右灸左，左灸右。千金不傳，耳病亦灸之。

To treat sudden wind strike with deviation of the mouth: Insert one end of a five cùn long handle of a writing brush[51] into the ear, wrap dough tightly around the handle [within the ear] to avoid letting qì [air] leak out; put a piece of mugwort [floss the size] of a bean in the other end and burn it. Apply seven cones of moxibustion to cure the disease. If the right side is affected, apply moxibustion to the left, if the left side is affected, apply moxibustion to the right. *Qiān Jīn*《千金》did not pass this on. You can also apply this moxibustion for ear diseases.

中風口喎：灸手交脈三壯。左灸右，右灸左。炷如鼠屎形，橫安兩頭下火。口喎，刺承泣（見目瞤）。

Wind stroke with deviation of the mouth: Apply three cones of moxibustion on the hand crossed vessel,[52] burn moxibustion on the right when left side is affected, and on the left when the right side is affected. The size of the cone equals the size of mice droppings. Put the moxa cones horizontally [on the crossed vessel] and light both ends. Needle Chéng Qì 承泣 (ST 1) for deviation of the mouth (see the section on twitching of the eyelids).

51. A brush handle is made from a hollow piece of bamboo.

52. Hand crossed vessel: The location of this is not clear. It could be Liè Quē 列缺 (LU 7).

## 口喎 591 4.26

## *Piān Fēng (Piān Kū, Bàn Shēn Bù Suì)*

# 偏風（偏枯　半身不遂）

## Hemilateral wind

**(Hemilateral withering, hemiplegia)**

岐伯答黃帝灸中風半身不遂（《明下》見中風）。

Qí Bó replied to the Yellow Emperor [on how to] apply moxibustion for wind stroke with hemiplegia (see the section on wind stroke in *Míng Xià*《明下》).

列缺治偏風口喎，手腕無力（《明下》作腕勞），半身不隨（《明》同），咳嗽，掌中熱，口噤不開（《銅》）。下關治偏風，口目喎，牙車脫臼。上關治偏風口眼喎（《明》云眼喎通睛），耳中如蟬聲《明》同）。

Liè Quē 列缺 (LU 7) treats hemilateral wind, deviation of the mouth, weakness of the wrists (*Míng Xià* says taxation of the wrists), hemiplegia (*Míng*《明》agrees), cough, heat in the palms, and clenched jaws (*Tóng*《銅》).

Xià Guān 下關 (ST 7) treats hemilateral wind, deviation of the mouth and eyes, and dislocation of the teeth carriage (jaw).

Shàng Guān 上關 (GB 3) treats hemilateral wind, deviation of the mouth and eyes (*Míng* says: deviation of the eyes, converging eyes [a kind of squint]), ringing in the ears like the sound of cicadas (*Míng* agrees).

完骨治偏風，口面喎，頸項痛不得顧，小便赤黃，喉痹頰腫。承漿療偏風口喎面腫（《明》同）。衝陽（見口喎）、地倉治偏風口喎（見口喎）。迎香治偏風口喎，面癢浮腫，風動葉葉，狀如蟲行；或唇腫痛（《明》同）。

Wán Gǔ 完骨 (GB 12) treats hemilateral wind, deviation of the mouth and face, pain of the neck and nape with inability to turn it, dark yellow urine, throat *bì*-impediment,[53] and swollen cheeks.

53. Throat *bì*-impediment is a disorder with sore throat or a dry itchy feeling in the throat.

Chéng Jiāng 承漿 (Rèn 24) treats hemilateral wind, deviation of the mouth, and facial swelling (*Míng*《 明 》agrees).

Chōng Yáng 衝陽 (ST 42) (see the section on deviation of the mouth [and eyes]) and Dì Cāng 地倉 (ST 4) treat hemilateral wind and deviation of the mouth (see the section on deviation of the mouth [and eyes]).

Yíng Xiāng 迎香 (LI 20) treats hemilateral wind with deviation of the mouth and itchy puffy swollen face [with sensations under the skin] as if wind were blowing leaves or insects were creeping; or painful swollen lips (*Míng* agrees).

環跳治冷風濕痹，風疹，偏風半身不遂，腰胯痛不得轉（《明下》同）。肩髃治偏風，半身不遂，熱風癮疹，手臂攣急（《明》云：手不得向頭），捉物不得，挽弓不開，臂細無力，筋骨酸疼。若灸偏風，可七七壯，不宜多。

Huán Tiào 環跳 (GB 30) treats cold, wind, and damp *bì*-impediment, wind papules, hemilateral wind, hemiplegia, and pain of the lower back and hips with inability to turn (*Míng Xià*《 明下 》agrees).

Jiān Yú 肩髃 (LI 15) treats hemilateral wind, hemiplegia, hot wind, dormant papules, hypertonicity of the arms (*Míng* says: the hands cannot [move] toward the head), inability to grasp things or draw a bow, thin weak arms, and aching sinews and bones. Apply seven times seven cones of moxibustion for hemilateral wind. It is not appropriate to burn more cones.

曲池療偏風，半身不遂，刺風疹疼痛冷緩，捉物不得，挽弓不開，屈身難隱，脈風，臂肘細無力。

Qū Chí 曲池 (LI 11) cures hemilateral wind and hemiplegia. Needle it for wind papules with pain, inability to grasp things or draw a bow, difficulty bending the body to hide, vessel wind [leprosy], and thin weak arms and elbows.

陽陵泉、環跳（並見膝痛）、曲池治偏風半身不遂（《明下》同）。照海治大風偏枯，半身不遂（《明》同）。上廉治偏風，腰腿手足不仁（並《銅》，《明下》同）。

Yáng Líng Quán 陽陵泉 (GB 34), Huán Tiào (GB 30) (for both, see the section on knee pain), and Qū Chí (LI 11) treat hemilateral wind and hemiplegia (*Míng Xià* agrees).

Zhào Hǎi 照海 (KI 6) treats great wind [leprosy], hemilateral withering, and hemiplegia (*Míng* agrees).

腰腳 542
口喎 591
腳弱 524
香港 519
濕痹 682
月水 735

Shàng Lián 上廉 (LI 9 or ST 37) treats hemilateral wind and numbness of the lower back, legs, hands and feet (for both, see *Tóng*《銅》; *Míng Xià*《明下》agrees).

下崑崙（見腰腳）、委中療半身不遂（《明》）。地倉（見口喎）、承山（見腳弱）、上廉（見香港腳）、下廉（見濕痹）療偏風。陰蹻療手足偏枯（見月水）。

Xià Kūn Lún 下崑崙 (UB 60) (see the section on low back and leg [pain]) and Wěi Zhōng 委中 (UB 40) cure hemiplegia (*Míng*《明》).

Dì Cāng 地倉 (ST 4) (see the section on deviation of the mouth [and eyes]), Chéng Shān 承山 (UB 57) (see the section on weak legs), Shàng Lián (ST 37) (see the section on leg qì), and Xià Lián 下廉 (ST 39) (see the section on damp *bì*-impediment) cure hemilateral wind.

Yīn Qiāo 陰蹻 (KI 6 or KI 8) cures hemilateral withering of the hands and feet (see the section on menstruation).

猥腿風，半身不遂，失音，灸百會（《千》見中風失音）。

For *wěi tuǐ fēng* 猥腿風 [flaccid leg wind], hemiplegia, and loss of voice: Apply moxibustion on Bǎi Huì 百會 (Dū 20) (see the section on wind stroke with loss of voice in *Qiān*《千》).

半身不遂，男女皆有此患，但男尤忌左，女尤忌右爾。若得此疾後，風藥不宜暫闕。常令身上有灸瘡可也。最忌房室，或能如道、釋修養，方能保其無他。

Anyone can suffer wind hemiplegia whether male or female. But males should especially dread its occurrence on the left side and females on the right side. It is important not to lack wind herbs when suffering this disease. It is also appropriate to make moxa sores on the body. Sexual activity should especially be avoided. No other [pathological changes] can be guaranteed only if [the patient practices] Dàoist or Buddhist self-cultivation.

若灸則當先百會、囟會，次風池、肩髃、曲池、合谷、環跳、風市、三里、絕骨，不必拘舊經病左灸右，病右灸左之說，但按酸疼處灸之。若兩邊灸亦佳，但當自上而下灸之。

First apply moxibustion on Bǎi Huì (Dū 20) and Xìn Huì 囟會 (Dū 22); then on Fēng Chí 風池 (GB 20), Jiān Yú 肩髃 (LI 15), Qū Chí 曲池 (LI 11), Hé Gǔ 合谷 (LI 4), Huán Tiào 環跳 (GB 30), Fēng Shì 風市 (GB 31), Sān Lǐ 三里 (ST 36), and Jué Gǔ 絕骨 (GB 39).

We do not have to follow the theory in the old classics of applying moxibustion on the right side for the diseases of the left, or applying moxibustion on the left side for the disease of the right. Only apply moxibustion to sites that ache when pressed. It is also good to apply moxibustion on both sides, but moxibustion should be burned from the upper body down to the lower body.

痃癖 433
傷寒 661
目眩 575
脊 555
膝痛 539

## 4.27

## *Tán Xián (Tán Yǐn, Tǔ Mò, Yú Jiàn Tuò)*

# 痰涎（痰飲　吐沫　餘見唾）

## Phlegm-drool

**(Phlegm-rheum, foaming at the mouth; for further discussion, see the section on spittle)**

巨闕治熱病，胸中痰飲，腹脹暴痛，恍惚不知人（《銅》）。通谷治結積留飲，胸滿，食不化。不容治痰癖（見痃癖）。少衝治痰冷（見傷寒）。率谷治膈胃寒痰，傷酒風發，腦兩角強痛，不能飲食，煩滿吐不止。浮白治痰沫胸中滿，不得喘息。本神治癲疾吐涎沫。絲竹空（見目眩）治涎沫。然谷、復溜（見脊）治涎出。陰谷（見膝痛）治涎下。

Jù Quē 巨闕 (Rèn 14) treats heat diseases, phlegm-rheum in the chest, distension and violent pain of the abdomen, abstraction, and unconsciousness (*Tóng* 《銅》).

Tōng Gǔ 通谷 (KI 20)[54] treats binds and accumulations, lodged rheum, chest fullness, and non-transformation of food.

Bù Róng 不容 (ST 19) treats phlegm aggregation (see the section on strings and aggregations).

Shào Chōng 少衝 (HT 9) treats cold phlegm (see the section on cold damage).

Shuài Gǔ 率谷 (GB 8) treats cold phlegm in the diaphragm and stomach, wind attack after becoming drunk, stiffness and pain at the corners of the head, inability to eat and drink, vexation and fullness, as well as incessant vomiting.

Fú Bái 浮白 (GB 10) treats foamy phlegm, chest fullness, and panting with inability to catch one's breath.

Běn Shén 本神 (GB 13) treats epilepsy and vomiting of drool and foam.

54. Tōng Gǔ 通谷 may refer to UB 66 or KI 20. Since here, the author discusses points of the abdomen first, it should be KI 20.

心脹 445
吐 274
泄 243
癲狂 345
癲癇 357
風癇 366
瘛瘲 354

Sī Zhú Kōng 絲竹空 (SJ 23) (see the section on dizzy vision) treats foamy drool.

Rán Gǔ 然谷 (KI 2) and Fù Liū 復溜 (KI 7) (see the section on [pain of the lower back and] spine) treat drooling.

Yīn Gǔ 陰谷 (KI 10) (see the section on knee pain) treats drooling.

膈俞療痰飲吐逆，汗出，寒熱骨痛，虛脹舌滿痰瘧（《明》）。膽俞療痰悶（見心脹）上管療痰多吐涎（《下》見吐）。

Gé Shù 膈俞 (UB 17) cures phlegm-rheum and spitting counterflow, sweating, [sensations of] cold and heat with pain of the bones, vacuity distention, tongue fullness, and phlegm malaria (*Míng*《明》).

Dǎn Shù 膽俞 (UB 19) cures oppression due to phlegm (see the discussion of heart distention).

Shàng Guǎn 上管 (Rèn 13) cures copious phlegm and vomiting of drool (see vomiting in *Xià*《下》).

結積留飲，灸通谷（《千》見腸癖）。

Apply moxibustion on Tōng Gǔ 通谷 (KI 20 or UB 66) for binds, accumulations and lodged rheum (see intestinal afflux in *Qiān*《千》).

下廉治涎出不覺（《銅》見泄）。少海（《明》同）、兌端（《下》同）、本神治吐沫（見癲狂）。

Xià Lián 下廉 (ST 39 or LI 8) treats uncontrollable drooling (see diarrhea in *Tóng*《銅》).

Shào Hǎi 少海 (HT 3) (*Míng* agrees), Duì Duān 兌端 (Dū 27) (*Xià* agrees), and Běn Shén 本神 (GB 13) treat spitting of foam (see the section on withdrawal and mania).

絲竹空、通谷、商丘主嘔沫（《千》見癲癇）。兌端等主嘔沫（見風癇）。

Sī Zhú Kōng (SJ 23), Tōng Gǔ (KI 20 or UB 66), and Shāng Qiū 商丘 (SP 5) govern retching of foam (see epilepsy and withdrawal in *Qiān*).

Duì Duān 兌端 (Dū 27), and so forth, govern retching of foam (see wind epilepsy).

溫溜治吐涎（《銅》見癲狂）。上關治沫出（見瘛瘲）。顱囟治小兒吐沫（見瘛瘲）。

Wēn Liū 溫溜 (LI 7) treats vomiting of drool (see withdrawal and mania in *Tóng*《銅》). 上氣 420

Shàng Guān 上關 (GB 3) treats foaming (see tugging and slackening). 少氣 426

Lú Xìn 顱囟 (SJ 19) treats foaming in children (see tugging and slackening).

彧中、雲門等主涎出多唾(《千》)。庫房等主多唾濁沫(並見上氣)。

Yù Zhōng 彧中 (KI 26), Yún Mén 雲門 (LU 2), and so forth govern drooling and copious spittle (*Qiān*《千》).

Kù Fáng 庫房 (ST 14) and so forth govern frequent spitting of turbid foam (for all these, see the section on counterflow qì).

廉泉治嘔沫(《銅》見上氣)。《明》云:療喘息嘔沫(見少氣)。

Lián Quán 廉泉 (Rèn 23) treats retching of foam (see counterflow qì in *Tóng*). *Míng*《明》says: It cures panting and retching of foam (see the section on qì shortage).

痰涎等證,不一而。惟勞瘵有痰為難治,最宜灸膏肓穴,壯數既多,當有所下。礱礱然流水之狀,蓋痰下也。餘當隨證治之。

[Author's notes:] Phlegm-drool has different kinds of symptoms. The phlegm of consumption is the most difficult to treat. It is appropriate to apply moxibustion on Gāo Huāng 膏肓 (UB 43). Something should descend after a lot of cones of moxibustion are applied. If it sounds like water flowing down, like something grinding, this must be the phlegm. Treat other symptoms according to their patterns.

凡人患水症,口中涌水,《經》謂之肺來乘腎,食後吐水:可灸肺俞,又灸三陰交、期門,瀉肺補腎也。各隨年壯。然則痰涎有類此者,又當如此法灸之。

In people suffering water infixation, water gushes into the mouth. The Classic says[55] this is the lungs overwhelming the kidneys. There is spitting of the water after eating: Apply moxibustion on Fèi Shù 肺俞 (UB 13), then Sān Yīn Jiāo 三陰交 (SP 6), and Qī Mén 期門 (LV 14); this drains the

55. The following phrase is also found in *Zhōng Zàng Jīng*《中藏經》(Classic of the Central Viscera). However, even though this book is attributed to Huá Tuó, it was written later by unknown authors. It is uncertain whether Wáng is referring to this book or some other source that is now lost.

lungs and supplements the kidneys. Burn the same number of the cones as the age of the patient. If there is phlegm-drool like this, follow this method and apply moxibustion.

## 4.28

## *Tuò Xuè (Ǒu Xuè, Tù Xuè, Yú Jiàn Tuò)*

# 唾血（嘔血　吐血　餘見唾）

## Spitting of blood

**(Retching of blood and vomiting blood; for further discussion, see the section on spittle)**

凡內損（又作傷），唾血不足，外無膏澤：地五會（《銅》同）主之。刺入三分，特忌灸（《千》）。

For all internal detriment (also written as damage) with incessant spitting of blood, and without a moist shiny body: Dì Wǔ Huì 地五會 (GB 42) (*Tóng*《銅》agrees) governs it. Needle 3 fēn deep. Moxibustion is especially contraindicated (*Qiān*《千》).

凡唾血，瀉魚際、補尺澤。然谷主咳唾有血。大淵（《明下》見胃痛）、神門主唾血振寒，嘔血上氣。

For spitting of blood, drain Yú Jì 魚際 (LU 10) and supplement Chǐ Zé 尺澤 (LU 5).

Rán Gǔ 然谷 (KI 2) governs coughing and spitting of blood.

Tài Yuān 太淵 (LU 9) (see stomach ache in *Míng Xià*《明下》) and Shén Mén 神門 (HT 7) govern spitting of blood, quivering with cold, retching of blood, and counterflow of qì.

胸堂、手心、脾俞、間使、胃管、天樞、肝俞、魚際、勞宮、肩俞、大溪主唾血吐血。心俞、肝俞、缺盆、巨闕、鳩尾主咳唾血。

Xiōng Táng 胸膛 (Dàn Zhōng 膻中 (Rèn 17)), Shǒu Xīn 手心 (Dà Líng 大陵 (PC 7)), Pí Shù 脾俞 (UB 20), Jiān Shǐ 間使 (PC 5), Wèi Guǎn 胃管 (Rèn 13), Tiān Shū 天樞 (ST 25), Gān Shù 肝俞 (UB 18), Yú Jì 魚際 (LU 10), Láo Gōng 勞宮 (PC 8), Jiān Shù 肩俞 (non-channel),[56] and Tài Xī 太溪 (KI 3) govern spitting of blood and vomiting blood.

56. Jiān Shù 肩俞 is a non-channel point. It is located between Jiān Yú 肩髃 (LI 15) and Yún Mén 云門 (LU 2).

Xīn Shù 心俞 (UB 15), Gān Shù 肝俞 (UB 18), Quē Pén 缺盆 (ST 12), Jù Quē 巨闕 (Rèn 14), and Jiū Wěi 鳩尾 (Rèn 15) govern coughing and spitting of blood.

庫房、中府、周榮、尺澤主咳逆上氣，呼吸多唾濁沫膿血。上管(《明下》同)、不容、大陵主嘔血。郄門主嘔血衄血。行間主短氣，嘔血，胸背痛。太衝主面唇色白，時時嘔血，女子漏血。

Kù Fáng 庫房 (ST 14), Zhōng Fǔ 中府 (LU 1), Zhōu Róng 周榮 (SP 20), and Chǐ Zé 尺澤 (LU 5) govern coughing counterflow qì and breathing with spitting of turbid foam, pus, and blood.

Shàng Guǎn 上管 (Rèn 13) (*Míng Xià*《明下》agrees), Bù Róng 不容 (ST 19), and Dà Líng 大陵 (PC 7) govern retching of blood.

Xī Mén 郄門 (PC 4) governs retching of blood and nosebleeds.

Xíng Jiān 行間 (LV 2) governs shortness of breath, retching of blood and pain of the chest and back.

Tài Chōng 太衝 (LV 3) governs pale face and lips, frequent retching of blood, and spotting of blood in women.

手少陰郄主吐血。三里主胸中瘀血，樁滿脅膈痛，不能久立，膝痿寒。上管主心膈下嘔血。不容主嘔血，肩脅痛，口乾，心痛與背相引，不可咳，咳引腎痛。太淵主唾血振寒嗌乾。太陵及郄門主嘔血。神門主嘔血上氣。虛勞吐血，灸胃管三百壯，亦主勞，嘔逆吐血，少食，多飽多唾(一作多睡)百病。

Hand Shàoyīn Xī 少陰郄 [Yīn Xī 陰郄 (HT 6)] governs vomiting blood.

Sān Lǐ 三里 (ST 36 or LI 10) governs blood stasis in the chest, propping fullness, pain of the rib-sides and diaphragm, inability to stand for long, and weak cold knees.

Shàng Guǎn (Rèn 13) governs retching of blood under the heart and diaphragm.

Bù Róng 不容 (ST 19) governs retching of blood, pain of the shoulders and rib-sides, dry mouth, heart pain radiating to the back, inability to cough, or cough that induces pain of the kidneys.

Tài Yuān 太淵 (LU 9) governs spitting of blood, quivering with cold, and dry throat.

Dà Líng (PC 7) and Xī Mén (PC 4) govern retching of blood.

Shén Mén 神門 (HT 7) governs retching of blood and counterflow qì.

肺氣 412
咳逆 417
腹脹 449
嗽 414
淋 222
狂走 345
胸脅 476
痰 399
心痛 312
心煩 335
風勞 371

Vacuity taxation with vomiting blood: Apply three hundred cones of moxibustion on Wèi Guǎn 胃管 (Rèn 12 or Rèn 13); this also governs the hundred diseases of taxation with retching counterflow, vomiting blood, reduced eating, and a lot of spitting (one source says a lot of sleeping) after overeating.

吐血：胸堂百壯，不針。吐血，腹痛雷鳴：天樞百壯。吐血唾血，上氣咳逆：肺俞隨年壯。吐血酸削：肝俞百壯。吐血嘔逆：灸手心主五十壯（《千金翼》云太陵，是）。凡口鼻出血不止，名腦衄：上星五十壯。

Vomiting blood: Apply a hundred cones of moxibustion on Xiōng Táng 胸膛 [Dàn Zhōng (Rèn 17)]; do not use acupuncture.

Vomiting blood, abdominal pain, and thunderous rumbling: Apply a hundred cones of moxibustion on Tiān Shū 天樞 (ST 25).

Vomiting blood, spitting of blood, counterflow qì and cough: Apply the same number of moxa cones as the age of the patient on Fèi Shù 肺俞 (UB 13).

Vomiting blood and extreme aching pain: Apply a hundred cones of moxibustion on Gān Shù 肝俞 (UB 18).

Vomiting blood and retching counterflow: Apply fifty cones of moxibustion on Shǒu Xīn Zhǔ 手心主 [Dà Líng 大陵 (PC 7)] (*Qiān Jīn Yì*《千金翼》says: Tài Líng 太陵 (PC 7). This is correct).

Incessant bleeding from the nose and mouth is called brain bleed: Apply fifty cones of moxibustion on Shàng Xīng 上星 (Dū 23).

膻中治唾膿（《銅》見肺氣）。肝俞（見咳逆）、承滿（腹脹）、肩中俞（見嗽）治唾血。大鐘（見淋）、然谷、心俞（狂走）治咳唾血。天突治咯唾膿血（見肺）。庫房治多唾濁沫膿血（見胸脅滿）。屋翳治多濁沫膿血（見痰）。巨闕治息賁，時唾血（《明下》云：療嘔血煩心）。太淵（見心痛）、神門（心煩）、行間、太衝、魚際治嘔血。曲泉治逆氣嘔血。五里治吐血（風勞）。太溪治咽腫唾血（並《銅》、《明下》療唾血及衄血不止）。

Dàn Zhōng 膻中 (Rèn 17) treats spitting pus (see the section on lung qì in *Tóng*《銅》).

Gān Shù 肝俞 UB 18) (see the section on coughing counterflow), Chéng Mǎn 承滿 (ST 20) (see the section on abdominal fullness), and Jiān Zhōng Shù 肩中俞 (SI 15) (see the section on cough) treat spitting of blood.

中風 379
唾 402
咳逆 417
心煩 335
肺 412

Dà Zhōng 大鐘 (KI 4) (see the section on dribbling), Rán Gǔ 然谷 (KI 2), and Xīn Shù 心俞 (UB 15) (see the section on manic walking) treat coughing and spitting of blood.

Tiān Tū 天突 (Rèn 22) treats expectoration of pus and blood (see the section on lung [qì]).

Kù Fáng 庫房 (ST 14) treats frequent spitting of turbid foam, pus, and blood (see the section on the chest and rib-side fullness).

Wū Yì 屋翳 (ST 15) treats copious turbid foam, pus and blood (see the discussion of phlegm).

Jù Quē 巨闕 (Rèn 14) treats rushing respiration[57] and frequent spitting of blood (*Míng Xià* 《明下》 says: It cures retching of blood and vexation of the heart).

Tài Yuān 太淵 (LU 9) (see the section on heart pain), Shén Mén 神門 (HT 7) (see the section on vexation of the heart), Xíng Jiān 行間 (LV 2), Tài Chōng 太衝 (LV 3), and Yú Jì 魚際 (LU 10) treat retching of blood.

Qū Quán 曲泉 (LV 8) treats counterflow qì and retching of blood.

Wǔ Lǐ 五里 (LV 10 or LI 13) treats vomiting blood (see the section on wind taxation).

Tài Xī 太溪 (KI 3) treats swollen throat and spitting of blood (*Tóng* 《銅》 and *Míng Xià* say: It cures spitting of blood and incessant nosebleeds).

巨骨療驚癎，破心吐血（《明》）。魚際療吐血唾血。肝俞（見中風）、紫宮（見唾）。石門（見咳逆）療吐血。孔最療吐血失音腫痛。曲澤療心痛出血嘔血（見心煩）。肺俞（見肺）療唾血（《千》）。承滿療膈氣吐血。

Jù Gǔ 巨骨 (LI 16) cures fright epilepsy, vomiting blood [as if] the heart has broken open (*Míng* 《明》).

Yú Jì 魚際 (LU 10) cures vomiting blood and spitting of blood.

Gān Shù 肝俞 (UB 18) (see the section on wind stroke), Zǐ Gōng 紫宮 (Rèn 19) (see the section on spitting), and Shí Mén 石門 (Rèn 5) (see the section on coughing counterflow) cure vomiting blood.

Kǒng Zuì 孔最 (LU 6) cures vomiting blood, loss of voice, swelling, and pain.

Qū Zé 曲澤 (PC 3) cures heart pain, bleeding and retching of blood (see the section on vexation of the heart).

---

57. *Xī bēn* 息賁 is a disease with the symptoms of gasping, cough, chest pain, spitting of blood, chills and fever, and cup-like masses under the lungs. It is due to blockage of lung qì and retention of phlegm-heat. It can transform into lung abscess.

瘧 301
心煩 335
肩背 486
痃癖 433
胸滿 470
淋 222
吐瀉 271
胸脅 476

Fèi Shù 肺俞 (UB 13) (see the section on the lung qì) cures spitting of blood (*Qiān*《千》).

Chéng Mǎn 承滿 (ST 20) cures diaphragm[58] qì and vomiting blood.

## 4.29
## *Chuǎn (Yú Jiàn Ké Sòu)*
# 喘（餘見咳嗽）
## Panting
**(for further discussion, see the section on cough)**

崑崙主腹痛喘暴滿（《千》）。

Kūn Lún 崑崙 (UB 60) treats abdominal pain, panting, and violent fullness (*Qiān*《千》).

崑崙（《千》同）治咳喘暴滿（《銅》）。三間治氣喘（見瘧）。神門（見心煩）、譩譆治喘逆（見肩背痛）。不容治喘咳（見痃癖）。商陽治喘咳支腫（見胸滿）。《明下》云：胸膈氣滿喘急。大鐘治胸張喘息（見淋）。期門治大喘不得臥（見吐瀉）。俞府治咳逆上喘（承滿同見腹脹），嘔吐胸滿，不得食（《明》同）。彧中治咳逆（《明下》作嗽），喘不能食（見胸脅滿）。

Kūn Lún (UB 60) (*Qiān* agrees) treats cough, panting and violent fullness (*Tóng*《銅》).

Sān Jiān 三間 (LI 3) treats panting (see the section on malaria).

Shén Mén 神門 (HT 7) (see the section on vexation of the heart) and Yī Xī 譩譆 (UB 45) treat panting counterflow (see the sections on shoulder and back pain).

Bù Róng 不容 (ST 19) treats cough and panting (see the section on strings and aggregations).

Shāng Yáng 商陽 (LI 1) treats panting and cough and propping swelling (see the section on chest pain). *Míng Xià*《明下》says: Qì fullness and rapid panting in the chest and diaphragm.

Dà Zhōng 大鐘 (KI 4) treats chest distention and panting (see the section on dribbling).

58. Diaphragm qì 膈氣 is *yē gé* 噎膈. It includes the symptoms of chest and abdominal oppression and difficulty swallowing.

胸滿 470
吐瀉 271
胸脅 476
月事 735
上氣 420

Qī Mén 期門 (LV 14) treats severe panting with inability to lie down (see the sections on vomiting and diarrhea).

Shù Fǔ 俞府 (KI 27) treats coughing counterflow as well as panting (the same as Chéng Mǎn 承滿 (ST 20); see the section on abdominal fullness), vomiting and chest fullness, and inability to eat (*Míng* 《 明 》 agrees).

Yù Zhōng 彧中 (KI 26) treats coughing counterflow (*Míng Xià* 《 明下 》 says cough), panting and inability to eat (see the section on fullness of the chest and rib-sides).

天府治逆氣，喘不得息。雲門（ 見胸滿 ）、人迎（ 見吐瀉 ）、神藏（ 《 明 》 同 ）治咳逆，喘不得息。氣戶治喘逆上氣。步郎治喘息不得舉臂（ 並見胸脅滿 ）。足臨泣（ 見月事 ）治喘。

Tiān Fǔ 天府 (LU 3) treats counterflow qì and panting with inability to breathe.

Yún Mén 雲門 (LU 2) (see the section on chest fullness), Rén Yíng 人迎 (ST 9) (see the section on vomiting and diarrhea), and Shén Cáng 神藏 (KI 25) (*Míng* agrees) treat coughing counterflow and panting with inability to breathe.

Qì Hù 氣戶 (ST 13) treats panting counterflow and qì ascent.

Bù Láng 步廊 (KI 22) treats panting and inability to raise the arms (for all, see the section on fullness of the chest and rib-sides).

Zú Lín Qì 足臨泣 (GB 41) (see the section on menstruation) treats panting.

魄戶、中府主喘氣相追逐（ 《 千 》 ）。天突、華蓋主喘暴。俞府、神藏主喘不得息。天容等主喘息嘔沫。曲澤主咳喘（ 並見上氣 ）。

Pò Hù 魄戶 (UB 42) and Zhōng Fǔ 中府 (LU 1) govern panting and qì chasing each other [shortness of breath] (*Qiān* 《 千 》).

Tiān Tū 天突 (Rèn 22) and Huá Gài 華蓋 (Rèn 20) govern violent panting.

Shù Fǔ 俞府 (KI 27) and Shén Cáng 神藏 (KI 25) govern panting and inability to breathe.

Tiān Róng 天容 (SI 17) and so forth govern panting and retching of foam.

Qū Zé 曲澤 (PC 3) governs cough and panting (for all, see the section on qì ascent).

背痛 483
咳逆 420
肺氣 412
寒熱 675
上氣 420

顱息療小兒癎，喘不得息，耳聾（《明》）。魄戶療咳逆上喘（見背痛）。浮白療不得喘息（見咳逆）。經渠療掌中熱生，咳逆上氣，喘數，久熱病汗不出，暴癉喘逆，心痛欲嘔。

Lú Xī 顱息 (SJ 19) cures epilepsy in children, panting, inability to breathe, and deafness (*Míng*《明》).

Pò Hù 魄戶 (UB 42) cures coughing counterflow as well as panting (see the section on back pain).

Fú Bái 浮白 (GB 10) cures inability to breathe (see the section on coughing counterflow).

Jīng Qú 經渠 (LU 8) cures heat in the palms, coughing counterflow with qì ascent, frequent panting, chronic heat diseases, absence of sweating, sudden pure-heat, panting and counterflow, and heart pain with desire to vomit.

中府（見肺氣）、魄戶（見背）、脅堂療喘逆（《下》）。璇璣療咳逆上喘，喉鳴。三間療傷寒氣熱，身熱喘。天突療咳逆氣喘（《下》）。肺俞（見肺）療肺喘。解溪療喘息急。魚際（見寒熱）療咳喘（《明》）。

Zhōng Fǔ 中府 (LU 1) (see the section on lung qì), Pò Hù (UB 42) (see the section on the back), and Xié Táng 脅堂 (non-channel)[59] cure panting and counterflow (*Xià*《下》).

Xuán Jī 璇璣 (Rèn 21) cures coughing counterflow, panting and throat rales.

Sān Jiān 三間 (LI 3) cures cold-damage and qì heat, general heat and panting.

Tiān Tū 天突 (Rèn 22) cures coughing counterflow and panting (*Xià*).

Fèi Shù 肺俞 (UB 13) (see the section on the lung qì) cures lung panting.

Jiě Xī 解溪 (ST 41) cures rapid breathing.

Yú Jì 魚際 (LU 10) (see the section on [sensations of] cold and heat) cures cough and panting (*Míng*).

膻中治咳嗽上喘（《銅》見肺）。水突治喘息不得。扶突治喘息如水雞鳴（並見上氣）。頭維主喘逆煩滿，嘔沫流汗（《千》）。

Dàn Zhōng 膻中 (Rèn 17) treats cough and panting (see the section on the lung qì in *Tóng*《銅》).

59. Xié Táng 脅堂 is located on the mid-axillary line, 2 cùn below the axilla.

肺氣 412
上氣 420

Shuǐ Tū 水突 (ST 10) treats panting with inability to breathe.

Fú Tū 扶突 (LI 18) treats breathing with frog-like rales (for all, see the section on qì ascent).

Tóu Wéi 頭維 (ST 8) governs panting counterflow, vexation, retching of foam, and sweating (*Qiān*《千》).

肺俞(《明下》見肺)、腎俞主喘咳少氣百病。俞府、神藏(見上氣)、天府主上氣喘不得息。扶突主咽中鳴喘。

Fèi Shù 肺俞 (UB 13) (see the section on the lung qì in *Míng Xià*《明下》) and Shèn Shù 腎俞 (UB 23) govern the hundred diseases of cough, panting, and qì shortage.

Shù Fǔ 俞府 (KI 27), Shén Cáng 神藏 (KI 25) (see the section on qì ascent), and Tiān Fǔ 天府 (LU 3) govern qì ascent and panting with inability to breathe.

Fú Tū (LI 18) governs panting and rales in the throat.

天突、華蓋主喘暴(並見上氣)。經渠主咳逆上氣喘，掌中熱。少商、大陵主咳逆喘。天突、華蓋主喘暴。太泉主咳逆胸滿，喘不得息。期門主喘逆，臥不安席，咳，脅下積聚。咳喘，曲澤出血立已。彧中等主呼吸喘。氣逆喘鳴，取天容(並見上氣)。

Tiān Tū 天突 (Rèn 22) and Huá Gài 華蓋 (Rèn 20) govern violent panting (for both, see the section on qì ascent).

Jīng Qú 經渠 (LU 8) governs coughing counterflow as well as panting and heat in the palms.

Shào Shāng 少商 (LU 11) and Dà Líng 大陵 (PC 7) govern coughing counterflow as well as panting.

Tiān Tū (Rèn 22) and Huá Gài (Rèn 20) govern violent panting.

Tài Quán 太泉 (LU 9) governs coughing counterflow, chest fullness, and panting with inability to breathe.

Qī Mén 期門 (LV 14) governs panting and counterflow, inability to lie peacefuly on the mat to sleep [unquiet sleep], cough, and accumulations and gatherings under the rib-sides.

Cough and panting: Bleed Qū Zé 曲澤 (PC 3) to cure the disease immediately.

Yù Zhōng 彧中 (KI 26) and so forth govern panting while breathing.

脅痛 476
上氣 420
咳逆 420
寒熱 675

Qì counterflow, panting, and rales: Needle Tiān Róng 天容 (SI 17) (for all, see the section on qì ascent).

上廉治喘息不能行（《銅》見脅痛）。經渠主喘（見上氣）。大陵等主喘。天府主喘不得息。廉泉治喘息（並見咳逆）。魚際療喘（見寒熱）。

Shàng Lián 上廉 (LI 9 or ST 37) treats panting with inability to walk (see the discussion of rib-side pain in *Tóng*《銅》).

Jīng Qú 經渠 (LU 8) governs panting (see the section on qì ascent).

Dà Líng 大陵 (PC 7) and so forth govern panting.

Tiān Fǔ 天府 (LU 3) governs panting with inability to breathe.

Lián Quán 廉泉 (Rèn 23) treats panting (for all, see the section on coughing counterflow).

Yú Jì 魚際 (LU 10) cures panting (see the section on [sensations of] cold and heat).

有貴人久患喘，夜臥不得而起行，夏月亦衣夾背心。予知是膏肓病也，令灸膏肓而愈。亦有暴喘者，予知是痰為梗，令細銼厚朴七八錢重，以薑七片，水小碗煎七分服，滓再煎服，不過數服愈。

[Author's notes:] A nobleman suffered panting for long time. At night, he could not lie down and had to get up to walk; in the summer, he also needed to wear a vest in addition to his clothes. I knew this was a disease in the Gāo Huāng [the area below the heart and above the diaphragm]. After I applied moxibustion on Gāo Huāng 膏肓 (UB 43), he was cured.

Another patient had violent panting. I knew it was due to phlegm retention. So I asked him to finely powder 7 or 8 *qián* of *hòu pò* 厚朴 [Magnoliae Officinalis Cortex] and cook it in small bowl of water with 7 slices of ginger, boiling it down to 70%. He was to re-cook the dregs and drink it again. The patient recovered after drinking it several times.

若不因痰而喘者，當灸肺俞。凡有喘與哮者，為按肺俞，無不酸疼。皆為謬刺肺俞，令灸而愈。亦有只謬刺不灸而愈，此病有淺深也。舍弟登山，為雨所搏，一夕氣悶幾不救，見昆季必泣，有欲別之意。予疑其心悲，為刺百會不效。按其肺俞，云其疼如錐刺。以火針微刺之即愈。因此與人治哮喘，只謬肺俞，不謬他穴。惟按肺俞不疼酸者，然後點其它穴云。

If panting is not due to the phlegm, apply moxibustion on Fèi Shù 肺俞 (UB 13). Those with panting or wheezing always have pain at Fèi Shù (UB 13) when pressed. After applying cross-needling technique (*miù cì*) and moxibustion on Fèi Shù (UB 13), the disease will be cured. One can also cure the disease by applying cross-needling only without moxibustion, depending on the severity of the disease. My younger brother was caught out in the rain when he climbed a mountain, and he soon suffered oppressed breathing and almost died. He would cry when he saw his brothers, as if he was going to depart [die]. I thought he was sad, so I needled Băi Huì 百會 (Dū 20) on him, but it did not work. I pressed Fèi Shù (UB 13) and he said it was so painful, just like he had been stabbed by an awl. When I applied a fire needle on it [Fèi Shù (UB 13)], the disease was immediately cured. So to treat people with wheezing and panting, apply cross-needling technique on Fèi Shù (UB 13) only, rather than on other points. Locate other points only if there is no aching pain upon pressure on Fèi Shù (UB 13).

上氣
420

# 4.30
## *Fèi Qì (Fèi Fēng)*
# 肺氣（肺風）
## Lung qì
**(Lung wind[60])**

肺脹，氣搶脅下，熱痛：灸陰都隨年壯。肺脹脅滿，嘔吐上氣等病：灸大椎並兩乳上第三肋間，各止七壯。肺與大腸俱實。中府主肺寒熱（見上氣）。

Lung distension and qì prodding the rib-sides with hot pain: Apply the same number of cones of moxibustion as the patient's age on Yīn Dū 陰都 (KI 19).

For the disease of lung distension, fullness of rib-sides, retching and vomiting, qì ascent, and so forth: Apply moxbustion on Dà Zhuī 大椎 (Dū 14) and the third intercostal space above the two nipples, stop at seven cones.

Lung and large intestine repletion[61]: Zhōng Fǔ 中府 (LU 1) governs cold and heat in the lungs (see the section on qì ascent).

膻中治肺氣咳嗽，上喘唾膿，不得下食，胸中如塞（《銅》）。天突治肺癰，咯唾膿血，咽乾，舌下急，喉生瘡。中府治肺系急，胸痛悚悚，膽熱，嘔逆上氣，咳唾濁涕，肩背痛，風汗出，腹脹，食不下。《明下》云：肺急胸滿，喘逆唾濁，善噎皮痛。太淵治肺脹滿膨膨。《明下》云：療胸中氣滿不得臥，肺脹滿膨膨。

Dàn Zhōng 膻中 (Rèn 17) treats lung qì and cough, panting with spitting of pus, inability to get food down, and feeling of blockage in the chest (*Tóng*《銅》).

Tiān Tū 天突 (Rèn 22) treats lung abscesses, expectoration and spitting of pus and blood [hemoptysis], dry throat, tension under the tongue, and sores in the throat.

60. Lung wind refers to lung diseases caused by wind invasion.

61. This phrase is the name of chapter 17 in *Qiān Jīn Yào Fāng*《千金要方》. Wáng Zhízhōng 王執中 must have accidently copied it here.

Zhōng Fǔ 中府 (LU 1) treats tension of the lung system, chest pain with terror, gallbladder heat, retching counterflow with qì ascent, coughing and spitting turbid snivel, shoulder and back pain, sweating during wind attack, abdominal distension, and difficulty getting food down. *Míng Xià* 《明下》 says: It treats lung tension, chest fullness, panting counterflow, spitting of turbidity, frequent dysphagia, and skin pain.

Tài Yuān 太淵 (LU 9) treats lung distension and fullness with a feeling of inflation. *Míng Xià* says: It cures qì fullness of the chest, inability to lie down, lung distension and fullness with a feeling of inflation.

肺俞療肺寒熱，肺痿，上喘咳嗽，嗽血，胸脅氣滿，不得臥，不嗜食，汗不出，及背急強（《明下》）。

Fèi Shù 肺俞 (UB 13) cures cold and heat in the lungs, lung wilting, panting and cough, coughing up blood, qì fullness of the chest and rib-sides, inability to lie down, no desire to eat, absence of sweating, and tension and stiffness of the back (*Míng Xià*).

凡肺風氣痿絕，四肢滿脹，喘逆胸滿，灸肺俞各二壯。

For all lung wind, qì wilting, fullness and distension of the limbs, panting counterflow, and chest fullness: Apply two cones of moxibustion on Fèi Shù (UB 13).

水溝療面腫唇動，葉葉肺風，狀如蟲行（《明》）。風池（見面腫）療肺風。

Shuǐ Gōu 水溝 (Dū 26) cures facial swelling, twitching of the lips, lung wind that appears like [the sensation of] wind moving the leaves and insects crawling [under the skin] (*Míng* 《明》).

Fēng Chí 風池 (GB 20) (see the section on facial swelling) cures lung wind.

寒熱 675
傳尸 188
心痛 312
逆氣 420
少氣 426
肺癰 412
喘 406

## 4.31
## *Ké Sòu (Yú Jiàn Ké Nì)*
# 咳嗽（餘見咳逆）

## Cough
**(for further discussion, see the section on coughing counterflow)**

三里主咳嗽多唾（《千》。）缺盆、膻中、巨闕主咳嗽。

Sān Lǐ 三里 (ST 36 or LI 10) governs cough with copious spittle (*Qiān*《千》).

Quē Pén 缺盆 (ST 12), Dàn Zhōng 膻中 (Rèn 17), and Jù Quē 巨闕 (Rèn 14) govern cough.

魚際療咳嗽喘（見寒熱），又療肺心痛，咳引尻溺出（《明》）。肺俞療肺嗽（見傳尸）。少澤、心俞（見心痛）、庫房（見逆氣）療咳嗽。天突療咳嗽，上氣噎，胸中氣，喉內如水聲。廉泉療咳嗽少氣（見少氣）。膻中（見肺癰）療咳嗽上氣。《下》云：療咳嗽氣短。經渠（見喘）療嗽逆上氣。天池療上氣咳嗽，胸中氣滿，喉鳴，四肢不舉，腋下腫（《下》）。解溪療上氣咳嗽，喘息急，腹中積氣上下行。

Yú Jì 魚際 (LU 10) cures cough and panting (see the section on [sensations of] cold and heat); it also cures pain of the lungs and heart, and cough-induced urination (*Míng*《明》).

Fèi Shù 肺俞 (UB 13) cures lung cough (see the discussion of corpse transmission [lung consumption]).

Shào Zé 少澤 (SI 1), Xīn Shù 心俞 (UB 15) (see the section on heart pain), and Kù Fáng 庫房 (ST 14) (see the section on qì counterflow) cure cough.

Tiān Tū 天突 (Rèn 22) cures cough, qì ascent and dysphagia, qì in the chest, and water sounds in the throat.

Lián Quán 廉泉 (Rèn 23) cures cough and qì shortage (see the section on qì shortage).

Dàn Zhōng (Rèn 17) (see the discussion of lung abscess) cures cough and qì ascent. *Xià*《下》says: It cures cough and shortage of qì.

Jīng Qú 經渠 (LU 8) (see the section on panting) cures coughing counterflow with qì ascent.

Tiān Chí 天池 (PC 1) cures qì ascent and cough, qì fullness of the chest, throat rales, inability to lift the four limbs, and swelling of the axilla (*Xià*《下》).

Jiě Xī 解溪 (ST 41) cures qì ascent, cough, panting, rapid breathing, and qì accumulation in the abdomen that is running up and down.

瘛瘲 354
喉痹 628
風勞 371
勞瘵 188
肺氣 412
上氣 420

魚際、列缺、少澤（見瘛瘲）、缺盆治咳嗽（《銅》）。尺澤治咳嗽唾濁（見喉痹）。肩中俞治咳嗽上氣唾血。大杼治風勞氣咳嗽（見風勞）。風門治喘氣臥不安（見風勞）。肺俞治肺痿咳嗽（見勞瘵）。膻中治肺氣咳嗽（見肺氣）。涌泉治婦人無子，咳嗽身熱（《明下》咳嗽氣短）。前谷治咳嗽衄血，項頸痛。太溪治痃癖咳嗽，不嗜食。

Yú Jì 魚際 (LU 10), Liè Quē 列缺 (LU 7), Shào Zé 少澤 (SI 1) (see the section on tugging and slackening), and Quē Pén 缺盆 (ST 12) treat cough (*Tóng*《銅》).

Chǐ Zé 尺澤 (LU 5) treats cough and spitting turbidity (see the section on throat *bì*-impediment).

Jiān Zhōng Shù 肩中俞 (SI 15) treats cough, qì ascent, and spitting of blood.

Dà Zhù 大杼 (UB 11) treats wind taxation qì[62] and cough (see the section on wind taxation).

Fēng Méng 風門 (UB 12) treats panting and unquiet sleep (see the section on wind taxation).

Fèi Shù 肺俞 (UB 13) treats lung wilting and cough (see the section on consumption).

Dàn Zhōng 膻中 (Rèn 17) treats lung qì cough[63] (see the section on lung qì).

Yǒng Quán 涌泉 (KI 1) treats infertility in women, cough, and generalized heat (*Míng Xià*《明下》says: cough and shortage of qì).

Qián Gǔ 前谷 (SI 2) treats cough, nosebleeds, and neck pain.

Tài Xī 太溪 (KI 3) treats strings and aggregations, cough, and no desire to eat.

上氣咳嗽：灸肺募五十壯（《千》見上氣）。嗽：灸手屈臂中，有橫文外，骨捻頭得痛處，十四壯良。嗽：灸兩乳下黑白際，各百壯，即瘥。又以蒲當乳頭周匝圍身，令前後正平，當脊骨解中，灸十壯云云。

62. Wind taxation qì has symptoms of weakness, poor appetite, emaciation, steaming fever, chills and fever, cough, and night sweating. It is caused by wind attacking when the constitution is weak.

63. Lung qì cough refers the severe cough with scant drool or foam.

上氣 420 Qì ascent and cough: Apply fifty cones of moxibustion on Fèi Mù 肺募 (LU 1) (see the section
不臥 340 on qì ascent in *Qiān*《千》).

Cough: Have the patient flex his arm and find the painful area when you pinch the end of the bone located at the lateral end of the transverse crease;[64] it is good to apply fourteen cones of moxibustion on it.

Cough: Apply a hundred cones of moxibustion on the border of dark and light skin below the nipples. This will cure the disease. Or wrap a piece of cattail around the body at the level of the nipples, making sure in is at the same level on the front and back; then locate the corresponding vertebral joint. Apply ten cones moxibustion on it.

廉泉、天井（並見上氣）、太淵治咳嗽（《銅》見不臥）。

Lián Quán 廉泉 (Rèn 23), Tiān Jǐng 天井 (SJ 10) (see the section on qì ascent), and Tài Yuān 太淵 (LU 9) treat cough (see the section on insomnia in *Tóng*《銅》).

久嗽最宜灸膏肓穴，其次則宜灸肺俞等穴。各隨證治之，若暴嗽則不必灸也。有男子忽氣出不絕聲，病數日矣，以手按其膻中穴而應，微以冷針頻頻刺之而愈。初不之灸，何其神也。

[Author's notes:] For enduring cough, it is the most appropriate to apply moxibustion on Gāo Huāng 膏肓 (UB 43), then Fèi Shù 肺俞 (UB 13), and so forth. Treat according to the pattern. Do not apply moxibustion when cough suddenly occurs. There was a man who suddenly suffered breath sounds that did not stop for several days. He responded when Dàn Zhōng 膻中 (Rèn 17) was pressed, and the disease was cured after it was needled frequently without moxibustion. [In this case], not applying moxibustion at the initial stage was miraculous.

《千翼》十二種風。風入肺，則咳逆短氣。又肝咳刺足太衝，心咳刺神門，脾咳刺太白，肺咳刺太泉，腎咳刺太溪，膽咳刺陽陵泉，又第五節下第六節上穴中間，隨年，並主上氣。

*Qiān Yì*《千翼》discusses twelve kinds of wind. Wind invades the lungs, [resulting in] cough, counterflow, and shortness of breath. Needle Foot Tài Chōng 太衝 (LV 3) for liver cough;[65]

64. This could be describing the location of Qū Chí 曲池 (LI 11).

65. Liver cough: cough with pain of the rib-sides and inability to turn to the sides.

needle Shén Mén 神門 (HT 7) for heart cough;[66] needle Tài Bái 太白 (SP 3) for spleen cough;[67] needle Tài Quán 太泉 (LU 9) for lung cough;[68] needle Tài Xī 太溪 (KI 3) for kidney cough;[69] needle Yáng Líng Quán 陽陵泉 (GB 34) for gallbladder cough;[70] or apply moxibustion on the area below the fifth vertebra and above the sixth vertebra to govern qì ascent. Burn the same number of cones as the patient's age.

## 4.32

## *Ké Nì (Yú Jiàn Ké Nì Shàng Chuǎn, Shāng Hán Ǒu Yuē)*

# 咳逆（餘見咳逆上喘　傷寒嘔噦）

## Coughing counterflow

**(for further discussion, see the sections on coughing counterflow and panting; and cold damage, retching and vomiting)**

然谷、天泉、陷谷、胸堂、章門、曲泉、天突、雲門、肺俞、臨泣、肩井、風門、行間、主咳逆(《千》)。維道主咳逆不止。大陵主咳逆，寒熱發。大陵、少商主咳逆喘。太泉主咳逆胸滿，喘不得息(《明下》同)。三里主咳逆多吐。中府主肺系急，咳輒胸痛。前谷主咳而胸滿。經渠、行間主喜咳。俠白主咳，乾嘔煩滿。支溝主咳，面赤而熱。咳唾，噫，善咳，氣無所出：先取三里，後取太白、章門(並《千》)。

Rán Gǔ 然谷 (KI 2), Tiān Quán 天泉 (PC 2), Xiàn Gǔ 陷谷 (ST 43), Xiōng Táng 胸膛 (Rèn 17), Zhāng Mén 章門 (LV 13), Qū Quán 曲泉 (LV 8), Tiān Tū 天突 (Rèn 22), Yún Mén 雲門 (LU 2), Fèi Shù 肺俞 (UB 13), Lín Qì 臨泣 (GB 41), Jiān Jǐng 肩井 (GB 21), Fēng Mén 風門 (UB 12), and Xíng Jiān 行間 (LV 2) govern coughing counterflow (*Qiān* 《千》).

Wéi Dào 維道 (GB 28) governs incessant cough.

Dà Líng 大陵 (PC 7) governs coughing counterflow and the onset of chills and fever.

66. Heart cough: cough with heart pain, sore throat, and feeling as if something were stuck in the throat.

67. Spleen cough: cough with pain of the right rib-side radiating to the back. The cough gets worse when the patient moves.

68. Lung cough: cough with panting or spitting up blood.

69. Kidney cough: cough with pain radiating through the back, as well as coughing up drool.

70. Gallbladder cough: coughing up bile.

心痛 312
喘 406
胸滿 470
臍痛 466
善噫 281

Dà Líng (PC 7) and Shào Shāng 少商 (LU 11) govern coughing counterflow and panting.

Tài Quán 太泉 (LU 9) governs coughing counterflow, chest fullness, and panting with inability to breathe (*Míng Xià*《明下》agrees).

Sān Lǐ 三里 (ST 36 or LI 10) governs cough, counterflow, and frequent vomiting.

Zhōng Fǔ 中府 (LU 1) governs tension of the lung tie[71] and chest pain when coughing.

Qián Gǔ 前谷 (SI 2) governs cough and chest fullness.

Jīng Qú 經渠 (LU 8) and Xíng Jiān 行間 (LV 2) govern tendency to cough.

Xiá Bái 俠白 (LU 4) governs cough, dry retching, vexation, and fullness.

Zhī Gōu 支溝 (SJ 6) governs cough with hot red face.

Cough, spitting, belching, frequent cough, qì has nowhere to go[72]: treat Sān Lǐ 三里 (ST 36) first, then Tài Bái 太白 (SP 3), and Zhāng Mén 章門 (LV 13) (all of this is in *Qiān*《千》).

孔最、天泉（見心痛）、太溪（見心痛）、行間、俞府（見喘）、神封（見胸滿）、腹結（見臍痛）、少商（見善噫）、浮白治咳逆（《銅》）。肝俞治咳引兩脅急痛，不得息，轉側難，橛脅下與脊相引而反折，目上視，目眩，循眉頭痛，驚狂鼽衄，起則目䀮䀮，目生白翳，咳引胸中痛，寒疝小腹痛，唾血短氣。《明下》云：療咳逆，兩脅滿悶。魚際治咳引尻痛。竅陰治脅痛，咳逆不得息。

Kǒng Zuì 孔最 (LU 6), Tiān Quán 天泉 (PC 2) (see the section on heart pain), Tài Xī 太溪 (KI 3) (see the section on heart pain), Xíng Jiān 行間 (LV 2), Shù Fǔ 俞府 (KI 27) (see the section on panting), Shén Fēng 神封 (KI 23) (see the section on chest fullness), Fù Jié 腹結 (SP 14) (see the section on umbilical pain), Shào Shāng 少商 (LU 11) (see the section on frequent belching), and Fú Bái 浮白 (GB 10) treat cough with counterflow (*Tóng*《銅》).

Gān Shù 肝俞 (UB 18) treats cough-induced acute pain of the rib-sides, inability to breathe, difficulty turning to the sides, pulling [sensation] and arched-back rigidity between the peg ribs [free rib region] and spine, upward staring eyes, dizzy vision, headache along the eyebrows, fright and mania, running nose and nosebleeds, blurred vision when getting up, white screens in the eyes, cough with

71. There are two ways to read this. *Xì jí* 系急 as a compound term means constraint, so this would read tension or constraint of the lungs. However, *fèi xì jí* 肺系急 can also be read tension of the lung tie. In *Shí Sì Jīng Fā Huī*《十四經發揮》(Elaboration on the Fourteen Channels), *Yuán* (元) Dynasty, 1341, Huá Shòu 滑壽 wrote " The lung tie means the throat. (肺繫，謂喉嚨也。)"
72. *Qì wú suǒ chū* 氣無所出 (qì has nowhere to go) means the qì is unable to descend.

pain radiating to the chest, cold *shàn*-mounting, pain of the smaller abdomen, spitting up blood, and shortness of breath. *Míng Xià*《明下》says: It cures coughing counterflow with fullness and oppression of the rib-sides.

Yú Jì 魚際 (LU 10) treats sacral pain induced by cough.

Qiào Yīn 竅陰 (GB 44) treats rib-side pain, cough, counterflow, and inability to breathe.

浮白療咳逆，疝積胸滿，不得喘息，胸痛（《明》）。太淵療咳逆煩心，不得臥（《下》）。

Fú Bái 浮白 (GB 10) cures cough, counterflow, *shàn*-mounting accumulations, chest fullness, inability to breathe, and chest pain (*Míng*《明》).

Tài Yuān 太淵 (LU 9) cures cough, counterflow, vexation of the heart, and inability to lie down (*Xià*《下》).

灸咳逆法：乳下一指許，正與乳相直骨間陷中，婦人即屈乳頭度之，乳頭齊處是穴。炷如小豆許，灸三壯。男左女右，只一處火到肌，即瘥。《良方》云：族中有霍亂吐痢垂困，忽發咳逆，遂至危殆。與鄜延陳中裕病傷寒，咳逆甚，氣已不屬，皆一灸而愈云。凡傷寒及久病，得咳逆，皆為惡候。投藥不效者，灸之必瘥。若不瘥，則多不救（《必用方》云：噦者克逆也，見嘔噦）。

Moxibustion method for coughing counterflow: [Find the point] one finger-breadth below the nipple, in the bony depression in line with the nipple, [or] measure the points by bending the women's nipple; the point is level with the nipple. Burn three cones of moxibustion the size of a small bean. Apply moxibustion on the left side for men and the right side for women, only on one site. Burning it down to the flesh will cure the disease. *Liáng Fāng*《良方》says: There was someone in the clan who suffered sudden turmoil [cholera], vomiting, and dysentery, and was very tired. He had sudden onset of coughing counterflow and was in critical condition. Chén Zhōngyù of Fūyán had cold damage with severe coughing counterflow, and his qì could not continue [breathing difficulty]. They both recovered after applying one cone of moxibustion [on this site]. For all cold damage and chronic illness, coughing counterflow are evil signs. If herbs do not work, moxibustion will cure the disease. If not, the disease is incurable. (*Bì Yòng Fāng*《必用方》says: Retching is coughing counterflow. See the section on retching).

咳病有十，曰風咳、寒咳、支咳、膽咳、厥陰咳、與五臟咳。《千金》載其刺法詳矣。而傷寒咳為惡證，施秘監尊人患傷寒咳甚，醫告技窮，施檢《灸經》，於結喉下灸三壯，即瘥。蓋天突穴也，神哉神哉。

齒噤
607 [Author's notes:] There are ten types of cough: wind cough, cold cough, propping cough, gallbladder cough, juéyīn cough and cough of the five viscera. *Qiān Jīn*《千金》records the needling methods for [these types of] cough in detail. Cold damage cough is a malign pattern. Supervisor Shī who was the director of the palace library[73] suffered severe cough due to cold damage. The doctor had exhausted his skills. Supervisor Shī checked the *Jiu Jīng*《灸經》, and then applied three cones of moxibustion below his laryngeal prominence [Adam's apple]. The disease was cured. This must be Tiān Tū 天突 (Rèn 22). It is divine.

## 4.33
## *Ké Nì Shàng Qì (Shàng Qì, Yòu Jiàn Ké Nì)*
# 咳逆上氣（上氣　又見咳逆）
### Coughing counterflow with qì ascent
**(for qì ascent, see also the section on coughing counterflow)**

魄戶、氣舍、譩譆（《甲乙》）、期門、右手屈臂中橫紋外骨上，主咳逆上氣（《千》）。天容等主咳逆上氣，喘息嘔沫（見齒噤）。魄戶、中府主肺寒熱，呼吸不得臥，咳逆上氣，嘔沫，喘，氣相追逐。天突、華蓋（《明》云：喘不能言）主咳逆上氣，喘暴。俞府（《明下》同）、神藏主咳逆上氣，喘不得息。

Pò Hù 魄戶 (UB 42), Qì Shě 氣舍 (ST 11), Yī Xī 譩譆 (UB 45) (*Jiă Yĭ*《甲乙》), Qī Mén 期門 (LV 14), and the point on the bone at the lateral side of the transverse crease when the right arm is flexed; they treat coughing counterflow with qì ascent (*Qiān*《千》).

Tiān Róng 天容 (SI 17) and so forth govern coughing counterflow with qì ascent, and panting and vomiting of foam (see the section on clenched jaws).

Pò Hù 魄戶 (UB 42) and Zhōng Fǔ 中府 (LU 1) govern cold and heat in the lungs, breathing with inability to lie down, coughing counterflow with qì ascent, vomiting of foam, panting, and qì chasing each other [shortness of breath].

Tiān Tū 天突 (Rèn 22) and Huá Gài 華蓋 (Rèn 20) (*Míng*《明》says: panting with inability to speak) govern coughing counterflow with qì ascent and violent panting.

---

73. *Mì jiān* 秘監 is short for *mì shū jiān* (秘書監), the director of the palace library in ancient times.

Shù Fǔ 俞府 (KI 27) (*Míng Xià*《明下》agrees) and Shén Cáng 神藏 (KI 25) govern coughing counterflow with qì ascent, and panting with inability to breathe.

胸脅 470
唾血 402
勞瘵 188

經渠主咳逆上氣喘，掌中熱。扶突主咳逆上氣，咽中鳴喘。咳喘，曲澤出血立已，又主卒咳逆，逆氣。紫宮、玉堂、太溪主咳逆上氣心煩（《明》云：紫宮、玉堂主咳逆）。彧中、石門主咳逆上氣，涎出多唾。彧中、雲門主咳逆上氣，涎出多唾，呼吸喘悸，坐不安席。庫房、中府、周榮、尺澤主咳逆上氣，呼吸多唾，濁沫膿血。

Jīng Qú 經渠 (LU 8) governs coughing counterflow with qì ascent, panting, and heat in the palms.

Fú Tū 扶突 (LI 18) governs coughing counterflow with qì ascent, panting, and rales in the throat.

Cough and panting: bleeding Qū Zé 曲澤 (PC 3) can cure the disease immediately; it also governs sudden coughing counterflow qì.

Zǐ Gōng 紫宮 (Rèn 19), Yù Táng 玉堂 (Rèn 18), and Tài Xī 太溪 (KI 3) govern coughing counterflow with qì ascent and vexation of the heart (*Míng*《明》says: Zǐ Gōng (Rèn 19) and Yù Táng (Rèn 18) govern coughing counterflow).

Yù Zhōng 彧中 (KI 26) and Shí Mén 石門 (Rèn 5) govern coughing counterflow with qì ascent, drooling, and copious spittle.

Yù Zhōng (KI 26) and Yún Mén 雲門 (LU 2) govern coughing counterflow with qì ascent, drooling, copious spittle, panting and palpitations when breathing, and inability to sit on the mat calmly.

Kù Fáng 庫房 (ST 14), Zhōng Fǔ 中府 (LU 1), Zhōu Róng 周榮 (SP 20), and Chǐ Zé 尺澤 (LU 5) govern coughing counterflow with qì ascent, breathing with spitting of turbidity, pus, and blood.

氣舍治咳逆上氣，瘤癭，喉痹咽腫，頸項強（《銅》）。水突治咳逆上氣，咽喉壅腫，呼吸短氣，喘息不得。厥陰俞治逆氣嘔吐，心痛留結，胸中煩悶。扶突治咳多唾上氣，咽引喘息，喉如水雞鳴。魄戶治背膊痛，咳逆上氣，嘔吐煩滿。庫房（見胸脅滿）、屋翳（見唾血）、膏肓俞治上氣咳逆（見勞瘵）。

Qì Shě 氣舍 (ST 11) treats coughing counterflow with qì ascent, goiter, throat *bì*-impediment, swollen throat, and stiffness of the neck and nape (*Tóng*《銅》).

Shuǐ Tū 水突 (ST 10) treats coughing counterflow with qì ascent, congestion and swelling of the throat, shortness of breath when breathing, and inability to breathe.

胸痛 469
肺氣 412
少氣 426

Jué Yīn Shù 厥陰俞 (UB 14) treats counterflow qì and vomiting, binding heart pain, vexation, and oppression of the chest.

Fú Tū 扶突 (LI 18) treats cough with copious spittle, qì ascent, panting induced by [a problem] in the throat, and frog-rales in the throat.

Pò Hù 魄戶 (UB 42) treats back and arm pain, coughing counterflow with qì ascent, and vomiting with vexation and fullness.

Kù Fáng 庫房 (ST 14) (see the section on fullness of the rib-sides), Wū Yì 屋翳 (ST 15) (see the section on spitting of blood), and Gāo Huāng Shù 膏肓俞 (UB 43) treat coughing counterflow with qì ascent (see the section on consumption).

天突治咳逆上氣，胸中氣噎，喉中如水雞聲。《下》云：胸中氣鯁鯁。天溪（見胸痛）、中府治吐逆上氣（見肺氣）。氣海治一切氣（見少氣）。《明下》云：療五臟氣逆上攻。經渠治咳嗽上氣，數欠。幽門治逆氣數咳，女子逆氣。

Tiān Tū 天突 (Rèn 22) treats coughing counterflow with qì ascent, qì blockage in the chest, and frog-rales in the throat. *Xià*《下》says: Qì stagnation in the chest [as if] a fishbone were stuck there.

Tiān Xī 天溪 (SP 18) (see the section on chest pain) and Zhōng Fǔ 中府 (LU 1) treat vomiting counterflow and qì ascent (see the section on lung qì).

Qì Hǎi 氣海 (Rèn 6) treats all qì [diseases] (see the section on qì shortage). *Míng Xià*《明下》says: It cures counterflow qì of the five viscera attacking upward.

Jīng Qú 經渠 (LU 8) treats cough with qì ascent, and frequent yawning.

Yōu Mén 幽門 (KI 21) treats counterflow qì, frequent cough, and qì counterflow in women.

魚際療短氣心痹，悲怒逆氣，狂惕，胃氣逆（《明》）。建里療嘔吐上氣，心痛身腫。厥陰俞療逆氣嘔逆，牙痛，留結胸滿。石門療身寒熱，咳逆上氣，嘔吐血（《下》）。

Yú Jì 魚際 (LU 10) cures shortness of breath, heart *bì*-impediment, sorrow, anger with qì counterflow, mania, fright, and stomach qì counterflow (*Míng*《明》).

Jiàn Lǐ 建里 (Rèn 11) cures vomiting with qì ascent, heart pain, and generalized swelling.

Jué Yīn Shù (UB 14) cures qì counterflow, retching counterflow, toothache, and binding chest fullness (*Xià*).

Shí Mén 石門 (Rèn 5) cures generalized [sensations of] cold and heat, coughing counterflow with qì ascent, and vomiting blood (*Xià*《下》).

庫房療胸脅滿，咳逆上氣，呼吸不至息。建里治嘔逆上氣。氣戶治喘逆上氣（見嗽）。

Kù Fáng 庫房 (ST 14) treats fullness of the chest and rib-sides, coughing counterflow with qì ascent, and breathing that cannot fulfill the breath (see the section on cough).

Jiàn Lǐ 建里 (Rèn 11) treats retching counterflow and qì ascent.

Qì Hù 氣戶 (ST 13) treats panting counterflow and qì ascent (see the section on cough).

凡上氣多有服吐藥得瘥，亦有針灸得除者，宜深體悟之（《千》）。上氣咳嗽，短氣，氣滿食不下：灸肺募五十壯。上氣咳逆，短氣，風勞百病：肩井二百壯。上氣短氣，咳逆，胸背痛：風門熱府百壯。上氣咳逆，短氣胸滿，多唾惡冷：肺俞五十壯。

Qì ascent can be cured by taking herbs that induce vomiting or needling and moxibustion. We should understand this deeply (*Qiān*《千》).

Qì ascent and cough, shortness of breath, qì fullness with difficulty getting food down: Apply fifty cones of moxibustion to Fèi Mù 肺募 (LU 1).

Coughing counterflow with qì ascent, shortness of breath, and the hundred diseases of wind taxation: Apply two hundred cones of moxibustion on Jiān Jǐng 肩井 (GB 21).

Qì ascent, shortness of breath, and coughing counterflow with chest and back pain: Apply a hundred cones of moxibustion on Fēng Mén Rè Fǔ 風門熱府 (UB 12).

Coughing counterflow with qì ascent, shortness of breath, chest fullness, frequent spitting, and malign cold: Apply fifty cones of moxibustion to Fèi Shù 肺俞 (UB 13).

上氣氣閉，咳逆咽冷，聲破，喉猜猜：天瞿五十壯。上氣胸滿，短氣咳逆：雲門五十壯。上氣咳逆，胸痹背痛：胸堂百壯，不針。上氣咳逆，膻中五十壯。上氣咳逆，胸滿短氣，牽背痛：巨闕、期門各五十壯。

Qì ascent, qì blockage, coughing counterflow, cold in the throat, broken sounds, and hoarse voice: Apply fifty cones of moxibustion to Tiān Qú 天瞿 (Rèn 22).

Qì ascent, chest fullness, shortness of breath, and coughing counterflow: Apply fifty cones of moxibustion to Yún Mén 雲門 (LU 2).

Qì ascent, coughing counterflow, chest *bì*-impediment, and back pain: Apply a hundred cones of moxibustion to Xiōng Táng 胸膛 (Rèn 17); acupuncture is contraindicated.

Qì ascent and coughing counterflow: Apply fifty cones of moxibustion to Dàn Zhōng 膻中 (Rèn 17).

Qì ascent, coughing counterflow, chest fullness, shortage of qì, and pain radiating to the back: Apply fifty cones of moxibustion to Jù Quē 巨闕 (Rèn 14) and Qī Mén 期門 (LV 14).

逆氣虛勞，寒損憂恚，筋骨攣痛，心中咳逆，泄注腹滿，喉痹，頸項強，腸痔逆氣，痔血陰急，鼻衄，骨痛，大小便澀，鼻中乾，煩滿狂走易氣。凡二十二病，皆灸絕骨五十壯。

Qì counterflow, vacuity taxation, cold detriment, anxiety and anger, hypertonicity and pain of the sinews and bones, coughing counterflow of the heart, outpour diarrhea, abdominal fullness, throat *bì*-impediment, stiffness of the neck and nape, intestinal hemorrhoids and qì counterflow, bleeding hemorrhoids, tension of the yīn,[74] nosebleeds, bone pain, difficult urination, difficult defecation, dry nose, vexation, fullness, manic walking, and tendency to get angry. For the twenty-two diseases above, apply fifty cones of moxibustion to Jué Gǔ 絕骨 (GB 39).

凡上氣冷發，腹中雷鳴轉叫，嘔逆不食：灸太衝，不限壯數。從痛至不痛，從不痛至痛止。上氣厥逆：灸胸堂百壯。穴在兩乳間。

Qì ascent occurring when cold, thunderous rumbling in the abdomen, and retching counterflow with inability to eat: Apply unlimited cones of moxibustion to Tài Chōng 太衝 (LV 3). If there was pain, stop when it disappears; if there was no pain, stop when there is pain.

Qì ascent and reverse counterflow: Apply a hundred cones of moxibustion to Xiōng Táng (Rèn 17). The point is located between the two nipples.

嘔吐上氣：灸尺澤，不三則七壯。肩俞主上氣。天府主上氣，喘不得息。天池主上氣喉鳴，陽氣大逆，上滿於胸中，憤瞋肩息。大氣逆上喘鳴，坐伏不得息，取之天容。上氣胸痛：取之廉泉（《甲乙》）。

Vomiting and qì counterflow: Apply either three or seven cones of moxibustion to Chǐ Zé 尺澤 (LU 5).

Jiān Shù 肩俞 (non-channel)[75] governs qì ascent.

74. This term has no immediate explanation. It could mean the two yīn, or the genitals alone.

75. Jiān Shù 肩俞 is located between Jiān Yú 肩髃 (LI 15) and Yún Mén 云門 (LU 2).

Tiān Fǔ 天府 (LU 3) governs qì ascent and panting with inability to breathe. 風勞 371

Tiān Chí 天池 (PC 1) governs qì ascent with throat rales, yáng qì strongly counterflowing upward filling up the chest, and raised-shoulder breathing. 胸滿 470 咳嗽 414

Qì counterflowing upward with panting rales and inability to breathe when sitting up or laying down: treat Tiān Róng 天容 (SI 17).

Qì ascent and chest pain: treat Lián Quán 廉泉 (Rèn 23) (*Jiǎ Yǐ* 《 甲乙 》).

天井治咳嗽上氣( 《 銅 》 )。廉泉治咳嗽上氣，喘息嘔沫 。風門治嘔逆上氣( 見風勞 )。肺俞治上氣嘔吐支滿( 《 明 》有脊強寒熱字 )，不嗜，汗不出 。

Tiān Jǐng 天井 (SJ 10) treats cough with qì ascent (*Tóng* 《 銅 》).

Lián Quán 廉泉 (Rèn 23) treats cough with qì ascent, panting, and retching of foam.

Fēng Mén 風門 (UB 12) treats retching counterflow and qì ascent (see the section on wind taxation).

Fèi Shù 肺俞 (UB 13) treats qì ascent with vomiting, and propping fullness (*Míng* 《 明 》 has the words 'spine stiffness with [sensations of] cold and heat'), no desire to eat, and absence of sweating.

玉堂治上氣( 見胸滿 )。雲門治氣上衝心( 見胸滿 )。氣衝治腸中大熱，不得安臥，腹有逆氣上攻，心腹脹滿淫濼 。

Yù Táng 玉堂 (Rèn 18) treats qì ascent (see the section on chest fullness).

Yún Mén 雲門 (LU 2) treats qì surging up into the heart (see the section on chest fullness).

Qì Chōng 氣衝 (ST 30) treats great heat in the intestines, inability to sleep quietly, counterflow qì in the abdomen surging upward, distention and fullness of heart and abdomen, as well as aching pain and weakness [of the body].

雲門療嘔逆氣上，胸脅徹背痛( 《 明 》 )。天突 、膻中 、天池 、解溪( 《 下 》 )、肩中俞療咳嗽上氣( 並見咳嗽 )。

Yún Mén (LU 2) cures retching counterflow, qì ascent, and pain of the chest and rib-sides that penetrates through the back (*Míng*).

憂悲 331
便赤 229
傷寒 661
胸脅 476
狂 345
勞瘵 188
淋 222
煩心 335

Tiān Tū 天突 (Rèn 22), Dàn Zhōng 膻中 (Rèn 17), Tiān Chí 天池 (PC 1), Jiě Xī 解溪 (ST 41) (*Xià*《下》), and Jiān Zhōng Shù 肩中俞 (SI 15) cure cough with qì ascent (see the section on cough).

## 4.34

## *Shǎo Qì (Duǎn Qì, Fá Qì, Jié Qì)*

# 少氣（短氣　乏氣　結氣）

## Qì shortage

**(Shortness of breath, lack of qì, bound up qì)**

然谷治喘呼少氣（《銅》）。上廉治臟氣（《明》云大腸氣）不足。三里治胃氣不足。氣海治臟氣虛憊，真氣不足，一切氣疾久不瘥者，皆灸之。少府（見憂悲）、膀胱俞、（見便赤）、少衝（見傷寒）、步郎（見胸脅滿）、間使（見狂）、腎俞（見勞瘵）、大鐘（見淋）治少氣。至陰治少氣難言（見寒熱）。神門治少氣不足（見煩心）。

Rán Gǔ 然谷 (KI 2) treats panting and qì shortage (*Tóng*《銅》).

Shàng Lián 上廉 (ST 37 or LI 9) treats visceral qì (*Míng*《明》says: large intestine qì) insufficiency.

Sān Lǐ 三里 (ST 36 or LI 10) treats insufficiency of stomach qì.

Qì Hǎi 氣海 (Rèn 6) treats visceral qì vacuity and fatigue [exhaustion], insufficiency of true qì and all qì diseases that cannot heal for a long time. Apply moxibustion on it.

Shào Fǔ 少府 (HT 8) (see the section on anxiety and sorrow [of the heart]), Páng Guāng Shù 膀胱俞 (UB 28) (see the discussion of red urine), Shào Chōng 少衝 (HT 9) (see the section on cold damage), Bù Láng 步廊 (KI 22) (see chest and rib-side fullness), Jiān Shǐ 間使 (PC 5) (see mania), Shèn Shù 腎俞 (UB 23) (see the section on consumption), and Dà Zhōng 大鐘 (KI 4) (see the section on dribbling) treat qì shortage.

Zhì Yīn 至陰 (UB 67) treats qì shortage and difficulty talking (see the section on [sensations of] cold and heat).

Shén Mén 神門 (HT 7) treats qì shortage (see the section on vexation of the heart).

腳氣 519
傷寒 690
咳逆 417
無子 721
風勞 371
中風 379

小腸俞（見腳氣）、魚際、大陵（見傷寒無汗）、肝俞（見咳逆）治短氣。膺窗治胸滿短氣。行間治癲疾短氣。

Xiǎo Cháng Shù 小腸俞 (UB 27) (see the section on leg qì), Yú Jì 魚際 (LU 10), Dà Líng 大陵 (PC 7) (see the discussion of cold and heat without sweating), and Gān Shù 肝俞 (UB 18) (see the section on coughing counterflow) treat shortness of breath.

Yīng Chuāng 膺窗 (ST 16) treats chest fullness and shortness of breath.

Xíng Jiān 行間 (LV 2) treats epilepsy and shortness of breath.

凡胸滿短氣，不得汗：皆針補手太陰以出汗（《千》）。涌泉主短氣（見無子）。膻中、華蓋主短氣不得息，不能言。步郎、安都主膈上不通，呼吸少氣，喘息。大包主大氣不得息。

Chest fullness, shortness of breath, and inability to sweat: Needle and supplement Shǒu Tàiyīn[76] to promote sweating (*Qiān*《千》).

Yǒng Quán 涌泉 (KI 1) governs shortness of breath (see the section on infertility).

Dàn Zhōng 膻中 (Rèn 17) and Huá Gài 華蓋 (Rèn 20) govern shortness of breath and inability to catch the breath or speak.

Bù Láng (KI 22) and Ān Dū 安都[77] govern blockage of the diaphragm, shortness of breath when breathing, and panting.

Dà Bāo 大包 (SP 21) governs inability to breathe.

廉泉療咳嗽少氣，喘息，嘔沫，噤齘。風門療氣短不安（見風勞）。肝俞（見中風）療短氣不食。伏兔療腹脹少氣。肝俞（《明下》）療氣短。

Lián Quán 廉泉 (Rèn 23) cures cough with qì shortage, panting, retching of foam, and clenched jaws.

Fēng Mén 風門 (UB 12) cures shortness of breath and restlessness (see the section on wind taxation).

Gān Shù 肝俞 (UB 18) (see the section on wind stroke) cures shortness of breath and inability to eat.

76. Shǒu Tàiyīn 手太陰: According to *Xiǎo Pǐn Fāng* 小品方 (Short Sketches), this point is located on the tip of the little finger.

77. Ān Dū 安都 should read Yīn Dū 陰都 (KI 19).

上氣 420 Fú Tù 伏兔 (ST 32) cures abdominal distention and qì shortage.

瘛瘲 354 Gān Shù 肝俞 (UB 18) (*Míng Xià*《明下》) cures shortness of breath.

心痛 312

驚 323 短氣：灸肩井二百壯（《千》見上氣）。短氣不得語：灸天井百壯；或大椎隨年壯；或肺俞；或肝俞；或尺澤；各百壯；或小指第四指間交脈上，七壯；或手十指頭，合十壯。

Shortness of breath: Apply two hundred cones of moxibustion to Jiān Jǐng 肩井 (GB 21) (see the section on qì ascent in *Qiān*《千》).

Shortness of breath with inability to speak: Apply a hundred cones of moxibustion to Tiān Jǐng 天井 (SJ 10); or burn the same number of cones of moxibustion as the patient's age on Dà Zhuī 大椎 (Dū 14); or apply a hundred cones of moxibustion on Fèi Shù 肺俞 (UB 13), or Gān Shù 肝俞 (UB 18), or Chǐ Zé 尺澤 (LU 5); or apply seven cones of moxibustion on the intersecting vessel between little finger and the fourth finger; or burn a total of ten cones of moxibustion on the tips of the ten fingers [one cone per finger].

少年房多短氣：灸鳩尾頭五十壯；又鹽灸臍孔中二七壯。乏氣，灸第五椎下隨年壯。短氣：灸巨闕等（見上氣）。雲門、風門熱府、肺募（見上氣）、巨闕等（見瘛瘲）、期門等主短氣（見心痛）。巨闕、解溪（並見驚）、然谷、尺澤主少氣（並見心痛）。巨闕（見驚）治少氣（《銅》）。

Young people suffering from shortness of breath after excessive sexual activity: Apply fifty cones of moxibustion on tip of xiphoid process; also apply two times seven cones of salt-moxibustion on the umbilicus.

Lack of qì: Apply the same number of cones of moxibustion as the age of the patient below the fifth vertebra.

Shortness of breath: Apply moxibustion on Jù Quē 巨闕 (Rèn 14) and so forth (see the section on qì ascent).

Yún Mén 雲門 (LU 2), Fēng Mén Rè Fǔ 風門熱府 (UB 12), Fèi Mù 肺募 (LU 1) (see the section on qì ascent), Jù Quē 巨闕 (Rèn 14), and so forth (see the section on tugging and slackening), Qī Mén 期門 (LV 14), and so forth, govern shortness of breath (see the section on heart pain).

Jù Quē (Rèn 14), Jiě Xī 解溪 (ST 41) (for both, see the section on [heart] fright and [fear]), Rán Gǔ 然谷 (KI 2), and Chǐ Zé (LU 5) govern qì shortage (for all, see the section on heart pain).

Jù Quē (Rèn 14) (see the section on [heart] fright [and fear]) treats qì shortage (*Tong*《銅》).

膽俞療心脹滿，吐逆短氣，痰悶，食難下不消（《明》）。 心痛 312 嘔 274

Dǎn Shù 膽俞 (UB 19) cures fullness and distention of the heart, vomiting counterflow, shortness of breath, oppression due to phlegm, and difficulty getting food down with non-transformation (*Míng*《明》).

心痛如錐刀刺，氣結：灸膈俞七壯（《千》）。氣結：灸太倉百壯（見心痛）。通谷治結積留飲（《銅》見痰）。心腹諸病，堅滿煩痛，憂憊結氣，寒冷霍亂，心痛吐下，食不消，腸鳴泄利：灸太倉百壯。結氣囊裡，針藥所不及：灸肓募隨年壯（並《千》）。中脘治寒癖結氣（《銅》），隔結（見嘔）。

Heart pain that feels like the piercing of an awl and qì binds: Apply seven cones of moxibustion to Gé Shù 膈俞 (UB 17) (*Qiān*《千》).

Qì binds: Apply a hundred cones of moxibustion to Tài Cāng 太倉 (Rèn 12) (see the section on heart pain).

Tōng Gǔ 通谷 (UB 66) treats accumulations and binds of lodged rheum (see the section on phlegm in *Tóng*《銅》).

All diseases in the heart and abdomen with hardness, fullness, vexation, pain, anxiety, fatigue, qì binds, cold and sudden turmoil disease [cholera], heart pain with vomiting and diarrhea, non-dispersion of food, intestinal rumbling, and diarrhea: Apply a hundred cones of moxibustion on Tài Cāng (Rèn 12).

For qì binds inside the sac [abdomen][78] when acupuncture and herbal medicine cannot reach it: Apply the same number of cones of moxibustion as the age of the patient on Huāng Mù 肓募 (non-channel)[79] (all this is in *Qiān*).

Zhōng Wǎn 中脘 (Rèn 12) treats cold aggregations and qì binds (*Tóng*), as well as diaphragm binds (see the section on retching).

78. *Náng* 囊 (sac) can also indicate the scrotum. But according to the context, the abdomen seems more appropriate here.

79. Huāng Mù 肓募: Measure half the distance between the nipples and the umbilicus; the point is located this distance directly below the nipples.

產
731
無子
721

# 4.35
## Bēn Tún Qì (Fú Liáng Qì, Xī Bēn)
# 賁豚氣（伏梁氣　息賁）

## Running-piglet qì
**(Deep-lying beam qì; rushing respiration)**

凡卒厥逆上氣，氣攻兩脅，心下痛滿，奄奄欲絕，此為賁豚氣。即急作湯，以浸兩手足，數數易之（《千》）。賁豚腹腫：灸章門百壯。賁豚：灸氣海百壯；或期門、或關元百壯。

Sudden reverse counterflow and qì ascent, qì attacking the rib-sides, pain and fullness under the heart, feeble breathing and about to expire: This is running-piglet qì. Immediately soak the hands and feet in hot water or a decoction, and change it frequently (*Qiān*《千》).

Running-piglet and abdominal swelling: Apply a hundred cones of moxibustion on Zhāng Mén 章門 (LV 13).

Running-piglet: Apply a hundred cones of moxibustion on Qì Hǎi 氣海 (Rèn 6), or Qī Mén 期門 (LV 14), or Guān Yuán 關元 (Rèn 4).

賁豚搶心不得息，灸中極五十壯。賁豚上下，腹中與腰相引痛，灸中府百壯。賁豚上下，灸四滿二七壯。期門（見產）、陰交、石門主賁豚（見無子）。賁豚腹腫，章門主之。賁豚氣上，腹髖痛，莖腫，先引腰，後引小腹、腰髖小痛、堅痛，下引陰中，不得小便，兩丸騫，石門主之。

Running-piglet prodding the heart with inability to breathe: Apply fifty cones of moxibustion on Zhōng Jí 中極 (Rèn 3).

Running-piglet [moving] up and down and pain of the abdomen that radiates to the low back: Apply a hundred cones of moxibustion on Zhōng Fǔ 中府 (LU 1).

Running-piglet [moving] up and down: Apply two times seven cones of moxibustion on Sì Mǎn 四滿 (KI 14).

Qī Mén (LV 14) (see the section on postpartum diseases), Yīn Jiāo 陰交 (Rèn 7), and Shí Mén 石門 (Rèn 5) govern running-piglet (see the section on infertility).

Running-piglet with abdominal swelling: Zhāng Mén 章門 (LV 13) can govern it. 霍亂 267

Running-piglet ascending, with pain of the abdomen and hip, and swollen penis; at first it radiates to the lower back; later it radiates to the smaller abdomen and lower back with fullness, dull pain, tenderness and hardness; it may also radiate down to the genitals with inability to urinate and retracted testicles: Shí Mén 石門 (Rèn 5) can govern it. 陰痛 202

賁豚氣上，腹䐜堅痛，引陰中，不得小便，兩丸騫：陰交主之（並《甲》）。章門、（《銅》同）、石門（《明下》同）、陰交主賁豚上氣。期門主賁豚上下（《銅》同，見霍亂）。中極主賁豚上搶心，甚則不得息。天樞主賁豚脹疝。歸來主賁豚，卵上入，引莖痛。天樞主氣疝，煩嘔面腫賁豚（《甲》）。關元、中極主婦人賁豚搶心。

Running-piglet qì ascending, abdomen fullness, tenderness, and hardness that radiates to the genitals with inability to urinate and retracted testicles: Yīn Jiāo 陰交 (Rèn 7) can govern it (for all, see *Jiă*《甲》).

Zhāng Mén (LV 13) (*Tóng*《銅》agrees), Shí Mén (Rèn 5) (*Míng Xià*《明下》agrees), and Yīn Jiāo (Rèn 7) govern ascent of running-piglet.

Qī Mén 期門 (LV 14) governs running-piglet [moving] up and down (*Tóng* agrees; see the section on sudden turmoil [cholera]).

Zhōng Jí 中極 (Rèn 3) governs running-piglet ascending and prodding the heart and inability to breathe when it is severe.

Tiān Shū 天樞 (ST 25) governs running-piglet and distended *shàn*-mounting.

Guī Lái 歸來 (ST 29) governs running-piglet and testicles retracting upward as well as pain radiating to the penis.

Tiān Shū (ST 25) governs qì *shàn*-mounting, vexation, retching, facial swelling, and running-piglet (*Jiă*).

Guān Yuán 關元 (Rèn 4) and Zhōng Jí (Rèn 3) govern running-piglet prodding the heart in women.

上管療心中煩，賁豚氣，脹滿不能食（《明》）。巨闕賁豚氣脹不能食（《銅》）。中脘治因讀書得奔豚氣上攻，伏梁心下，狀如覆杯，寒癖結氣（《明》云：賁豚氣如悶，伏梁氣如覆杯）。歸來治小腹賁豚。《千》云：主賁豚（並見陰痛）。中極治賁豚搶心，甚則不得息，恍惚尸厥。

勞 188 產後 731 月事 735 無子 721

Shàng Guǎn 上管 (Rèn 13) cures vexation, running-piglet qì, fullness and distention, and inability to eat (*Míng*《明》).

Jù Quē 巨闕 (Rèn 14) treats running-piglet qì with distention and inability to eat (*Tóng*《銅》).

Zhōng Wǎn 中脘 (Rèn 12) treats running-piglet qì attacking upward due to [excessive] studying, deep-lying beams under the heart that are shaped like an overturned cup, cold aggregations and qì binds (*Míng* says: running-piglet qì that feels like oppression; deep-lying beam qì appears like an overturned cup).

Guī Lái 歸來 (ST 29) treats running-piglet in the smaller abdomen. *Qiān*《千》says: It treats running-piglet (for all, see the section on pain of the penis).

Zhōng Jí 中極 (Rèn 3) treats running-piglet prodding the heart with inability to breathe when it is severe, and abstraction with corpse-like reversal.

關元療賁豚，寒氣入小腹（《千》同），時欲嘔，溺血，小便黃，腹泄不止（《明下》）。氣海療賁豚腹堅（見勞）。期門主賁豚（見產後）。氣穴治賁氣上下，引腰脊痛（見月事）。

Guān Yuán 關元 (Rèn 4) cures running-piglet, cold qì entering the smaller abdomen (*Qiān* agrees), frequent retching, bloody or yellow urine, and incessant diarrhea.

Qì Hǎi 氣海 (Rèn 6) cures running-piglet with abdominal hardness (see the section on taxation).

Qī Mén 期門 (LV 14) governs running-piglet (see the section on post-partum diseases).

Qì Xué 氣穴 (KI 13) treats running-piglet [moving] up and down with pain radiating to the lower back and spine (see the section on menstruation).

關元、中極、陰交、石門、四滿（《千》並見無子）、期門（見產後疾）主婦人賁豚。上管治伏梁氣，狀如覆杯（《銅》與《明》同）。中管治伏梁氣（見《上》）。

Guān Yuán (Rèn 4), Zhōng Jí (Rèn 3), Yīn Jiāo 陰交 (Rèn 7), Shí Mén 石門 (Rèn 5), Sì Mǎn 四滿 (KI 14) (for all, see the section on infertility in *Qiān*), and Qī Mén (LV 14) (see the section on post-partum diseases) govern running-piglet in women.

Shàng Guǎn 上管 (Rèn 13) treats deep-lying beam qì which is shaped like an overturned cup (*Tóng* and *Míng* agree).

Zhōng Guǎn 中管 (Rèn 12) treats deep-lying beam qì (see *Shàng*《上》).

期門、缺盆（《千》見胸滿）、鳩尾（心痛）主息賁（肺之積曰息賁，在右脅下，大如杯）。

Qī Mén (LV 14), Quē Pén 缺盆 (ST 12) (see the section on chest fullness in *Qiān*《千》), and Jiū Wěi 鳩尾 (Rèn 15) (heart pain) govern rushing respiration. (Accumulations in the lungs are called rushing respiration; this is located under the right rib-side and is the size of a cup.)

胸滿 470
心痛 312
腹脹 449
腹痛 441

# 4.36
## *Xuán Pǐ*
## 痃癖
## Strings and aggregations

膈俞療痃癖，氣塊膈痛（《明》）。小兒癖：灸兩乳下一寸，各三壯（《千》）。

Gé Shù (UB 17) 膈俞 cures strings and aggregations and qì lumps and pain of the diaphragm (*Míng*《明》). For aggregations in children: Apply three cones of moxibustion on [the site] one cùn below the two nipples (*Qiān*).

三陰交治痃癖腹寒，膝股內痛，氣逆，小便不利（《銅》）。膈俞治熱病汗不出，腹中積癖，默默嗜臥，四肢怠惰，不欲動，身常濕不能食，食則心痛，周痹，身皆痛。脾俞治痃癖積聚（見腹脹）。中脘治寒癖結氣。下脘治癖塊（見腹痛）。《明》云：療腹堅硬癖塊，脈厥厥動。

Sān Yīn Jiāo 三陰交 (SP 6) treats strings and aggregations, cold in the abdomen, pain of the inner aspect of the knees and thighs, qì counterflow, and inhibited urination (*Tóng*《銅》).

Gé Shù 膈俞 (UB 17) treats heat diseases with absence of sweating, accumulations and aggregations in the abdomen, quietness and somnolence, fatigued limbs, no desire to move, the body is constantly damp with inability to eat or heart pain after eating, or generalized *bì*-impediment and pain.

Pí Shù 脾俞 (UB 20) treats strings and aggregations, accumulations and gatherings (see the section on abdominal fullness).

嗽 414 Zhōng Wǎn 中脘 (Rèn 12) treats cold aggregations and qì binds.

痹疼 377 Xian Wan 下脘 (Rèn 13) treats aggregations and lumps (see the section on abdominal pain). *Míng*《明》says: It cures abdominal hardness, aggregations and lumps, and strong pulsations of the [abdominal] vessels. 腎虛 193

不容治腹滿痃癖，不嗜食，腹虛鳴嘔吐，胸背相引痛，喘咳口乾，痰癖，脅下痛，重肋疝瘕。漏谷治痃癖冷氣，心腹脹滿，食飲不為肌膚。三里、太溪（見嗽）治痃癖（《明下》云：癥癖）。府舍治疝癖（見痹疼），灸小腸氣、痃癖氣，發時腹痛若刀刺不可忍者，並婦女本臟氣血癖，走疰刺痛（見腎虛）。

Bù Róng 不容 (ST 19) treats abdominal fullness, strings and aggregations, no desire to eat, vacuity rumbling in the abdomen, vomiting, pain radiating between chest and back, panting, coughing with dry mouth, phlegm aggregations, pain below the rib-sides, heavy sensation in the ribs, *shàn*-mounting, and conglomerations.

Lòu Gǔ 漏谷 (SP 7) treats strings and aggregations, cold qì, and distention and fullness of the heart and abdomen; food and drink is not [transformed into] sinews and skin.

Sān Lǐ 三里 (ST 36) and Tài Xī 太溪 (KI 3) (see the section on cough) treat strings and aggregations (*Míng Xià*《明下》says: concretions and aggregations).

Fǔ Shě 府舍 (SP 13) treats *shàn*-mounting and conglomerations (see the section on *bì*-impediment pain). Apply moxibustion on the point to treat small intestine qì, strings and aggregation qì with unbearable abdominal pain during onset that feels like a knife stabbing; as well as qì and blood aggregations of the viscera in women, and wandering infixation[80] with stabbing pain (see the section on kidney vacuity).

80. *Zǒu zhù* 走疰 (wandering infixation) refers to migrating pain in women due to qì and blood vacuity with wind invasion.

溏泄 247
疝瘕 220
痃癖 433
帶下 739

# 4.37
## *Zhēng Pǐ (Yú Jiàn Shàn Jiǎ)*
## 癥癖（餘見疝瘕）
## Concretions and conglomerations[81]
**(for further discussion, see the sections on *shàn*-mounting and conglomerations)**

癥瘕：灸內踝後宛中，隨年壯，又氣海百壯（《千》）。久冷及婦人癥瘕，腸鳴泄利，繞臍絞痛：天樞百壯，三報之，勿針。地機主溏瘕（見溏泄）。陰陵泉、太溪、太陰郄主疝瘕（見疝瘕）。

Concretions and conglomerations: Apply moxibustion in the depression posterior to the medial malleolus; burn the same number of cones as the age of the patient; or apply a hundred cones of moxibustion on Qì Hǎi 氣海 (Rèn 6) (*Qiān*《千》).

Enduring cold, concretions and conglomerations in women, rumbling intestines and diarrhea, and colicky pain around the umbilicus: Apply a hundred cones of moxibustion on Tiān Shū 天樞 (ST 25); repeat three times; acupuncture is not allowed.

Dì Jī 地機 (SP 8) governs sloppy conglomerations (see the section on sloppy diarrhea).

Yīn Líng Quán 陰陵泉 (SP 9), Tài Xī 太溪 (KI 3), and Tài Yīn Xì 太陰郄 (SP 8) govern *shàn*-mounting and conglomerations (see the section on *shàn*-mounting and conglomerations).

不容（見痃癖）、中極（見疝）治疝瘕。關元（見帶下）治婦人瘕聚（明云：療瘕聚諸病）。膀胱俞治女子瘕聚（《明》同），腳膝無力。曲泉（漏谷同）治女子血瘕，按之如湯滾股內（《千》同見無子）。

Bù Róng 不容 (ST 19) (see the section on strings and aggregations) and Zhōng Jí 中極 (Rèn 3) (see the section on *shàn*-mounting) treat *shàn*-mounting and conglomerations.

Guān Yuán 關元 (Rèn 4) (see the section on leucorrhea) treats concretions and conglomerations in women (*Míng*《明》says: It treats various diseases with conglomerations and gatherings).

81. Concretions and conglomerations are abdominal masses. Concretions are fixed masses with a definite shape and are related to the viscera and blood; conglomerations are movable masses without a definite shape and are related to the bowels and qì.

Páng Guāng Shù 膀胱俞 (UB 28) treats concretions and conglomerations in women (*Míng*《明》agrees) and weakness in the knees and legs.

Qū Quán 曲泉 (LV 8) (the same as Lòu Gǔ 漏谷 (SP 7)) treats blood conglomerations in women. When pressed, it feels like boiling water rolling along the inner thigh (*Qiān*《千》agrees; see the section on infertility).

小腹堅大如盤，胸腹脹滿，飲食不消，婦人瘕聚瘦瘠：三焦俞百壯（三報）；內踝後宛宛中，隨年壯；又氣海百壯。久冷及婦人癥癖，腸鳴泄痢，繞臍絞痛：天樞百壯（三報，勿針）。治瘕癖（患左灸左，患右灸右）：第一屈肋頭近第二肋下是灸處；第二肋頭近第三肋頭下向肉翅前，亦是灸處，初日灸三，次日五，後七，周而復始，至十止（唯忌大蒜）；又關元五十壯，臍上四指五十壯。積聚堅滿痛：章門一百壯。

The smaller abdomen is as big and hard as a plate with distention and fullness of the chest and abdomen, non-dispersion of food, concretions and conglomerations in women, and emaciation: Apply a hundred cones of moxibustion on Sān Jiāo Shù 三焦俞 (UB 22) (repeat three times); or burn the same number of cones as the patient's age in the depression posterior to the medial malleolus; or apply a hundred cones of moxibustion on Qì Hǎi 氣海 (Rèn 6).

Enduring cold, concretions and conglomerations in women, intestinal rumbling and diarrhea, and colicky pain around the umbilicus: Apply a hundred cones of moxibustion on Tiān Shū 天樞 (ST 25) (repeat three times; acupuncture is not allowed).

To treat conglomerations and aggregations (apply moxibustion on the left side for the diseases on the left side; apply moxibustion on the right side for the diseases on the right side): Apply moxibustion on the site below the head of the first curved rib, near the second rib; or on the site below the head of the second rib, near the head of the third rib, anterior to the flesh wings.[82] Burn three cones of moxibustion on the first day; then five cones on the second day; and seven cones on the day after. Keep up this cycle continuously until ten sessions are given (just avoid [eating] garlic). Also apply fifty cones of moxibustion on Guān Yuán 關元 (Rèn 4); and four fingers breadth above the umbilicus.

Accumulations and gatherings with hardness and distending pain: Apply a hundred cones of moxibustion on Zhāng Mén 章門 (LV 13).

82. *Ròu chì* 肉翅, literally the flesh wings: This seems to be an anatomical term, but its meaning is unknown. Perhaps it is the latissimus dorsi muscles.

# 4.38
## *Jī Jù*
## 積聚
## Accumulations and gatherings

腹痛
441

衝門主腹中積聚疼痛（《千》）。膈俞、陰谷（見腹痛）主積聚。上管主心下堅，積聚冷脹。懸樞主腹中積，上下行。商曲主腹中積聚。太陰郄主腹滿積聚。膀胱俞主堅結積聚。積聚堅滿：灸脾募百壯，穴在章門季肋端。心下堅，積聚冷脹：灸上管百壯，三報之。積聚堅大如盤，冷脹：灸胃管二百壯，三報之。

Chōng Mén 衝門 (SP 12) governs accumulations and gatherings with pain of the abdomen (*Qiān*《千》).

Gé Shù 膈俞 (UB 17) and Yīn Gǔ 陰谷 (KI 10) (see the section on abdominal pain) govern accumulations and gatherings.

Shàng Guǎn 上管 (Rèn 13) governs hardness below the heart, accumulations and gatherings, and cold distention.

Xuán Shū 懸樞 (Dū 5) governs abdominal accumulations that move up and down.

Shāng Qū 商曲 (KI 17) governs accumulations and gatherings in the abdomen.

Tài Yīn Xì 太陰郄 (SP 8) governs abdominal fullness, accumulations, and gatherings.

Páng Guāng Shù 膀胱俞 (UB 28) governs hard binds, accumulations, and gatherings.

Accumulations and gatherings with hardness and fullness: Apply a hundred cones of moxibustion on Pí Mù 脾募 (spleen alarm) (LV 13). This is Zhāng Mén 章門 (LV 13) and is located at the end of the free rib.

Hardness below the heart, accumulations and gatherings, and cold distention: Apply a hundred cones of moxibustion on Shàng Guǎn (Rèn 13) and repeat three times.

Accumulations and gatherings as big and hard as a plate and cold distention: Apply two hundred cones of moxibustion on Wèi Guǎn 胃管 (Rèn 12 or Rèn 13) and repeat three times.

腹脹 449
脾疼 309
腹痛 441
痃癖 433
痰 399

衝門（見腹滿）、府舍（見脾疼）治腹滿積聚（《銅》）。膈俞、陰谷（見腹痛）主積聚（《千》）。

Chōng Mén 衝門 (SP 12) (see the section on abdominal fullness) and Fǔ Shě 府舍 (SP 13) (see the section on spleen pain) treat abdominal fullness, accumulations, and gatherings (*Tóng*《銅》).

Gé Shù 膈俞 (UB 17) and Yīn Gǔ 陰谷 (KI 10) (see the section on abdominal pain) govern accumulations and gatherings (*Qiān*《千》).

懸樞治積聚上下行水穀不化，下利，腹中留積（《銅》）。《明下》云：積氣上下行，（解溪同），腹中盡痛。脾俞治積聚（見痃癖）。商曲治腹中積聚（《千》同），腸中切痛，不嗜食。四滿治臍下積聚，疝瘕，腸澼切痛，振寒，大腹有水。通谷治結積留飲（見痰）。

Xuán Shū 懸樞 (Dū 5) treats accumulations and gatherings that move up and down, non-transformation of food, diarrhea, and accumulations in the abdomen (*Tóng*). *Míng Xià*《明下》says: It treats accumulations of qì moving up and down (the same as Jiě Xī 解溪 (ST 41)), and pain of the abdomen.

Pí Shù 脾俞 (UB 20) treats accumulations and gatherings (see the section on strings and aggregations).

Shāng Qū 商曲 (KI 17) treats accumulations and gatherings in the abdomen (*Qiān* agrees), cutting pain of the intestines, and no desire to eat.

Sì Mǎn 四滿 (KI 14) treats accumulations and gatherings below the umbilicus, *shàn*-mounting and conglomerations, intestinal afflux with cutting pain, quivering with cold, and water in the greater abdomen.

Tōng Gǔ 通谷 (KI 20) treats binds, accumulations, and lodged rheum (see the section on phlegm).

章門療積聚氣（《明》）。中極療冷氣積聚，時上衝心，飢不能食（《下》）。脾俞治積聚（《銅》見腹脹）。

Zhāng Mén 章門 (LV 13) cures accumulations and gatherings of qì (*Míng*《明》).

Zhōng Jí 中極 (Rèn 3) cures cold qì accumulations and gatherings that sometimes surge upward to the heart, and hunger with inability to eat (*Xià*《下》).

Pí Shù (UB 20) treats accumulations and gatherings (see the section on abdominal fullness in *Tóng*).

中管主積聚（《千》見腹脹）。積聚：灸肺俞，或三焦俞（見腹脹）。脾俞療黄膽積聚，（見黄膽）。臟腑積聚：灸三焦俞。心腹積聚：灸肝俞（並見腹脹）。期門主喘逆，臥不安席，咳，脅下積聚（《千》）。

腹脹 449
黄膽 668

Zhōng Guǎn 中管 (Rèn 12) governs accumulations and gatherings (see the section on abdominal fullness in *Qiān*《千》).

Accumulations and gatherings: Apply moxibustion on Fèi Shù 肺俞 (UB 13) or Sān Jiāo Shù 三焦俞 (UB 22) (see the section on abdominal fullness).

Pí Shù 脾俞 (UB 20) cures jaundice, accumulations, and gatherings (see the section on jaundice).

Accumulations and gatherings in the viscera and bowels: Apply moxibustion on Sān Jiāo Shù (UB 22).

Accumulations and gatherings in the heart and abdomen: Apply moxibustion on Gān Shù 肝俞 (UB 18) (for all, see the section on abdominal distention).

Qī Mén 期門 (LV 14) governs panting counterflow, inability to lie peacefuly on the mat to sleep, cough, and accumulations and gatherings under the rib-sides (*Qiān*).

吐瀉 271
咳嗽 414
積聚 437
臍痛 466
腹堅 455
腹痛 441
鼓脹 457

# 4.39
# *Jī Qì*
# 積氣

## Accumulation of qì

梁門治脅下積氣（ 期門同，見吐瀉 ），食飲不思，大腸滑泄，穀不化《 銅 》。解溪（ 見咳嗽 ）、懸樞治積氣上下行（ 見積聚 ）。關門治積氣，腸鳴卒痛，泄利，不欲食，腹中氣游走，夾臍急 。氣海治氣結成塊，狀如覆杯（ 見臍痛 ）。

Liáng Mén 梁門 (ST 21) treats qì accumulation below the rib-sides (same as Qī Mén 期門 (LV 14); see the section on vomiting and diarrhea), no desire to eat, efflux diarrhea of the large intestine, and non-transformation of food (*Tóng*《 銅 》).

Jiě Xī 解溪 (ST 41) (see the section on cough) and Xuán Shū 懸樞 (Dū 5) treat accumulation of qì that moves up and down (see the section on accumulations and gatherings).

Guān Mén 關門 (ST 22) treats accumulation of qì, intestinal rumbling with acute pain, diarrhea, no desire to eat, qì wandering in the abdomen, and tension around the umbilicus.

Qì Hăi 氣海 (Rèn 6) treats qì accumulating into a lump that appears like an over-turned cup (see the section on umbilical pain).

陰交療氣痛如刀攪，作塊如覆杯（ 《 明 》見便赤 ）。章門療積聚氣（ 見積聚 ）。膻中，岐伯云：療積氣成噎（ 《 下 》 ）。三里（ 見腹堅 ）、不容療積氣（ 見腹痛 ）。章門療積氣如石（ 見鼓脹 ）。梁門主胸下積氣 。

Yīn Jiāo 陰交 (Rèn 7) cures qì pain that feels like a knife is stirring; or lumps that appear like an overturned cup (see the discussion of red stools in *Míng*《 明 》).

Zhāng Mén 章門 (LV 13) cures accumulations and gatherings of qì (see the section on accumulations and gatherings).

Dàn Zhōng 膻中 (Rèn 17): Qí Bó said that this cures accumulations of qì that become dysphagia (*Xià*《 下 》).

Sān Lǐ 三里 (ST 36 or LI 10) (see the section on hardness [and enlargement] of the abdomen) and Bù Róng 不容 (ST 19) cure accumulation of qì (see the section on abdominal pain).

Zhāng Mén 章門 (LV 13) cures stone-like accumulation of qì (see the section on drum distention).

Liáng Mén 梁門 (ST 21) governs accumulation of qì under the chest.

## 4.40
## *Fù Tòng (Yú Jiàn Xīn Tòng)*
# 腹痛（餘見心痛）
## Abdominal pain
**(for further discussion, see the section on heart pain)**

氣海主小腹疝氣，游行五臟，腹中切痛（《千》）。膈俞、陰谷主腹脹，胃管暴痛，及腹積聚，肌肉痛。高曲（一名商曲）主腹中積聚，時切痛。衝門主寒氣滿，腹中積痛，癃淫濼。四滿主腹僻切痛。天樞、外陵主腹中盡疼，崑崙主腹痛，喘暴滿。

Qì Hǎi 氣海 (Rèn 6) governs *shàn*-mounting qì in the smaller abdomen that wanders among the five viscera and cutting pain of the abdomen (*Qiān*《千》).

Gé Shù 膈俞 (UB 17) and Yīn Gǔ 陰谷 (KI 10) govern abdominal distention, violent pain of the stomach duct, accumulations and gatherings in the abdomen, and pain of the flesh.

Gāo Qū 高曲 (KI 17) (another name for Shāng Qū 商曲 (KI 17)) governs accumulations and gatherings in the abdomen, occasionally with cutting pain.

Chōng Mén 衝門 (SP 12) governs fullness due to cold qì, abdominal accumulations with pain, dribbling urination, and aching weakness [of the body].

Sì Mǎn 四滿 (KI 14) governs abdominal masses (*pì* 僻) with cutting pain.

Tiān Shū 天樞 (ST 25) and Wài Líng 外陵 (ST 26) govern pain of the entire abdomen.

Kūn Lún 崑崙 (UB 60) governs abdominal pain, panting, and violent fullness.

吐 274 復溜主腹厥痛。巨闕、上管、石門、陰蹻主腹中滿，暴痛汗出。太溪主腹中相引痛。豐隆主胸痛如刺，腹若刀切痛（《銅》同，《明》見厥逆）。鳩尾主腹皮痛瘙癢。肓俞主腹切痛。氣衝主身熱，腹痛。中極主腹中熱痛。行間主腹痛而熱，上柱心，心下滿。

Fù Liū 復溜 (KI 7) governs reversal pain of the abdomen.

Jù Quē 巨闕 (Rèn 14), Shàng Guǎn 上管 (Rèn 13), Shí Mén 石門 (Rèn 5), and Yīn Jiāo 陰交 (Rèn 7) govern abdominal fullness with violent pain, and sweating.

Tài Xī 太溪 (KI 3) governs pain radiating into the abdomen.

Fēng Lóng 豐隆 (ST 40) governs piercing chest pain and pain of the abdomen that feels like a knife cutting (*Tóng*《銅》agrees; see the discussion of reverse counterflow in *Míng*《明》).

Jiū Wěi 鳩尾 (Rèn 15) governs itching and pain of the abdominal skin.

Huāng Shù 肓俞 (KI 16) governs cutting pain of the abdomen.

Qì Chōng 氣衝 (ST 30) governs generalized heat and abdominal pain.

Zhōng Jí 中極 (Rèn 3) governs hot pain of the abdomen.

Xíng Jiān 行間 (LV 2) governs abdominal pain with heat like a column up to the heart, and fullness below the heart.

分水療腹腫不能食，腸堅腹痛，胃脹不調，堅硬（《明》）。大杼療腹痛。腎俞療寒熱腹痛雷鳴，氣逆心痛。不容療腹弦急，不得食，腹痛如刀刺，內脅積氣膨膨（《下》）。上管療腹疞刺痛（見吐）。

Fēn Shuǐ 分水 (Rèn 9) cures abdominal swelling and inability to eat, hardness in the intestines and abdominal pain, and stomach distention with disharmony and hardness (*Míng*).

Dà Zhù 大杼 (UB 11) cures abdominal pain.

Shèn Shù 腎俞 (UB 23) cures cold and hot pain of the abdomen with thunderous rumbling, qì counterflow, and heart pain.

Bù Róng 不容 (ST 19) cures bowstring tension of the abdomen, inability to eat, abdominal pain like a knife stabbing, accumulation of qì, and an inflated feeling inside the rib-sides (*Xià*《下》).

Shàng Guǎn 上管 (Rèn 13) cures colicky pain of the abdomen (see the section on vomiting).

霍亂 267
胃 287
水腫 459
痃癖 433
腹脹 449
月事 735
無子 721

太白（見霍亂）、溫溜、三里（見胃）、陷谷（見水腫）治腹痛。腹哀治大便膿血，寒中，食不化，腹中痛（《銅》）。魚際治腹痛不下食。肓俞治大腹寒疝，大便燥，腹切痛。地機（見水腫）治腹脅氣脹。外陵治腹痛心如懸，下引臍腹痛。下脘治腹痛，六腑之氣寒，穀不轉，不嗜食，小便赤，腹堅硬，癖塊，臍上厥氣動，日漸瘦（《銅》）。

Tài Bái 太白 (SP 3) (see the section on sudden turmoil [cholera]), Wēn Liū 溫溜 (LI 7), Sān Lǐ 三里 (ST 36 or LI 10) (see the section on stomach ache), and Xiàn Gǔ 陷谷 (ST 43) (see the section on edema) treat abdominal pain.

Fù Āi 腹哀 (SP 16) treats pus and blood in the stool, cold strike with non-transformation of food, and pain of the abdomen (*Tóng* 《銅》).

Yú Jì 魚際 (LU 10) treats abdominal pain with inability to get food down.

Huāng Shù 肓俞 (KI 16) treats cold *shàn*-mounting in the greater abdomen, dry stools, and cutting pain of the abdomen.

Dì Jī 地機 (SP 8) (see the section on edema) treats qì distention of the abdomen and rib-sides.

Wài Líng 外陵 (ST 26) treats abdominal pain, a feeling like the heart is suspended, and pain radiating into the umbilical region.

Xià Wǎn 下脘 (Rèn 10) treats abdominal pain, cold qì in six bowels, non-transformation of food, no desire to eat, reddish urine, abdominal hardness, aggregations and lumps, reverse qì moving in the umbilicus and gradual emaciation day by day (*Tóng*).

脾俞治腹痛不嗜食（見痃癖）。三焦俞治腹痛欲泄（見腹脹）。膀胱俞治腹痛（《明下》同）。天樞治女人腹痛（見月事）。石關治婦人惡血上衝，腹痛不可忍（見無子）。胃俞治腹痛（見腹脹）。中管主腹中甚痛，作膿（《千》見腹脹）。

Pí Shù 脾俞 (UB 20) treats abdominal pain with no desire to eat (see the section on strings and aggregations).

Sān Jiāo Shù 三焦俞 (UB 22) treats abdominal pain and diarrhea (see the section on abdominal fullness).

Páng Guāng Shù 膀胱俞 (UB 28) treats abdominal pain (*Míng Xià* 《明下》 agrees).

Tiān Shū 天樞 (ST 25) treats abdominal pain in women (see the section on menstruation).

Shí Guān 石關 (KI 18) treats malign blood surging upward in women and insufferable abdominal pain (see the section on infertility).

Wèi Shù 胃俞 (UB 21) treats abdominal pain (see the section on abdominal fullness).

Zhōng Guǎn 中管 (Rèn 12) governs severe pain of the abdomen with suppuration (see the section on abdominal fullness in *Qiān*《千》).

小兒卒患肚皮青黑，不急治，須臾即死，酒和胡粉塗，乾則再塗之。又灸臍四邊各半寸，並鳩尾骨下一寸，各三壯（《集效》）。

A child suddenly suffering with a green-blue and black belly will die if he does not get treatment immediately. Mix liquor with processed galenite powder and apply it [on the belly]; apply it again when it dries. Also burn three cones of moxibustion on the sites that are a half cùn away from the four sides of the umbilicus; as well as the site one cùn below the xiphoid process (*Jí Xiào*《集效》).

# 4.41

## *Fù Mǎn (Xīn Mǎn Zhàng)*

## 腹滿（心滿脹）

噫 281
産 731
腸澼 259
大便 235

### Abdominal fullness

**(Fullness and distention of the heart)**

凡腹滿痛不得息：正仰臥，屈一膝伸一腳，並氣衝針入三寸，氣至瀉之（《千》）。大鐘主腹滿便難。陷谷（見噫）、懸鐘主腹滿（《千》云：小兒腹滿不食）。陰市主腹中滿，痿厥少氣。

Whenever there is abdominal fullness and pain with inability to breathe: Lie supine, flex one knee and extend the other leg; needle Qì Chōng 氣衝 (ST 30) 3 cùn deep, and drain after qì arrives (*Qiān*《千》).

Dà Zhōng 大鐘 (KI 4) governs abdominal fullness and difficult defecation.

Xiàn Gǔ 陷谷 (ST 43) (see the section on belching) and Xuán Zhōng 懸鐘 (GB 39) govern abdominal fullness (*Qiān* says: pediatric abdominal fullness and inability to eat).

Yīn Shì 陰市 (ST 33) governs abdominal fullness, wilting reversal, and qì shortage.

太陰郄主腹滿積聚。衝門主寒氣腹滿，腹中積聚痛。隱白主腹滿喜嘔。三里、行間、曲泉主腹䐜滿。商丘主腹中滿，向向然不便，心下有寒痛。漏谷主腸鳴，強欠，心悲，氣逆，腹䐜滿急。巨闕、上管、石門、陰蹻主腹中滿，暴痛汗出。期門主傷食腹滿（見産）。通谷主結積留飲癖（見腸澼）。石關主心堅滿（見大便不通）。陰都主心滿氣逆腸鳴。

Tàiyīn Xì 太陰郄 (SP 8) governs abdominal fullness, accumulations, and gatherings.

Chōng Mén 衝門 (SP 12) governs cold qì, abdominal fullness, and abdominal pain from accumulations and gatherings.

Yǐn Bái 隱白 (SP 1) governs abdominal fullness and frequent retching.

Sān Lǐ 三里 (ST 36), Xíng Jiān 行間 (LV 2), and Qū Quán 曲泉 (LV 8) govern abdominal fullness.

積聚 437
尸厥 531
痃癖 433
上氣 420
腹痛 441
腹脹 449

Shāng Qiū 商丘 (SP 5) governs abdominal fullness, a feeling of inflation, inability to defecate, and coldness and pain below the heart.

Lòu Gǔ 漏谷 (SP 7) governs intestinal rumbling, belching, sorrowful heart, qì counterflow, and abdominal fullness and tension.

Jù Quē 巨闕 (Rèn 14), Shàng Guǎn 上管 (Rèn 13), Shí Mén 石門 (Rèn 5), and Yīn Qiāo 陰蹻 (KI 6 or KI 8) govern abdominal fullness, violent pain, and sweating.

Qī Mén 期門 (LV 14) governs food damage and abdominal fullness (see the section on postpartum diseases).

Tōng Gǔ 通谷 (UB 66) governs binding accumulations, lodged rheum, and aggregations (see the section on intestinal afflux).

Shí Mén (Rèn 5) governs hardness and fullness of the heart (see the section on fecal stoppage [constipation]).

Yīn Dū 陰都 (KI 19) governs fullness of the heart, qì counterflow, and intestinal rumbling.

聽宮（《明》同）治心腹滿（《銅》）。衝門治腹寒氣滿（見積聚）。大都治熱病汗不出，手足逆冷，腹滿善嘔，煩熱悶亂，吐逆目眩。厲兌（見尸厥）、漏谷（見痃癖）治心腹脹滿。

Tīng Gōng 聽宮 (SI 19) (*Míng*《明》agrees) treats fullness of the heart and abdomen (*Tóng*《銅》).

Chōng Mén 衝門 (SP 12) treats cold in the abdomen and qì fullness (see the section on accumulations and gatherings).

Dà Dū 大都 (SP 2) treats heat disease with absence of sweating, reversal cold of the hands and feet, abdominal fullness, frequent retching, vexation heat, oppression and derangement, vomiting counterflow, and dizzy vision.

Lì Duì 厲兌 (ST 45) (see the section on deathlike reversal) and Lòu Gǔ 漏谷 (SP 7) (see the section on strings and aggregations) treat distention and fullness of the heart and abdomen.

腹滿：灸絕骨（《千》見上氣）。巨闕等主腹滿。崑崙主腹暴滿（並見腹痛）。太白等主腹大滿（見腹脹）。

Abdominal fullness: Apply moxibustion on Jué Gǔ 絕骨 (GB 39) (see the section on qì ascent in *Qiān*《千》).

Jù Quē 巨闕 (Rèn 14) and so forth govern abdominal fullness.

Kūn Lún 崑崙 (UB 60) governs sudden onset of abdominal fullness (for all, see the section on abdominal pain).

Tài Bái 太白 (SP 3), and so forth govern severe abdominal fullness (see the section on abdominal fullness).

上氣 420
水腫 459
肩痛 491
傷寒 661
無子 721
腹痛 441
腹脹 449

譩譆（在鼻衄門）、三里療腹滿（《明》見腹大）。中管治心下脹滿，傷飽，食不化，霍亂，出泄不自知，心痛（《銅》）。心腹諸病心痛：灸太倉（《千》）。心腹痞痛：灸肝俞。膽俞療心脹滿（《明》見上氣）。府舍治腹滿（《銅》）。四滿治大腹有水（見水腫）。

Yī Xī 譩譆 (UB 45) (see the section on nosebleeds) and Sān Lǐ 三里 (ST 36 or LI 10) cure abdominal fullness (see the discussion of enlarged abdomen in *Míng*《明》).

Zhōng Guǎn 中管 (Rèn 12) treats distention and fullness under the heart, damage from overeating, non-transformation of food, sudden turmoil [cholera] with uncontrollable diarrhea, and heart pain (*Tóng*《銅》).

All diseases of the heart and abdomen, heart pain: Apply moxibustion on Tài Cāng 太倉 (Rèn 12) (*Qiān*《千》).

Pain occurring in the heart and abdomen: Apply moxibustion on Gān Shù 肝俞 (UB 18).

Dǎn Shù 膽俞 (UB 19) cures distention and fullness of the heart (see the section on qì ascent in *Míng*).

Fǔ Shě 府舍 (SP 13) treats abdominal fullness (*Tóng*).

Sì Mǎn 四滿 (KI 14) treats water in the greater abdomen (see the section on edema).

神堂治胸腹滿（見肩痛）。魚際（《銅》同）等治腹滿（見傷寒）。石門主腹滿疝積，（《千》見無子）。分水療腹腫不能食（見腹痛）。意舍治腹滿虛脹（見腹脹）。

Shén Táng 神堂 (UB 44) treats fullness of the abdomen and chest (see the section on shoulder pain).

Yú Jì 魚際 (LU 10) (*Tóng* agrees) and so forth treat abdominal fullness (see the section on cold damage).

Shí Mén 石門 (Rèn 5) governs abdominal fullness and *shàn*-mounting accumulations (see the section on infertility in *Qiān*).

Fēn Shuǐ 分水 (Rèn 9) cures abdominal swelling and inability to eat (see the section on abdominal pain).

Yì Shě 意舍 (UB 49) treats abdominal fullness and vacuity distention (see the section on abdominal fullness).

人有心腹滿脹者，予只多以厚朴與之，令每服細銼七八錢重（幼小量減）。用生薑七片水小碗煎至七分服，滓再煎服，不過五六服，脹滿脫去。針灸之效，未必如此速也，因識於此。

[Author's notes:] For people suffering with fullness and distention of the heart and abdomen, I usually just treat them with *hòu pò* 厚朴 (Officinal Magnolia). Use 7 to 8 *qián* [21 to 24 grams] of finely filed herb per decoction (reduce the dosage in children). Cook with 7 slices of ginger in a small bowl of water, boil it down to seventy percent [of the volume], and take it. Cook the dregs again and take it. The distention and fullness will disappear after taking five to six doses. The results of acupuncture will not be as fast as this, so I record it here.

腹痛，按之痛，重按卻不痛，此是氣痛 。重按愈痛而堅，有積也 。氣痛不可下，下之愈痛，虛寒證也，小建中湯治腹痛如神（《良方》）。

In abdominal pain, when there is pain with pressure but no pain when pressed heavily, it is qì pain. If pain and hardness get worse when pressed heavily, it is an accumulation. Precipitation cannot be used for qì pain or else the pain will worsen. This is a pattern of vacuity cold. Treat abdominal pain with *Xiǎo Jiàn Zhōng Tāng* 小建中湯 (Minor Center-Fortifying Decoction). It will have divine effects (*Liáng Fāng*《良方》).

腹痛
441
腸鳴
263

# 4.42

## *Fù Zhàng*

*(Xiōng Xié Zhàng Fù, Xīn Zhàng, Yú Jiàn Xīn Fù Mǎn Zhàng)*

# 腹脹

## (胸脅脹附　心脹　餘見心腹滿脹)

## Abdominal distention

**(with appendices on distention of the chest and rib-sides and distention of the heart; for further discussion, see the section on fullness and distention of the heart and abdomen)**

膈俞等（見腹痛）主腹脹（《千》）。脾俞、大腸俞主腹中氣脹，引脊痛，食飲多而身羸瘦。中極主寒中腹脹。上管主心下堅，積聚冷脹。隱白主腹脹逆息，又主腹中寒冷氣脹喘。尺澤主腹脹喘振栗。天樞主腹脹，氣衝胸（見腸鳴）。中管主腹脹不通疰，大便堅，憂思損傷，氣積聚，腹中甚痛，作膿腫，往來上下。

Gé Shù 膈俞 (UB 17) and so forth (see the section on abdominal pain) govern abdominal distention (*Qiān*《千》).

Pí Shù 脾俞 (UB 20) and Dà Cháng Shù 大腸俞 (UB 25) govern qì distention of the abdomen with pain radiating to the spine, and generalized emaciation even when eating a lot.

Zhōng Jí 中極 (Rèn 3) governs cold strike with abdominal distention.

Shàng Guǎn 上管 (Rèn 13) governs hardness below the heart and accumulations and gatherings with cold distention.

Yǐn Bái 隱白 (SP 1) governs abdominal distention, counterflow breathing, cold and qì distention of the abdomen, as well as panting.

Chǐ Zé 尺澤 (LU 5) governs abdominal distention, panting, and shivering.

Tiān Shū 天樞 (ST 25) governs abdominal distention and qì surging into the chest (see the section on intestinal rumbling).

Zhōng Guǎn 中管 (Rèn 12) governs abdominal distention with stoppage and infixation, hard stool, anxiety and thought damage, accumulations and gatherings of qì, abdominal pain with an abscess, or [qì] moving up and down.

痢 249
中風 379
漏下 728
腸鳴 263

太溪主腹中脹腫。京門主寒熱䐜脹。三里、章門、京門、厲兑、內庭、陰谷、絡卻、崑崙、商丘、陰陵、曲泉主腹脹滿不得息。氣衝主腹中大熱不安，腹有大氣，暴腹脹(《明下》云：又臍下堅)，滿癃淫濼。期門主腹大堅不得息，脹痹滿，小腹尤大。巨闕、上管主腹脹心腹滿。五里主心下脹滿而痛，上氣。太白(又見痢)、公孫主腹脹食不化，鼓脹，腹中氣大滿。

Tài Xī 太溪 (KI 3) governs distention and swelling of the abdomen.

Jīng Mén 京門 (GB 25) governs [sensations of] cold and heat as well as distention.

Sān Lǐ 三里 (ST 36 or LI 10), Zhāng Mén 章門 (LV 13), Jīng Mén (GB 25), Lì Duì 厲兑 (ST 45), Nèi Tíng 內庭 (ST 44), Yīn Gǔ 陰谷 (KI 10), Luò Què 絡卻 (UB 8), Kūn Lún 崑崙 (UB 60), Shāng Qiū 商丘 (SP 5), Yīn Líng [Quán] 陰陵[泉] (SP 9), and Qū Quán 曲泉 (LV 8) govern abdominal distention with inability to breathe.

Qì Chōng 氣衝 (ST 30) governs great heat and disquiet of the abdomen, great qì of the abdomen, sudden onset of abdominal distention (*Míng Xià*《明下》says: hardness under the umbilicus), dribbling blockage, aching pain, and weakness.

Qī Mén 期門 (LV 14) governs enlarged and hard abdomen with inability to breath, and distending *bì*-impediment and fullness especially in the smaller abdomen.

Jù Quē 巨闕 (Rèn 14) and Shàng Guǎn 上管 (Rèn 13) govern abdominal distention, and fullness of the heart and abdomen.

Wǔ Lǐ 五里 (LV 10 or LI 13) governs pain, distention, and fullness under the heart as well as qì ascent.

Tài Bái 太白 (SP 3) (also see the section on dysentery) and Gōng Sūn 公孫 (SP 4) govern abdominal distention, non-transformation of food, [a feeling of] inflation, and great fullness of qì in the abdomen.

陰陵泉主腹中脹，不嗜食，脅下滿，腹中盛水，脹逆不得臥。凡頭目癰腫，胸脅支滿：刺陷谷出血立已。大鐘主胸喘息脹。關元、期門、少商主脅下脹。石門治腹脹堅硬，水腫支滿(《銅》)。解溪(見中風)、血海(見漏下)、商丘(見腸鳴)治腹脹。膽俞治心腹脹滿，嘔則食無所出，口苦舌乾，咽痛，食不下。

Yīn Líng Quán 陰陵泉 (SP 9) governs abdominal distention, no desire to eat, fullness below the rib-sides, water overflowing in the abdomen, distention with counterflow, and inability to lie down.

For all welling-abscesses, swelling of the head and eyes, and propping fullness of the chest and rib-sides: Bleed Xiàn Gǔ 陷谷 (ST 43) to cure these diseases immediately.

Dà Zhōng 大鐘 (KI 4) governs chest distention and panting.

Guān Yuán 關元 (Rèn 4), Qī Mén 期門 (LV 14), and Shào Shāng 少商 (LU 11) govern distention under the rib-sides.

Shí Mén 石門 (Rèn 5) treats abdominal distention and hardness, edema, and propping fullness (*Tóng*《銅》).

Jiě Xī 解溪 (ST 41) (see the section on wind stroke), Xuè Hǎi 血海 (SP 10) (see the section on spotting of blood), and Shāng Qiū 商丘 (SP 5) (see the section on intestinal rumbling) treat abdominal distention.

Dǎn Shù 膽俞 (UB 19) treats distention and fullness of the heart and abdomen; vomiting with no food coming out; bitter taste in the mouth, dry tongue, sore throat, and difficulty getting food down.

消渴 195
肩背 486
嘔吐 274
勞瘵 188
胃 287
膝攣 536

中膂俞（見消渴）、譩譆（見肩背痛）、膈俞治腹脹（見嘔吐）。脾俞治腹脹引胸背痛，食飲倍多，身漸羸瘦（《明下》同），黄膽，善欠，脅滿泄利，體重，四肢不收，痃癖腹痛，不嗜食。

Zhōng Lǚ Shù 中膂俞 (UB 29) (see the section on wasting and thirsting), Yī Xī 譩譆 (UB 45) (see the discussion of shoulder and back pain), and Gé Shù 膈俞 (UB 17) treat abdominal distention (see the section on vomiting).

Pí Shù 脾俞 (UB 20) treats abdominal distention with pain radiating to the chest and back, overeating, gradual emaciation (*Míng Xià*《明下》agrees), jaundice, frequent yawning, fullness of the rib-sides, diarrhea, heavy body, loss of use of the limbs, strings and aggregations, abdominal pain, and no desire to eat.

胃俞治胃寒腹脹，不嗜食（《明》同），羸瘦，腸鳴腹痛，胸脅支滿，脊痛筋攣。三焦俞治腸鳴腹脹，水穀不化，腹痛欲泄注，目眩頭痛，吐逆，飲食不下。腎俞治心腹膨脹（見勞瘵）。三里（見胃）、懸鐘治心腹脹滿（見膝攣）。大腸俞治腹脹繞臍切痛，大小便不利，洞泄食不化，脊強不得俯仰。中髎治腹脹下利。

Wèi Shù 胃俞 (UB 21) treats stomach cold with abdominal distention, no desire to eat (*Míng*《明》agrees), emaciation, intestinal rumbling, abdominal pain, propping fullness of the chest and rib-sides, spine pain, and hypertonicity of the sinews.

Sān Jiāo Shù 三焦俞 (UB 22) treats intestinal rumbling and abdominal distention, non-transformation of food, abdominal pain with outpour diarrhea, dizzy vision and headache, vomiting counterflow, and difficulty getting drink and food down.

肺氣 412

Shèn Shù 腎俞 (UB 23) treats inflation of the heart and abdomen (see the section on consumption).

Sān Lǐ 三里 (ST 36) (see the section on the stomachache) and Xuán Zhōng 懸鐘 (GB 39) treat distention and fullness of the heart and abdomen (see the section on [hypertonicity of the legs and] knees).

Dà Cháng Shù 大腸俞 (UB 25) treats abdominal distention with cutting pain around the umbilicus, inhibited defecation and urination, throughflux diarrhea, non-transformation of food, stiffness of the spine, and inability to bend forward and backward.

Zhōng Liáo 中髎 (UB 33) treats abdominal distention and diarrhea.

陽綱治腹滿脹，大便泄利(《明下》同)，小便赤澀，身熱目黃。太白治身熱煩滿，腹脹，食不化，嘔吐，泄膿血。意舍治腹滿虛脹，大便滑泄，背痛惡風寒，食飲不下，嘔吐消渴，目黃。胃倉治腹虛脹，水腫，食飲不下，惡寒，背脊不得俯仰。中府治腹脹食不下(見肺氣)。

Yáng Gāng 陽綱 (UB 48) treats abdominal fullness and distention, diarrhea (*Míng Xià*《明下》agrees), inhibited urination with red urine, generalized heat, and yellow eyes.

Tài Bái 太白 (SP 3) treats generalized heat, vexation and fullness, abdominal distention, non-transformation of food, vomiting, and diarrhea with pus and blood.

Yì Shě 意舍 (UB 49) treats abdominal fullness and vacuity distension, efflux diarrhea, back pain and aversion to wind-cold, difficulty getting food and drink down, vomiting with wasting-thirst, and yellow eyes.

Wèi Cāng 胃倉 (UB 50) treats vacuity distention of the abdomen, edema, difficulty getting food and drink down, aversion to cold, and inability of the spine to bend forward and backward.

Zhōng Fǔ 中府 (LU 1) treats abdominal distention and difficulty getting food down (see the section on lung qì).

中脘治傷寒飲水過多，腹脹氣喘。陰谷治腹脹滿不得息，小便黃，男如蠱，女如妊娠。承滿治腸鳴腹脹，上喘氣逆，食飲不下，肩息唾血。大敦治腹脹滿。三陰交治脾病身重，四肢不舉，腹脹，腸鳴溏泄，食不化。隱白治腹脹喘滿，不得臥，嘔吐，食下暴泄。

Zhōng Wǎn 中脘 (Rèn 12) treats cold damage, drinking too much water, abdominal distention, and panting.

Yīn Gǔ 陰谷 (KI 10) treats abdominal distention and fullness, inability to breathe, and yellow urine. In men, [the abdomen] looks like *gǔ* 蠱; while in women, it looks like she is pregnant.

Chéng Mǎn 承滿 (ST 20) treats intestinal rumbling, abdominal distention, panting ascent and qì counterflow, difficulty getting food and drink down, raised-shoulder breathing, and spitting of blood.

Dà Dūn 大敦 (LV 1) treats abdominal distention and fullness.

Sān Yīn Jiāo 三陰交 (SP 6) treats spleen diseases, generalized heaviness, inability to lift the limbs, abdominal distention, intestinal rumbling and diarrhea, and non-transformation of food.

Yǐn Bái 隱白 (SP 1) treats abdominal distention, panting and fullness, inability to lie down, and vomiting and violent diarrhea after eating.

隱白療腹中有寒熱起，氣喘，衄血不止，腹中脹逆，脛寒熱不得臥，氣滿胸中熱，暴泄，膈中嘔吐，不欲食（《明下》）。上管（見吐）療腹脹。

Yǐn Bái (SP 1) cures [sensations of] cold and heat arising in the abdomen, panting, incessant nosebleeds, distention and counterflow of the abdomen, [sensations of] cold and heat in the lower legs with inability to lie down, qì fullness and heat in the chest, violent diarrhea, [occlusion] in the diaphragm[83] with vomiting, and no desire to eat (*Míng Xià*《明下》).

Shàng Guǎn 上管 (Rèn 13) (see the section on vomiting) cures abdominal distention.

臚脹，脅腹滿：灸膈俞百壯，三報（《千》）。胸滿，心腹積聚痞痛：灸肝俞百壯，三報。脹滿水腫：脾俞隨年壯，三報。腹中氣脹，引脊痛，食飲多，身羸瘦，名曰食晦。先取脾俞，後取季肋。臟腑積聚脹滿，羸瘦，不能飲食：三焦俞隨年壯。脹滿雷鳴：大腸俞百壯，三報。

Abdominal distention and fullness of the rib-sides and abdomen: Apply a hundred cones of moxibustion on Gé Shù 膈俞 (UB 17) and repeat three times (*Qiān*《千》).

Chest fullness, accumulations and gatherings, pain from concretions of the heart and abdomen: Apply a hundred cones of moxibustion on Gān Shù 肝俞 (UB 18) and repeat three times.

Distention and edema: Apply the same number of cones of moxibustion as the patient's age on Pí Shù 脾俞 (UB 20) and repeat three times.

83. *Gé zhōng* 膈中 ([occlusion] in the diaphragm) is a disorder with vomiting right after eating. It is a type of dysphagia-occlusion and is usually caused by spleen deficiency.

Distention of the abdomen with pain radiating to the spine and eating a lot but emaciated: This is called *shí huì* 食晦.[84] Treat Pí Shù (UB 20) first, then Jì Xié 季脅 (LV 13).

Accumulations and gatherings in the viscera and bowels with distention and fullness, emaciation, and inability to eat: Apply the same number of cones of moxibustion as the patient's age on Sān Jiāo Shù 三焦俞 (UB 22).

[Abdominal] distention and fullness and thunderous rumbling: Apply a hundred cones of moxibustion on Dà Cháng Shù 大腸俞 (UB 25) and repeat three times.

脹滿，氣聚寒冷：胃管百壯，三報，在鳩尾下三寸。腹脹滿，繞臍結痛堅，不能食：中守百壯，在臍上一寸，一名水分。脹滿瘕聚，滯下疼：氣海百壯，忌針。脹滿氣如水腫狀，小腹堅如石：膀胱募百壯，在中極，臍下四寸。脹滿腎冷，瘕聚泄利：天樞百壯。

[Abdominal] distention and fullness and qì gatherings with a cold feeling: Apply a hundred cones of moxibustion on Wèi Guǎn 胃管 (Rèn 12 or Rèn 13) and repeat three times. It is located 3 cùn below the xiphoid process.

Abdominal distention and fullness, gripping pain and hardness around the umbilicus, and inability to eat: Apply a hundred cones of moxibustion on Zhōng Shǒu 中守 (Rèn 9). It is located 1 cùn above the umbilicus and is also named Shuǐ Fēn 水分 (Rèn 9).

[Abdominal] fullness, conglomerations and gatherings, and dysentery with pain: Apply a hundred cones of moxibustion on Qì Hǎi 氣海 (Rèn 6). Needling is contraindicated.

[Abdominal] distention and fullness with qì that appears like water swelling [edema]; the smaller abdomen is as hard as a stone: Apply a hundred cones of moxibustion on the *Mù* 募 of the urinary bladder, which is Zhōng Jí 中極 (Rèn 3), 4 cùn below the umbilicus.

[Abdominal] distention and fullness with cold kidneys, conglomerations and gatherings, and diarrhea: Apply a hundred cones of moxibustion on Tiān Shū 天樞 (ST 25).

84. *Shí huì* 食晦 is hard to translate. It is a type of wasting disease with the symptoms listed here. *Shí* means food or to eat. *Huì* is the last day of the lunar month, when the moon has reached end-stage decline.

# 4.43

## *Xīn Fù Jiān Dà (Yú Lùn Jiàn Fù Mǎn)*

# 心腹堅大（餘論見腹滿）

霍亂
267
腹脹
449
水腫
459
腹痛
441

## Hardness and enlargement of the heart and abdomen

**(for further discussion, see the section on abdominal fullness)**

下管療腹胃不調，腹痛不能食，小便赤，腹堅硬癖塊，脈厥厥動（《明》）。衝陽治腹堅大，不嗜食，振寒（《銅》）。期門治腹堅硬（見霍亂）。次髎治心下堅脹。石門治腹（《明》有痛字）堅硬（見腹脹）。肓門治心下肓大堅。水分治腹堅如鼓（見水腫）。志室治腹堅急。陰陵泉、地機（並見水腫），下脘治腹堅硬（見腹痛）。

Xià Guǎn 下管 (Rèn 10) cures irregularities of the abdomen and stomach, abdominal pain with inability to eat, reddish urination, abdominal hardness with glomus lumps, and strong pulsations of the [abdominal] vessels (*Míng*《明》).

Chōng Yáng 衝陽 (ST 42) treats hardness and enlargement of the abdomen with no desire to eat and quivering with cold (*Tóng*《銅》).

Qī Mén 期門 (LV 14) treats hardness of the abdomen (see the section on sudden turmoil [cholera]).

Cì Liáo 次髎 (UB 32) treats hardness and distention below the heart.

Shí Mén 石門 (Rèn 5) treats abdominal (*Míng* also has pain [and]) hardness (see the section on abdominal fullness).

Huāng Mén 肓門 (UB 51) treats severe hardness below the heart and in the *Huāng* 肓.[85]

Shuǐ Fēn 水分 (Rèn 9) treats drum-like hardness of the abdomen (see the section on edema).

Zhì Shì 志室 (UB 52) treats abdominal hardness and tension.

Yīn Líng Quán 陰陵泉 (SP 9), Dì Jī 地機 (SP 8) (for both, see the section on edema), and Xià Wǎn (Rèn 10) treat hardness of the abdomen (see the section on abdominal pain).

85. *Huāng* 肓 indicates the region below the heart and above the diaphragm.

腹脹 449
漏下 728
水腫 459
腹痛 441
大便 235
積聚 437

膀胱俞主堅結積聚(《千》)。上管主心下堅，積聚冷脹。肓門主心下大堅。丘墟主大疝腹堅。期門主腹大堅(見腹脹)。衝陽主腹大，不嗜食。解溪主腹大下重，又主厥氣上柱腹大。

Páng Guāng Shù 膀胱俞 (UB 28) governs hard binds, accumulations, and gatherings (*Qiān*《千》).

Shàng Guǎn 上管 (Rèn 13) governs hardness below the heart, accumulations and gatherings, and cold distention.

Huāng Mén 肓門 (UB 51) governs great hardness below the heart.

Qiū Xū 丘墟 (GB 40) governs great *shàn*-mounting and abdominal hardness.

Qī Mén 期門 (LV 14) governs enlarged and hard abdomen (see the section on abdominal fullness).

Chōng Yáng 衝陽 (ST 42) governs abdomen enlargement with no desire to eat.

Jiě Xī 解溪 (ST 41) governs abdomen enlargement and lower body heaviness; it also governs reverse qì ascent and blockage with abdomen enlargement.

三里療腹滿堅塊，不能食，胃氣不足，反胃，胸脅腹積氣(《明》)。天樞療腹大堅(《下》見漏下)。小兒腹大，灸分水(見水腫)。分水療腹痛，胃脹堅硬(《明》見腹痛)。石關主心堅滿(《千》見大便不通)，積如盤(積聚)。

Sān Lǐ 三里 (ST 36 or LI 10) cures abdominal fullness with hard lumps, inability to eat, insufficiency of stomach qì, stomach reflux, and qì accumulation in the chest, rib-sides and abdomen (*Míng*《明》).

Tiān Shū 天樞 (ST 25) cures enlarged and hard abdomen (see the section on spotting of blood in *Xià*《下》).

Enlarged abdomen in children: Apply moxibustion on Fēn Shuǐ 分水 (Rèn 9) (see the section on edema).

Fēn Shuǐ (Rèn 9) cures abdominal pain, and stomach distention and hardness (see the section on abdominal pain in *Míng*).

Shí Guān 石關 (KI 18) cures hardness and fullness of the heart (see the section on constipation in *Qiān*) and accumulations that appear like a plate (accumulations and gatherings).

水腫 459
陰縮 198
腹脹 449

# 4.44
## *Gŭ Zhàng (Yú Jiàn Fù Zhàng)*
## 鼓脹（餘見腹脹）

### Drum distention
**(for further discussion, see the section on abdominal fullness)**

水分治腹堅如鼓，水腫腹（《明》作腸）鳴，胃虛脹不嗜食，繞臍痛，衝胸不息（《銅》）。神闕（見水腫）、公孫治腹虛脹如鼓。水分治腹堅如鼓。《明下》云：療鼓脹（見水腫）。復溜治腹中雷鳴，腹脹如鼓，四肢腫，十水病（《明下》同）。

Shuǐ Fēn 水分 (Rèn 9) treats drum-like hardness of the abdomen, edema and abdominal (*Míng*《明》says intestinal) rumbling, vacuity distention of the stomach, no desire to eat, pain around the umbilicus, and [qì] surging upward into the chest with inability to breathe (*Tóng*《銅》).

Shén Quē 神闕 (Rèn 8) (see the section on edema) and Gōng Sūn 公孫 (SP 4) treat drum-like abdominal distention due to vacuity.

Shuǐ Fēn (Rèn 9) treats drum-like abdominal hardness. *Míng Xià*《明下》says: It treats drum distention (see the section on edema).

Fù Liū 復溜 (KI 7) treats thunderous rumbling in the abdomen, drum-like abdominal distention, swollen extremities, and the ten water diseases[86] (*Míng Xià* agrees).

章門療身黃羸瘦，四肢怠惰，腹脹如鼓，兩脅積氣如卵石（《明下》）。中封、四滿主鼓脹（《千》見陰縮）。太白、公孫主腹鼓脹，腹中氣大滿（見腹脹）。三陰交、石門主水脹，小腹皮敦敦然（見水腫）。

Zhāng Mén 章門 (LV 13) cures yellow body, emaciation, fatigued limbs, drum-like abdominal distention, and accumulations of qì under both rib-sides that appear like pebbles (*Míng Xià*).

Zhōng Fēng 中封 (LV 4) and Sì Mǎn 四滿 (KI 14) govern drum distention (see the section on wilted and retracted genitals in *Qiān*《千》).

86. The ten water diseases refer to ten kinds of edema, related to various organs.

水腫
459

Tài Bái 太白 (SP 3) and Gōng Sūn 公孫 (SP 4) govern drum distention of the abdomen and great fullness of qì in the abdomen (see the section on abdominal fullness).

Sān Yīn Jiāo 三陰交 (SP 6) and Shí Mén 石門 (Rèn 5) govern water distention and thickening of the skin of smaller abdomen (see the section on edema).

甄權云：分水主鼓脹腸鳴（ 水腫 ）。鼓脹：中封二百壯 。賁豚冷氣，心間伏梁，狀如覆杯，冷結諸氣：針中管八分，留七呼，瀉五吸，疾出針；須灸，日二七壯，至四百止，忌房室 。心腹諸病堅滿煩痛，憂思結氣，寒冷霍亂，心痛吐下，食不消，腸鳴泄利：太倉中管百壯 。心下堅，積聚冷熱腹脹：上管百壯（ 《 千翼 》 ）。

Zhēn Quán said: Fēn Shuǐ 分水 (Rèn 9) governs drum distention and intestinal rumbling (see the section on edema).

Drum distention: Apply two hundred cones of moxibustion on Zhōng Fēng 中封 (LV 4).

Running-piglet cold qì, deep-lying beams in the heart shaped like an overturned cup; all qì binds and coldness: needle Zhōng Guǎn 中管 (Rèn 12) 8 fēn deep; retain the needle for seven respirations, drain for five respirations; remove the needle immediately. Moxibustion also is needed: Apply two times seven cones of moxibustion daily and stop at four hundred cones. Sexual activities should be avoided.

All diseases of the heart and abdomen with hardness, fullness, vexation, and pain; anxiety and [excessive] thought, with qì binds, coldness and sudden turmoil, heart pain with vomiting and diarrhea, non-dispersion of food, intestinal rumbling and diarrhea: Apply a hundred cones of moxibustion on Tài Cāng Zhōng Guǎn 太倉中管 (Rèn 12).

Hardness below the heart, accumulations and gatherings, cold and heat, and abdominal distention: Apply a hundred cones of moxibustion on Shàng Guǎn 上管 (Rèn 13) (*Qiān Yì*《 千翼 》).

## 4.45

## *Shuǐ Zhǒng (Zá Zhǒng, Sì Zhī Zhǒng, Shí Shuǐ)*

# 水腫（雜腫　四肢腫　石水）

## Edema

**(Miscellaneous swelling, swollen limbs, stone water)**

水通身腫：灸足第二指上一寸，隨年壯；又灸兩手大指縫頭七壯（《千》）。虛勞浮腫：灸太衝百壯，又灸腎俞。凡頭目癰腫，留飲胸脅支滿：刺陷谷，出血立已。陷谷、列缺主面目癰腫。陽陵泉、公孫主頭面腫。完骨、巨窌主頭面氣，胕腫。天樞、豐隆、厲兌、陷谷、衝陽主面浮腫。中府、間使、合谷主面腹腫。

Generalized edema: Apply the same number of cones of moxibustion as the patient's age on the site that is 1 cùn above [proximal to] the second toe; also apply seven cones of moxibustion at the end of the crease of the thumbs (*Qiān*《千》).

Vacuity-taxation with puffy swelling: Apply a hundred cones of moxibustion on Tài Chōng 太衝 (LV 3) and Shèn Shù 腎俞 (UB 23).

All swollen welling-abscesses on the head and eyes, with lodged rheum, and propping fullness of the chest and rib-sides: needle and bleed Xiàn Gǔ 陷谷 (ST 43) to cure the disease immediately.

Xiàn Gǔ (ST 43) and Liè Quē 列缺 (LU 7) govern swollen welling-abscesses on the face and eyes.

Yáng Líng Quán 陽陵泉 (GB 34) and Gōng Sūn 公孫 (SP 4) govern head and facial swelling.

Wán Gǔ 完骨 (GB 12) and Jù Liáo 巨窌 (ST 3) govern head and facial qì [swelling] and swelling of the skin.

Tiān Shū 天樞 (ST 25), Fēng Lóng 豐隆 (ST 40), Lì Duì 厲兌 (ST 45), Xiàn Gǔ (ST 43), and Chōng Yáng 衝陽 (ST 42) govern puffy facial swelling.

Zhōng Fǔ 中府 (LU 1), Jiān Shǐ 間使 (PC 5), and Hé Gǔ 合谷 (LI 4) govern swelling of the face and abdomen.

腹脹 449 解溪主風水，面腫，顏黑。氣舍主肩腫不得顧。三里主水，腹脹，皮腫。曲
瘰歷 泉主腹腫。陰谷主寒熱腹偏腫。大敦主大腹腫脹，臍腹邑邑。陰交、石門主
702 水脹，水氣行皮中，小腹皮敦敦然，小便黃，氣滿。屋翳主身腫，皮痛不可近衣。關門主身腫身重。天府主身脹逆息不得臥，風汗身腫，喘息多唾。

Jiě Xī 解溪 (ST 41) governs wind-water, facial swelling and dark complexion.

Qì Shě 氣舍 (ST 11) governs shoulder swelling with inability to turn the head.

Sān Lǐ 三里 (ST 36 or LI 10) governs water, abdominal distention, and swelling of the skin.

Qū Quán 曲泉 (LV 8) governs abdominal swelling.

Yīn Gǔ 陰谷 (KI 10) governs [sensations of] cold and heat and unilateral abdominal swelling.

Dà Dūn 大敦 (LV 1) governs swelling and distention in the larger abdomen, the umbilicus and abdomen are level with each other [due to swelling of the umbilicus].

Yīn Jiāo 陰交 (Rèn 7) and Shí Mén 石門 (Rèn 5) govern water distention with water qì flowing under the skin, thickening of the skin of smaller abdomen, yellow urine, and qì fullness.

Wū Yì 屋翳 (ST 15) governs generalized swelling and skin pain that cannot bear being touched by the clothes.

Guān Mén 關門 (ST 22) governs generalized swelling and heaviness.

Tiān Fǔ 天府 (LU 3) governs generalized distention, counterflow of the breath with inability to lie down, wind sweating, generalized swelling, panting, and frequent spitting.

上星治頭風面虛腫（《銅》）。囟會治目眩面腫。前頂治目眩，面赤腫，小兒頂腫。腦戶治目黃頭腫。水溝治水氣遍身腫（《明》云：若是水氣，唯得針此。若針餘穴，水盡即死。）。胃倉治水腫（見腹脹）。缺盆治水氣（見瘰歷）。屋翳治身體腫，皮膚痛不可近，及淫濼瘛瘲不仁。

Shàng Xīng 上星 (Dū 23) treats head wind and vacuity swelling of the face (*Tóng*《銅》).

Xìn Huì 囟會 (Dū 22) treats dizzy vision and facial swelling.

Qián Dǐng 前頂 (Dū 21) treats dizzy vision, red swollen face, and swelling of the vertex in children.

Nǎo Hù 腦戶 (Dū 17) treats yellow eyes and swollen head.

Shuǐ Gōu 水溝 (Dū 26) treats water qì and generalized swelling (*Míng*《明》says: if there is water qì, needle this point only; needling other points exhausts water and leads to death).

Wèi Cāng 胃倉 (UB 50) treats edema (see the section on abdominal fullness).

Quē Pén 缺盆 (ST 12) treats water qì (see the section on scrofula).

Wū Yì 屋翳 (ST 15) treats swelling of the body, skin pain that cannot bear being touched, aching and weakness, and tugging and slackening as well as numbness.

腎俞治身腫（見勞瘵）。建里治腹脹身腫。神闕治水腫鼓脹，腸鳴如流水聲。

勞瘵 188
腹脹 449
積聚 437
鼓脹 457
嘔吐 274

Shèn Shù 腎俞 (UB 23) treats generalized swelling (see the section on consumption).

Jiàn Lǐ 建里 (Rèn 11) treats abdominal distention and generalized swelling.

Shén Quē 神闕 (Rèn 8) treats edema, drum distention, and intestinal rumbling with sounds like flowing water.

中極、石門治水腫（見腹脹）。四滿治大腹有水（見積聚）。章門治腹腫，脊強，四肢傷惰。涌泉治男子如蠱，女子如妊娠，五指端盡痛，足不得踐地（陰谷同上）。三里治水氣（《明》同）。復溜治十水病（見鼓脹）。維道治水腫，不嗜食（見嘔吐）。地機治丈夫溏泄腹脅脹，水腫腹堅，不嗜食，小便不利。陰陵泉治腹中寒，不嗜食，脇下滿，水脹腹堅，喘逆不得臥，腰痛難俯仰。

Zhōng Jí 中極 (Rèn 3) and Shí Mén 石門 (Rèn 5) treat edema (see the section on abdominal fullness).

Sì Mǎn 四滿 (KI 14) treats water in the greater abdomen (see the section on accumulations and gatherings).

Zhāng Mén 章門 (LV 13) treats abdominal swelling, stiffness of the spine, and fatigued limbs.

Yǒng Quán 涌泉 (KI 1) treats [abdominal distention] in males that appears like *gǔ* 蠱; while in females it appears like pregnancy; pain at the tips of all the toes so the feet cannot step on the ground (Yīn Gǔ 阴谷 (KI 10) is the same).

Sān Lǐ 三里 (ST 36 or LI 10) treats water qì (*Míng*《明》agrees).

Fù Liū 復溜 (KI 7) treats the ten water diseases (see the section on drum distention).

Wéi Dào 維道 (GB 28) treats edema with no desire to eat (see the section on vomiting).

Dì Jī 地機 (SP 8) treats sloppy diarrhea in males as well as distention of the abdomen and rib-sides, edema, hardness of the abdomen, no desire to eat, and inhibited urination.

鼓脹 457 無子 721 Yīn Líng Quán 陰陵泉 (SP 9) treats cold in the abdomen, no desire to eat, fullness below the diaphragm, water distention, abdominal hardness, panting counterflow with inability to lie down, and lower back pain with inability to bend forward and backward.

陷谷治面目浮腫，及水病善噫，腸鳴腹痛。分水療腹腫不能食。若是水病，灸大良，《明下》云：療水病腹腫，繞臍痛，衝胸不得息。甄權云：主水氣浮腫，鼓脹，腸鳴如雷聲，時上衝心(《銅》見鼓脹)。曲骨療水病脹滿(《下》)。小兒水氣，四肢盡腫，及腹大：灸分水三壯。胃倉主水腫臚脹，食飲不下，惡寒(《千》)。

Xiàn Gŭ 陷谷 (ST 43) treats puffy swelling of the face and eyes, water disease, frequent belching, intestinal rumbling, and abdominal pain.

Fēn Shuĭ 分水 (Rèn 9) cures abdominal swelling with no desire to eat. If it is water disease, moxibustion is better. *Míng Xià*《明下》says: It cures water disease with abdominal swelling, pain around the umbilicus, [qì] surging into the chest, and inability to breathe. Zhēn Quán said: It governs water qì, puffy swelling, drum distention, intestinal rumbling with sounds like thunder, and [water qì] frequently surging upward into the heart (see the section on drum distention in *Tóng*《銅》).

Qū Gŭ 曲骨 (Rèn 2) cures water diseases with distention and fullness (*Xià*《下》).

Water qì in children, with swelling of the limbs and greater abdomen: Apply three cones of moxibustion on Fēn Shuĭ (Rèn 9).

Wèi Cāng 胃倉 (UB 50) governs edema, distention of the abdomen, difficulty getting food and drink down, and aversion to cold (*Qiān*《千》).

水溝主水腫，人中滿。關元主婦人小腹滿，石水(見無子)。章門主身潤，石水身腫。關元主小腹滿，石水。四滿、然谷主大腹石水。氣衝主大氣石水。豐隆主四肢腫，身濕(《銅》同)。豐隆、復溜主風逆四肢腫。列缺主汗出四肢腫。復溜治四肢腫(《銅》見鼓脹)。

Shuĭ Gōu 水溝 (Dū 26) governs edema and fullness of the philtrum.

Guān Yuán 關元 (Rèn 4) governs fullness of the smaller abdomen in women and stone water (see the section on infertility).

Zhāng Mén 章門 (LV 13) governs moistness of the body, stone water, and generalized swelling.

Guān Yuán (Rèn 4) governs fullness of the smaller abdomen and stone water.

Sì Mǎn 四滿 (KI 14) and Rán Gǔ 然谷 (KI 2) govern stone water in the greater abdomen.

Qì Chōng 氣衝 (ST 30) governs great qì and stone water.

Fēng Lóng 豐隆 (ST 40) govern swollen extremities and dampness of the body (*Tóng*《銅》agrees).

Fēng Lóng (ST 40) and Fù Liū 復溜 (KI 7) govern wind counterflow and swelling of the extremities.

Liè Quē 列缺 (LU 7) governs sweating and swelling of the limbs.

Fù Liū (KI 7) treats swollen limbs (see the section on drum distention in *Tóng*).

水腫惟得針水溝，若針餘穴，水盡即死，此《明堂》、《銅人》所戒也。庸醫多為人針水分，殺人多矣。若其它穴，亦有針得瘥者，特幸焉耳，不可為法也。或用藥，則禹餘糧元為第一（見《既效方》）。予屢見人服驗，故書於此。然灸水分，則最為要穴也。有裡醫為李生治水腫，以藥飲之，久之不效，以受其延待之勤。一日忽為灸水分與氣海穴，翌早顴面如削矣，信乎水分之能治水腫也。《明堂》固云：若是水病灸大良，蓋以此穴能分水，不使妄行云焉耳。但不知《明堂》又云針四分者，豈治其它病當針四分耶？

[Author's notes:] Only needle Shuǐ Gōu 水溝 (Dū 26) for edema; if other points are needled, people will die after water becomes exhausted. This is the contraindication from *Míng Táng*《明堂》and *Tóng Rén*《銅人》. Vulgar healers usually needle Shuǐ Fēn 水分 (Rèn 9) on patients, so they have killed a lot of people. If other points are needled, it will be very lucky for these people to recover afterwards. This cannot be set as the standard principle.

When using herbs, *yú yú liáng* 禹餘糧 (Limonite) is the first choice (see *Jì Xiào Fāng*《既效方》). I have always seen its effectiveness after people take it, so I put it here.

But the most important thing is to apply moxibustion on Shuǐ Fēn (Rèn 9). There was fellow doctor who treated Lǐ Shēng for edema. There was no effect after using herbs for a long time, but [Lǐ Shēng's family] still retained his services. One day, the doctor applied moxibustion on Shuǐ Fēng (Rèn 9) and Qì Hǎi 氣海 (Rèn 6). The next morning, the bones were more visible in Lǐ Shēng's face. Don't you believe that Shuǐ Fēng (Rèn 9) can treat edema? *Míng Táng*《明堂》says: It is better to apply moxibustion for water disease. This is because this point can separate water and does not let the water flow improperly. But I do not know why *Míng Táng* also says to needle it 4 fēn deep. Is needling it 4 fēn deep for treating other diseases?

百病水腫：腎俞百壯，胃倉隨年。水腫：陷谷隨年。水腫上下：陰交百壯。水腫脹：曲骨百壯。大腹：陰市隨年。人中滿唇腫，及水腫大水：臍中、石門百壯。風水：上廉隨年。水腫不得臥：陰陵泉百壯。石水：灸然谷、氣衝、四滿、章門。水分主水腫，腹滿不能食，堅硬；日七壯至四百止，忌針，針水盡即死，水病灸至瘥止（《千翼》）。

The hundred diseases with edema: Apply a hundred cones of moxibustion on Shèn Shù 腎俞 (UB 23); or apply the same number of cones of moxibustion as the patient's age on Wèi Cāng 胃倉 (UB 50).

Edema: Apply the same number of cones of moxibustion as the patient's age on Xiàn Gǔ 陷谷 (ST 43).

Edema above and below: Apply a hundred cones of moxibustion on Yīn Jiāo 陰交 (Rèn 7).

Edema with distention: Apply a hundred cones of moxibustion on Qū Gǔ 曲骨 (Rèn 2).

Greater abdomen: Apply the same number of cones of moxibustion as the patient's age on Yīn Shì 陰市 (ST 33).

Fullness of the philtrum, swollen lips, and severe edema: Apply a hundred cones of moxibustion on Qí Zhōng 臍中 (Rèn 8) and Shí Mén 石門 (Rèn 5).

Wind-water: Apply the same number of cones of moxibustion as the patient's age on Shàng Lián 上廉 (ST 37 or LI 9).

Edema with inability to lie down: Apply a hundred cones of moxibustion on Yīn Líng Quán 陰陵泉 (SP 9).

Stone water: Apply moxibustion on Rán Gǔ 然谷 (KI 2), Qì Chōng 氣衝 (ST 30), Sì Mǎn (KI 14), and Zhāng Mén 章門 (LV 13).

Shuǐ Fēn 水分 (Rèn 9) governs edema, abdominal fullness, inability to eat, and [abdominal] hardness. Apply seven cones of moxibustion daily and stop at four hundred cones. Needling is contraindicated. People will die after needling it because this exhausts the water. Keep applying moxibustion on it until the disease is cured (*Qiān Yì*《千翼》).

# *Zhēn Jiǔ Zī Shēng Jīng*
# 《針灸資生經·第五》

淋
222
瘧
301
水腫
459
瀉
243
疝
213

# 5.01
## *Qí Tòng*
# 臍痛
## Umbilical pain

中極療臍下塊如覆杯（《明》見淋）。《銅》云：結如覆杯（見淋）。關元治臍下疞痛，小便赤澀，不覺遺瀝，小便處痛狀如散火，溺血，暴疝痛，臍下結血，狀如覆杯（《明》同），轉胞不得（《銅》）。陰交治臍下疞痛，女子月事不絕，帶下，產後惡露不止，繞臍冷痛。中封（見瘧）、水分（見水腫）、神闕（見瀉）治繞臍痛。曲泉主痛引臍中（《千》見疝）。

Zhōng Jí 中極 (Rèn 3) cures lumps below the umbilicus that appear like an overturned cup (see the section on dribbling in *Míng*《明》). *Tóng*《銅》 says: gatherings that appear like an overturned cup (see the section on dribbling).

Guān Yuán 關元 (Rèn 4) treats colicky pain below the umbilicus, inhibited urination with red urine, uncontrollable dribbling after urination, pain of the genital area that feels like scattered fire, bloody urine, violent *shàn*-mounting pain, gatherings of blood below the umbilicus that appear like an overturned cup (*Míng* agrees), and shifted bladder with inability [to urinate] (*Tóng*).

Yīn Jiāo 陰交 (Rèn 7) treats colicky pain below the umbilicus, incessant menstruation in women, abnormal vaginal discharge, persistent flow of lochia after childbirth, and cold pain around the umbilicus.

Zhōng Fēng 中封 (LV 4) (see the section on malaria), Shuǐ Fēn 水分 (Rèn 9) (see the section on edema), and Shén Quē 神闕 (Rèn 8) (see the section on diarrhea) treat pain around the umbilicus.

Qū Quán 曲泉 (LV 8) governs pain radiating to the umbilicus (see the section on *shàn*-mounting in *Qiān*《千》).

予舊苦臍中疼則欲溏瀉。常以手中指按之，少止。或正瀉下，亦按之，則不疼。它日灸臍中，遂不疼矣。後又嘗溏利不已，灸之則止。凡臍疼者，宜灸神闕。

In the past I suffered pain of my umbilicus and had sloppy diarrhea. The pain was less when I pressed my umbilicus with my middle finger. Or the pain would stop when I pressed my umbilicus during the diarrhea. The pain stopped one day after I applied moxibustion on the umbilicus. The sloppy diarrhea occurred again later and stopped after moxibustion. So it is appropriate to apply moxibustion on Shén Quē 神闕 (Rèn 8) for pain of the umbilicus.

積氣 440
腹痛 441
冷氣 678
瀉 243
脅痛 476
積聚 437

關門治氣游走，夾臍急（見積氣）。下脘治臍上厥氣動（見腹痛）。氣海治臍下冷氣上衝心，血結成塊，狀如覆杯，小便赤澀。腹結治繞臍痛，上搶心（《千》同），腹寒，泄利咳逆。天樞治夾臍切痛，時上衝心煩滿，嘔吐霍亂。《明下》云：冷氣臍痛（見冷氣）。《千》云：冬感寒臍痛（見瀉）。

Guān Mén 關門 (ST 22) treats qì that wanders with tension around the umbilicus (see the section on accumulation of qì).

Xià Wǎn 下脘 (Rèn 10) treats reverse qì moving in the umbilicus (see the section on abdominal pain).

Qì Hǎi 氣海 (Rèn 6) treats qì that accumulates into a lump that appears like an over-turned cup and inhibited urination with red urine.

Fù Jié 腹結 (SP 14) treats pain around the umbilicus that surges up to the heart (*Qiān*《千》 agrees), cold abdomen, diarrhea, and coughing counterflow.

Tiān Shū 天樞 (ST 25) treats cutting pain around the umbilicus sometimes surging up to the heart, vexation of the heart and fullness, vomiting and sudden turmoil [cholera]. *Míng Xià*《明下》says: It treats cold qì and umbilical pain (see the discussion of cold qì). *Qiān* says: It treats umbilical pain due to cold invading in winter (see the section on diarrhea).

外陵主心如懸，下引臍腹痛（《千》見腹痛）。上廉治夾臍腹痛（見脅痛）。四滿治臍下切痛（見積聚）。分水療水腫繞臍痛（《明下》）。小兒臍腫：灸腰後對臍骨節間三壯。然谷主兒臍風口不開（《銅》同），善驚。

Wài Líng 外陵 (ST 26) governs a feeling like the heart is suspended with pain radiating into the umbilical region (see the section on abdominal pain in *Qiān*).

Shàng Lián 上廉 (ST 37 or LI 9) treats abdominal pain around the umbilicus (see the section on pain of the chest and rib-side pain).

Sì Mǎn 四滿 (KI 14) treats cutting pain below the umbilicus (see the section on accumulations and gatherings).

Fēn Shuǐ 分水 (Rèn 9) cures edema and pain around the umbilicus (*Míng Xià*).

癥瘕 435
腹寒 678
疝 213

Swollen umbilicus in children: Apply three cones of moxibustion on the space between the joint of the lower back at the level of the umbilicus.

Rán Gǔ 然谷 (KI 2) governs clenched jaws in children due to umbilical wind (*Tóng*《銅》agrees) and susceptibility to fright.

繞臍絞痛：灸天樞百壯(《千》見癥瘕)。臍下絞痛：灸關元百壯(見腹寒熱)。臍中、石門等主疝繞臍。臍中、石門、天樞主臍疝繞臍。蠡溝療臍中積氣(《千》並見疝)。

Colicky pain around the umbilicus: Apply a hundred cones of moxibustion on Tiān Shū 天樞 (ST 25) (*Qiān*《千》see the section on concretions and conglomerations).

Colicky pain below the umbilicus: Apply a hundred cones of moxibustion on Guān Yuán 關元 (Rèn 4) (see the section on [sensations of] cold and heat in abdomen).

Qí Zhōng 臍中 (Rèn 8), Shí Mén 石門 (Rèn 5) and so forth govern *shàn*-mounting around the umbilicus.

Qí Zhōng (Rèn 8), Shí Mén (Rèn 5), and Tiān Shū (ST 25) govern *shàn*-mounting around the umbilicus.

Lí Gōu 蠡溝 (LV 5) cures accumulated qì in the umbilicus (also see the section on prominent *shàn*-mounting in *Qiān*)

心煩 335
胸脅 476

# 5.02
## *Yīng Tòng*
## 膺痛
## Chest pain

玉堂療胸滿膺痛（見心煩）。玉堂治胸膺骨疼。紫宮治胸膺骨疼。天溪治乳腫賁膺（並見胸脅痛）。

Yù Táng 玉堂 (Rèn 18) cures chest fullness and pain (see the section on vexation of the heart).

Yù Táng (Rèn 18) treats bone pain of the anterior chest.

Zǐ Gōng 紫宮 (Rèn 19) treats bone pain of the anterior chest.

Tiān Xī 天溪 (SP 18) treats breast swelling and [qì] rushing into the chest (see the section on pain of the chest and rib-sides).

霍亂
267

# 5.03

## *Xiōng Mǎn (Xiōng Xié Mǎn, Guī Xiōng)*

## 胸滿（胸脅滿　龜胸）

## Chest fullness

**(Fullness of the chest and rib-sides, pigeon chest)**

凡胸滿短氣，不得汗：皆針補手太陰以出汗（《千》又見霍亂）。神堂主胸腹滿。三間主胸滿腸鳴。陽溪、天容主胸滿不得息。曲池、人迎、神道、章門、中府（《明下》同）、臨泣、天池、璇璣、府俞主胸中滿。陽交主胸滿腫。鳩尾主胸滿咳逆。大泉主胸滿噭呼，胸膺痛。巨闕、間使主胸中淡淡。

Chest fullness and shortness of breath without sweating: Needle and supplement hand tàiyīn 手太陰 to produce sweating (also see the section on sudden turmoil [cholera] in *Qiān*《千》).

Shén Táng 神堂 (UB 44) governs fullness of the abdomen and chest.

Sān Jiān 三間 (LI 3) governs chest fullness and intestinal rumbling.

Yáng Xī 陽溪 (LI 5) and Tiān Róng 天容 (SI 17) govern chest fullness and inability to breathe.

Qū Chí 曲池 (LI 11), Rén Yíng 人迎 (ST 9), Shén Dào 神道 (Dū 11), Zhāng Mén 章門 (LV 13), Zhōng Fǔ 中府 (LU 1) (*Míng Xià*《明下》agrees), Lín Qì 臨泣 (GB 41 or GB 15), Tiān Chí 天池 (PC 1), Xuán Jī 璇璣 (Rèn 21), and Fǔ Shù 府俞 (KI 27)[1] govern fullness of the chest.

Yáng Jiāo 陽交 (GB 35) governs chest fullness and swelling.

Jiū Wěi 鳩尾 (Rèn 15) governs chest fullness and coughing counterflow.

Dà Quán 大泉 (LU 9)[2] governs chest fullness, crying out, and pain of the anterior chest.

Jù Quē 巨闕 (Rèn 14) and Jiān Shǐ 間使 (PC 5) govern a rolling sensation in the chest.

1. Fǔ Shù 府俞 is a mistake which is repeated in multiple versions of the source text. The proper name for KI 27 is Shù Fǔ 俞府.

2. Dà Quán 大泉 is a mistake also. The proper name for LU 9 is Tài Quán 太泉.

梁門主胸下積氣。期門、缺盆主胸中熱，息賁，脅下氣上。雲門主胸中暴逆。心俞、大杼主胸中鬱鬱。然谷主胸中寒，脈代，時不至寸口，小腹脹，上搶心。胸脅滿：灸期門（見心痛）。玉堂（見心煩）療胸滿膺痛（《明》）。三間療胸滿腹鳴。膻中（見肺癰）療胸中氣滿如塞。乳根療胸下滿悶。

心痛 312
心煩 335
肺癰 694
膝痛 539
腋腫 496
尸厥 531
喘 406
背痛 483

Liáng Mén 梁門 (ST 21) governs accumulation of qì under the chest.

Qī Mén 期門 (LV 14) and Quē Pén 缺盆 (ST 12) govern heat in the chest, rushing respiration, and qì ascent below the rib-sides.

Yún Mén 雲門 (LU 2) governs sudden counterflow in the chest.

Xīn Shù 心俞 (UB 15) and Dà Zhù 大杼 (UB 11) govern oppression of the chest.

Rán Gǔ 然谷 (KI 2) governs cold in the chest, intermittent pulse that sometimes cannot reach the *cùn kǒu* 寸口 area, and distention of the smaller abdomen that ascends to prod the heart.

Fullness of the chest and rib-sides: Apply moxibustion on Qī Mén 期門 (LV 14) (see the section on heart pain).

Yù Táng 玉堂 (Rèn 18) (see the section on vexation of the heart) cures chest fullness and pain (*Míng*《明》).

Sān Jiān 三間 (LI 3) cures chest fullness and abdominal rumbling.

Dàn Zhōng 膻中 (Rèn 17) (see the discussion of welling-abscess of the lungs) cures qì fullness of the chest with a stuffy feeling.

Rǔ Gēn 乳根 (ST 18) cures fullness and oppression below the chest.

陽交（見膝痛）、臨泣（見腋腫）治胸滿。委陽治胸滿膨膨（《銅》見尸厥）。璇璣治胸皮滿痛（《明》同）。《下》云：胸脅支滿。俞府治胸滿（見喘）。商陽治胸中氣滿，喘咳支腫。膈關治胸中噎悶（見背痛）。陽溪、神封治胸滿不得息，咳逆。肺俞治胸中氣滿，背僂如龜，腰強頭目眩，令人失顏色。輒筋治胸中暴滿，不得臥，喘息。

Yáng Jiāo 陽交 (GB 35) (see the section on knee pain) and Lín Qì 臨泣 (GB 41) (see the section on swelling of the axilla) treat chest fullness.

Wěi Yáng 委陽 (UB 39) treats chest fullness with a feeling of inflation (see the section on death-like reversal in *Tóng*《銅》).

Xuán Jī 璇璣 (Rèn 21) treats fullness and pain of the skin of the chest (*Míng* agrees). *Xià*《下》says: It treats propping fullness of the chest and rib-sides.

嘔吐 274
腹脹 449
肩痛 486
膈痛 481

Shù Fǔ 俞府 (KI 27) treats chest fullness (see the section on panting).

Shāng Yáng 商陽 (LI 1) treats qì fullness of the chest, panting and cough with propping swelling.

Gé Guān 膈關 (UB 46) treats dysphagia and oppression in the chest (see the section on back pain).

Yáng Xī 陽溪 (LI 5) and Shén Fēng 神封 (KI 23) treat chest fullness with inability to breathe and coughing counterflow.

Fèi Shù 肺俞 (UB 13) treats qì fullness of the chest, a turtle-like hump on the back, stiffness of the lower back, and dizziness in the head and eyes which makes the person lose his normal color [look pale].

Zhé Jīn 輒筋 (GB 23) treats sudden fullness of the chest, inability to sleep, and panting.

膈俞治胸滿支腫（見嘔吐）。胃俞治胸脅支滿（見腹脹）。涌泉、神堂治胸腹滿（見肩痛）。中庭治胸脅支滿，噎塞食不下，嘔吐，食還出。雲門治喉痹，胸煩滿，氣上衝心，咳喘不得息，胸脅短氣，肩痛，不得舉臂。天池治胸中有聲（見膈痛）。曲池治胸中煩滿。胸鄉治胸脅滿，引胸背痛，不得（《明下》有臥字）轉側。周榮治胸脅滿，不得俯仰，食不下，咳唾稠膿（《明下》同）。

Gé Shù 膈俞 (UB 17) treat chest fullness and propping swelling (see the section on vomiting).

Wèi Shù 胃俞 (UB 21) treats propping fullness of the chest and rib-sides (see the section on abdominal fullness).

Yǒng Quán 涌泉 (KI 1) and Shén Táng 神堂 (UB 44) treat fullness of the chest and abdomen (see the section on aching pain of the shoulders [and back]).

Zhōng Tíng 中庭 (Rèn 16) treats propping fullness of the chest and rib-sides, dysphagia with difficulty getting food down, and vomiting with the food coming out again.

Yún Mén 雲門 (LU 2) treats throat *bì*-impediment, vexation and fullness of the chest, qì surging upward to the heart, cough and panting with inability to breathe, shortness of breath in the chest and rib-sides, and shoulder pain with inability to lift the shoulders.

Tiān Chí 天池 (PC 1) treats sounds in the chest (see the section on pain of the diaphragm).

Qū Chí 曲池 (LI 11) treats vexation and fullness of the chest.

Xiōng Xiāng 胸鄉 (SP 19) treats fullness of the chest and rib-sides with pain radiating to the chest and back, and inability to turn to the sides (*Míng Xià*《明下》has while lying down).

腸鳴 263
心痛 312
上氣 420
喘 406
心煩 335
反胃 289

Zhōu Róng 周榮 (SP 20) treats fullness of the chest, inability to bend forward or backward, difficulty getting food down, and coughing and spitting sticky pus (*Míng Xià*《明下》agrees).

彧中治胸脅支滿，咳逆喘，不能食(《明》同)。神藏治胸脅支滿，咳逆喘不得息，嘔吐，胸滿，不嗜食(《明》同)。氣戶治胸脅支滿，喘逆上氣，胸背急，不得息，不知食味。

Yù Zhōng 彧中 (KI 26) treats propping fullness of the chest, coughing counterflow, panting, and inability to get the food down (*Míng*《明》agrees).

Shén Cáng 神藏 (KI 25) treats propping fullness of the chest and rib-sides, coughing counterflow, panting with inability to breathe, vomiting and retching, chest fullness, and no desire to eat (*Míng* agrees).

Qì Hù 氣戶 (ST 13) treats propping fullness of the chest and rib-sides, panting counterflow and qì ascent, tension of the chest and back, inability to breathe, and food seems to have no taste.

食竇治胸脅支滿，膈間雷鳴。靈墟治胸脅支滿，痛引胸不得息，咳逆嘔吐，胸滿，不嗜食(《明》同)。步郎治支滿，鼻塞不通，呼吸少氣，喘息，不得舉臂(《明》同)。章門治胸脅支滿(見腸鳴)。

Shí Dòu 食竇 (SP 17) treats propping fullness of the chest and rib-sides and thunderous rumbling in diaphragm.

Líng Xū 靈墟 (KI 24) treats propping fullness of the chest and rib-sides, pain radiating to the chest with inability to breathe, coughing counterflow and vomiting, chest fullness, and no desire to eat (*Míng* agrees).

Bù Láng 步郎 (KI 22) treats propping fullness, nasal blockage, qì shortage while breathing, panting, and inability to lift the arms (*Míng* agrees).

Zhāng Mén 章門 (LV 13) treats propping fullness of the chest and rib-sides (see the section on intestinal rumbling).

庫房治胸脅支滿，咳逆上氣，多唾濁沫膿血。期門治產後胸脅支滿(見心痛)。外丘治胸脅脹滿。俠溪治胸脅支滿，寒熱汗不出。雲門療胸脅徹背痛(見上氣)。華蓋療胸脅滿痛引胸(《明》見喘)。紫宮(見心煩)、中庭(見反胃)、涌泉治胸脅支滿。通谷、章門、曲泉、膈俞、期門、食竇(《明下》同)、陷谷、石門主胸脅支滿(《千》)。

上氣 420

Kù Fáng 庫房 (ST 14) treats propping fullness of the chest and rib-sides, coughing counterflow with qì ascent, and spitting of turbid foam, pus, and blood.

Qī Mén 期門 (LV 14) treats propping fullness of the chest and rib-sides after childbirth (see the section on heart pain).

Wài Qiū 外丘 (GB 36) treats distention and fullness of the chest and rib-sides.

Xiá Xī 俠溪 (GB 43) treats propping fullness of the chest and rib-sides and [sensations of] cold and heat with absence of sweating.

Yún Mén 雲門 (LU 2) cures pain of the chest and rib-sides that penetrates through the back (see the section on qì ascent).

Huá Gài 華蓋 (Rèn 20) cures fullness and pain of the chest and rib-sides that radiates through the chest (see the section on panting in *Míng*《明》).

Zǐ Gōng 紫宮 (Rèn 19) (see the section on vexation of the heart), Zhōng Tíng 中庭 (Rèn 16) (see the section on stomach reflux), and Yǒng Quán 涌泉 (KI 1) treat propping fullness of the chest and rib-sides.

Tōng Gǔ 通谷 (KI 20), Zhāng Mén 章門 (LV 13), Qū Quán 曲泉 (LV 8), Gé Shù 膈俞 (UB 17), Qī Mén 期門 (LV 14), Shí Dòu 食竇 (SP 17) (*Míng Xià*《明下》agrees), Xiàn Gǔ 陷谷 (ST 43), and Shí Mén 石門 (Rèn 5) govern propping fullness of the chest and rib-sides (*Qiān*《千》).

胃俞、三里、紫宮、華蓋、中庭、神藏、靈墟、俠溪、步廊、商陽、上廉、氣戶、周榮、上管、勞宮、涌泉、陽陵泉主胸脅柱滿。膽俞(《明下》同)、章門主脅痛不得臥，胸滿，嘔無所出。前谷主咳而胸滿。陽氣逆上滿胸：取天容(見上氣)。肺俞、巨闕主胸滿(見上氣)。

Wèi Shù 胃俞 (UB 21), Sān Lǐ 三里 (ST 36), Zǐ Gōng 紫宮 (Rèn 19), Huá Gài 華蓋 (Rèn 20), Zhōng Tíng 中庭 (Rèn 16), Shén Cáng 神藏 (KI 25), Líng Xū 靈墟 (KI 24), Xiá Xī 俠溪 (GB 43), Bù Láng 步郎 (KI 22), Shāng Yáng 商陽 (LI 1), Shàng Lián 上廉 (LI 9), Qì Hù 氣戶 (ST 13), Zhōu Róng 周榮 (SP 20), Shàng Guǎn 上管 (Rèn 13), Láo Gōng 勞宮 (PC 8), Yǒng Quán 涌泉 (KI 1), and Yáng Líng Quán 陽陵泉 (GB 34) govern fullness stiffness and distention of the chest and rib-sides.

Dǎn Shù 膽俞 (UB 19) (*Míng Xià* agrees) and Zhāng Mén 章門 (LV 13) govern rib-side pain with inability to lie down, chest fullness, and vomiting with nothing come out [dry vomiting].

Qián Gǔ 前谷 (SI 2) governs cough and chest pain.

Yáng qì counterflow ascending to fill in the chest: Treat Tiān Róng 天容 (SI 17) (see the section on qì ascent).

Fèi Shù 肺俞 (UB 13) and Jù Quē 巨闕 (Rèn 14) govern chest fullness (see the section on qì ascent).

心痛 312
肩背 486
咳 414
尸厥 531

太泉治胸脅支滿(《銅》見心痛 )。天髎治胸中煩悶( 見肩背 )。肝俞療兩脅滿(《明》見咳 )。浮白療胸滿 。庫房療胸腹兩脅滿( 見咳 )。天池治寒熱，胸膈煩滿，頭痛，四肢不舉，腋下腫，上氣，胸中有聲，喉鳴 。膺窗治胸滿短氣 。

Tài Quán 太泉 (LU 9) propping fullness of the chest and rib-sides (see the section on heart pain in *Tóng*《銅》).

Tiān Liáo 天髎 (SJ 15) treats vexation and oppression of the chest (see the section on the aching pain of the shoulders [and back]).

Gān Shù 肝俞 (UB 18) cures fullness of both rib-sides (see the section on cough in *Míng*《明》).

Fú Bái 浮白 (GB 10) cures chest fullness.

Kù Fáng 庫房 (ST 14) cures fullness of the chest, abdomen, and both rib-sides (see the section on cough).

Tiān Chí 天池 (PC 1) treats [sensations of] cold and heat, vexation and fullness of the chest and diaphragm, headache, inability to lift the limbs, swelling of the axilla, qì ascent, sounds in the chest, and throat rales.

Yīng Chuāng 膺窗 (ST 16) treats chest fullness and shortness of breath.

魂門療胸背痛( 見尸厥 )。小兒龜胸，緣胎熱脹滿，攻胸膈所生；又緣乳母食熱面五辛 。胸轉起高：灸兩乳前各寸半，上兩行三骨罅間，六處各三壯 。春夏從下灸上，秋冬從上灸下 。若不依此法灸，十不愈一二 。

Hún Mén 魂門 (UB 47) cures pain of the chest and back (see the section on deathlike reversal).

Pigeon chest in children is due to fetal heat causing distention and fullness, and attacking the chest and diaphragm; or due to the wet nurse eating hot noodles and the five acrid foods. The [child's] chest becomes high: Apply three cones of moxibustion on each of the six sites that are 1.5 cùn medial to the nipples, moving up in two lines in the crevices [intercostals spaces] between the three

腹痛
441

[rib] bones.[3] Apply moxibustion from the bottom to the top during the spring and summer and from the top to the bottom during the fall and winter. If people do not follow this method of applying moxibustion, there is only ten to twenty percent rate of effectiveness.

# 5.04

## *Xiōng Xié Tòng (Xiōng Bì Tòng, Yú Jiàn Xiōng Mǎn)*

## 胸脅痛（胸痹痛　餘見胸滿）

## Pain of the chest and rib-sides

**(Chest *bì*-impediment pain; for further discussion, see the section on chest fullness)**

本神、顱息主胸脅相引，不得傾側（《千》）。太白主胸脅脹切痛。陽輔主胸脅痛。環跳、至陰主胸脅痛無常處，腰脅相引急痛。大包主胸脅中痛。豐隆（又見腹痛）、丘墟主胸痛如刺。胸脅滿心痛：灸期門隨年壯。乳根主胸下滿痛。膻中（百壯）、天井主胸痹心痛。大泉主胸膺痛。

Běn Shén 本神 (GB 13) and Lú Xī 顱息 (SJ 19) govern [pain] radiating between the chest and rib-sides and inability to turn over (*Qiān*《千》).

Tài Bái 太白 (SP 3) governs distention and cutting pain of the chest and rib-sides.

Yáng Fǔ 陽輔 (GB 38) governs pain of the chest and rib-sides.

Huán Tiào 環跳 (GB 30) and Zhì Yīn 至陰 (UB 67) govern wandering pain of the chest and rib-sides and acute pain between the lower back and rib-sides.

Dà Bāo 大包 (SP 21) governs pain of the chest and rib-sides.

Fēng Lóng 豐隆 (ST 40) (also see the section on abdominal pain) and Qiū Xū 丘墟 (GB 40) govern piercing chest pain.

Fullness of the chest and rib-sides with heart pain: Burn the same number of cones of moxibustion as the patient's age on Qī Mén 期門 (LV 14).

3. The description of the location is hard to understand. Here is a description in plain English: The first point is 1.5 cùn medial to the nipples, in the fourth intercostal space. There are two more points directly above the first point, in the third and second intercostal spaces. Since these points are bilateral, the text says there are six sites in all.

咳逆 417 傷寒 661 肺急 412

Rǔ Gēn 乳根 (ST 18) governs fullness and pain under the chest.

Dàn Zhōng 膻中 (Rèn 17) (a hundred cones) and Tiān Jǐng 天井 (SJ 10) govern chest *bì*-impediment with heart pain.

Dà Quán 大泉 (LU 9) governs pain of the anterior chest.

肺俞、雲門、中府、隱白、期門、魂門、大陵主胸中痛。少衝主胸痛，口熱。胸中痛引腰背，心下嘔逆，面無滋潤：灸上門隨年壯，穴在俠巨闕兩邊相去各半寸（一云一寸）。經渠、丘墟主胸背急，胸中膨膨。

Fèi Shù 肺俞 (UB 13), Yún Mén 雲門 (LU 2), Zhōng Fǔ 中府 (LU 1), Yǐn Bái 隱白 (SP 1), Qī Mén 期門 (LV 14), Hún Mén 魂門 (UB 47), and Dà Líng 大陵 (PC 7) govern pain of the chest.

Shào Chōng 少衝 (HT 9) governs chest pain and heat in the mouth.

Chest pain radiating to the lower and upper back, retching counterflow under the heart, and lack of moisture on the face: Apply the same number of cones of moxibustion as the patient's age on Shàng Mén 上門 (KI 20). The point is located 0.5 cùn (one source says 1.0 cùn) away from Jù Quē 巨闕 (Rèn 14) bilaterally.

Jīng Qú 經渠 (LU 8) and Qiū Xū 丘墟 (GB 40) govern tension of the chest and back and a feeling of inflation in the chest.

天溪治胸滿痛，乳腫賁膺，咳逆上氣，喉中作聲（《銅》）。肝俞治咳引胸痛（見咳逆）。少衝（見傷寒）、中府治胸痛（見肺急）。乳根治胸滿痛。華蓋治胸脅支滿，痛引胸中，咳逆上氣，喘不能言（《明下》同）。紫宮治胸脅支滿，胸膺骨疼，飲食不下，嘔逆，上氣煩心。

Tiān Xī 天溪 (SP 18) treats chest fullness and pain, breast swelling and [qì] rushing to the chest, coughing counterflow and qì ascent, and sounds in the throat (*Tóng*《銅》).

Gān Shù 肝俞 (UB 18) treats pain of the chest induced by coughing (see the section on coughing counterflow).

Shào Chōng 少衝 (HT 9) (see the section on cold damage) and Zhōng Fǔ 中府 (LU 1) treat chest pain (see the discussion of lung tension).

Rǔ Gēn (ST 18) treats chest fullness and pain.

Huá Gài 華蓋 (Rèn 20) treats propping fullness of the chest and rib-sides, pain radiating to the chest, coughing counterflow and qì ascent, and panting with inability to speak (*Míng Xià*《明下》agrees).

四肢 528
咳逆 417
上氣 420
咳 414

Zǐ Gōng 紫宮 (Rèn 19) treats propping fullness of the chest and rib-sides, bone pain of the anterior chest, difficulty getting drink and food down, retching counterflow, qì ascent, and vexation of the heart.

玉堂治胸滿不得喘息，胸膺骨疼，嘔吐寒痰，上氣煩心。幽門治胸中引痛，心下煩悶，逆氣裏急，支滿不嗜食，數咳，健忘。豐隆治厥逆，胸痛如刺，腹切痛。《明》云：氣刺不可忍（見四肢厥）。太淵治胸痹，逆氣寒厥，善噦嘔，飲水咳嗽，煩怒不得臥。

Yù Táng 玉堂 (Rèn 18) treats chest fullness with inability to breathe, bone pain of the anterior chest, vomiting of cold phlegm, qì ascent, and vexation of the heart.

Yōu Mén 幽門 (KI 21) treats pain radiating in the chest, vexation and oppression under the heart, counterflow qì with internal tension, propping fullness with no desire to eat, frequent cough, and forgetfulness.

Fēng Lóng 豐隆 (ST 40) treats reverse counterflow, piercing chest pain, and cutting pain of the abdomen. *Míng*《明》says: It treats an intolerable [sensation] of qì pricking (see the section on limb reversal).

Tài Yuān 太淵 (LU 9) treats chest *bì*-impediment, qì counterflow and reversal cold, frequent hiccups and retching, coughing when drinking water, vexation, and anger with inability to sleep.

胸痹引背，時寒：間使主之（《千》）。間使主胸痹，背相引。臨泣主胸痹不得息。魚際主痹走胸，不得息。浮白療胸滿胸痛（《明》見咳逆）。俞府療胸中痛（《下》）。胸痹心痛不得息，痛無常處：臨泣主之。胸痹：灸胸堂（見上氣）。廉泉（見上氣）、中府（見咳）主胸痛。

Chest *bì*-impediment radiating to the back and frequent coldness: Jiān Shǐ 間使 (PC 5) can govern it (*Qiān*《千》).

Jiān Shǐ (PC 5) governs chest *bì*-impediment that radiates to the back.

Lín Qì 臨泣 (GB 41 or GB 15) governs chest *bì*-impediment and inability to breathe.

Yú Jì 魚際 (LU 10) governs *bì*-impediment running through the chest and inability to breathe.

Fú Bái 浮白 (GB 10) cures chest fullness and pain (see the section on coughing counterflow in *Míng*).

Shù Fǔ 俞府 (KI 27) cures pain of the chest (*Xià*《下》).

Chest *bì*-impediment with heart pain, inability to breathe, and pain without a fixed location: Lín Qì (GB 41 or GB 15) can govern it.

乾嘔 279
太息 334
上氣 420
嘔吐 274
消渴 195
咳逆 417
寒熱 513

Chest *bì*-impediment: Apply moxibustion on Xiōng Táng 胸堂 (Rèn 17) (see the section on qì ascent).

Lián Quán 廉泉 (Rèn 23) (see the section on qì ascent) and Zhōng Fǔ 中府 (LU 1) (see the section on coughing) govern chest pain.

膽俞治胸脅不能轉（《銅》）。《明》云：胸脅滿（見乾嘔）。丘墟治胸脅滿痛，不得息。《明下》云：胸滿（見太息）。下廉治胸脅小腹痛。大包治胸脅痛（見上氣）。腎俞主兩脅引痛（《千》）。肝俞、脾俞、志室主兩脅急痛。支溝主脅腋急痛。中管、承滿主脅下堅痛。腕骨、陽谷主脅痛不得息。膽俞、章門主脅痛不得臥。竅陰主脅痛咳逆。

Dǎn Shù 膽俞 (UB 19) treats chest and rib-side [pain] with inability to turn (*Tóng*《銅》). *Míng*《明》says: It treats fullness of the chest and rib-sides (see the section on dry retching).

Qiū Xū 丘墟 (GB 40) treats fullness and pain of the chest and rib-sides and inability to breathe. *Míng Xià*《明下》says: It treats chest fullness (see the section on sighing).

Xià Lián 下廉 (LI 8 or ST 39) treats pain of the chest, rib-sides, and smaller abdomen.

Dà Bāo 大包 (SP 21) treats pain of the chest and rib-sides (see the section on qì ascent).

Shèn Shù 腎俞 (UB 23) governs pain radiating between both rib-sides (*Qiān*《千》).

Gān Shù 肝俞 (UB 18), Pí Shù 脾俞 (UB 20), and Zhì Shì 志室 (UB 52) govern acute pain in both rib-sides.

Zhī Gōu 支溝 (SJ 6) governs acute pain of the rib-sides and axilla.

Zhōng Guǎn 中管 (Rèn 12) and Chéng Mǎn 承滿 (ST 20) govern pain and hardness under the rib-sides.

Wàn Gǔ 腕骨 (SI 4) and Yáng Gǔ 陽谷 (SI 5) govern pain of the rib-sides and inability to breathe.

Dǎn Shù 膽俞 (UB 19) and Zhāng Mén 章門 (LV 13) govern pain of the rib-sides and inability to sleep.

Qiào Yīn 竅陰 (GB 44 or GB 11) govern pain of the rib-sides and coughing counterflow.

尺澤、少澤主短氣，脅痛心煩。關元、期門、少商主脅下脹。極泉治脅下滿痛（《銅》）。膈俞（見嘔吐）、中膂俞（見消渴）、竅陰（見咳逆）、陽谷、顱囟治脅痛（見寒熱）。肝俞治兩脅急痛（見咳逆）。腕骨治脅下痛，不得息。

勞瘵 188 胸滿 470

Chǐ Zé 尺澤 (LU 5) and Shào Zé 少澤 (SI 1) govern shortness of breath, pain of the rib-sides, and vexation of the heart.

Guān Yuán 關元 (Rèn 4), Qī Mén 期門 (LV 14) and Shào Shāng 少商 (LU 11) govern distention under the rib-sides.

Jí Quán 極泉 (HT 1) treats fullness and pain under the rib-sides (*Tóng*《銅》).

Gé Shù 膈俞 (UB 17) (see the section on vomiting), Zhōng Lǚ Shù 中膂俞 (UB 29) (see the section on wasting-thirst), Qiào Yīn 竅陰 (GB 44 or GB 11) (see the section on coughing counterflow), Yáng Gǔ 陽谷 (SI 5), and Lú Xìn 顱囟 (SJ 19) treat pain of the rib-sides (see the section on [sensations of] cold and heat).

Gān Shù 肝俞 (UB 18) treats acute pain in both rib-sides (see the section on coughing counterflow).

Wàn Gǔ 腕骨 (SI 4) treats pain of the rib-sides and inability to breathe.

腎俞治脅滿引小腹痛（見勞瘵）。上廉治飧泄，腹脅痛滿，狂走，俠臍腹痛，食不化，喘息不能行。太溪治腹脅痛連脊，手足厥冷。雲門療胸脅徹背痛。華蓋療胸脅痛（見胸滿）。三里主脅膈痛。

Shèn Shù 腎俞 (UB 23) treats rib-side fullness with pain radiating to the smaller abdomen (see the section on consumption).

Shàng Lián 上廉 (LI 9 or ST 37) treats swill diarrhea, pain and fullness of the abdomen and rib-sides, manic walking, abdominal pain around the umbilicus, non-transformation of food, and panting with inability to walk.

Tài Xī 太溪 (KI 3) treats pain of the abdomen and rib-sides radiating to the spine and reversal cold of the hands and feet.

Yún Mén 雲門 (LU 2) cures pain of the chest and rib-sides that penetrates through the back.

Huá Gài 華蓋 (Rèn 20) cures pain of the chest and rib-sides (see the section on chest fullness).

Sān Lǐ 三里 (ST 36 or LI 10) governs pain of the rib-sides and diaphragm.

## 5.05

## *Gé Tòng (Wǔ Yē, Qì Gěng)*

痰癖
433
喘
406
嘔吐
274

# 膈痛（五噎　氣哽）

## Pain of the diaphragm

**(The five chokings, qì dysphagia)**

承滿、乳根療膈氣（《明》見噎）。膻中療胸膈悶，咳嗽氣短，喉鳴（《下》）。膈俞療膈痛（見痰癖）。商陽療胸膈氣滿（見喘）。足臨泣療胸膈滿悶（《下》見頰痛）。胸中膈氣聚痛，好吐：灸厥陰俞隨年壯（《千》）。隱白（見嘔吐）、巨闕主膈中不利（《明下》同）。

Chéng Mǎn 承滿 (ST 20) and Rǔ Gēn 乳根 (ST 18) cure diaphragm qì [dysphagia] (see the discussion of dysphagia in *Míng*《明》).

Dàn Zhōng 膻中 (Rèn 17) cures oppression of the chest and diaphragm, coughing and shortness of breath, and throat rales (*Xià*《下》).

Gé Shù 膈俞 (UB 17) cures pain of the diaphragm (see the discussion of phlegm aggregations).

Shāng Yáng 商陽 (LI 1) cures qì fullness of the chest and diaphragm (see the section on panting).

Zú Lín Qì 足臨泣 (GB 41) cures fullness and oppression of the chest and diaphragm (see the discussion of cheek pain in *Xià*).

Diaphragm qì [dysphagia] with accumulated pain of the chest and frequent vomiting: Apply the same number of cones of moxibustion as the patient's age on Jué Yīn Shù 厥陰俞 (UB 14) (*Qiān*《千》).[4]

Yǐn Bái 隱白 (SP 1) (see the section on vomiting) and Jù Quē 巨闕 (Rèn 14) govern inhibited diaphragm (*Míng Xià*《明下》agrees).

4. This section says *xiōng zhōng gé qì jù tòng* 胸中膈氣聚痛 literally "In the chest - diaphragm qì accumulation pain." A few paragraphs down, the text says *xiōng gé zhōng qì* 胸膈中氣 literally "In the chest diaphragm qì." The meaning of these two phrases is a little unclear, as if perhaps one or both of them are corrupted. In both cases the treatment is applying the same number of cones as the age of the patient on Jué Yīn Shù 厥陰俞 (UB 14), so these must be two versions of the same treatment. If we assume the text is corrupted and try to make sense out of the two together, perhaps the solution is this: *xiōng gé zhōng qì jù tòng* 胸膈中氣聚痛 "Qì accumulation in the chest and diaphragm causing pain." However, it may also mean "Diaphragm qì [dysphagia] with pain."

痰 399
嘔吐 274
喉鳴 626
頭項 653
積氣 440
淋 222
霍亂 267
咳逆 420
嗽 414
吐瀉 271
脊 555
肺氣 412

食竇（《銅》同）主膈中雷鳴，察察隱隱，常有水聲（《明下》云：療膈間鳴，滀陸常有水聲）。胸膈中氣：灸闕俞隨年壯。天池治胸膈煩滿（《銅》見胸滿）。膻中治膈氣，嘔吐涎沫。率谷（見痰）、膈俞治膈胃寒痰（見嘔吐）。扶突等主氣哽（《千》見喉鳴）。

Shí Dòu 食竇 (SP 17) (*Tóng*《銅》agrees) governs thunderous rumbling in the diaphragm which is sometimes clear and sometimes indistinct with constant water sounds (*Míng Xià*《明下》says: It cures rumbling in the diaphragm with constant water sounds in *chù lù*).[5]

Qì [accumulation] in the chest and diaphragm: Apply the same number of cones of moxibustion as the patient's age on Jué Shù 厥俞 (UB 14).

Tiān Chí 天池 (PC 1) treats vexation and fullness of the chest and diaphragm (see chest fullness in *Tóng*《銅》).

Dàn Zhōng 膻中 (Rèn 17) treats diaphragm qì [dysphagia] and vomiting of drool and foam.

Shuài Gǔ 率谷 (GB 8) (see the section on phlegm [drool]) and Gé Shù 膈俞 (UB 17) treat cold phlegm in the diaphragm and stomach (see the section on vomiting).

Fú Tū 扶突 (LI 18) and so forth govern qì choking (see throat rales in *Qiān*《千》).

天突療氣鯁鯁（《明下》見頭項腫）。章門療噎（見積氣）。中庭治胸脅支滿噎塞（《銅》）。大鐘治食噎不下（見淋）。關衝（見霍亂）、天突治胸中氣噎（見咳逆上氣）。膻中治胸中如塞（《明下》，岐伯云：積氣成干噎）。天突（見嗽）、關衝（吐瀉）治氣噎（《明》）。乳根療膈氣，不下食，噎病。譩譆療久瘧，背氣滿悶，胸中氣噎（《下》）。神堂（見脊）、中府（見肺氣）療善噎（《下》）。

Tiān Tū 天突 (Rèn 22) cures qì dysphagia (see the discussion of swelling of the head and neck in *Míng Xià*).

Zhāng Mén 章門 (LV 13) cures choking (see the section on accumulation of qì).

Zhōng Tíng 中庭 (Rèn 16) treats propping fullness of the chest and rib-sides as well as dysphagia (*Tóng*).

Dà Zhōng 大鐘 (KI 4) treats choking on food with inability to get food down (see the section on dribbling).

Guān Chōng 關衝 (SJ 1) (see sudden turmoil [cholera]) and Tiān Tū (Rèn 22) treat qì dysphagia in the chest (see the section on coughing counterflow and qì ascent).

5. No definition or explanation has been found for these characters.

Dàn Zhōng 膻中 (Rèn 17) treats a feeling of blockage in the chest (in *Míng Xià*《 明下 》, Qí Bó said: accumulations of qì becoming dry choking).

Tiān Tū 天突 (Rèn 22) (see the section on cough) and Guān Chōng 關衝 (SJ 1) (see the section on vomiting and diarrhea) treat qì dysphagia (*Míng*《 明 》).

Rǔ Gēn 乳根 (ST 18) cures diaphragm qì [dysphagia], inability to get food down, and dysphagia disease.

Yī Xī 譩譆 (UB 45) cures enduring malaria, choking with fullness and oppression, and qì dysphagia in the chest (*Xià*《 下 》).

Shén Táng 神堂 (UB 44) (see the section on [pain of the lower back and] spine) and Zhōng Fǔ 中府 (LU 1) (see the section on lung qì) cure frequent dysphagia (*Xià*).

## 5.06

## *Bèi Tòng (Xiōng Bèi, Bèi Jǐ, Yú Jiàn Jiān Bèi Láo Zhài)*

# 背痛（胸背　背脊　餘見肩背勞瘵）

## Back pain

**(Chest and back; back and spine; for further discussion see the sections on shoulders and back, and consumption)**

經渠、丘墟主胸背急（《千》）。附分主背痛引頭（《明下》引頷）。膈關、秩邊、京骨主背惡寒痛，脊強難俯仰。崑崙主脊強，背尻骨重。膈俞治背痛惡寒，脊強俯仰難，食飲不下，嘔噦，多涎唾，胸噎悶（《銅》）。意舍治（《明下》有胸脅脹滿）背痛惡風寒，食不下，嘔吐。

Jīng Qú 經渠 (LU 8) and Qiū Xū 丘墟 (GB 40) govern tension of the chest and back (*Qiān*《 千 》).

Fù Fēn 附分 (UB 41) governs back pain radiating to the head (*Míng Xià* says radiating to chin).

Gé Guān 膈關 (UB 46), Zhì Biān 秩邊 (UB 54), and Jīng Gǔ 京骨 (UB 64) govern aversion to cold, pain of the back, and stiffness of the spine with difficulty bending forward and backward.

Kūn Lún 崑崙 (UB 60) governs stiffness of the spine, and a heavy sensation of the back and sacrum.

上氣 420
肩痛 486
胸脅滿 470
痃癖 433
瘧 301
寒熱 673

Gé Shù 膈俞 (UB 17) treats back pain with aversion to cold, stiffness of the spine with difficulty bending forward and backward, difficulty getting food and drink down, retching, and copious drool and spittle, dysphagia and a feeling of oppression in the chest (*Tóng*《銅》).

Yì Shě 意舍 (UB 49) treats (*Míng Xià*《明下》has distention and fullness of the chest and rib-sides) back pain, aversion to wind-cold, difficulty getting food down, and vomiting.

巨骨治背膊痛，胸中有瘀血，肩背不得屈伸而痛。魄戶治背膊痛（見上氣）。神堂治背脊強急（見肩痛）。氣戶治胸背急（見胸脅滿）。大椎治氣疰背膊拘急。承筋治腰背拘急。不容治胸背相引痛（見痃癖）。經渠治胸背拘急，胸滿膨膨（見瘧）。魚際治痹走胸背痛（見寒熱）。

Jù Gǔ 巨骨 (LI 16) treats back and arm pain, blood stasis in the chest, and back and shoulder pain with inability to flex and stretch.

Pò Hù 魄戶 (UB 42) treats back and arm pain (see the section on qì ascent).

Shén Táng 神堂 (UB 44) treats stiffness and tension of the back and spine (see the section on shoulder pain).

Qì Hù 氣戶 (ST 13) treats tension of the chest and back (see the section on fullness of the chest and rib-sides).

Dà Zhuī 大椎 (Dū 14) treats qì infixation and hypertonicity of the back and arms.

Chéng Jīn 承筋 (UB 56) treats hypertonicity of the lower and upper back.

Bù Róng 不容 (ST 19) treats pain radiating between the chest and back (see the section on strings and aggregations).

Jīng Qú 經渠 (LU 8) treats hypertonicity of the chest and back and chest fullness with a feeling of inflation (see the section on malaria).

Yú Jì 魚際 (LU 10) treats *bì*-impediment inducing pain of the chest and back (see the section on [sensations of] cold and heat).

魄戶療背胛悶（《明》見勞，《下》同）。《下》云：療肩膊間背，氣不能引顧，咳逆上喘。胃俞療背中氣上下行，脊痛腹鳴（《下》）。志室療背痛俯仰不得。背痛：灸巨闕等，或灸胸堂（《千》並上氣）。肺俞治背僂如龜背，生時被客風拍著脊骨達於髓所致：灸肺俞、心俞、膈俞各三壯。

Pò Hù 魄戶 (UB 42) cures oppression of the back and scapulae (see the section on taxation in *Míng*《明》; *Xià*《下》agrees). *Xià* says: It cures inability of qì to move between the shoulders and arms on the back and coughing counterflow with panting ascent [of qì].

Wèi Shù 胃俞 (UB 21) cures qì moving up and down in the back and pain of the spine with abdominal rumbling (*Xià*《下》).

Zhì Shì 志室 (UB 52) cures back pain and inability to bend forward and backward.

Back pain: Apply moxibustion on Jù Quē 巨闕 (Rèn 14) and so forth; or Xiōng Táng 胸堂 (Rèn 17) (also see the section on qì ascent in *Míng*《明》).

Fèi Shù 肺俞 (UB 13) treats hunchback that looks like a turtle's back. It is caused by visiting wind intruding into the spinal vertebrae that reaches into the marrow during childbirth: Apply three cones of moxibustion each on Fèi Shù 肺俞 (UB 13), Xīn Shù 心俞 (UB 15), and Gé Shù 膈俞 (UB 17).

譩譆療溫瘧、寒瘧、病瘧，背悶氣滿，腹脹氣眩（《明》），胸中痛引腰背（《千》見胸脅）。列缺主胸背寒栗（見肩痹）。魚際治痹走胸背痛（《銅》見寒熱）。雲門療胸脅徹背痛（《明》見上氣）。

Yī Xī 譩譆 (UB 45) cures warm malaria, cold malaria, malarial disease, a feeling of oppression and qì fullness on the back, abdominal qì distention with dizziness (*Míng*), and chest pain radiating to the lower and upper back (see the discussion of the chest and rib-sides in *Qiān*《千》).

Liè Quē 列缺 (LU 7) governs cold shivering in the chest and back (see the section on shoulder *bì*-impediment).

Yú Jì 魚際 (LU 10) treats *bì*-impediment inducing pain of the chest and back (see the section on [sensations of] cold and heat in *Tóng*《銅》).

Yún Mén 雲門 (LU 2) cures pain of the chest and rib-sides that penetrates through the back (see the section on qì ascent in *Míng*).

背疼乃作勞所致。技藝之人，與士女刻苦者，多有此患（士之書學，女之針指，皆刻苦而成背疼矣）。色勞者亦患之，晉之景公是也，惟膏肓為要穴。予嘗於膏肓之側，去脊骨四寸半，隱隱微疼，按之則疼甚。謾以小艾灸三壯，即不疼。它日復連肩上疼，卻灸肩疼處愈。方知千金方之阿是穴猶信云。（予每遇熱，膏肓穴所在多出冷汗，數年矣，因灸而愈。）

Back pain is caused by hard physical labor. Craftsmen and hard-working palace maids usually suffer this disease (the studying of scholars and the needlework of ladies both require painstaking work which can cause back pain). People who overindulge in sex can also suffer it. Duke Jǐng of *Jìn* was one of them. Gāo Huāng 膏肓 (UB 43) is the essential point. Once I had mild pain to the side of Gāo Huāng 膏肓 (UB 43), 4.5 cùn lateral to the vertebra; the pain was worse when pressed.

鼻衄 620 肺氣 412 腠理 557

It disappeared after casually applying three small cones of moxibustion. The pain occurred again another day and radiated to the shoulder. This was cured after applying moxibustion on the painful area of the shoulder. So I knew the *ā shì* 阿是 points mentioned in the *Qiān Jīn Fāng* are reliable.[6] (For several years, every time I encountered a fever, I had cold sweating at Gāo Huāng (UB 43). This was cured after moxibustion was applied.)

## 5.07

## *Jiān Bèi Suān Tòng (Jiān Bó, Jiān Bì, Yú Jiàn Bèi Tòng)*

# 肩背酸痛（肩膊　肩臂　餘見背痛）

### Aching pain of the shoulders and back

**(Shoulders and arms; for further discussion see the section on back pain)**

浮白治肩背不舉（《銅》）。神堂療肩背連胸痛，不可俯仰（《明下》）。商陽治肩背急，引缺盆痛（見鼻衄）。中府治肩背痛（見肺氣）。附分治肩背急（見腠理）。神堂治肩痛，胸腹滿，灑淅寒熱，脊背急（《明》同）。三焦俞治肩背急，腰脊強，不得俯仰。

Fú Bái 浮白 (GB 10) treats inability to raise the shoulders and back (*Tóng*《銅》).

Shén Táng 神堂 (UB 44) cures pain between the shoulders, back, and chest, and inability to bend forward and backward (*Míng Xià*《明下》).

Shāng Yáng 商陽 (LI 1) treats tension of the shoulders and back that induces pain of the empty basin [supraclavicular fossa] (see the section on nosebleeds).

Zhōng Fǔ 中府 (LU 1) treats pain of the shoulders and back (see the section on lung qì).

Fù Fēn 附分 (UB 41) treats tension of the back and shoulders (see the section on interstices).

Shén Táng 神堂 (UB 44) treats shoulder pain, fullness of the chest and abdomen, shivering with [sensations of] cold and heat, and tension of the spine and back (*Míng*《明》agrees).

Sān Jiāo Shù 三焦俞 (UB 22) treats tension of the shoulders and back, stiffness of the low back and spine, and inability to bend forward and backward.

6. *Qiān Jīn Fāng*《千金方》was the first book to mention *ā shì* 阿是 or ouch points.

涌泉主肩背頸項痛（《千》）。天牖、缺盆、神道、大杼、天突、水道、巨骨主肩背痛。膈俞、譩譆、京門、尺澤主肩背寒痙，肩胛內廉痛。天柱治肩背痛欲折（《銅》）。肝俞（見腰痛）療肩疼（《明》）。曲垣治肩痛，周痹（《明》同）氣注，肩膊拘急疼悶（《銅》）。 胸滿 470 風痹 377

Yǒng Quán 涌泉 (KI 1) governs pain of the shoulders, back, neck, and nape (*Qiān*《千》).

Tiān Yǒu 天牖 (SJ 16), Quē Pén 缺盆 (ST 12), Shén Dào 神道 (Dū 11), Dà Zhù 大杼 (UB 11), Tiān Tū 天突 (Rèn 22), Shuǐ Dào 水道 (ST 28), and Jù Gǔ 巨骨 (LI 16) govern pain of the shoulders and back.

Gé Shù 膈俞 (UB 17), Yī Xī 譩譆 (UB 45), Jīng Mén 京門 (GB 25), and Chǐ Zé 尺澤 (LU 5) govern cold and spasms of the shoulders and back, and pain of the medial aspect of the scapula.

Tiān Zhù 天柱 (UB 10) treats pain of the shoulders and back, feeling like they are broken (*Tóng*《銅》).

Gān Shù 肝俞 (UB 18) (see lower back pain) cures shoulder pain (*Míng*《明》).

Qū Yuán 曲垣 (SI 13) treats shoulder pain, generalized *bì*-impediment (*Míng* agrees), qì pooling,[7] and hypertonicity of the shoulders and arms with pain and a feeling of oppression (*Tóng*).

肩外俞治肩痹熱痛，而寒至肘（《明》同）。《下》云：療肩痛發寒熱，引項強。肩井治頸項不得顧，肩膊悶，兩手不得向頭，或因撲傷。雲門（見胸滿）、秉風治肩痛不能舉。肩貞治肩中熱痛（見風痹）。天宗治肩胛痛。天窗（《明下》同）治肩痛引項不得顧。前谷療膊胛小指痛。

Jiān Wài Shù 肩外俞 (SI 14) treats shoulder *bì*-impediment with hot pain, and cold moving down to the elbows (*Míng* agrees). *Xià*《下》says: It cures shoulder pain with fever and chills that induces hypertonicity of the nape.

Jiān Jǐng 肩井 (GB 21) treats inability to turn the neck and nape, oppressed feeling in the shoulders and arms, hands unable to move toward the head, or injury due to a fall.

Yún Mén 雲門 (LU 2) (see the section on chest fullness) and Bǐng Fēng 秉風 (SI 12) treat shoulder pain with inability to raise the arms.

Jiān Zhēn 肩貞 (SI 9) treats hot pain of the shoulders (see wind *bì*-impediment).

7. Qì pooling or qì wandering *qì zhù* 氣注 is one of nine poolings or wanderings. It is caused by wind attacking lung qì. The lungs control qì, and their qì travels externally and internally. Evils can exploit lung qì vacuity so right and evil contend with each other. Then the evils follow the lung qì and induce pain that has no fixed location (wandering pain).

Tiān Zōng 天宗 (SI 11) (*Míng Xià*《明下》agrees) treats shoulder pain radiating to the nape that prevents the head from turning.

Tiān Chuāng 天窗 (SI 16) (*Míng Xià*《明下》agrees) treats shoulder pain radiating to the nape that prevents the head from turning.

Qián Gǔ 前谷 (SI 2) cures pain of the arms, scapula, and little finger.

養老療肩欲折（《下》見臂）。青靈療肩不舉，不能帶衣。肩髎療肩重不舉（見臂）。養老、天柱主肩痛欲折。天井主肩痛不可屈伸。曲池、天窌主肩重痛不舉。巨骨主肩中痛，不能動搖（《明下》同）。肩外俞主肩甲痛而寒至肘。後溪主肩臑痛。前腋主肩腋前痛，與胸相引。天髎治肩肘痛引頸項急，寒熱缺盆中痛，汗不出，胸中煩悶（《銅》）。

Yǎng Lǎo 養老 (SI 6) cures shoulder [pain that] feels like it is broken (see the discussion of arms in *Xià*《下》).

Qīng Líng 青靈 (HT 2) cures inability to raise the shoulders and put on clothing.

Jiān Liáo 肩髎 (SJ 14) cures heavy shoulders with inability to raise them (see the section on the arm [pain]).

Yǎng Lǎo 養老 (SI 6) and Tiān Zhù 天柱 (UB 10) govern shoulder pain that feels like it is broken.

Tiān Jǐng 天井 (SJ 10) governs shoulder pain with inability to flex and stretch.

Qū Chí 曲池 (LI 11) and Tian Liáo 天窌 (SJ 15) govern heavy painful shoulders with inability to lift.

Jù Gǔ 巨骨 (LI 16) governs pain of the shoulders and inability to move them (*Míng Xià* agrees).

Jiān Wài Shù 肩外俞 (SI 14) governs pain of the scapula and cold moving down to the elbow.

Hòu Xī 後溪 (SI 3) governs pain of the shoulders and arms.

Qián Yè 前腋 (non-channel)[8] governs pain on the anterior aspect of the shoulder and axilla that radiates to the chest.

Tiān Liáo 天髎 (SJ 15) treats pain of the shoulders and elbows that induces tension of the neck and nape, [sensations of] cold and heat, pain of the the empty basin [supraclavicular fossa], absence of sweating, and vexation and oppression in the chest (*Tóng*《銅》).

8. Qián Yè 前腋 is located on the anterior aspect of the shoulder, between two sinews. Perhaps this is the same as Jiān Qián 肩前.

背痛 483
手痛 492
腋 496

章門治厥逆，肩臂不舉。青靈治肩臂不舉，不能帶衣。肩髎治肩重不能舉臂肘。巨骨治肩臂不得屈伸（見背痛）。居髎治肩引胸臂急（見手痛）。臑俞治寒熱肩腫，引胛中痛，臂酸無力。支溝療肩臂酸重（見腋）。

Zhāng Mén 章門 (LV 13) treats reverse counterflow, inability to lift the shoulders and arms.

Qīng Líng 青靈 (HT 2) treats inability to lift the shoulders and arms as well as put on clothing.

Jiān Liáo 肩髎 (SJ 14) treats heavy shoulders with inability to lift the shoulders and elbows.

Jù Gǔ 巨骨 (LI 16) treats inability to flex and stretch the shoulders and arms (see the section on back pain).

Jū Liáo 居髎 (GB 29) treats tension of the shoulders radiating to the chest and arms (see the section on arm pain).

Nào Shù 臑俞 (SI 10) treats [sensations of] cold and heat, shoulder swelling that induces pain of the scapula, and aching weak arms.

Zhī Gōu 支溝 (SJ 6) cures aching heavy shoulders and arms (see the section on [swelling of] the axilla).

關衝主肩臂酸重。腕骨主肩臂疼。天宗主肩重臂痛。章門治厥逆，肩臂不舉（《銅》）。青靈治肩臂不舉，不能帶衣。肩髎治肩重不能舉臂肘。巨骨治肩臂不得屈伸（見背痛）。[9]

Guān Chōng 關衝 (SJ 1) cures aching heavy shoulders and arms.

Wàn Gǔ 腕骨 (SI 4) governs pain of the shoulders and arms.

Tiān Zōng 天宗 (SI 11) governs heavy shoulders and painful arms.

Zhāng Mén (LV 13) treats reverse counterflow and inability to lift the shoulders and arms (*Tóng* 《銅》).

Qīng Líng (HT 2) treats inability to lift the shoulders and arms, as well as put on clothing.

Jiān Liáo 肩髎 (SJ 14) treats heavy shoulders with inability to lift shoulders and elbows.

Jù Gǔ (LI 16) treats inability to flex and stretch the shoulders and arms (see the section on back pain).

9. This paragraph from Zhāng Mén 章門 (LV 13) to Jù Gǔ 巨骨 (LI 16) is duplicated from above in error.

肘痛 499 勞 351

關衝主肩臂酸重。支溝療肩臂酸重（《明下》見腋）。列缺主肩背寒栗，少氣不足以息，寒厥交兩手而瞀。凡實則肩背熱，背汗出，四肢暴腫，虛則肩寒栗，氣不足以息。天井療頸項及肩背痛（見肘痛）。腰背痛：灸三焦俞。大椎治背膊急（見勞）。下焦俞療背痛身熱。

Guān Chōng 關衝 (SJ 1) governs aching heavy shoulders and arms.

Zhī Gōu 支溝 (SJ 6) cures aching heavy shoulders and arms (see the section on [swelling of] the axilla in *Míng Xià*《明下》).

Liè Quē 列缺 (LU 7) governs cold shivering of the shoulders and back, and shortness of breath with inability to breathe. When there is cold reversal, the patient crosses both his arms over his chest and has visual distortion. In repletion, there is heat in the shoulders and back, sweating on the back, and sudden swelling of the limbs; in vacuity, there is cold shivering of the shoulders and shortness of breath with inability to breathe.

Tiān Jǐng 天井 (SJ 10) cures pain of the neck and nape as well as the shoulders and back (see elbow pain).

Lower and upper back pain: Apply moxibustion on Sān Jiāo Shù 三焦俞 (UB 22).

Dà Zhuī 大椎 (Dū 14) treats back and arm tension (see taxation).

Xià Jiāo Shù 下焦俞 (unknown) cures back pain and generalized heat.

肩背酸疼，諸家針灸之詳矣，當隨病證針灸之。或背上先疼，遂牽引肩上疼者，乃是膏肓為患。《千金》、《外臺》固云：按之自覺牽引於肩中是也，當灸膏肓俞，則肩背自不疼矣。予嘗肩背痛，已灸膏肓，肩痛猶未已，遂灸肩井三壯而愈。以此知雖灸膏肓而他處亦不可不灸云。

All doctors have the details on acupuncture and moxibustion for aching pain of the shoulders and back. We should treat according to the disorder. If the pain is in the back first, and then radiates to the shoulders, there is something wrong at Gāo Huāng 膏肓 (UB 43). *Qiān Jīn*《千金》and *Wài Tái*《外臺》say: If the pain radiates to the shoulders when pressed, it is appropriate to apply moxibustion on Gāo Huāng Shù 膏肓俞 (UB 43) so the pain of the shoulders and back will disappear. I had pain on my shoulders and back before. The shoulder pain did not go away when I applied moxibustion on Gāo Huāng (UB 43), so I applied three cones of moxibustion on Jiān Jǐng 肩井 (GB 21) and the pain was cured. Then I knew, we should apply moxibustion on other points as well as Gāo Huāng (UB 43).

# 5.08

## *Jiān Bì Tòng (Bù Rén Bù Jǔ)*

肘痛 499
肩背 486

# 肩痹痛（不仁不舉）

## ***Bì*-impediment pain of the shoulders**

**(Numbness, inability to lift)**

天井主肩痛，痿痹不仁，不可屈伸，肩肉麻木。曲垣主肩甲周痹。肩貞、肩髎、關衝主肩中熱，頭不可顧。曲池、天髎主肩重痛不舉。清冷泉（《明》同）、陽谷主肩不舉，不得帶衣。天井療肘痛引肩，不屈伸（見肘）。肩外俞治肩痹。曲垣治肩痛周痹（並見肩背）。

Tiān Jǐng 天井 (SJ 10) governs shoulder pain, wilting and *bì*-impediment with numbness, inability to flex and stretch, and numbness of the shoulder sinews.

Qū Yuán 曲垣 (SI 13) governs generalized *bì*-impediment of the scapula.

Jiān Zhēn 肩貞 (SI 9), Jiān Liáo 肩髎 (SJ 14), and Guān Chōng 關衝 (SJ 1) govern heat in the shoulders, and inability to turn the head.

Qū Chí 曲池 (LI 11) and Tiān Liáo 天髎 (SJ 15) govern heavy painful shoulders with inability to lift.

Qīng Lěng Quán 清冷泉 (SJ 11) (*Míng*《明》agrees) and Yáng Gǔ 陽谷 (SI 5) govern inability to raise the shoulders and put on clothing.

Tiān Jǐng (SJ 10) cures elbow pain radiating to the shoulder, and inability to flex and stretch (see the section on elbow [pain]).

Jiān Wài Shù 肩外俞 (SI 14) treats shoulder *bì*-impediment.

Qū Yuán 曲垣 (SI 13) treats shoulder pain and generalized *bì*-impediment (for all see the section on [aching pain of the] shoulders and back).

兩肩頭冷疼，尤不可忽。予屢見將中風人臂骨脫臼，不與肩相連接，多有治不愈者。要之，才覺肩上冷疼，必先灸肩髎等穴，毋使至于此極可也。予中年每遇寒月，肩上多冷，常以手掌心撫摩之，夜臥則多

瘰癧 702 肘痛 499

以被擁之，僅能不冷。後灸肩髃，方免此患。蓋肩髃系兩手之安否，環跳系兩足之安否，不可不灸也。

Cold pain in both shoulders cannot be ignored. I frequently see people who are suffering wind strike with dislocation of the humerus that cannot be reconnected to the shoulder. It is incurable. To summarize, people should apply moxibustion on Jiān Liáo 肩髎 (SJ 14) and so forth when they first feel cold pain of the shoulders. They cannot wait until the disease reaches its summit. I had cold shoulders during the cold months when I was middle aged. I usually massaged them with my palms and covered my shoulders with quilts at night while sleeping. That was the only way I was not cold anymore. The disease never came back after I applied moxibustion on Jiān Yú 肩髃 (LI 15). It might because Jiān Yú (LI 15) is related to the health of the arms while Huán Tiào 環跳 (GB 30) is related to the health of the legs. So moxibustion must be applied.

# 5.09
## *Bì Tòng (Bèi Wú Lì)*
## 臂痛（臂無力）
### Arm pain
**(Weak arms)**

曲池療肘臂偏細（《明下》見肘）。肩髎療臂細無力酸疼，臂冷而緩（《明》）。臂臑、肩髃療臂細無力，手不得向頭。少海（見瘰癧）、乳根、聽宮療臂痛。中渚、孔最、肘髎療肘臂酸痛（見肘痛）。間使療臂腫痛，屈伸難（《下》）。肩髎療肩重不舉，臂痛。扁骨（即肩髃）療肩中熱，指臂痛。

Qū Chí 曲池 (LI 11) cures thin arms and elbows (see the section on the elbow [pain] in *Míng Xià*《明下》).

Jiān Liáo (SJ 14) cures thin weak arms with aching pain and cold weak arms (*Míng*《明》).

Bì Nào 臂臑 (LI 14) and Jiān Yú (LI 15) cure thin weak arms with inability to make the hands face the head.

Shào Hǎi 少海 (HT 3) (see the section on scrofula), Rǔ Gēn 乳根 (ST 18), and Tīng Gōng 聽宮 (SI 19) cure arm pain.

Zhōng Zhǔ 中渚 (SJ 3), Kǒng Zuì 孔最 (LU 6), and Zhǒu Liáo 肘髎 (LI 12) cure aching pain of the elbows and arms. 瘰癧 702

Jiān Shǐ 間使 (PC 5) cures swelling and pain of the arms with difficulty in flexing and stretching (*Xià*《下》). 肘痛 499

Jiān Liáo 肩髎 (SJ 14) cures heaviness of the shoulders with inability to lift [the arms] and arm pain. 咽腫 624 肩痛 486

Biǎn Gǔ 扁骨 (meaning Jiān Yú 肩髃 (LI 15)) cures heat of the shoulders and pain of the arms and fingers.

乳根治臂腫(《銅》)。太淵治臂內廉痛。居髎治腰引小腹痛，肩引胸臂攣急，手臂不得舉而至肩。臂臑(見瘰癧)、肘髎治臂痛不舉(見肘)。聽宮治臂痛。孔最治臂厥痛，可針。陽谷治臂腕外側痛不舉。液門(見咽腫)、前谷治臂不得舉。陽池治因折傷手腕，捉物不得，肩臂痛不舉。極泉治臂肘厥寒。

Rǔ Gēn 乳根 (ST 18) treats swollen arms (*Tóng*《銅》).

Tài Yuān 太淵 (LU 9) treats pain of the medial aspect of the arms.

Jū Liáo 居髎 (GB 29) treats low back pain radiating to the smaller abdomen, hypertonicity between the shoulders and chest, and inability to lift the arms to shoulder level.

Bì Nào 臂臑 (LI 14) (see the section on scrofula) and Zhǒu Liáo 肘髎 (LI 12) treat pain and inability to lift the arms (see the section on elbow [pain]).

Tīng Gōng 聽宮 (SI 19) treats arm pain.

Kǒng Zuì (LU 6) treats reversal pain of the arms. Acupuncture is applicable.

Yáng Gǔ 陽谷 (SI 5) treats pain on the lateral aspect of the wrists with inability to lift them.

Yè Mén 液門 (SJ 2) (see the discussion of swollen throat) and Qián Gǔ 前谷 (SI 2) treat inability to lift the arms.

Yáng Chí 陽池 (SJ 4) treats wrist injury due to fractures, inability to grasp things, arm and shoulder pain with inability to lift [the arms].

Jí Quán 極泉 (HT 1) treats reversal cold of the arms and elbows.

清冷淵治臑從肩臂不舉，不得帶衣。養老治肩欲折，臂如拔，臂(《明下》作手)痛不能自上下。臑俞治臂酸無力(見肩痛)。章門治厥逆，肩臂不舉。巨骨治肩臂不得屈伸而痛(見肩痛)。臑會治臂痛不能舉，氣腫痓痛。

偏風 396 肘痛 499

肩髃治手臂攣急（見偏風）。尺澤、肩貞治風痹手臂不舉。合谷治痿臂。陽溪治臂不舉（見肘）。

Qīng Lěng Yuān 清冷淵 (SJ 11) treats inability to lift the arms and put on clothing.

Yǎng Lǎo 養老 (SI 6) treats shoulder [pain that] feels like it is broken, arm [pain] as if it is dislocated, and arm (*Míng Xià*《明下》says hand) pain with inability to move it up and down.

Nào Shù 臑俞 (SI 10) treats aching weak arms (see the section on aching pain of the shoulders [and back]).

Zhāng Mén 章門 (LV 13) treats reverse counterflow and inability to lift the arms and shoulders.

Jù Gǔ 巨骨 (LI 16) treats inability to flex and stretch the arms and shoulders, as well as pain (see the section on aching pain of the shoulders [and back]).

Nào Huì 臑會 (SJ 13) treats pain and inability to lift the arms, qì swelling, and pain due to hypertonicity.

Jiān Yú 肩髃 (LI 15) treats hypertonicity of the arms (see the section on hemilateral wind).

Chǐ Zé 尺澤 (LU 5) and Jiān Zhēn 肩貞 (SI 9) treat wind *bì*-impediment with inability to lift the arms.

Hé Gǔ 合谷 (LI 4) treats wilting of the arms.

Yáng Xī 陽溪 (LI 5) treats inability to lift the arms (see the section on the elbow [pain]).

天宗、五里等治臂痛。後溪治臂急。竅陰等、腕骨治臂不伸。附分治臂不仁（並肘）。巨骨、前谷主臂不舉。尺澤、關衝、外關、竅陰主臂不及頭。前腋主臂攣急，手不上舉。神門、少海主臂攣。顏色焦枯，勞氣失精，肩臂痛不得上頭：肩髃百壯。

Tiān Zōng 天宗 (SI 11), Wǔ Lǐ 五里 (LI 13) and so forth treat arm pain.

Hòu Xī 後溪 (SI 3) treats tension of the arms.

Qiào Yīn 竅陰 (GB 44) and so forth, and Wàn Gǔ 腕骨 (SI 4) treat inability to stretch the arms.

Fù Fēn 附分 (UB 41) treats numbness of the arms (also see the section on elbow [pain]).

Jù Gǔ (LI 16) and Qián Gǔ 前谷 (SI 2) govern inability to lift the arms.

Chǐ Zé (LU 5), Guān Chōng 關衝 (SJ 1), Wài Guān 外關 (SJ 5), and Qiào Yīn (GB 44) govern inability of the arms to reach the head

Qián Yè 前腋 (non-channel) [see footnote above] governs hypertonicity of the arms and inability to lift the arms. 肩背痛 486 肘痛 499

Shén Mén 神門 (HT 7) and Shào Hǎi 少海 (HT 3) govern hypertonicity of the arms.

Dried up withered complexion, qì taxation, loss of essence, and shoulder and arm pain with inability to reach the head: Apply a hundred cones of moxibustion to Jiān Yú 肩髃 (LI 15).

液門主臂痛。肩髃、天宗、陽谷主臂痛。前谷、後溪、陽溪主臂重痛肘攣。太泉、經渠主臂內廉痛。腕骨、曲池、前谷、陽谷主臂腕急，腕外側痛脫如拔。腕骨、天宗主肩臂痛（見肩背痛）。列缺主手臂身熱。後溪、三里、曲池療臂痛（明見肘痛）。

Yè Mén 液門 (SJ 2) governs arm pain.

Jiān Yú (LI 15), Tiān Zōng 天宗 (SI 11), and Yáng Gǔ 陽谷 (SI 5) govern arm pain.

Qián Gǔ 前谷 (SI 2), Hòu Xī 後溪 (SI 3), and Yáng Xī 陽溪 (LI 5) govern heavy pain of the arms and hypertonicity of the elbows.

Tài Quán 太泉 (LU 9) and Jīng Qú 經渠 (LU 8) govern pain of the medial aspect of the arms.

Wàn Gǔ 腕骨 (SI 4), Qū Chí 曲池 (LI 11), Qián Gǔ (SI 2), and Yáng Gǔ (SI 5) govern hypertonicity of the arms and wrists, and pain of the lateral aspect of the wrists that feels like they have been dislocated.

Wàn Gǔ (SI 4) and Tiān Zōng 天宗 (SI 11) govern pain of the arms and shoulders (see the section on aching pain of the shoulders and back).

Liè Quē 列缺 (LU 7) governs heat in the arms and body.

Hòu Xī (SI 3), Sān Lǐ 三里 (LI 10), and Qū Chí (LI 11) cure arm pain (see the section on elbow pain in *Míng* 《明》).

憂悲 331
膈痛 481
尸厥 531
膝痛 536
狂 345

## 5.10
## *Yè Tòng (Yè Zhǒng)*
## 腋痛（腋腫）
## **Pain of the axilla**
**(Swelling of the axilla)**

足臨泣治胸滿，缺盆中及腋下腫（《明下》同），馬刀瘍瘻，善嚙唇，天牖中腫，淫濼胻酸，目眩，枕骨合顱痛，灑淅振寒（《銅》）。丘墟治腋下腫，痿厥，坐不能起，髀樞中痛，目生翳膜，腿胻酸，轉筋卒疝，小腹堅，寒熱頸腫。

Zú Lín Qì 足臨泣 (GB 41) treats chest fullness, swelling of the empty basin (supraclavicular fossa) and under the axilla (*Míng Xià*《明下》agrees), saber lumps and fistulas, frequently biting one's lips, swelling under Tiān Yǒu 天牖 (SJ 16), aching and weakness of the lower legs, dizzy vision, pain of the occiput and Hé Lú 合顱 (Dū 17), and quivering with cold as if after a soaking (*Tóng*《銅》).

Qiū Xū 丘墟 (GB 40) treats swelling of the axilla, wilting and reversal, inability to get up when sitting, pain of the hip joint, screens and membranes in the eyes, aching lower legs, cramping and sudden *shàn*-mounting, hardness of the smaller abdomen, and [sensations of] cold and heat with neck swelling.

譩譆治腋拘攣，暴脈急引脅痛。少府治股腋攣急（見憂悲）。少海治肘腋腫，小腹痛。小海治肘攣，腋脅下痛，四肢不舉。支溝治肩臂酸重，脅腋痛，四肢不舉。天池（見膈痛）、臑俞、委陽（見尸厥）、陽輔（見膝痛）治腋下腫。間使治掌中熱，腋腫肘攣（見狂）。

Yī Xī 譩譆 (UB 45) treats hypertonicity of the axilla, sudden vessel tension radiating into the rib-sides with pain.

Shào Fǔ 少府 (HT 8) treats hypertonicity of the thighs and axilla[10] (see the section on anxiety and sorrow [of the heart]).

---

10. This should say *zhǒu yè* 肘腋 (elbows and axilla) according to *Tóng Rén Tú Jīng*《銅人圖經》(The Illustrated Classic of the Bronze Statue).

痿 511 瘰癧 702 痔 254

Shào Hǎi 少海 (HT 3) treats swollen elbow and axilla and pain of the smaller abdomen.

Xiǎo Hǎi 小海 (SI 8) treats hypertonicity of the elbows, pain under the rib-sides and axilla, and inability to lift the four limbs.

Zhī Gōu 支溝 (SJ 6) treats aching heavy shoulders and arms, pain of the rib-sides and axilla, and inability to lift the arms.

Tiān Chí 天池 (PC 1) (see the section on pain of the diaphragm), Dǎn Shù 膽俞 (UB19), Wěi Yáng 委陽 (UB 39) (see the section on deathlike reversal), and Yáng Fǔ 陽輔 (GB 38) (see the section on knee pain) treat swelling of the axilla.

Jiān Shǐ 間使 (PC 5) treats heat in the palms, swelling of the axilla, and hypertonicity of the elbows (see the section on mania).

地五會、陽輔、申脈、委陽、天池、臨泣、俠溪等（見痿）主腋下腫。大陵主肘攣腋腫。臨泣主腋下腫，胸中滿。丘墟、陽蹻主腋下腫，寒熱頸腫。少海療腋下瘰癧（見瘰癧）。承筋等主腋腫（見痔）。

Dì Wǔ Huì 地五會 (GB 42), Yáng Fǔ (GB 38), Shēn Mài 申脈 (UB 62), Wěi Yáng 委陽 (UB 39), Tiān Chí (PC 1), Lín Qì 臨泣 (GB 41), Xiá Xī 俠溪 (GB 43) and so forth (see the discussion of wilting) govern swelling of the axilla.

Dà Líng 大陵 (PC 7) governs hypertonicity of the elbows and swelling of the axilla.

Lín Qì (GB 41) governs swelling of the axilla and chest fullness.

Qiū Xū 丘墟 (GB 40) and Yáng Qiāo 陽蹻 (UB 62) govern swelling of the axilla and [sensations of] cold and heat with neck swelling.

Shào Hǎi (HT 3) cures scrofula under the axilla (see the section on scrofula).

Chéng Jīn 承筋 (UB 56) and so forth govern swelling of the axilla (see the section on hemorrhoids).

腋下腫痛，最不可忽。予屢見患瘡癬人腋下或發瘡，有至於不可救者，可不早治之乎？

Pain and swelling under the axilla cannot be ignored. I frequently see people who suffer skin ulcers or boils and have sores under the axilla whose life cannot be saved. Can't they get the treatment earlier?

手掣
505

# 5.11
## Wàn Láo
# 腕勞
## Taxation of the wrists

曲池、腕骨等主腕急(《千》見臂痛)。陽溪療臂腕外側痛不舉(《明》)。列缺療腕勞(《上》同),臂肘痛。《銅》云:手腕無力(《下》)。偏歷療臂膊肘腕酸痛,難伸屈。外關療肘腕酸重。後溪療肘臂腕重(並見手掣)。通里療肘腕酸重。

Qū Chí 曲池 (LI 11), Wàn Gǔ 腕骨 (SI 4) and so forth govern tension of the wrists (see arm pain in *Qiān*《千》).

Yáng Xī 陽溪 (LI 5) cures pain on the lateral aspect of the arms and wrists with inability to lift them (*Míng*《明》).

Liè Quē 列缺 (LU 7) cures wrist taxation (*Shàng*《上》 agrees) and arm and elbow pain. *Tóng*《銅》 says: [It treats] weakness of the wrists (*Xià*《下》).

Piān Lì 偏歷 (LI 6) cures aching pain in arms, elbows and wrists, with difficulty flexing and stretching.

Wài Guān 外關 (SJ 5) cures aching heaviness of the elbows and wrists.

Hòu Xī 後溪 (SI 3) cures heavy elbows, arms and wrists (for all this, see the section on hypertonicity of the hands).

Tōng Lǐ 通里 (HT 5) cures aching heaviness of the elbows and wrists.

# 5.12
## *Zhǒu Tòng (Zhǒu Luán, Bù Rén)*

臂 492
肩背痛 486
四肢厥 528

# 肘痛（肘攣　不仁）

## Elbow pain
**(Hypertonicity of the elbows, numbness)**

前谷、後溪、陽溪主肘攣。魚際、靈道主肘攣柱滿。大陵主肘攣腋腫。中膂俞、譩譆主腋攣。曲池主肘中痛（見臂）。曲池、腕骨、臑會、支溝、肘髎主肘節痹，臂酸重，腋急痛，肘難屈伸。中衝等主肘痛（見臂痛）。

Qián Gǔ 前谷 (SI 2), Hòu Xī 後溪 (SI 3), and Yáng Xī 陽溪 (LI 5) govern hypertonicity of the elbows.

Yú Jì 魚際 (LU 10) and Líng Dào 靈道 (HT 4) govern hypertonicity of the elbows with stiffness and distention.

Dà Líng 大陵 (PC 7) governs hypertonicity of the elbows and swelling of the axilla.

Zhōng Lǚ Shù 中膂俞 (UB 29) and Yī Xī 譩譆 (UB 45) govern hypertonicity of the axilla.

Qū Chí 曲池 (LI 11) governs pain of the elbows (see the section on the arm [pain]).

Qū Chí (LI 11), Wàn Gǔ 腕骨 (SI 4), Nào Huì 臑會 (SJ 13), Zhī Gōu 支溝 (SJ 6), and Zhǒu Liáo 肘髎 (LI 12) govern *bi*-impediment of the elbow joint, aching heavy arms, acute pain of the axilla, and difficulty flexing and stretching the elbows.

Zhōng Chōng 中衝 (PC 9) and so forth govern elbow pain (see the section on arm pain).

關衝主肘疼，不能自帶衣。間使主肘內廉痛。曲池、三里、關衝、中渚、陽谷、尺澤主肘痛時寒。曲池主肘痛（見四肢厥）。肩外俞主肘寒（見肩背痛）。天宗治臂肘外後廉痛（《銅》）。天髎治肩肘痛（見肩背痛）。

Guān Chōng 關衝 (SJ 1) governs elbow pain with inability to put on clothing.

Jiān Shǐ 間使 (PC 5) governs pain on the medial aspect of the elbows.

心痛 312
腋 496
風痹 377
中風 379
喉痹 629
風勞 371

Qū Chí 曲池 (LI 11), Sān Lǐ 三里 (LI 10), Guān Chōng 關衝 (SJ 1), Zhōng Zhǔ 中渚 (SJ 3), Yáng Gǔ 陽谷 (SI 5) and Chǐ Zé 尺澤 (LU 5) govern painful elbows that sometimes feel cold.

Qū Chí (LI 11) governs elbow pain (see the section on limb reversal).

Jiān Wài Shù 肩外俞 (SI 14) governs cold elbows (see the section on aching pain of the shoulders and back).

Tiān Zōng 天宗 (SI 11) treats pain of the lateral and posterior aspect of the elbows and arms (*Tóng*《銅》).

Tiān Liáo 天髎 (SJ 15) governs shoulder and elbow pain (see the section on aching pain of the shoulders and back).

肘髎治肘節風痹，臂痛不可舉，屈伸攣急。《明下》云：臂酸重，麻痹不仁。魚際治肘攣支滿。靈道（見心痛）、尺澤、少海（見腋）治肘攣（見風痹）。支正、內關（見中風）、陽溪治驚掣，肘臂不舉。

Zhǒu Liáo 肘髎 (LI 12) treats wind *bì*-impediment of the elbows, arm pain with inability to lift them, and hypertonicity when flexing and stretching. *Míng Xià*《明下》says: It treats aching heavy arms and numbness.

Yú Jì 魚際 (LU 10) treats hypertonicity of the elbows and propping fullness.

Líng Dào 靈道 (HT 4) (see the section on heart pain), Chǐ Zé (LU 5), and Shào Hǎi 少海 (HT 3) (see the section on [swelling of] the axilla) treat hypertonicity of the elbows (see the section on wind *bì*-impediment).

Zhī Zhèng 支正 (SI 7), Nèi Guān 內關 (PC 6) (see the section on wind stroke), and Yáng Xī 陽溪 (LI 5) treat fright pulling[11] and inability to lift the arms and elbows.

極泉治臂肘厥寒。竅陰（見喉痹）、手三里治手臂肘攣不伸。後溪治臂肘攣急。附分治臂肘不仁（見風勞）。腕骨治偏枯，臂肘不得屈伸。五里（見風勞）、天井（見風痹）、下廉治臂肘痛。

Jí Quán 極泉 (HT 1) treats reversal cold of the arms and elbows.

Qiào Yīn 竅陰 (GB 44) (see the section on throat *bì*-impediment) and Shǒu Sān Lǐ 手三里 (LI 10) treat hypertonicity of the arms and elbows and inability to stretch.

11. This probably means one of the signs of fright wind - pulling means a drawing together of the shoulders. Fright wind is generally equivalent to infantile convulsions.

口喎 591
腕 498
手掣 505

Hòu Xī 後溪 (SI 3) treats hypertonicity of the arms and elbows.

Fù Fēn 附分 (UB 41) treats numbness of the arms and elbows (see the section on wind taxation).

Wàn Gǔ 腕骨 (SI 4) treats hemilateral withering and inability to flex and stretch the arms and elbows.

Wǔ Lǐ 五里 (LI 13) (see the section on wind taxation), Tiān Jǐng 天井 (SJ 10) (see the section on wind *bì*-impediment), and Xià Lián 下廉 (LI 8) treat arm and elbow pain.

衝陽（見口喎）、曲池治肘中痛。魚際療肘攣支滿，喉中焦乾渴，瘲上氣。偏歷（見腕）、三里療肘臂酸重，屈伸難（《下》）。中渚療肘臂酸痛（見手掣）。太淵療肘痛。曲池療肘痛屈伸難，手不得舉，偏風半身不遂，捉物不得，挽弓不開，肘臂偏細。

Chōng Yáng 衝陽 (ST 42) (see the section on deviation of the mouth) and Qū Chí 曲池 (LI 11) treat elbow pain.

Yú Jì 魚際 (LU 10) cures hypertonicity of the elbows, propping fullness, dryness and thirst in the throat, spasms, and qì ascent.

Piān Lì 偏歷 (LI 6) (see the section on taxation of the wrists) and Sān Lǐ 三里 (ST 36 or LI 10) cure aching heavy elbows and arms with difficulty flexing and stretching (*Xià*《下》).

Zhōng Zhǔ 中渚 (SJ 3) cures aching pain of the elbows and arms (see the section on pulling [pain] of the hands).

Tài Yuān 太淵 (LU 9) cures elbow pain.

Qū Chí (LI 11) cures elbow pain, difficulty flexing and stretching, inability to lift the arms, hemilateral wind, hemiplegia, inability to grasp things and draw a bow, and thin arms and elbows.

孔最療肘臂厥痛屈伸難，手不及頭，不握。支正療肘臂攣，難屈伸，手不握，十指盡痛。肘髎療肘臂酸重，不可屈伸，麻痹不仁。天井療肘痛引肩，不可屈伸，頸項及肩背痛，臂痿不仁。液門療肘痛不能上下。列缺主肘中痛。

Kǒng Zuì 孔最 (LU 6) cures reversal pain of the elbows and arms, difficulty flexing and stretching, inability of the hands to reach the head, and inability to grasp things.

Zhī Zhèng 支正 (SI 7) cures hypertonicity of the elbows and arms, difficulty flexing and stretching, inability to grasp things, and pain in all ten fingers.

Zhǒu Liáo 肘髎 (LI 12) cures aching heaviness of the elbows and arms, difficulty flexing and stretching, and numbness.

Tiān Jǐng 天井 (SJ 10) cures elbow pain radiating to the shoulder, difficulty flexing and stretching, pain of the neck, nape, shoulders and back, and wilting of the arms with numbness.

Yè Mén 液門 (SJ 2) cures elbow pain with inability to move them up and down.

Liè Quē 列缺 (LU 7) governs elbow pain.

《甲乙經》云：五里在肘上三寸大脈中。《玉篇》說肘云臂節也。此臂之下節也。宓子賤使書吏書而掣其肘，蓋其臂節也。當以此求之。

*Jiǎ Yǐ Jīng*《甲乙經》says: Wǔ Lǐ 五里 (LI 13) is located at the big vessel 3 cùn above the elbow. *Yù Piān*《玉篇》says that the elbow is the arm joint. This is the lower joint of the arms. Mì Zǐjiān 宓子賤[12] asked two scribes to write but pushed their elbows, which should mean the arm joint. We should confirm the meaning based on this.

12. Mì Zǐjiān 宓子賤 was a student of Kǒng Zǐ 孔子 (Confucius).

# 5.13
## *Shǒu Má Bì Bù Rén (Bù Jǔ)*

# 手麻痹不仁（不舉）

## Numbness of the hands
**(Inability to lift them)**

中封治身體不仁（《銅》見痹）。少商主手不仁（《千》）。肩貞主手麻小不舉。內庭主四厥手足悶。列缺主四肢厥，喜笑。曲池、支溝、臑會、腕骨、肘髎主節痹。曲池、天井、外關主臂痿不仁。白環俞療手足不仁（明下見脊）。曲池主手不舉，又主手不可舉重，腕急，肘中痛，難屈伸。

Zhōng Fēng 中封 (LV 4) treats numbness of the body (*bì*-impediment in *Tóng*《銅》).

Shào Shāng 少商 (LU 11) governs numbness of the hands (*Qiān*《千》).

Jiān Zhēn 肩貞 (SI 9) governs numbness of the hands and mild inability to lift things.

Nèi Tíng 內庭 (ST 44) governs reversal cold of the limbs and a feeling of oppression of the hands and feet.

Liè Quē 列缺 (LU 7) governs limb reversal and frequent laughter.

Qū Chí 曲池 (LI 11), Zhī Gōu 支溝 (SJ 6), Nào Huì 臑會 (SJ 13), Wàn Gǔ 腕骨 (SI 4), and Zhǒu Liáo 肘髎 (LI 12) govern *bì*-impediment of the joints.

Qū Chí (LI 11), Tiān Jǐng 天井 (SJ 10) and Wài Guān 外關 (SJ 5) govern wilting of the arms with numbness.

Bái Huán Shù 白環俞 (UB 30) cures numbness of the hands and feet (see the section on [pain of the lower back and] the spine).

Qū Chí (LI 11) governs inability to lift the hands; it also governs inability to lift heavy things, tension of the wrists, and elbow pain with difficulty flexing and stretching.

間使主手痛。陽溪主臂腕外側痛不舉。中衝、少衝（《明》同）、勞宮、太泉、經渠、列缺主手掌熱，肘中痛。勞宮療手掌厚，瘡痹（《銅》云手痹）

，手皮白屑起（《明》）。勞宮治手痹（《銅》）。附分治肘臂不仁（《銅》見風勞）。上廉治手足不仁（見偏風）。肘髎、天井療肘臂不仁（《明下》見肘痛）。

Jiān Shǐ 間使 (PC 5) governs pain of the hands.

Yáng Xī 陽溪 (LI 5) governs pain on the lateral aspect of the arms and wrists and inability to lift things.

Zhōng Chōng 中衝 (PC 9), Shào Chōng 少衝 (HT 9) (*Míng*《明》agrees), Láo Gōng 勞宮 (PC 8), Tài Quán 太泉 (LU 9), Jīng Qú 經渠 (LU 8), and Liè Quē 列缺 (LU 7) govern heat in the palms and elbow pain.

Láo Gōng (PC 8) cures thick palms, sore *bì*-impediment (*Tóng*《銅》says *bì*-impediment of the hands), and white scaling of the skin of the hands (*Míng*).

Láo Gōng (PC 8) treats *bì*-impediment of the hands (*Tóng*).

Fù Fēn 附分 (UB 41) treats numbness of the elbows and arms (see the section on wind taxation in *Tóng*).

Shàng Lián 上廉 (LI 9) treats numbness of the hands and feet (see the section on hemilateral wind). Zhǒu Liáo 肘髎 (LI 12), Tiān Jǐng 天井 (SJ 10) cure numbness of the elbow and arm (see the section on elbow pain in *Míng Xià*《明下》).

有貴人手中指攣，已而，無名指小指亦攣。醫為灸肩髃、曲池、支溝而愈。支溝在腕後三寸。或灸風疾，多有不灸支溝，只灸合谷云。

A noble person suffered from hypertonicity of the middle finger; after that, the ring finger and little finger also had hypertonicity. The doctor applied moxibustion on Jiān Yú 肩髃 (LI 15), Qū Chí 曲池 (LI 11), and Zhī Gōu 支溝 (SJ 6) to cure the disease. Zhī Gōu (SJ 6) is located 3 cùn proximal to the wrist. Perhaps one should apply moxibustion on Hé Gǔ 合谷 (LI 4) rather than on Zhī Gōu (SJ 6) for wind diseases.

轉筋
267

# 5.14

## *Shǒu Zhǐ Luán (Shǒu Chè Tòng, Yú Lùn Jiàn Shǒu Má)*

# 手指攣（手掣痛　餘論見手麻）

## Hypertonicity of the fingers

**(Pulling pain of the hands; for further discussion, see the section on numbness of the hands)**

養老主手不得上下（《千》）。陰交主手足拘攣。大陵主手攣不伸。心俞、肝俞主筋急手相引（見轉筋）。少商治手攣指痛（《銅》）。少府治掌中熱，股腋攣急，胸中痛，手卷不伸。少衝療手卷不得伸（《明堂上》云：治手攣不伸，引眼痛）。外關療肘腕酸重，屈伸難，十指痛不得握（《明下》）。《銅人》云：治肘臂不得屈伸，五指痛，不能握物。

Yǎng Lǎo 養老 (SI 6) governs inability of the hands to move up and down (*Qiān*《千》).

Yīn Jiāo 陰交 (Rèn 7) governs hypertonicity of the hands and feet.

Dà Líng 大陵 (PC 7) governs hypertonicity of the hands and inability to stretch.

Xīn Shù 心俞 (UB 15) and Gān Shù 肝俞 (UB 18) govern tension of the sinews with pulling of the hands (see the section on cramping).

Shào Shāng 少商 (LU 11) treats hypertonicity of the hand and pain of the fingers (*Tóng*《銅》).

Shào Fǔ 少府 (HT 8) treats heat in the palms, hypertonicity of the thighs and axilla, chest pain, and curled hands that are unable to stretch.

Shào Chōng 少衝 (HT 9) cures curling hands with inability to stretch (*Míng Táng Shàng*《明堂上》says: treats hypertonicity of the hands with inability to stretch and radiating eye pain).

Wài Guān 外關 (SJ 5) cures aching heaviness of the elbows and wrists, difficulty flexing and stretching, and pain of the ten fingers with inability to grip things (*Míng Xià*《明下》). *Tóng Rén*《銅人》says: inability to flex and stretch the elbows and arms, pain of the five fingers, and inability to grasp things.

後溪療肘臂腕重，難屈伸，五指盡痛，不可掣。中渚療肘臂酸痛，手五指不握，盡痛。《銅人》云：治咽腫肘臂痛，五指不得屈伸。腕骨、中渚主五指掣，不可屈伸。大陵主手掣小偏。尺澤主掣痛，手不可伸。治手足指掣痛不可忍：灸指端七壯，立瘥。腕骨治瘈瘲，五指掣(《銅》)。扁骨療指臂痛(《明下》見臂痛)。

Hòu Xī 後溪 (SI 3) cures heavy elbows, arms, and wrists, difficulty flexing and stretching, pain in all five fingers, and inability to pull things.

Zhōng Zhǔ 中渚 (SJ 3) cures aching pain in elbows and arms and pain in all five fingers with inability to grasp things. *Tóng Rén*《銅人》says: swollen throat, elbow and arm pain, and the five fingers cannot flex and stretch.

Wàn Gǔ 腕骨 (SI 4) and Zhōng Zhǔ (SJ 3) govern pulling of the five fingers and inability to flex and stretch.

Dà Líng 大陵 (PC 7) governs pulling of the hands with slight deviation.

Chǐ Zé 尺澤 (LU 5) governs pulling pain and inability to stretch the hands.

To treat intolerable pulling pain of the fingers and toes: Apply seven cones of moxibustion on the tip of the fingers and toes. It will cure the disease immediately.

Wàn Gǔ (SI 4) treats tuggling and slackening and pulling of the five fingers (*Tóng*《銅》).

Biǎn Gǔ 扁骨 (LI 15) cures pain of the arms and fingers (see the section on arm pain in *Míng Xià*《明下》).

# 5.15

## *Shǒu Rè (Shǒu Hán, Shǒu Qīng, Shǒu Xīn Rè)*

# 手熱（手寒　手清　手心熱）

## Heat in the hands

**(Cold hands, cool hands, heat in the palms)**

小兒食時頭痛，及五心熱，灸譩譆各一壯（《明下》）。內關主手中風熱（《千》）。中衝、少衝、太泉（《明下》同）、勞宮、經渠、列缺主手掌熱，肘痛。太溪主手足寒至節。曲澤主手清逆氣。巨闕主手清。經渠、列缺（見偏風）、少衝（見傷寒）、中衝、（見心痛）、間使（見狂）、太淵治掌中熱。

Headache in children when eating and five center heat: Apply one cone of moxibustion on Yī Xī 譩譆 (UB 45) (*Míng Xià*《明下》).

Nèi Guān 內關 (PC 6) governs wind heat in the hands (*Qiān*《千》).

Zhōng Chōng 中衝 (PC 9), Shào Chōng 少衝 (HT 9), Tài Quán 太泉 (LU 9) (*Míng Xià* agrees), Láo Gōng 勞宮 (PC 8), Jīng Qú 經渠 (LU 8), and Liè Quē 列缺 (LU 7) govern heat in the palms and elbow pain.

Tài Xī 太溪 (KI 3) governs hands and feet become cold up to the joints.

Qū Zé 曲澤 (PC 3) governs cold hands and reverse flow.

Jù Quē 巨闕 (Rèn 14) governs cold hands.

Jīng Qú 經渠 (LU 8), Liè Quē 列缺 (LU 7) (see the section on hemilateral wind), Shào Chōng 少衝 (HT 9) (see the section on cold damage), Zhōng Chōng (PC 9) (see the section on heart pain), Jiān Shǐ 間使 (PC 5) (see the section on mania), and Tài Yuān 太淵 (LU 9) treat heat in the palms.

偏風 396
傷寒 661
心痛 312
狂 345
無汗 690
膝 536
腹滿 445
指攣 505
尸厥 531
胸脅痛 476

間使治掌中熱（見狂）。中衝治掌熱（見傷寒無汗）。陽陵泉治腳冷（見膝）。大都治手足逆冷（見腹滿）。少商治掌熱（見指攣）。豐隆治厥逆（見尸厥）。內庭、章門治厥逆。行間治四肢冷。曲池等、肩外俞主肘寒（《千》見肘）。太溪治手足冷（見胸脅痛）。

Jiān Shǐ 間使 (PC 5) treats heat in the palms (see the section on mania).

Zhōng Chōng 中衝 (PC 9) treats heat in the palms (see the section on cold damage with absence of sweating).

Yáng Líng Quán 陽陵泉 (GB 34) treats cold legs (see the section on the knee pain).

Dà Dū 大都 (SP 2) treats counterflow cold of the extremities (see the section on abdominal fullness).

Shào Shāng 少商 (LU 11) treats heat in the palms (see the section on hypertonicity of the fingers).

Fēng Lóng 豐隆 (ST 40) treats reverse counterflow (see deathlike reversal).

Nèi Tíng 内庭 (ST 44) and Zhāng Mén 章門 (LV 13) treat reverse counterflow.

Xíng Jiān 行間 (LV 2) treats cold extremities.

Qū Chí 曲池 (LI 11) and so forth and Jiān Wài Shù 肩外俞 (SI 14) govern cold elbows (see the section on elbow [pain] in *Qiān*《千》).

Tài Xī 太溪 (KI 3) treats cold extremities (see the section on pain of the chest and rib-sides).

**五心之熱，小兒傷食證也。大人亦然。若手足寒清過節，證惡可知，當早隨證針炙之，毋使至於此極方可。清，猶寒也。《禮記》言：冬溫而夏清，是已。針炙法見四肢厥。**

Five center heat is a sign of food damage in children and also in adults. If the extremities are cold and cool beyond the joints, it is known as a malign sign. It is appropriate to treat this with acupuncture and moxibustion according to the symptoms described above. Do not wait until the symptoms reach their peak. *Cool* [*clear*] means same as cold. *Lǐ Jì*《禮記》[13] says: Warm up in the winter and keep cool [clear] in the summer. That is it. For the methods of acupuncture and moxibustion, see the section on reversal of the extremities.

13. *Lǐ Jì*《禮記》(The Book of Rites) is one of the Five Classics that constitute the core of the traditional Confucian canon. It describes the social forms, administration, and ceremonial rites of the *Zhōu* (周) Dynasty as it was understood during the Spring and Autumn Period.

足雜病
515

# 5.16
## *Zú Má Bì Bù Rén*

# 足麻痹不仁

## Numbness of the legs[14]

至陰主風寒從足小指起，脈痹上下（《千》）。陰陵泉主足痹痛。中都主足濕痹不能行。陽輔、陽交、陽陵泉主髀樞膝骨痹不仁。陽關、環跳、承筋主脛痹不仁。腰俞、風府主足不仁。膀胱俞、太溪、次髎主足清不仁。陽關主脛痹不仁（見足雜病）。

Zhì Yīn 至陰 (UB 67) governs wind-cold starting from the little toe and inducing vessel *bì*-impediment above and below (*Qiān*《千》).

Yīn Líng Quán 陰陵泉 (SP 9) governs *bì*-impediment pain of the feet.

Zhōng Dū 中都 (LV 6) governs damp *bì*-impediment of the legs with inability to walk.

Yáng Fǔ 陽輔 (GB 38), Yáng Jiāo 陽交 (GB 35), and Yáng Líng Quán 陽陵泉 (GB 34) govern bone *bì*-impediment and numbness of the thigh pivot and knees.

Yáng Guān 陽關 (GB 33), Huán Tiào 環跳 (GB 30), and Chéng Jīn 承筋 (UB 56) govern *bì*-impediment and numbness of the lower legs.

Yāo Shù 腰俞 (Dū 2), Fēng Fǔ 風府 (Dū 16) govern numbness of the feet.

Páng Guāng Shù 膀胱俞 (UB 28), Tài Xī 太溪 (KI 3), and Cì Liáo 次髎 (UB 32) govern coldness and numbness of the feet.

Yáng Guān (GB 33) governs *bì*-impediment and numbness of the lower legs (see the section on miscellaneous disorders of the legs).

14. *Zú* 足: Before the *Qín* (秦) and *Hàn* (漢) Dynasties - *zú* 足 and *zhǐ* 趾 both indicated the feet, while *jiǎo* 脚 indicated the legs; after the *Jìn* (晉) Dynasty, these three words all indicated the feet. Since this book records information from different dynasties, *zú* 足 could mean legs or feet, depending on the period of the source text.

腰腳
542

浮郄治髀樞不仁（《銅》見足雜病）。膀胱俞治腳足不仁（見腰腳）。白環俞療手足不仁（《明下》見脊）。上廉治手足不仁（《銅》見偏風）。犢鼻、髀關、陽陵泉主膝不仁（《千》見腰痛）。

Fú Xī 浮郄 (UB 38) treats numbness of the thigh pivot [great trochanter] (see the section on miscellaneous disorders of the legs in *Tóng*《銅》).

Páng Guāng Shù 膀胱俞 (UB 28) treats numbness of the feet and legs (see the section on lower back and leg [pain]).

Bái Huán Shù 白環俞 (UB 30) cures numbness of the hands and feet (see the section on the spine in *Míng Xià*《明下》).

Shàng Lián 上廉 (ST 37) treats numbness of the hands and feet (see the section on hemilateral wind in *Tóng*).

Dú Bí 犢鼻 (ST 35), Bì Guān 髀關 (ST 31), and Yáng Líng Quán 陽陵泉 (GB 34) govern numbness of the knees (see the section on lower back pain in *Qiān*《千》).

《列子》載偃師造倡云：廢其腎則足不能行。是足之不能行，蓋腎有病也，當灸腎俞。或一再灸而不效，宜灸環跳、風市、犢鼻、膝關、陽陵泉、陰陵泉、三里、絕骨等穴。但按略酸疼，即是受病處，灸之無不效也。

Liè Zǐ 列子[15] records that Master Yǎn made a [mechanical] entertainer[16]: When its kidneys were destroyed, it was unable to walk. So the inability to walk must be caused by kidney disorders. It is appropriate to apply moxibustion to Shèn Shù 腎俞 (UB 23). If applying moxibustion again is not effective, it is appropriate to apply moxibustion to Huán Tiào 環跳 (GB 30), Fēng Shì 風市 (GB 31), Dú Bí 犢鼻 (ST 35), Xī Guān 膝關 (LV 7), Yáng Líng Quán 陽陵泉 (GB 34), Yīn Líng Quán 陰陵泉 (SP 9), Sān Lǐ 三里 (ST 36), Jué Gǔ 絕骨 (GB 39), and so forth. The sites with aching pain when pressed are the diseased sites. Applying moxibustion is always effective.

15. Liè Zǐ 列子 (Master Liè) Western scholars believe it was compiled around the 4th century CE. It was honorifically entitled the *Chōng Xū Zhēn Jīng* 衝虛真經 (True Classic of Simplicity and Vacuity), also known as the Classic of the Perfect Emptiness.

16. Master Yǎn 偃 was a highly skilled craftsman of the *Zhōu* (周) Dynasty. He made a puppet that could mimic a professional singer. He showed this puppet to the King Mù 穆 of *Zhōu* (周), but the puppet made the king angry because his concubine was so attracted to it. The King thought the puppet was actually a real person, so Master Yǎn had to remove its internal organs to show the king it was made by craft.

# 5.17
## *Zú Bù Néng Xíng (Bù Néng Lì, Bù Shōu)*

脅痛 476
腰脊 551
腰腳 542
足寒熱 513

# 足不能行 （不能立 不收）

## Inability to walk
**(Inability to stand, loss of use [of legs])**

三陰交療不能行（《明下》）。上廉治喘息不能行（見脅痛）。合陽（見腰脊）治履步難。天柱、行間主足不任身（《千》與《銅》同）。京門主腰痛不能立。然谷治胻酸不能久立（《銅》見失精）。承山治戰栗不能立（見腰腳）。

Sān Yīn Jiāo 三陰交 (SP 6) cures inability to walk (*Míng Xià*《明下》).

Shàng Lián 上廉 (ST 37) treats panting with inability to walk (see the section on pain of the [chest and] rib-sides).

Hé Yáng 合陽 (UB 55) (see the section on [pain of] the lower back and spine) treats difficulty walking.

Tiān Zhù 天柱 (UB 10) and Xíng Jiān 行間 (LV 2) govern inability of the feet to bear the body (*Qiān*《千》and *Tóng*《銅》agree).

Jīng Mén 京門 (GB 25) governs lower back pain with inability to stand.

Rán Gǔ 然谷 (KI 2) treats aching of the lower legs with inability to stand for long (see the discussion of seminal loss in *Tóng*).

Chéng Shān 承山 (UB 57) treats shivering with inability to stand (see the section on lower back and leg [pain]).

漏谷療不能久立（《明下》見足寒熱）。飛揚療體重起坐不能，步履不收，腳腨酸重戰栗，不能久立坐。跗陽療不能久立，坐不能起（見腰腳）。申脈治胻寒不能久立，坐如在舟車中（《銅》見腰腳）。中都主不能行（光明同）立。三里主不能立（並見足寒熱）。

乳癰 718
四肢厥 528
唾血 402
虛損 174

Lòu Gǔ 漏谷 (SP 7) cures inability to stand for long (see the section on [sensations of] cold and heat in the legs in *Míng Xià*《 明下 》).

Fēi Yáng 飛揚 (UB 58) cures heaviness of the body with inability to get up or sit, loss of use of the legs, aching, heaviness and shivering of the calves, and inability to stand or sit for a long time.

Fù Yáng 跗陽 (UB 59) cures inability to stand for long and inability to get up when sitting (see the section on lower back and leg [pain]).

Shēn Mài 申脈 (UB 62) treats cold lower legs with inability to stand for long and a a sensation as if sitting in a boat or wagon (see the section on lower back and leg [pain] in *Tóng*《 銅 》).

Zhōng Dū 中都 (LV 6) governs inability to walk (the same as Guāng Míng 光明 (GB 37)) and stand.

Sān Lǐ 三里 (ST 36) governs inability to stand (for all, see the section on [sensations of] cold and heat in the legs).

浮白主足緩不收(《千》)。三里、衝陽、僕參、飛揚、復溜、完骨主足痿失履不收。下廉主驚痹跗不收(見乳癰)。豐隆(見四肢厥)、脾俞治四肢不收(《銅》見腹脹)。支溝等治四肢不舉。曲泉、大巨(《銅》同)等主四肢不收(並見四肢厥)。三里主不能久立(見唾血虛損)。

Fú Bái 浮白 (GB 10) governs loss of use of the feet (*Qiān*《 千 》).

Sān Lǐ 三里 (ST 36), Chōng Yáng 衝陽 (ST 42), Pū Cān 僕參 (UB 61), Fēi Yáng (UB 58), Fù Liū 復溜 (KI 7), and Wán Gǔ 完骨 (GB 12) govern wilting of the feet and inability to walk.

Xià Lián 下廉 (ST 39) governs fright, *bì*-impediment, and loss of use of the feet (see the section on mammary welling-abscess).

Fēng Lóng 豐隆 (ST 40) (see the section on limb reversal) and Pí Shù 脾俞 (UB 20) treat loss of use of the limbs (see the section on abdominal fullness).

Zhī Gōu 支溝 (SJ 6) and so forth treat inability to lift the four limbs.

Qū Quán 曲泉 (LV 8), Dà Jù 大巨 (ST 27) (*Tóng* agrees) and so forth govern loss of use of the limbs (for all, see the section on limb reversal).

Sān Lǐ (ST 36) governs inability to stand for long (see the sections on spitting of blood and vacuity detriment).

## 5.18

### *Zú Hán Rè (Jìng Hán, Yòu Jiàn Zú Zá Bìng)*

# 足寒熱 (脛寒　又見足雜病)

### [Sensations of] cold and heat in the legs

**(Cold lower legs, also see the section on miscellaneous disorders of the legs)**

不能立 511
腹滿 445
尸厥 531
小便 226
瘧 301
膝痛 536

至陰主風寒從足小指起，脈痹上下。腎俞、京骨、然谷主足寒。陰市主膝上伏兔中寒。行間主厥，足下熱。中都主足下熱，脛寒不能久立，濕痹不能行。三里、條口、承山、承筋主足下熱，不能久立。委中治足熱厥逆滿，取其經血立愈(《銅》)。

Zhì Yīn 至陰 (UB 67) governs wind-cold starting from the little toe, then inducing vessel *bì*-impediment above and below (*Qiān*《千》).

Shèn Shù 腎俞 (UB 23), Jīng Gǔ 京骨 (UB 64) and Rán Gǔ 然谷 (KI 2) govern cold feet.

Yīn Shì 陰市 (ST 33) governs cold in the crouching rabbit [area] (anterior thighs) above the knees.

Xíng Jiān 行間 (LV 2) governs reversal and heat on the bottom of the feet.

Zhōng Dū 中都 (LV 6) governs heat on the bottom of the feet, cold lower legs with inability to stand for long, and damp *bì*-impediment with inability to walk.

Sān Lǐ 三里 (ST 36), Tiáo Kǒu 條口 (ST 38), Chéng Shān 承山 (UB 57) and Chéng Jīn 承筋 (UB 56) govern heat on the bottom of the feet and inability to stand for long.

Wěi Zhōng 委中 (UB 40) treats heat reversal of the feet and counterflow fullness. Drain blood from the channel to cure the disorder immediately (*Tóng*《銅》).

涌泉治足下熱，喘滿，乃熱厥也。齊王患此，針之愈。至陰治下熱。然谷治足一寒一熱(見不能立)。大都(見腹滿)治手足逆冷。隱白(見尸厥)、太衝治足寒(見小便不利)。中封治足逆冷(見瘧)。陽陵泉治足冷無血色(見膝痛)。復溜主胻寒，不能自溫(《千》)。漏谷療足熱腿冷疼，不能久立，麻痹不仁(《明下》)。

Yǒng Quán 涌泉 (KI 1) treats heat on the bottom of the feet, panting, and fullness; this is heat reversal. King Qí suffered this disorder and was cured after needling this point.

Zhì Yīn 至陰 (UB 67) treats heat on the bottom of the feet.

Rán Gǔ 然谷 (KI 2) treats cold in one foot and heat in the other (see the section on inability to stand).

Dà Dū 大都 (SP 2) (see the section on abdominal fullness) treats counterflow cold of the extremities.

Yǐn Bái 隱白 (SP 1) (see the section on deathlike reversal) and Tài Chōng 太衝 (LV 3) treat cold feet (see the section on inhibited urination).

Zhōng Fēng 中封 (LV 4) treats reversal cold of the feet (see the section on malaria).

Yáng Líng Quán 陽陵泉 (GB 34) treats cold feet without the color of blood [pale] (see the section on knee pain).

Fù Liū 復溜 (KI 7) governs cold in the lower legs with inability to warm up naturally (*Qiān*《千》).

Lòu Gǔ 漏谷 (SP 7) cures heat in the feet and cold painful legs, inability to stand for long, and numbness (*Míng Xià*《明下》).

《史記》：濟北王阿母足熱而懣，太倉公曰：熱厥也。刺其足心各三所，案之無出血，病旋已。病得之飲酒大醉。

*Shǐ Jì*《史記》(The Records of the Grand Historian) says: The wet nurse of King Jì Běi suffered hot feet and oppression. Master Tài Cāng said it was heat reversal. He pricked three places in the center of each of the soles. According to the record, there was no blood-letting, but the disease was cured. The disease was caused by drinking too much liquor and drunkenness.)

風痹 377
歷節風 707
轉筋 267

# 5.19

## *Zú Zá Bìng*

*(Gēn Gǔ, Xíng Jìng Shuàn Tuǐ, Bì Shū, Yú Jiàn Jiǎo Xī Luán)*

## 足雜病

## （跟股　胻脛腨腿　髀樞　餘見腳膝攣）

## Miscellaneous disorders of the legs

**(Heels and thighs, lower legs, calves, thigh pivot; for further discussion, see the section on hypertonicity of the legs and knees)**

僕參治足跟痛，不得履地，腳痿轉筋（《銅》）。浮郄治腳股筋急，髀樞不仁。跗陽治髀樞股胻痛（見風痹）。飛揚治足指不屈伸（見歷節風）。經渠治足心痛（《銅》見熱病無汗）。築賓治足腨痛。承筋治腳腨酸（見轉筋）。涌泉療心中結熱，腳底白肉際不得履地。《明下》云：療足指盡疼，不得履地。《千》云：涌泉、然谷主五指盡痛，足不履地。

Pū Cān 僕參 (UB 61) treats heel pain, inability to step on the ground, and wilting of the legs with cramping (*Tóng*《銅》).

Fú Xī 浮郄 (UB 38) treats sinew tension of the legs and thighs, and numbness of the thigh pivot [great trochanter].

Fū Yáng 跗陽 (UB 59) treats pain of the thigh pivot, thigh, and lower leg (see the section on wind *bì*-impediment).

Fēi Yáng 飛揚 (UB 58) treats inability to flex and stretch the toes (see the section on joint running wind).

Jīng Qú 經渠 (LU 8) treats pain of the soles (see the section on heat disease without sweating in *Tóng*).

Zhù Bīn 筑賓 (KI 9) treats painful feet and calves.

Chéng Jīn 承筋 (UB 56) treats aching legs and calves (see the section on cramping).

Yǒng Quán 涌泉 (KI 1) cures heat bind in the center of the heart [of the feet] while there is inability of the border of the white flesh on the bottom of the feet to step on the ground [due to pain].

腳氣 519
膝腳痛 536
足寒熱 513
中風 379

*Míng Xià*《明下》says: It cures pain in all the toes when they cannot step on the ground. *Qiān*《千》says: Yǒng Quán 涌泉 (KI 1) and Rán Gǔ 然谷 (KI 2) govern pain in all five toes with inability of the feet to step on the ground.

三陰交療不能行(《千》)。三陰交療足痿不能行(見膝腳痛)。上廉療腳重不得履地(見腳氣)。崑崙療腳重不得履地。崑崙治踹腫不得履地。然谷治足跗腫,不得履地。中都主脛寒(見足寒熱)。絕骨:灸百壯,治風身重脛寒(見中風)。

Sān Yīn Jiāo 三陰交 (SP 6) cures inability to walk (*Qiān*).

Sān Yīn Jiāo (SP 6) cures wilting legs with inability to walk (see the section on leg and knee pain).

Shàng Lián 上廉 (ST 37) cures heavy legs with inability to step on the ground (see the section on leg qì).

Kūn Lún 崑崙 (UB 60) cures heavy legs with inability to step on the ground.

Kūn Lún (UB 60) treats calf swelling with inability to step on the ground.

Rán Gǔ (KI 2) treats swelling of the instep with inability to step on the ground.

Zhōng Dū 中都 (LV 6) governs coldness of the lower legs (see the section on [sensations of] cold and heat in the legs).

Jué Gǔ 絕骨 (GB 39): Apply a hundred cones of moxibustion on it to treat wind, generalized heaviness, and coldness of the lower legs (see the section on wind stroke).

條口(太溪同)療脛寒(《明》見足麻)。梁丘療大驚脛痛,冷痹膝痛,不屈伸。

Tiáo Kǒu 條口 (ST 38) (Tài Xī 太溪 (KI 3) is the same) cures coldness of the lower legs (see the section on numbness of the legs in *Míng*《明》).

Liáng Qiū 梁丘 (ST 34) cures great fright, pain of the lower legs, cold *bì*-impediment, and knee pain with inability to flex and stretch.

《難經疏》云:足脛寒者,腎主骨,有病先脛冷也。當以此求之。

*Nàn Jīng Shū*《難經疏》says: Coldness of the lower legs - since the kidneys govern the bones, if they have disease, the lower legs will feel cold first. People should follow this theory.

然谷主足不能安，脛酸不能久立（《千》）。涌泉、太衝主脛酸。至陽主脛疼，四肢重，少氣難言。承山、承筋（又見轉筋）主腳脛酸，腳急跟痛，腳筋急痛。環跳、內庭主脛痛，不可屈伸。陽關主脛痹不仁。至陽主脛酸（《銅》見寒熱）。膀胱俞治脛寒拘急，不得屈伸。 轉筋 267 足麻痹 509

Rán Gŭ 然谷 (KI 2) governs restless legs and aching lower legs with inability to stand for long (*Qiān*《千》).

Yŏng Quán 涌泉 (KI 1) and Tài Chōng 太衝 (LV 3) govern aching of the lower legs.

Zhì Yáng 至陽 (Dū 9) governs pain of the lower legs, heavy limbs, qì shortage, and difficulty talking.

Chéng Shān 承山 (UB 57) and Chéng Jīn 承筋 (UB 56) (also see the section on cramping) govern aching of the lower legs, leg tension, heel pain, and acute pain of the leg sinews.

Huán Tiào 環跳 (GB 30) and Nèi Tíng 內庭 (ST 44) govern pain of the lower legs with inability to flex and stretch.

Yáng Guān 陽關 (GB 33) governs *bì*-impediment and numbness of the lower legs.

Zhì Yáng (Dū 9) governs aching of the lower legs (see the section on [sensations of] cold and heat in *Tóng*《銅》).

Páng Guāng Shù 膀胱俞 (UB 28) treats coldness and hypertonicity of the lower legs with inability to flex and stretch.

丘墟療足腕不收，足脛偏細（《明》）。復溜主脛寒（《千》見足寒）。環跳、束骨、交信、陰交、陰谷主髀樞中痛不可舉。臨泣、三陰交主髀中痛，不得行走，外皮痛。凡髀樞中痛不可舉：以毫針，寒而留之，以月生死為數，立已。丘墟主髀樞腳痛。陽輔等主髀樞不仁（見足麻痹）。

Qīu Xū 丘墟 (GB 40) cures loss of use of the legs and ankles, while the lower legs tend to be thin (*Míng*《明》).

Fù Liū 復溜 (KI 7) governs coldness of the lower legs (see the section on cold legs in *Qiān*).

Huán Tiào 環跳 (GB 30), Shù Gŭ 束骨 (UB 65), Jiāo Xìn 交信 (KI 8), Yīn Jiāo 陰交 (Rèn 7), and Yīn Gŭ 陰谷 (KI 10) govern pain of the thigh pivot with inability to lift [the legs].

Lín Qì 臨泣 (GB 41) and Sān Yīn Jiāo 三陰交 (SP 6) govern pain of the thighs and inability to walk with painful skin.

Pain of the thigh pivot and inability to lift [the legs]: Apply acupuncture with a filiform needle. Retain the needles for cold retention, and count the number of insertions according to the phase of the moon. This will cure the disease immediately.

Qiū Xū 丘墟 (GB 40) governs pain of the thigh pivot and legs.

Yáng Fǔ 陽輔 (GB 38) and so forth govern numbness of the thigh pivot (see the section on numbness of the legs).

膝以上病：宜灸環跳、風市。膝及膝下病：宜灸犢鼻、膝關、三里、陽陵泉。足踝以上病：宜灸三陰交、絕骨、崑崙。足踝以下病：宜灸照海、申脈。然須按其穴酸疼處灸之，方效。

For diseases above the knees: it is appropriate to apply moxibustion on Huán Tiào 環跳 (GB 30) and Fēng Shì 風市 (GB 31).

For diseases of the knees or below the knees: it is appropriate to apply moxibustion on Dú Bí 犢鼻 (ST 35), Xī Guān 膝關 (LV 7), and Yáng Líng Quán 陽陵泉 (GB 34).

For diseases above the ankles: it is appropriate to apply moxibustion on Sān Yīn Jiāo 三陰交 (SP 6), Jué Gǔ 絕骨(GB 39), and Kūn Lún 崑崙 (UB 60).

For diseases below the ankles: it is appropriate to apply moxibustion on Zhào Hǎi 照海 (KI 6) and Shēn Mài 申脈 (UB 62).

This will only be effective when moxibustion is applied to sites that ache when pressed.

## 5.20
## *Jiǎo Qì*
# 腳氣
## Leg qì

世有勤工力學之士，一心注意於事，久坐、行立於濕地，不時動轉。冷風來擊，入於經絡，不覺成病。故風毒中人，或先中手足十指，因汗毛孔開，腠理疏通，風如擊箭。或先中足心，或先中足趺，或先中膝以下腨脛表里者。若欲使人不成病者，初覺即灸所覺處三二十壯。因此即愈，不復發（《千》）。

There are people who work and study hard; they are always concentrating on doing things. They sit or walk and stand for a long time on the damp ground, and do not move frequently. When a cold wind strikes, it enters the channels and network vessels, and induces disease before the person realizes it. When wind toxins attack someone, it attacks the ten fingers or toes first; this is because the pores are open, the interstices are unlocked, and the wind shoots in like an arrow. The wind can also attack the soles first, or attack the instep first, or attack the tibia and calves below the knees. If someone does not want disease to form, he needs to apply twenty or thirty cones of moxibustion on the reactive sites when they are first perceived. This will cure the disease, and the disease will not reoccur (*Qiān*《千》).

凡腳氣初得腳弱，便速灸之，並服竹瀝湯。灸訖，可服八風散，無不瘥者，惟急速治之。若人但灸而不能服散，服散而不灸者，半瘥半死。雖得瘥者，或至一二年後更發動。覺得便依此法速灸之，及服散者，治十十愈。此病輕者，登時雖不即惡，治之不當，根源不除，久久殺人，不可不以為意。初灸風市，次灸伏兔，次犢鼻，次膝兩眼（一法忌灸），次三里，次上廉，次下廉，次絕骨。

When people initially come down with leg qì and the legs are weak, apply moxibustion immediately and ask them to drink *Zhú Lì Tāng* 竹瀝湯 (Bambusa Succus Decoction) at the same time. Once the moxibustion is complete, *Bā Fēng Sǎn* 八風散 (Eight Wind Powder) can be offered. The disease will be cured like this, but immediate treatment is necessary. If people use moxibustion only without taking the powder, or if they take the powder only without using moxibustion, half will recover, and half will die. Even if they are cured, the disease will reoccur in one or two years.

If people follow this method and receive moxibustion as soon as they realize they have the disease, taking the powder at the same time, they will all be cured. In a mild case of this disease, it will not become malign right away; but if there is no proper treatment, the root will not be removed and it will kill them after a long while. More attention must be given to it.

Apply moxibustion on Fēng Shì 風市 (GB 31) first, then on Fú Tù 伏兔 (ST 32), then on Dú Bí 犢鼻 (ST 35), then on the two eyes of the knees (another method forbids moxibustion [on this point]), then Sān Lǐ 三里 (ST 36), then Shàng Lián 上廉 (ST 37), then Xià Lián 下廉 (ST 39), and then Jué Gǔ 絕骨 (GB 39).

凡灸八處：一、風市百壯，多亦任人，輕者不可減百壯，重乃至一處五六百壯，勿令頓灸，三報之佳。二、伏兔百壯，亦可五十壯。三、犢鼻五十壯，有至百壯。四、膝眼。五、三里百壯。六、上廉百壯。七、下廉百壯。八、絕骨。凡此諸穴，不必一頓灸盡壯數，可日日報灸之，三日之中，灸令盡壯數為佳。

Apply moxibustion on these eight sites: first, burn a hundred cones of moxibustion on Fēng Shì (GB 31); more is also allowed. In mild cases, burn no less than a hundred cones; in severe cases, burn five or six hundred cones on one site. Do not apply all the cones of moxibustion at once, but burn all the cones over three sessions.

Second, burn a hundred cones of moxibustion on Fú Tù (ST 32); fifty cones also is good.

Third, burn fifty cones of moxibustion on Dú Bí (ST 35), up to a hundred cones.

Fourth, Xī Yǎn 膝眼 (non-channel).

Fifth, burn a hundred cones of moxibustion on Sān Lǐ 三里 (ST 36).

Sixth, burn a hundred cones of moxibustion on Shàng Lián (ST 37).

Seventh, burn a hundred cones of moxibustion on Xià Lián (ST 39).

Eighth, Jué Gǔ (GB 39).

For all the points above, all the cones must not be burned at once, rather give moxibustion in daily sessions. It is best to complete burning all the cones in three days.

凡病一腳，則灸一腳；病兩腳，則灸兩腳；凡腳弱病，皆灸兩腳。一方云：如覺腳惡，便灸三里及絕骨各一處。兩腳惡者，合四處灸之，多少隨病輕重。大要，雖輕不可減百壯；不差，速以次灸之，多多益佳。一說灸絕骨最要。人有患此腳弱不即治，及入腹，腹腫大上氣。於是乃須大法灸。隨諸俞及諸管關節腹背盡灸之，並服八風散，往往得瘥。覺病入腹，若病人不堪痛，不能盡作大灸，但灸胸中心腹諸穴，及兩腳諸穴。亦有得好瘥者，亦依支法存舊法。梁丘、犢鼻、三里、上廉、下廉、解溪、太衝、陽陵泉、絕骨、崑崙、陰陵泉、三陰交、足太陰、復溜、然谷、涌泉、承山、束骨等凡十八穴。

When one leg is diseased, apply moxibustion on one leg; if two legs are diseased, apply moxibustion on both; for weak legs, apply moxibustion on both legs. One formula says: When someone perceives that a leg is malign, apply moxibustion on one site each of Sān Lǐ 三里 (ST 36) and Jué Gǔ 絕骨 (GB 39). When two legs are malign, apply moxibustion on all four sites. The number of the cones of moxibustion depend on severity of the disease. To summarize, even if the disease is mild, the number of the cones cannot be less than a hundred; if the disease is not cured, immediately apply moxibustion on these points in order, the more the better. In another theory, applying moxibustion on Jué Gǔ (GB 39) is the most important.

When people suffer from weak legs with this [leg qì], but they do not get treatment immediately, the disease will enter the abdomen, and will develop into abdominal swelling and qì ascent. Strong moxibustion should be followed. Apply moxibustion on all the points, ducts, joints, abdomen, and back; also ask the patient to take *Bā Fēng Sǎn* 八風散 (Eight Wind Powder). It will cure the disease. If someone feels that the disease has entered the abdomen but they cannot bear pain, strong moxibustion cannot be offered; in that case just apply moxibustion on the points located on the chest, heart region, and abdomen, as well as on the two legs. For those who get better after treatment, we need to follow the old method of *Zhī Fǎcún* 支法存.[17] [Apply moxibustion on] Liáng Qiū 梁丘 (ST 34), Dú Bí 犢鼻 (ST 35), Sān Lǐ (ST 36), Shàng Lián 上廉 (ST 37), Xià Lián 下廉 (ST 39), Jiě Xī 解溪 (ST 41), Tài Chōng 太衝 (LV 3), Yáng Líng Quán 陽陵泉 (GB 34), Jué Gǔ (GB 39), Kūn Lún 崑崙 (UB 60), Yīn Líng Quán 陰陵泉 (SP 9), Sān Yīn Jiāo 三陰交 (SP 6), Zú Tài Yīn 足太陰, Fù Liū 復溜 (KI 7), Rán Gǔ 然谷 (KI 2), Yǒng Quán 涌泉 (KI 1), Chéng Shān 承山 (UB 57), and Shù Gǔ 束骨 (UB 65). This is eighteen points.

舊法多灸百會、風府，五臟六腑俞募。頃來灸者，悉覺引氣向上，所以不取其法。氣不上者可用之。其要，病已成，恐不救者，悉須灸之其足十指去指奇一分。兩足凡八穴，曹氏名曰八衝。極下氣有效。其足十指端，名曰氣端，日灸三壯，並大神要。其八衝可日灸七壯，氣下即止。凡灸八衝，艾柱小作。病者非深相委悉，勿為灸。上廉療偏風腲腿，腳不隨重不得履地，腳氣刺風痺風腳冷（《明》）。肩井治腳氣上攻（《銅》）。

The old method is to apply moxibustion on Bǎi Huì 百會 (Dū 20), Fēng Fǔ 風府 (Dū 16) and the transport and alarm points of the five viscera and six bowels. Some people who have this moxibustion feel qì is conducted upward, so this method should not be used. For those whose qì does not run upward, this method can be used.

17. Zhī Fǎcún 支法存 was a monk doctor during the *Jìn* (晉) Dynasty. He was an expert at treating weakness of the legs.

To summarize, for those whose disease has already formed, it is feared that they cannot be saved; we should apply moxibustion on their ten toes, 1 *fēn* away from the nail. There are eight points on the two legs; Master Cáo called them Bā Chōng 八衝. They are the utmost for descending qì and are very effective. The points on the tips of the toes are named Qì Duān 氣端. Apply three cones of moxibustion daily, and this is very important. It is appropriate to apply seven cones of moxibustion on Bā Chōng, stopping when qì descends. When applying moxibustion on Bā Chōng, burn small cones. Do not apply moxibustion if the patient does not understand the details.

Shàng Lián 上廉 (ST 37) cures hemilateral wind and weak legs, legs that cannot support the weight with inability to step on the ground, leg qì, prickly wind,[18] wind disease, and cold legs (*Míng*《明》).

Jiān Jǐng 肩井 (GB 21) treats leg qì attacking upward (*Tóng*《銅》).

《千金》云：腳氣一病最宜針。若針而不灸，灸而不針，非良醫也。針灸而不藥，藥不針灸，亦非良醫也，此論甚當。

*Qiān Jīn*《千金》says: For leg qì, acupuncture is the most appropriate. If acupuncture is used without moxibustion; or moxibustion is used without acupuncture – this is not a good doctor. Applying acupuncture and moxibustion but not herbs, or using herbs without acupuncture and moxibustion, – this is not a good doctor either. This discussion is extremely appropriate.

若始覺腳氣，速灸風市、三里各一二百壯，以瀉風濕毒氣。若覺悶熱者，不得灸。以本有熱，灸之則大助風生。食物大忌酒面海鮮，及忌房勞。不爾，服藥無益（《指》）。

When people start to feel leg qì, apply one or two hundred cones of moxibustion on Fēng Shì 風市 (GB 31) and Sān Lǐ 三里 (ST 36) immediately to drain wind-damp and toxic qì. When people feel oppression and heat, do not apply moxibustion; because there is heat already, moxibustion will generate wind. Foods which are seriously contraindicated are liquor, noodles, and sea food; sexual taxation also must be contraindicated. Otherwise, there is no use in taking herbs (*Zhǐ*《指》).

有同舍為予言，史載之謂腳氣有風濕二種，宜瀉不宜補。只宜以沉香湯瀉（見《既效方》），而不許其灸。《千金方》乃載灸法，如此其詳，豈虛人患腳氣方可灸耶。故《指迷方》云：若覺悶熱不得灸，蓋

18. *Cì fēng* 刺風 (prickly wind) is caused by wind-cold attacking the skin, blocking the circulation of qi and blood, and then generating heat. Cold and heat contend with each other and stay under the skin. This results in painful skin that feels like the pricking of a needle.

有所見也。凡灸腳氣，三里、絕骨為要穴，而以愛護為第一。予舊有此疾，不履濕則數歲不作；若履濕則頻作。自後常忌履濕，凡有水濕，不敢著鞋踐之；或立潤地，亦不敢久，須頻移足而後無患。此亦愛護之第二義也。有達官久患腳氣，多服八味丸愈。亦以腳氣衝心，惟此藥能治之。

A colleague told me that Shǐ Zaǐzhī[19] said: there are two types of leg qì: wind and damp. It is appropriate to drain, [but is] not appropriate to supplement. It is appropriate to drain with *Chén Xiāng Tāng* 沉香湯 (Aquilaria Decoction) (see *Jì Xiào Fāng*《既效方》), but moxibustion is contraindicated.

*Qiān Jīn Fāng*《千金方》recorded a method of moxibustion. It is so detailed that moxibustion may be given not only to people with vacuity. *Zhǐ Mí Fāng*《指迷方》says: Moxibustion is contraindicated when people feel oppression and heat. Such opinions may have existed.

When applying the moxibustion for leg qì, Sān Lǐ 三里 (ST 36) and Jué Gǔ 絕骨 (GB 39) are the important points, but taking care [of the body] is the first thing. I suffered this disease in the past, it wouldn't occur for several years if I did not step on the damp ground; but it occured frequently if I stepped on the damp ground. So I have avoided stepping on the damp ground since then. If there is water, I am afraid to tread on it even when wearing shoes. If I stand on the moist ground, I dare not stand for a long time, so I have to move about frequently. In this way I won't suffer the disease. This is the other meaning of taking care. There was a high ranking officer who suffered leg qì for a long time. He took *Bā Wèi Wán* 八味丸 (Eight Ingredients Pill) and the disease was cured. Leg qì can rush into the heart; only this pill can treat that.

19. Shǐ Zaǐzhī 史載之, also named Shǐ Kān 史堪, was a doctor during the *Sòng* (宋) Dynasty. He is the author of *Shǐ Zaǐzhī Fāng*《史載之方》(Formulas of Shǐ Zaǐzhī).

# 5.21

## *Jiǎo Ruò (Jiǎo Bì)*

## 脚弱（脚痹）

## Weak Legs

**(*Bì*-impediment of the legs)**

委中療腳弱無力，風濕痹，筋急，半身不遂(《明》)。三里療腳弱。承山療腳弱無力，腳重，偏風不遂。委中療腳弱無力，腰尻重，曲脉中筋急，半身不遂(《下》)。

Wěi Zhōng 委中 (UB 40) cures weak legs, wind-damp *bì*-impediment, sinew tension, and hemiplegia (*Míng*《明》).

Sān Lǐ 三里 (ST 36) cures weak legs.

Chéng Shān 承山 (UB 57) cures weak legs, heavy legs, and hemilateral wind and paralysis.

Wěi Zhōng (UB 40) cures weak legs, heaviness of the low back, sacrum, and coccyx, sinew tension of the curved part of the knees [popliteal fossa], and hemiplegia (*Xià*《下》).

有人舊患脚弱且瘦削，後灸三里、絕骨，而脚如故。益知黄君針灸圖所謂絕骨治脚疾神信也。同官以脚腫灸承山，一穴瘡即干，一穴數月不愈，不曉所謂，豈亦失之將攝耶？是未可知也。

Someone suffered weak thin legs; after applying moxibustion on Sān Lǐ (ST 36) and Jué Gǔ 絕骨 (GB 39), the legs looked like they did before he became sick. I knew what was said in the Acupuncture Diagrams by Master Huáng, that Jué Gǔ 絕骨 (GB 39) treats leg diseases and can be trusted like a god. My colleague applied moxibustion on Chéng Shān (UB 57) for swelling of the legs; on one side, the moxa sore dried, but the other did not heal for several months. He did not know why. It is not because of bad care. The reason is unknown.

《單方歌》云：風毒腳弱痹，肩井及大椎，風市與三里，百壯不須疑。

*Dān Fāng Gē*《單方歌》(Single Formula Rhymes) says: for wind toxins, weak legs and *bì*-impediment, Jiān Jǐng 肩井 (GB 21) and Dà Zhuī 大椎 (Dū 14), Fēng Shì 風市 (GB 31), and Sān Lǐ 三里 (ST 36), do not doubt [the effectiveness of] a hundred cones.

《千金》灸腳弱凡八穴，病一腳則灸一腳，兩腳病則灸兩腳。凡腳弱病，皆灸兩腳（見腳氣）。或未能盡灸，且先灸風市、犢鼻、三里、絕骨亦效。或不效，當如其法灸之（但肩井不可多灸爾）。

*Qiān Jīn*《千金》applies moxibustion on eight points for weakness of the legs: if one leg is diseased, apply moxibustion on one leg; if two legs are diseased, apply moxibustion on both. For leg weakness, apply moxibustion on both legs (see the section on leg qì). If the moxibustion [prescription] cannot be completed, applying moxibustion on Fēng Shì (GB 31), Dú Bí 犢鼻 (ST 35), Sān Lǐ (ST 36) and Jué Gǔ 絕骨 (GB 39) first is also effective. If it is not effective, the method of moxibustion [applying moxibustion on all eight points described above] should be followed (However, do not apply too much moxibustion on Jiān Jǐng (GB 21)).

腰脚
542

# 5.22
## *Jiǎo Zhǒng*
# 脚腫
## Swelling of the legs

陽蹻療脚氣腎氣（《明》）。上崑崙療惡血風氣腫痛，脚腫。承山治脚氣膝腫（見腰脚）。小腸俞治脚腫，短氣，不嗜食（《明》云：不食，煩熱胻痛）。然谷治足跗腫，不得履地。

Yáng Qiāo 陽蹻 (UB 62) cures leg qì and kidney qì (*Míng*《明》).

Shàng Kūn Lún 上崑崙 (upper UB 60) cures malign blood, swelling and pain due to wind qì, and swelling of the legs.

Chéng Shān 承山 (UB 57) treats leg qì and swelling of the knees (see the section on lower back and leg [pain]).

Xiǎo Cháng Shù 小腸俞 (UB 27) treats swelling of the legs, shortness of breath, and no desire to eat (*Míng* says: inability to eat, vexation heat, and leg pain).

Rán Gǔ 然谷 (KI 2) treats swelling of the instep and inability to step on the ground.

執中母氏常久病，夏中脚忽腫。舊傳夏不理足，不敢著艾。謾以針置火中令熱，於三里穴刺之，微見血。凡數次，其腫如失去。執中素患脚腫，見此奇效，亦以火針刺之。翌日，腫亦消。何其速也，後亦常灸之。凡治脚腫，當先三里而後陽蹻等穴可也。又予患脚氣指縫爛，每以茶末滲之愈。他日復爛而腫，用茶末不效，漸腫至脚背上，予以為脚氣使然，竊憂之，策杖而後敢行。偶賣藥僧者見之，云可取床荐下塵滲之，如其言滲之而愈。此物不值一錢，而能愈可憂之疾，其可忽哉。

My mother frequently suffered enduring diseases; she suddenly developed swelling of the legs in the middle of the summer. An old tradition says 'do not regulate the legs in the summer,' so I was afraid to apply moxibustion on her legs. Instead, I just held the needle in the fire to make it hot, punctured Sān Lǐ 三里 (ST 36), and let a little blood. The swelling disappeared after several treatments. I often suffer swelling of the legs. After seeing this divine effect, I also punctured myself with a fire needle. The swelling disappeared the next day. It was so fast. Later, I frequently applied moxibustion. When treating swelling of the legs, it is appropriate to treat Sān Lǐ 三里 (ST 36) first, then Yáng Qiāo 陽蹻 (UB 62), and so forth.

I also suffered leg qì with erosion between my toes; it was cured by sprinkling them with tea powder. The toes eroded again and became swollen later on, and the tea powder was not effective anymore. The swelling gradually reached the dorsum of the foot. I thought this was caused by leg qì and started to worry about it. I was afraid to walk without using a walking stick. By chance, a monk who sold herbs saw me and told me that I could use the dust from under the straw bed mat to sprinkle between my toes. I followed what he said and the disease was cured. This substance has no value, but it can cure a disease that makes people worry, so we cannot ignore it.

寒熱 675
水腫 459
痃癖 433
悲愁 331
腹脹 449
腋痛 496
風痹 377
膈痛 481
小腹脹 211
勞瘵 188
喉痹 629
無汗 690

# 5.23

## *Sì Zhī Jué (Shǒu Zú Bù Jǔ, Yú Jiàn Shǒu Zú Má Bì)*

## 四肢厥
## （手足不舉　餘見手足麻痹）

## Limb reversal

**(Inability to lift the limbs; for further discussion, see the section on numbness of the limbs)**

內庭治四肢厥逆，腹脹，數欠（《銅》）。至陽治四肢重（《明下》同）痛（見寒熱）。章門治厥逆，四肢惰（見水腫）。膈俞治四肢怠惰（見痃癖）。極泉、日月（見悲愁）、脾俞治四肢不收（見腹脹）。支溝（見腋痛）、小海、跗陽（見風痹）、天池（見膈痛）、三陰交治四肢不舉（見腹脹）。

Nèi Tíng 內庭 (ST 44) treats reverse counterflow of the limbs, abdominal distention, and frequent yawning (*Tóng*《銅》).

Zhì Yáng 至陽 (Dū 9) treats heaviness of the limbs (*Míng Xià*《明下》agrees) and pain (see the section on [sensations of] cold and heat).

Zhāng Mén 章門 (LV 13) treats reverse counterflow and lazy limbs (see the section on edema).

Gé Shù 膈俞 (UB 17) treats fatigued limbs (see the section on strings and aggregations).

Jí Quán 極泉 (HT 1), Rì Yuè 日月 (GB 24) (see the section on sorrow and anxiety [of the heart]), and Pí Shù 脾俞 (UB 20) treat loss of use of the limbs (see the section on abdominal fullness).

Zhī Gōu 支溝 (SJ 6) (see the section on pain of the axilla), Xiǎo Hǎi 小海 (SI 8), Fū Yáng 跗陽 (UB 59) (see the section on wind *bì*-impediment), Tiān Chí 天池 (PC 1) (see the section on pain of the diaphragm), and Sān Yīn Jiāo 三陰交 (SP 6) treat inability to lift the limbs (see the section on abdominal fullness).

大巨治偏枯，四肢不舉（見小腹脹）。腎俞治腰中四肢淫濼（見勞瘵）。尺澤治四肢暴腫，臂寒短氣（見喉痹）。三里治四肢腫滿。大都療手足逆冷腫（見傷寒無汗）。豐隆療厥逆，胸痛氣刺不可忍，腹中如刀疞，大小便難，四肢不收，身體怠惰，腿膝酸痹，屈伸難（《明下》）。

Dà Jù 大巨 (ST 27) treats hemilateral withering and inability to lift the four limbs (see the section on distention [and fullness] of the smaller abdomen). 胸脅痛 476

Shèn Shù 腎俞 (UB 23) treats soreness and weakness of the low back and four limbs (see the section on consumption). 傷寒 661 腹滿 445

Chǐ Zé 尺澤 (LU 5) treats sudden swelling of the limbs, cold arms, and shortness of breath (see the section on throat *bì*-impediment).

Sān Lǐ 三里 (ST 36) treats swelling and fullness of the limbs.

Dà Dū 大都 (SP 2) cures swelling and reversal cold of the limbs (see the section on cold damage with absence of sweating).

Fēng Lóng 豐隆 (ST 40) cures reverse counterflow, unbearable stabbing chest pain due to qì accumulation, gripping colic in the abdomen that feels like a knife, difficult urination and defecation, loss of use of the limbs, fatigue, aching and *bì*-impediment of the knees and legs, and difficulty flexing and stretching (*Míng Xià*《明下》).

內庭主四肢厥手足悶(《千》)。太溪主手足寒至節。內庭主四肢厥，手足悶者，久持之。厥熱腦痛，腹脹皮痛者，使人久持之。列缺主四肢厥，喜笑。章門主四肢懈惰，喜怒。照海主四肢淫濼。曲泉、跗陽、天池、大巨、小海(《明下》作少海)、支溝、絕骨、前谷主四肢不舉。

Nèi Tíng 內庭 (ST 44) governs limb reversal and a feeling of oppression of the hands and feet (*Qiān*《千》).

Tài Xī 太溪 (KI 3) governs hands and feet become cold up to the joints.

Nèi Tíng (ST 44) governs limb reversal, oppression and contraction of the extremities, heat reversal, brain pain, and abdominal distention with painful skin that make the patient feel tension.

Liè Quē 列缺 (LU 7) governs limb reversal and frequent laughter.

Zhāng Mén 章門 (LV 13) governs sluggish limbs and frequent anger.

Zhào Hǎi 照海 (KI 6) governs pain and weakness of the limbs.

Qū Quán 曲泉 (LV 8), Fū Yáng 跗陽 (UB 59), Tiān Chí 天池 (PC 1), Dà Jù 大巨 (ST 27), Xiǎo Hǎi 小海(SI 8) (*Míng Xià*《明下》says Shào Hǎi 少海 (HT 3)), Zhī Gōu 支溝(SJ 6), Jué Gǔ 絕骨 (GB 39), and Qián Gǔ 前谷 (SI 2) govern inability to lift the limbs.

五里、三陽絡、厲兌、天井主嗜臥，四肢不欲動搖。行間治四肢逆冷(《銅》)。太溪治手足厥冷(見胸脅痛)。四逆取俠溪(見傷寒)。大都治手足逆冷(見腹滿)。

Wǔ Lǐ 五里 (LI 13 or LV 10), Sān Yáng Luò 三陽絡 (SJ 8), Lì Duì 厲兌 (ST 45), and Tiān Jǐng 天井 (SJ 10) govern somnolence and inability to move the limbs.

Xíng Jiān 行間 (LV 2) treats cold limb reversal (*Tóng*《 銅 》).

Tài Xī 太溪 (KI 3) treats cold limb reversal (see the section on pain of the chest and rib-sides).

Limb reversal: Treat Xiá Xī 俠溪 (GB 43) (see the section on cold damage).

Dà Dū 大都 (SP 2) treats cold limb reversal (see the section on abdominal fullness).

有士人患陰證傷寒，手足冷甚，以火溫之，亦不暖。予與理中湯服，即得汗而病愈，手足自溫矣。若其他手足厥者，當隨證灸之。

A scholar suffered yīn pattern cold damage; his limbs were very cold and fire did not warm him up. I gave him *Lǐ Zhōng Wán* 理中丸 (Center Rectifying Pill), he sweated, and the disease was cured. His limbs also naturally became warm. For other types of limb reversal, moxibustion should be applied according to the pattern.

四厥脈沉絕：灸手間使便通，起死法（ 乾嘔 ）。四厥：灸乳根（ 轉筋 ）。

Limb reversal with a pulse that is deep and expiring: Apply moxibustion on Jiān Shǐ 間使 (PC 5) to unblock the vessels. This is a method of raising the dead (dry heaves).

Limb reversal: Apply moxibustion on Rǔ Gēn 乳根 (ST 18) (cramping).

人病狂痴手足厥，作狂病治不效。《名醫錄》曰：此驚恐憂思所得。大驚傷心，大恐傷腎，大憂思傷神志，神不足則狂痴，志不足則恐怖，恐怖則腎氣留積。足不收，亦因積驚恐氣傷腎也。（鬼擊卒死：菖蒲根搗汁灌立瘥）。

Someone suffered mania with limb reversal. Treating it as mania was not effective. *Míng Yī Lù*《名醫錄》says: This is caused by fright, fear, anxiety, and preoccupation. Severe fright damages the heart, severe fear damages the kidneys, severe anxiety and preoccupation damage the spirit and will. Insufficient spirit causes mania, insufficient will causes fear, and fear makes kidney qì accumulate. Loss of use of the legs is also due to kidney damage from accumulated fright and fear qì. (For sudden death due to ghost strike: Pound the root of *chāng pǔ* 菖蒲 to make juice and pour it into the patient to cure the disease immediately.

# 5.24
# *Shī Jué*
# 尸厥
## Deathlike reversal

百會、玉枕主卒起僵仆，惡見風寒（《千》）。通天（《明》同）、絡卻主暫起僵仆。大杼主僵仆不能久立，煩滿里急，身不安席。隱白、大敦主卒尸厥不知人，脈動如故。金門主尸厥暴死。中極、僕參主恍惚尸厥，煩痛。內庭主四厥，手足悶者，久持之，厥熱腦痛，腹脹皮痛者，使人久持之。

Bǎi Huì 百會 (Dū 20) and Yù Zhěn 玉枕 (UB 9) govern sudden collapse after getting up and aversion to wind-cold (*Qiān*《千》).

Tōng Tiān 通天 (UB 7) (*Míng*《明》agrees) and Luò Què 絡卻 (UB 8) govern collapse when attempting to stand up.

Dà Zhù 大杼 (UB 11) governs sudden collapse with inability to stand for long, vexation and fullness, internal tension, and inability to lie down.

Yǐn Bái 隱白 (SP 1) and Dà Dūn 大敦 (LV 1) govern sudden deathlike reversal and unconsciousness but the vessels pulsate as usual.

Jīn Mén 金門 (UB 63) governs deathlike reversal and sudden death.

Zhōng Jí 中極 (Rèn 3) and Pū Cān 僕參 (UB 61) govern abstraction, deathlike reversal, and vexation pain.

Nèi Tíng 內庭 (ST 44) governs limb reversal, oppression and contraction of the extremities, heat reversal, brain pain, and abdominal distention with painful skin which make the patient feel tension.

列缺主四肢厥，喜笑，邪客於手足少陰、太陰、足陽明之絡。此五絡者，皆會於耳中，上絡左角。五絡俱竭，令人身脈動如故，其形無所知，其狀若尸。刺足大指內側爪甲上，去端如韭葉；後刺足心；後取足中指爪甲上各一；後取手大指之內，去爪甲如韭葉；後刺手心主少陰兌骨之端各一痏，立已。不已，以筒吹其兩耳中立已。不已，拔其左角發方寸燔治，飲以淳酒一杯，不能飲者，灌之立已。

Liè Quē 列缺 (LU 7) governs reversal cold of the limbs, frequent laughter, and evils settling in the network vessels of hand and foot shàoyīn, tàiyīn and foot yángmíng. These five network vessels all meet in the ears and connect to the left corner of the head. Expiry of the five networks allows a person's vessels to pulsate as usual, but their body cannot perceive anything, so they appear like a corpse. Needle the site that is the distance of a leek leaf from the nail, on the medial aspect of the big toe; then needle the sole; then bilaterally needle the site above the nail of the middle toe; then the site that is the distance of a leek leaf away from the nail, on the medial aspect of the thumb; then needle the site located at the end of the sharp bone of the hand pericardium and shàoyīn. This will immediately cure the disease. If not, blow into the ear with a tube; this will cure the disease immediately. If not, pull out a square-*cùn* size patch of hair on the left corner of the head and burn it; drink it with one cup of pure liquor. If the patient is unable to drink, pour it into him. It will cure the disease immediately.

豐隆主厥逆，足卒青痛如刺，腹若刀切之狀，大便難，煩心，狂見鬼好笑，卒面四肢腫。旁廷在腋下四肋間，高下正與乳相當，乳後二寸陷中，俗名注市，舉掖取之，刺入五分，灸五十壯。主卒中惡，飛尸遁注，胸脅滿。九曲中府在旁廷注市下三寸，刺入五分，灸三十壯。主惡風邪氣遁尸，內有瘀血。天府主卒中惡風邪氣，飛尸惡注，鬼語遁下（並《千》）。

Fēng Lóng 豐隆 (ST 40) governs reverse counterflow, sudden green color and pricking pain of the feet, abdominal pain that feels like a knife cutting, difficult defecation, vexation of the heart, mania, seeing ghosts, frequent laughter, and sudden swelling of the face and limbs.

Páng Tíng 旁廷 (non-channel) is located below the axilla in the fourth intercostal space, 2 cùn posterior to and level with the nipples. Its common name is Zhù Shì 注市. Locate the point while lifting the axilla. Needle it 5 fēn deep; apply fifty cones of moxibustion. It governs sudden malignity strike, flying corpse, *dùn zhù* 遁注,[20] and fullness of the chest and rib-sides.

Jiǔ Qū Zhōng Fǔ 九曲中府 (non-channel) is located 3 cùn below Páng Tíng 旁廷 (Zhù Shì 注市). Needle it 5 fēn deep; apply thirty cones of moxibustion. It governs malign wind evil qì retreating corpse, and internal blood stasis.

Tiān Fǔ 天府 (LU 3) governs sudden malign wind and evil qì strike, flying corpse, malignity infixation, ghost speech, and hiding (together with *Qiān*《千》).

20. *Dùn zhù* 遁注 is hard to translate. Perhaps it is something like 'fleeing influx.' It is the name of a disease that is caused by a strike from toxic qì when the person is weak. The toxic qì remains and hides inside the channels or organs. When the disease occurs, the patient suffers intermittent heaviness of the limbs and stabbing pain of the abdomen.

隱白治卒尸厥不識人（《明》同），足寒，不能溫（《銅》）。中極治恍惚尸厥（見賁豚）。《明下》云：尸厥不知人。大敦治尸厥狀如死。僕參治尸厥如中惡狀，霍亂癲癇，狂言見鬼。厲兌治尸厥，口噤氣絕，狀如中惡，心腹脹滿。《明》云：尸厥如死，不知人。 賁豚 430 狂 345

Yǐn Bái 隱白 (SP 1) treats sudden deathlike reversal and loss of consciousness (*Míng*《明》agrees), cold feet, and inability to feel warm (*Tóng*《銅》).

Zhōng Jí 中極 (Rèn 3) treats abstraction and deathlike reversal (see the section on running-piglet). *Míng Xià*《明下》said: deathlike reversal with unconsciousness.

Dà Dūn 大敦 (LV 1) treats deathlike reversal, appearing to be dead.

Pū Cān 僕參 (UB 61) treats deathlike reversal that appears like malignity strike, sudden turmoil, withdrawal and epilepsy, manic raving as if seeing ghosts.

Lì Duì 厲兌 (ST 45) treats deathlike reversal, clenched jaws, qì expiry that appears like malignity strike, and distention and fullness of the heart and abdomen. *Míng* says: deathlike reversal and appearing to be dead with unconsciousness.

金門治癲癇，尸厥，暴疲。委陽治腋腫膨膨，失志身熱，飛尸遁注，痿厥不仁。魂門療尸厥走疰，胸背連痛（《明下》）。僕參療癲疾，尸厥，霍亂，馬癇。攢竹（見狂）、禾髎療尸厥。天府療卒中惡，鬼疰，不得安臥，禁灸（《銅》）。

Jīn Mén 金門 (UB 63) treats withdrawal and epilepsy, deathlike reversal, and acute fatigue.

Wěi Yáng 委陽 (UB 39) treats axillary swelling with a feeling of inflation, loss of will, generalized heat, flying corpse, *dùn zhù* 遁注, wilting, reversal, and numbness.

Hún Mén 魂門 (UB 47) cures deathlike reversal, wandering infixation, and pain radiating between the chest and back (*Míng Xià*).

Pū Cān (UB 61) cures withdrawal disease, deathlike reversal, sudden turmoil, and horse epilepsy.

Zǎn Zhú 攢竹 (UB 2) (see the section on mania) and Hé Liáo 禾髎 (LI 19) cure deathlike reversal.

Tiān Fǔ 天府 (LU 3) cures sudden malignity attack, ghost infixation, and inability to sleep. Moxibustion is contraindicated (*Tóng*).

凡尸厥而死，脈動如故，此陽脈下墜，陰脈上爭，氣閉故也。針百會，入三分補之，灸、熨斗熨兩脅下。又竈突墨彈丸大，漿水和飲之。又針足中指頭，去甲如韭葉。又刺足大指甲下內側，去甲三分（《千》）。水溝治卒中惡（《銅》）。

Deathlike reversal and dead, yet the vessels are still pulsating as usual: This is because the yáng vessels are falling downward and the yīn vessels are rushing upward, so the qì is blocked. Needle Bǎi Huì 百會 (Dū 20) 3 fēn deep and supplement; apply moxibustion, iron by pressing a flatiron below the rib-sides. Or get some *zào tū mò* 竈突墨[21] the size of a pebble, mix it with sour millet water, and drink it. Or needle the site at the tip of the middle toe, the distance of a leek leaf away from the nail. Or needle the site 3 fēn away from the nail of the big toe, on the medial aspect (*Qiān*《千》).

Shuĭ Gōu 水溝 (Dū 26) treats sudden malignity strike (*Tóng*《銅》).

凡五尸者，飛尸、遁尸、風尸、沉尸、尸疰也。今皆取一方兼治之。其狀腹痛脹急，不得氣息，上衝心胸，旁攻兩脅，或累塊踴起，或攣引腰背。治之法：灸乳後三寸，男左女右，可二七壯。不止者，多其壯，取愈止（《千》）。又兩手大拇指頭，各七壯；又心下三寸十壯；又乳下一寸，隨病左右，多其壯數；又以細繩量患人兩乳頭內，即裁斷中屈之，又從乳頭向外量，使當肋罅於繩頭灸三壯，或七壯，男左女右。

The five corpses are flying corpse, retreating corpse, wind corpse, sinking corpse and corpse infixation. Just use one formula treats them all. The symptoms are: abdominal pain, distention and tension, inability to breathe, qì surging upward into the chest and heart that attacks both rib-sides on the sides; or lumps accumulating and popping up; or hypertonicity radiating to the lower and upper back.

The method of treatment: Apply moxibustion 3 cùn posterior to the nipples; burn two times seven cones on left side for males, and on the right side for females. If the symptoms do not go away, burn more cones until they are all gone (*Qiān*). Or apply seven cones of moxibustion each on the tips of both thumbs; or burn ten cones of moxibustion on the site 3 cùn below the heart; or 1 cùn below the nipple. Apply moxibustion on the affected side and burn a lot of cones.

Measure the space between patient's nipples with a thin string, cut the string [to that length] and fold it at the center. Measure with this string from the nipple to the side. Apply three or seven cones of moxibustion at the end of the string in the intercostal space. Apply moxibustion on the left side for males and on the right side for females.

卒疰忤攻心胸，灸第七椎隨年；又心下一寸三壯；又手肘交隨年壯。一切病食疰，灸手小指頭隨年壯，男左女右。五毒疰，不能飲食百病，灸心下三寸，胃管十壯。水疰口中涌水。

21. *Zào tū mò* 竈突墨 is the ash from burning grass that is found inside a stovepipe or chimney.

Sudden infixation attacking the heart and chest: Apply the same number of cones as the patient's age on the seventh vertebra ($C_7$); or burn three cones of moxibustion on the site 1 cùn below the heart; or burn the same number of cones as the patient's age on the junction of the arm and the elbow.

All diseases of food infixation[22]: apply the same number of cones as the patient's age on the tip of the little finger. Apply moxibustion on the left side for males and on the right side for females.

The five toxic infixations and the hundred diseases with inability to eat: Apply ten cones of moxibustion on Wèi Guǎn 胃管 (Rèn 12 or Rèn 13) which is 3 cùn below the heart.

Water infixation has water gushing from the mouth.

《經》云：肺來乘腎，食後吐水，灸肺俞，又灸三陰交，又灸期門，瀉肺補腎也，各隨年壯。一切疰無新久，先仰臥，灸兩乳邊斜下三寸第三肋間，隨年壯，可至三百壯。又治諸氣神良，一名注市。間使，岐伯云：療鬼神，邪（《明下》）。《銅》云：可灸鬼邪卒死。陰囊下第一橫理十四。

*Jīng*《經》says: when the lungs overact on the kidneys, there is vomiting of water after eating: Apply moxibustion on Fèi Shù 肺俞 (UB 13) and Qī Mén 期門 (LV 14). Drain the lungs and supplement the kidneys. Burn the same number of cones as the age of the patient.

For all infixation diseases, regardless of whether they are acute or chronic, ask the patient to lie supine and apply moxibustion in the third intercostal space, 3 cùn obliquely inferior to the nipples. Burn the same number of cones as the age of the patient, up to three hundred cones. This is divinely good for treating all qì diseases. Another name is Zhù Shì 注市.

As for Jiān Shǐ 間使 (PC 5), Qí Bó said it cures [diseases caused by] ghosts, spirits, and evils (*Míng Xià*《明下》). *Tóng*《銅》says: Apply moxibustion on it to treat ghost evils and sudden death. Burn fourteen cones of moxibustion on the site at the first transverse crease below the scrotum.

有貴人內子產後暴卒，急呼其母為辦後事。母至，為灸會陰、三陰交各數壯而蘇。母蓋名醫女也。

The wife of a nobleman died suddenly after childbirth. He anxiously asked her mother to make funeral arrangements. Her mother came and applied several cones of moxibustion on Huì Yīn 會陰 (Rèn 1) and Sān Yīn Jiāo 三陰交 (SP 6) and she woke up. Her mother must have been the daughter of a famous doctor.

22. *Shí zhù* 食疰 (food infixation) is one of ten infixations. The symptoms include pain under the heart that radiates to the back.

凡溺死，一宿尚可救，解死人衣，灸臍中，即活（《集效》）。

Someone who has drowned can still be rescued after one night. Untie the clothes of the dead person and apply moxibustion on Qí Zhōng 臍中 (the center of the umbilicus). The drowning victim will revive (*Jí Xiào*《集效》).

## 5.25

## *Jiǎo Xī Tòng (Luán Jí Bù Shōu Bù Rén)*

# 脚膝痛（攣急不收不仁）

## Leg and knee pain

**(Hypertonicity, loss of use, numbness)**

委中治膝不得屈伸，取其經血立愈（《銅》見腰脊）。腎俞治腳膝拘急，足寒如水（見《明》）。髀關療膝寒不仁，痹痿，不屈伸。梁丘療脛痛冷痹，膝痛，不能屈伸。懸鐘療腿膝連膝脛麻痹，屈伸難（《下》）。又云膝脛連腰痛，筋攣急，足不收履，坐不能起。

Wěi Zhōng 委中 (UB 40) treats inability to flex the knees. Draining blood from the channel cures the disease immediately (see the section on [pain of] the lower back and spine in *Tóng*《銅》).

Shèn Shù 腎俞 (UB 23) treats hypertonicity of the legs and knees with feet as cold as water (see *Míng*《明》).

Bì Guān 髀關 (ST 31) cures cold knees with numbness, *bì*-impediment, wilting, and inability to flex and stretch.

Liáng Qiū 梁丘 (ST 34) cures pain and cold *bì*-impediment of lower legs, knee pain, and inability to flex and stretch.

Xuán Zhōng 懸鐘 (GB 39) cures numbness of the legs, knees, and lower legs with inability to stretch and flex (*Xià*《下》). It is also said: [Xuán Zhōng (GB 39)] treats pain from the knees and lower legs connected to the lower back, hypertoncity of the sinews, loss of use of the feet, and inability to get up when sitting.

蠡溝療足寒脛酸，屈伸難（見疝）。巨虛療腳脛酸痛，屈伸難，不能久立。 疝 213
甄權云：主大氣不足，偏風腲腿，腳不相隨。風市療脛麻膝痛（見腰腳）。 腰腳 542
三里療四肢腫滿，腿膝酸痛。三陰交療膝內廉痛，小便不利，身重，足痿不能行（《下》）。

Lí Gōu 蠡溝 (LV 5) cures cold legs, aching lower legs, and difficulty flexing and stretching (see the section on prominent *shàn*-mounting).

Jù Xū 巨虛 (ST 37 or ST 39) cures aching pain of the lower legs, difficulty flexing and stretching, and inability to stand for long. Zhēn Quán said: It governs great qì insufficiency, hemilateral wind, and weak legs, as well as hemiplegia of the legs.

Fēng Shì 風市 (GB 31) cures numbness of the lower legs and knee pain (see the section on lower back and leg [pain]).

Sān Lǐ 三里 (ST 36) cures swelling and fullness of the limbs and aching pain of the legs and knees.

Sān Yīn Jiāo 三陰交 (SP 6) cures pain of the inner aspect of the knees, inhibited urination, generalized heaviness, and wilting legs with inability to walk (*Xià*《下》).

京骨療腿膝脛痿，腳攣不得伸，癲病狂走，自嚙，膝脛寒。跗陽療腿膝脛酸（見腰腳）。承山療腳酸膝重（見腰腳）。陽陵泉療膝股內外廉痛不仁，屈伸難。風市主兩膝攣痛，引脅拘急，或青或焦，或枯或黧如腐木。絕骨主膝脛骨搖，酸痹不仁。

Jīng Gǔ 京骨 (UB 64) cures wilting thighs, knees, and lower legs, hypertonicity of the lower legs with inability to stretch, epilepsy, frenetic walking, biting oneself, and cold knees and lower legs.

Fū Yáng 跗陽 (UB 59) cures aching thighs, knees, and lower legs (see the section on lower back and leg [pain]).

Chéng Shān 承山 (UB 57) cures aching legs and heaviness of the knees (see the section on lower back and leg [pain]).

Yáng Líng Quán 陽陵泉 (GB 34) cures pain of the inner and outer aspect of the thighs and knees with numbness and difficulty flexing and stretching.

Fēng Shì (GB 31) governs hypertonicity and pain of the knees radiating to become hypertonicity of the rib-sides; the color could be green or withered, dry or dark, and appears like rotten wood.

Jué Gǔ 絕骨 (GB 39) governs shaking bones of the knees and lower legs with aching and numbness.

足雜病 515

髀關主寒不仁，痿痹，不得屈伸（《明》同）。犢鼻主膝不仁，難跪。光明主痿，坐不能起。《明下》云：膝脛酸痹不仁，手足偏小，坐不能久。膝關主膝內廉痛引臏，不可屈伸。曲泉主膝不可屈伸。曲泉、梁丘、陽關主筋攣膝不得屈伸，不可行。

Bì Guān 髀關 (ST 31) governs coldness and numbness, wilting and *bì*-impediment, and inability to stretch and flex (*Míng*《明》agrees).

Dú Bí 犢鼻 (ST 35) governs numbness of the knees and difficulty kneeling down.

Guāng Míng 光明 (GB 37) governs wilting and inability to get up when sitting. *Míng Xià*《明下》says: It treats aching and numbness of the knees and lower legs, small hands and feet, and inability to sit for a long time.

Xī Guān 膝關 (LV 7) governs pain of the inner aspect of the knees radiating to the patella and inability to stretch and flex the knees.

Qū Quán 曲泉 (LV 8) governs inability to stretch and flex the knees.

Qū Quán (LV 8), Liáng Qiū 梁丘 (ST 34), and Yáng Guān 陽關 (GB 33) govern hypertonicity of the sinews, inability to stretch and flex the knees, and inability to walk.

解溪、條口、丘墟、太白主膝股腫，胻酸轉筋。上廉主風水膝腫（《千》）。中封主膝腫（見身濕）。解溪治膝股胻腫（《銅》見風）。復溜主腳後廉急，不可前卻。承山、承筋主腳筋急痛。崑崙主腳如結，踝如別（《銅》作裂）。京骨、承山、承筋、商丘主腳攣。膀胱俞治拘急（見足雜病）。

Jiě Xī 解溪 (ST 41), Tiáo Kǒu 條口 (ST 38), Qiū Xū 丘墟 (GB 40), and Tài Bái 太白 (SP 3) govern swollen knees and thighs, and aching and cramping of the lower legs.

Shàng Lián 上廉 (ST 37) governs wind-water and knee swelling (*Qiān*《千》).

Zhōng Fēng 中封 (LV 4) governs knee swelling (see the discussion of general dampness).

Jiě Xī (ST 41) treats swollen knees, thighs, and lower legs (see the discussion of wind in *Tóng*《銅》).

Fù Liū 復溜 (KI 7) governs tension of the posterior aspect of the legs and inability to move backward and forward.

Chéng Shān 承山 (UB 57) and Chéng Jīn 承筋 (UB 56) govern acute pain of the leg sinews.

Kūn Lún 崑崙 (UB 60) governs a knotted feeling in the legs and a splitting feeling in the ankles (*Tóng* says breaking).

Jīng Gǔ 京骨 (UB 64), Chéng Shān 承山 (UB 57), Chéng Jīn 承筋 (UB 56), and Shāng Qiū 商丘 (SP 5) govern hypertonicity of the legs.

Páng Guāng Shù 膀胱俞 (UB 28) treats hypertonicity (see the section on miscellaneous diseases of the legs).

## 5.26
## *Xī Tòng (Yú Jiàn Jiǎo Xī)*
# 膝痛（餘見腳膝）

### Knee pain
**(for further discussion, see the section on the legs and knees)**

三里治膝胻酸痛（《銅》）。陽交治喉痹，面腫，寒痹，膝胻不收。條口治膝胻寒，足緩履不收，濕痹足下熱。陰谷治膝痛如錐，不得屈伸。膀胱俞治腳膝無力（見瘕癖）。合陽主膝股重。陰交治腰膝拘攣。髀關治膝寒（《明》同），不仁痿厥，股內筋絡急。

Sān Lǐ 三里 (ST 36) treats aching pain of the knees and calves (*Tóng*《銅》).

Yáng Jiāo 陽交 (GB 35) treats throat *bì*-impediment, facial swelling, cold *bì*-impediment, and loss of use of the knees and calves.

Tiáo Kǒu 條口 (ST 38) treats cold knees and calves, sluggish legs with loss of ability to step, damp *bì*-impediment, and heat beneath the soles.

Yīn Gǔ 陰谷 (KI 10) treats knee pain that feels like the piercing of an awl and inability to flex and stretch.

Páng Guāng Shù 膀胱俞 (UB 28) treats weakness in the knees and legs (see the section on conglomerations and aggregations).

Hé Yáng 合陽 (UB 55) governs heavy knees and thighs.

Yīn Jiāo 陰交 (Rèn 7) treats hypertonicity of the low back and knees.

Bì Guān 髀關 (ST 31) treats cold knees (*Míng*《明》agrees), numbness, wilting reversal, and tension of the sinews and network vessels of the inner aspect of the thighs.

痃癖 433
疝 213
風痹 377
風勞 371
尸厥 531

陽陵泉治膝伸不得屈，冷腳不仁，偏風半身不遂，腳冷無血色。京骨治膝痛不得屈伸。梁丘治寒痹，膝不能屈伸。陽關治膝外痛，不可屈伸，風痹不仁。犢鼻治膝中痛不仁，難跪起，膝臏癰腫，不潰可治，潰者不治。

Yáng Líng Quán 陽陵泉 (GB 34) treats inability to flex the knees after stretching, coldness and numbness of the legs, hemilateral wind, hemiplegia, and cold legs without the color of blood.

Jīng Gǔ 京骨 (UB 64) treats knee pain with inability to flex and stretch.

Liáng Qiū 梁丘 (ST 34) treats cold *bì*-impediment and inability to flex and stretch the knees.

Yáng Guān 陽關 (GB 33) treats pain of the outer aspect of the knees, inability to flex and stretch, wind *bì*-impediment, and numbness.

Dú Bí 犢鼻 (ST 35) treats pain in the knee with numbness, inability to kneel down and get up, and abscesses and swelling of the patella; it is curable if it does not ulcerate and incurable if it ulcerates.

三陰交治膝股內痛（見痃癖）。交信治膝脛內廉痛。曲泉（見疝）、膝關治痛（見風痹）。懸鐘治心腹脹滿，胃熱不嗜食，膝胻痛，筋攣，足不收履，坐不能久。膝眼療膝冷痛不已（《明》忌灸）。伏兔療膝冷（見風勞）。豐隆療腿膝酸痹（見尸厥）。

Sān Yīn Jiāo 三陰交 (SP 6) treats pain of the inner aspect of the knees and thighs (see the section on strings and aggregations).

Jiāo Xìn 交信 (KI 8) treats pain of the inner aspect of the knees and lower legs.

Qū Quán 曲泉 (LV 8) (see the section on prominent *shàn*-mounting) and Xī Guān 膝關 (LV 7) treat pain (see the section on wind *bì*-impediment).

Xuán Zhōng 懸鐘 (GB 39) treats distention and fullness of the heart and abdomen, stomach heat with no desire to eat, pain of the knees and lower legs, hypertonicity of the sinews, loss of use of the feet, and inability to sit for a long time.

Xī Yǎn 膝眼 (non-channel) cures incessant cold pain of the knees (*Míng*《明》says moxibustion is contraindicated).

Fú Tù 伏兔 (ST 32) cures cold knees (see the section on wind taxation).

Fēng Lóng 豐隆 (ST 40) cures aching and *bì*-impediment of the knees and legs (see the section on deathlike reversal).

合陽（ 見脊 ）治膝股重（ 《 千 》 ）。《 銅 》云：注膝胻酸 。俠溪 、陽關主膝外廉痛 。膝關主膝內廉痛引髕，不可屈伸，連腹引喉痛 。中封主膝腫，內踝前痛 。太衝主膝內踝前痛 。犢鼻主膝中痛不仁 。光明主膝痛脛熱不能行，手足偏小 。《 明下 》云療膝脛酸痹不仁 。

脊 551
月事 735
唾血 402
腰腳 542

Hé Yáng 合陽 (UB 55) (see the section on [pain of the lower back and] the spine) treats heavy knees and thighs (*Qiān* 《 千 》). *Tóng* 《 銅 》 says: It governs aching knees and lower legs.

Xiá Xī 俠溪 (GB 43) and Yáng Guān 陽關 (GB 33) govern pain of the outer aspect of the knees.

Xī Guān 膝關 (LV 7) governs pain of the inner aspect of the knees radiating to the patella, inability to flex and stretch, and pain connected to the abdomen that radiates to the throat.

Zhōng Fēng 中封 (LV 4) governs swelling of the knees and pain of the anterior aspect of the medial ankle.

Tài Chōng 太衝 (LV 3) governs pain of the inner aspect of the knees and the anterior aspect of the medial ankle.

Dú Bí 犢鼻 (ST 35) governs pain in the knees with numbness.

Guāng Míng 光明 (GB 37) governs knee pain, heat in the lower legs, inability to walk, and small hands and feet. *Míng Xià* 《 明下 》 says: It cures aching, *bì*-impediment, and numbness of the knees and tibia.

氣衝治腰痛不得俯仰（ 見月事 ）。三里主膝痿痛（ 見唾血 ）。風市療膝酸 。承山療膝重（ 並見腰腳 ）。

Qì Chōng 氣衝 (ST 30) treats lower back pain with inability to bend backward and forward (see the section on menstruation).

Sān Lǐ 三里 (ST 36) governs wilting and pain of the knees (see the section on spitting of blood).

Fēng Shì 風市 (GB 31) cures aching knees.

Chéng Shān 承山 (UB 57) cures heaviness of the knees (for all, see the section on lower back and leg [pain]).

舍弟行一二里路，膝必酸疼不可行，須坐定，以手撫摩久之，而後能行。後因多服附子而愈。予冬月膝亦酸疼，灸犢鼻而愈。以此見藥與灸不可偏廢也。若灸膝關、三里亦得，但按其穴酸疼，即是受病處，灸之不拘。

My younger brother suffered aching pain of the knees after walking one or two *lǐ*, and could not walk any more. He had to sit down and rub his knees for a long time; then he could walk again. The disease was cured after he took a lot of *fù zǐ* 附子 (Aconiti Radix Lateralis Praeparata). I had aching pain of the knees during the winter; after I applied moxibustion on Dú Bí 犢鼻 (ST 35), it was cured. Because of this, it can be seen that herbs and moxibustion cannot be abandoned. It is also appropriate to apply moxibustion on Xī Guān 膝關 (LV 7) and Sān Lǐ 三里 (ST 36). If the point aches when pressed, it is the affected site. Apply moxibution on it without limiting [the number of cones].

## 5.27

## *Yāo Jiǎo Tòng (Yú Jiàn Yāo Xī)*

# 腰腳痛 （餘見腰膝）

## Lower back and leg pain

**(for further discussion, see the section on the low back and knees)**

凡腰腳重痛，刺委中出血 。久固宿疹，亦皆立已 。次髎主腰下至足不仁（ 並《 千 》 ）。陰市療腰腳如冷水（ 《 明 》見疝 ）。承山治腰背痛，腳腨重，戰栗不能立，腳氣，膝下腫 。申脈治腰痛不能舉體，足胻寒，不能久立，坐如在舟車中 。崑崙治腰尻痛（ 《 千 》作踵 ），足腨（ 《 千 》作跟 ）腫，不得履地 。

For heavy pain of the low back and legs, bleed Wěi Zhōng 委中 (UB 40). This also immediately cures intractable papules.

Cì Liáo 次髎 (UB 32) governs numbness from the low back down to the feet (for all, see *Qiān*《千》).

Yīn Shì 陰市 (ST 33) cures a feeling like cold water in the low back and legs (see the section on prominent *shàn*-mounting in *Míng*《明》).

Chéng Shān 承山 (UB 57) treats lower and upper back pain, heaviness of the legs and calves, shivering with inability to stand, leg qì, and swelling below the knees.

Shēn Mài 申脈 (UB 62) treat lower back pain, inability to raise the body, coldness of the lower legs, inability to stand for long, and a sensation as if sitting in a boat or wagon.

Kūn Lún 崑崙 (UB 60) treats pain of the low back and sacrum (*Qiān*《千》says heel), swollen calves (*Qiān* says heel), and inability to step on the ground.

下崑崙療腰疼，偏風半身不遂，腳重痛不得履地(《明》)。膀胱俞療腰足不仁(見脊)。僕參療腰痛不可舉，承山下重，腳痿(《下》)。地機療腰痛不可俯仰，足痹痛，屈伸難。風市療冷痹，腳脛麻，腿膝酸痛，腰尻重，起坐難。

Xià Kūn Lún 下崑崙 [this may be UB 60 or it may be 1 cùn below lateral malleolus] cures lower back pain, hemilateral wind and hemiplegia, heavy pain of the legs, and inability to step on the ground (*Míng*《明》).

Páng Guāng Shù 膀胱俞 (UB 28) cures numbness of the low back and legs (see the discussion of the spine).

Pū Cān 僕參 (UB 61) cures lower back pain, inability to get up, heaviness below Chéng Shān 承山 (UB 57), and wilting of the legs (*Xià*《下》).

Dì Jī 地機 (SP 8) cures lower back pain, inability to bend backward and forward, *bì*-impediment pain of the legs, and difficulty flexing and stretching.

Fēng Shì 風市 (GB 31) cures cold *bì*-impediment, numbness of the feet and lower legs, aching pain of the legs and knees, heaviness of the low back, sacrum, and coccyx, and difficulty getting up when sitting.

承山療腳酸痛，不能久立，腰膝重，起坐難，筋攣急，不可屈伸。張仲文療腰重痛，不可轉，起坐難，及冷痹腳筋攣，不可屈伸：灸曲脷兩紋頭，左右腳四處，各三壯。每灸一腳，二火齊下，燒纔到肉。初覺痛，使用二人兩邊齊吹，至火滅。午時著艾，至人定，自行動臟腑一兩回，或臟腑轉如雷聲，立愈。神效。

Chéng Shān (UB 57) cures aching pain of the legs, inability to stand for long, heaviness of the low back and knees, difficulty getting up when sitting, hypertonicity of the sinews, and inability to flex and stretch.

Zhāng Zhòngwén treated heavy pain of the low back, inability to turn, difficulty getting up when sitting, cold *bì*-impediment, hypertonicity of the sinews of the legs, and inability to flex and stretch by applying moxibustion on both ends of the curved crease [popliteal crease], four sites in total on both legs. Burn three cones of moxibustion on each site. Each time applying moxibustion on one leg, burn the two fires at the same time on each side of the crease. When the fire burns down to the flesh and the patient first starts to feel pain, have two people simultaneously blow on the moxa

偏風 396 疝 213

cones from both sides until the fire burns out. Apply this moxibustion at *wǔ* double-hour [11am-1pm]. Later at night, the patient will have one or two movements of the organs or rumbling in the organs that sounds like the thunder. The disease will be immediately cured. It is divinely effective.

上廉治腰腿手足不仁（見偏風）。陽輔治腰溶溶坐水中，膝下膚腫筋攣，諸節盡痛無常處，腋腫瘻，馬刀喉痹，膝胻酸，風痹不仁。陰交治腰膝拘攣（見疝）。

Shàng Lián 上廉 (ST 37) treats numbness of the low back, legs, hands, and feet (see the section on hemilateral wind).

Yáng Fǔ 陽輔 (GB 38) treats lower back weakness with a feeling like sitting in water, skin swelling, hypertonicity of the sinews below the knees, pain migrating to all the joints, swollen armpits with fistulas, saber lumps,[23] throat *bì*-impediment, aching knees and lower legs, and numbness due to wind *bì*-impediment.

Yīn Jiāo 陰交 (Rèn 7) treats hypertonicity of the low back and knees (see the section on prominent *shàn*-mounting).

仁壽宮備身患腳，奉敕針環跳、陽陵泉、巨虛下廉、陽輔，即起。大理趙卿患風，腰腳不隨，不得跪起。針上窌、環跳、陽陵泉、巨虛下廉各二穴，即得跪起。治冷痹脛膝痛，腰足攣急，足冷氣上，不能久立，手足沉重，日覺羸瘦，此名復連病：宜灸懸鐘（絕骨），一灸即愈（見身濕痹，《千金》）。

An imperial bodyguard of the Rénshòu Palace suffered a disease of the legs, according to imperial order, [Zhēn Quán] treated him and needled Huán Tiào 環跳 (GB 30), Yáng Líng Quán 陽陵泉 (GB 34), Jù Xū Xià Lián 巨虛下廉 (ST 39) and Yáng Fǔ 陽輔 (GB 38). He got up right away.

Judge Zhào suffered from wind with paralysis of his low back and legs and could not get up from kneeling. After needling Shàng Liáo 上窌 (UB 31), Huán Tiào (GB 30), Yáng Líng Quán (GB 34), and Jù Xū Xià Lián (ST 39) bilaterally, he could get up from kneeling.

To treat cold *bì*-impediment, pain of the lower legs and knees, hypertonicity of the low back and legs, cold legs with qì ascent, inability to stand for long, heavy limbs, and becoming more emaciated day by day - this is named *Fù Lán* 復連 disease. It is appropriate to apply moxibustion on Xuán Zhōng 懸鐘 (Jué Gǔ 絕骨 (GB 39)). This will cure the disease right after one application of moxibustion (see the discussion of generalized damp *bì*-impediment in *Qiān Jīn*《千金》).

23. *Mǎ dāo* 馬刀 (saber lumps) are a type of scrofula occurring in the armpits. They form a shape like a saber.

《千金翼》溫腎湯主腰脊膝腳浮腫不隨（茯苓、乾薑、澤瀉各二兩，桂心三兩銼，每服四五錢重，水二盞，煎八分盞服。日三二服。）。然則腰腳等病，亦當服藥，不可專恃灸云。

*Wēn Shèn Tāng* 溫腎湯 (Warm the Kidney Decoction) from *Qiān Jīn Yì*《千金翼》governs puffy swelling of the low back, spine, knees, and legs with paralysis (two *liǎng* of *fú líng* 茯苓 [Poria], *gān jiāng* 乾薑 [Zingiberis Rhizoma], and *zé xiè* 澤瀉 [Alismatis Rhizoma]; three *liǎng* of filed *guì xīn* 桂心 [Cinnamomi Cortex Rasus]; take four to five *qián* for each dose, add two bowls of water and boil it down to 80% of one bowl and drink it two to three times a day). So for the diseases of the low back and legs, people should also take herbs, not just receive moxibustion.

# 5.28

# *Yāo Tòng (Yāo Jiàng, Yāo Qū)*

# 腰痛（腰強　腰屈）

## Lower back pain

**(Lower back stiffness, bent low back)**

陰包治腰尻引小腹痛（《明下》云：腰痛連小腹腫，小便不利），遺溺不禁（《銅》）。居髎治腰引小腹痛（見手痛）。胞肓治腰痛惡寒，小腹堅急，癃閉重不得，小便澀痛，腰背卒痛。秩邊治腰痛不能俯仰，小便赤澀，腰尻重不能舉（《明》同）。

Yīn Bāo 陰包 (LV 9) treats pain of the low back, sacrum, and coccyx that radiates to the smaller abdomen (*Míng Xià*《明下》says: Lower back pain with smaller abdomen swelling and inhibited urination), and incontinence of urine (*Tóng*《銅》).

Jū Liáo 居髎 (GB 29) treats pain of the low back pain radiating to the smaller abdomen (see the section on arm pain).

Bāo Huāng 胞肓 (UB 53) treats lower back pain, aversion to cold, hardness and tension of the smaller abdomen, dribbling urinary block with an insufferable sensation of heaviness, difficult painful urination, and sudden pain of the lower and upper back.

Zhì Biān 秩邊 (UB 54) treats lower back pain with inability to bend forward and backward, inhibited urination with red urine, heaviness of the low back, sacrum, and coccyx, and inability to rise (*Míng*《明》agrees).

腰脊 551
瘛瘲 354
膝痛 536
疝 213

委中治腰重不舉體（ 見腰脊 ）。白環俞治腰髖疼，腳膝不遂 。肩井治因撲傷腰髖疼 。腰俞治腰髖疼，脊強不得轉 。命門主腰腹相引痛（ 見瘛瘲 ）。肺俞治腰背強痛 。陰陵泉（ 水腫 ）、大腸俞治腰痛（ 《 明 》同 ）。下髎治腰痛不得轉側 。

Wěi Zhōng 委中 (UB 40) treats heaviness of the lower back with inability to raise the body (see the section on [pain of] the low back and spine).

Bái Huán Shù 白環俞 (UB 30) treats pain of the low back and hips and paralysis of the legs and knees.

Jiān Jǐng 肩井 (GB 21) treats pain of the low back and hips due to a fall.

Yāo Shù 腰俞 (Dū 2) treats pain of the low back and hips and stiffness of the spine with inability to turn.

Mìng Mén 命門 (Dū 4) governs pulling pain between the low back and abdomen (see the section on tugging and slackening).

Fèi Shù 肺俞 (UB 13) treats stiffness and pain of the lower and upper back.

Yīn Líng Quán 陰陵泉 (SP 9) (edema), and Dà Cháng Shù 大腸俞 (UB 25) treat lower back pain (*Míng* 《 明 》 agrees).

Xià Liáo 下髎 (UB 34) treats lower back pain with inability to turn to the sides.

陽輔治腰如坐水（ 見膝痛 ）。《 明下 》：陰市療腰如冷水（ 見疝 ）。陰市療腰腳如冷水（ 見疝 ）。涌泉治腰痛大便難 。京門治腰痛不得俯仰，寒熱䐜脹，引背不得息 。肝俞療腰痛肩疼（ 《 明 》 ）。

Yáng Fǔ 陽輔 (GB 38) treats lower back pain that feels like sitting in the water (see the section on knee pain). *Míng Xià* 《 明下 》 says: Yīn Shì 陰市 (ST 33) cures a feeling like cold water in the low back (see the section on prominent *shàn*-mounting).

Yīn Shì (ST 33) cures a feeling like cold water in the low back and legs (see the section on prominent *shàn*-mounting).

Yǒng Quán 涌泉 (KI 1) treats lower back pain and difficult defecation.

Jīng Mén 京門 (GB 25) treats lower back pain with inability to bend forward and backward, [sensations of] cold and heat with distention radiating to the back, and inability to breathe.

Gān Shù 肝俞 (UB 18) cures lower back pain and shoulder pain (*Míng*).

腎俞（見勞）、氣海俞、中膂俞（見脊）療腰痛。關元俞、膀胱俞療風勞腰痛。胞肓療惡氣腰背卒痛。《下》云：腰痛不可忍，俯仰難，惡寒，小便澀。崑崙療腰尻重不欲起，俯仰難，惡聞人音（《下》）。風市療腰尻重，起難（見腰腳）。

勞 188
脊 555
腰腳 542

Shèn Shù 腎俞 (UB 23) (see the section on taxation), Qì Hǎi Shù 氣海俞 (UB 24), and Zhōng Lǚ Shù 中膂俞 (UB 29) (see the section on [pain of] the spine) cure lower back pain.

Guān Yuán Shù 關元俞 (UB 26), Páng Guāng Shù 膀胱俞 (UB 28) cures wind taxation and lower back pain.

Bāo Huāng 胞肓 (UB 53) cures malign qì and sudden pain of the lower and upper back. *Xià*《下》says: insufferable lower back pain, difficulty bending forward and backward, aversion to cold, and inhibited urination.

Kūn Lún 崑崙 (UB 60) cures heaviness of the low back, sacrum, and coccyx, no desire to get up, difficulty bending forward and backward, and a dislike for hearing people talk (*Xià*).

Fēng Shì 風市 (GB 31) cures heaviness of the low back, sacrum, and coccyx and difficulty getting up (see section on the low back and leg [pain]).

腎俞療腰痛不可俯仰，轉側難（《下》）。腰俞療腰疼不能久立，腰以下至足不仁，坐起難，腰脊急強，不可俯仰，腰重如石，難舉動。張仲文灸腰痛（見腰腳），四肢寒熱，腰疼不得俯仰，身黃腹滿食嘔，舌根直：灸第十一椎上及左右各一寸五分，三處各七壯《千》）。

Shèn Shù (UB 23) cures lower back pain, inability to bend forward and backward, and difficulty turning to the sides (*Xià*).

Yāo Shù 腰俞 (Dū 2) cures lower back pain, inability to stand for long, numbness from low back down to the legs, difficulty getting up when sitting, acute stiffness of the low back and spine, inability to bend forward and backward, heaviness of the low back that feels like stone, and difficulty moving.

Zhāng Zhòngwén's moxibustion treatment for lower back pain (see the section on low back and leg [pain]), with [sensations of] cold and heat in the limbs, lower back pain with inability to bend forward and backward, yellow body (jaundice), abdominal fullness, vomiting after eating, and stiff root of the tongue: Apply moxibustion on eleventh vertebra ($T_{11}$) and on the site that is 1.5 cùn lateral on both sides. Burn seven cones of moxibustion on each of these three sites (*Qiān*《千》).

腰俞、膀胱俞、長強、氣衝、上窌、下窌、居髎主腰痛。三里、陰市、陽輔、蠡溝主腰痛不可顧。申脈、太衝、陽蹻主腰痛不能舉。委陽、殷門、太白、陰陵泉、行間（《銅》同）主腰痛不可俯仰。《甲》云：委陽、殷門主腰痛得俯不得仰。

Yāo Shù 腰俞 (Dū 2), Páng Guāng Shù 膀胱俞 (UB 28), Cháng Qiáng 長強 (Dū 1), Qì Chōng 氣衝 (ST 30), Shàng Liáo 上窌 (UB 31), Xià Liáo 下窌 (UB 34), and Jū Liáo 居髎 (GB 29) govern lower back pain.

Sān Lǐ 三里 (ST 36), Yīn Shì 陰市 (GB 33), Yáng Fǔ 陽輔 (GB 38), and Lí Gōu 蠡溝 (LV 5) govern lower back pain with inability to turn to the sides.

Shēn Mài 申脈 (UB 62), Tài Chōng 太衝 (LV 3), and Yáng Qiāo 陽蹻 (UB 62) govern lower back pain and inability to lift things.

Wěi Yáng 委陽 (UB 39), Yīn Mén 殷門 (UB 37), Tài Bái 太白 (SP 3), Yīn Líng Quán 陰陵泉 (SP 9), and Xíng Jiān 行間 (LV 2) (*Tóng*《銅》agrees) govern lower back pain with inability to bend forward and backward. *Jiă*《甲》says: Wěi Yáng (UB 39) and Yīn Mén (UB 37) govern lower back pain with inability to bend backward.

束骨、飛揚、承筋主腰痛如折。陽輔主腰痛如錘居中，腫痛不可咳，咳則筋縮急，諸節痛上下無常，寒熱。涌泉主腰痛，大便難（《甲》）。京門主腰痛不可久立（《甲》），腰背痛：宜針決膝腰勾畫中青赤絡脈，出血便瘥（《千》）。

Shù Gŭ 束骨 (UB 65), Fēi Yáng 飛揚 (UB 58), and Chéng Jīn 承筋 (UB 56) govern lower back pain that feels like it is broken.

Yáng Fǔ 陽輔 (GB 38) governs lower back pain that feels like an awl is inside, pain and swelling with inability to cough, acute contraction of the sinews while coughing, migrating pain of all the joints, and [sensations of] cold and heat.

Yǒng Quán 涌泉 (KI 1) governs lower back pain and difficulty defecating (*Jiă*).

Jīng Mén 京門 (GB 25) governs lower back pain and inability to stand for a long time (*Jiă*).

Lower and upper back pain: it is appropriate to needle and dredge the green and red network vessels between the low back and knees. The disease will be cured after bleeding (*Qiān*《千》).

腰痛不得俯仰者，令患人正立，以竹拄地，度至臍斷竹，乃以度度背脊，灸竹上頭處隨年壯。灸訖藏竹，勿令人得知。腰痛：灸腳跟上橫紋中白肉際十壯，良；又灸足巨陽七壯，巨陽在外踝下；又灸腰目窌七壯，在尻上約左右是；又灸八窌及外踝上骨約中。

For lower back pain with inability to bend forward and backward: Ask the patient to stand erect, stand a bamboo stick on the ground, measure up to the umbilicus, and break it. Then measure the same height on the spine with this bamboo. Apply the same number of cones as the patient's age on the site at the tip of the bamboo. Store the bamboo after the moxibustion is complete and do not let people know.

For lower back pain: Apply ten cones of moxibustion on the border of the white flesh of the transverse crease of the heel; the results will be good. Or apply seven cones of moxibustion on Zú Jù Yáng 足巨陽. Jù Yáng 巨陽 is located below the lateral malleolus. Or apply seven cones of moxibustion on Yāo Mù Liáo 腰目窌 (Yāo Yǎn 腰眼) which is located right above the tail bone. Or apply moxibustion on Bā Liáo 八窌[24] and on the bone above the lateral malleolus.

腰卒痛：灸窮骨上一寸七壯，左右一寸，各灸七壯。腰脊痛：灸小腸俞五十壯（見虛損）。腰背痛：灸三焦俞隨年（見勞）。

Sudden lower back pain: Apply seven cones of moxibustion each on the site one cùn above and one cùn lateral to Qióng Gǔ 窮骨 (Dū 1).

Pain of the low back and spine: Apply fifty cones of moxibustion on Xiǎo Cháng Shù 小腸俞 (UB 27) (see the section on vacuity detriment).

Lower and upper back pain: Apply the same number of cones as the patient's age on Sānjiāo Shù 三焦俞 (UB 22) (see the section on taxation).

有婦人久病而腰甚疼，腰眼忌灸。醫以針置火中令熱，謬刺痛處，初不深入，既而疼止。則知火不負人之說猶信云。

A lady was sick for a long time and developed severe lower back pain but moxibustion on Yāo Yǎn 腰眼 was contraindicated for her. The doctor heated a needle over a fire and applied cross needling on the painful area. He did not needle deeply at first. Afterwards, the pain stopped. I know that fire does not betray people and the theory is still reliable.

許知可因淮南大水，忽腹中如水吼，調治得愈，自此腰痛不可屈伸。思之，此必腎經感水氣而得，乃灸腎俞三七壯，服麋茸丸愈（予謂腰痛不可屈伸：灸腎俞自效，不服麋茸丸亦可）。舍弟腰疼，出入甚艱。予用火針微微頻刺腎俞，則行履如故，初不灸也。屢有人腰背傴僂來覓點灸，予意其是筋病使然，為點陽陵泉，令歸灸即愈。筋會陽陵泉也，然則腰疼又不可專泥腎俞，不灸其他穴也。

24. This is the same as the Bā Liáo 八髎 points.

胸滿 470 腰脊 551 Xǔ Zhīkě[25] suddenly had a feeling like water roaring in his abdomen due to flooding of the South Huái River. It was cured after treatment. But since then he had lower back pain with inability to bend forward and backward. He thought this must due to water qì attacking the kidney channel. After applying three times seven cones of moxibustion on Shèn Shù 腎俞 (UB 23) and taking *Mí Róng Wán* 麋茸丸 (Pilose Antler of Elk Pill), the disease was cured (I think applying moxibustion on Shèn Shù 腎俞 (UB 23) would be effective for lower back pain with inability to bend forward and backward; *Mí Róng Wán* (Pilose Antler of Elk Pill) is not necessary).

My younger brother had lower back pain with difficulty working and resting. I frequently used a fire needle on Shèn Shù 腎俞 (UB 23) and he walked normally as before. I did not apply moxibustion in the beginning. Someone repeatedly came for moxibustion to treat his stooped lower back. I thought it was due to sinew disease so I marked Yáng Líng Quán 陽陵泉 (GB 34) on him, and asked him to apply moxibustion after he went home. He recovered. Yáng Líng Quán (GB 34) is the meeting [influential] point of the sinews. We cannot apply moxibustion only [only] on Shèn Shù (UB 23) for lower back pain, and not on other points as well.

風池治腰傴僂引項筋無力不收（《銅》）。肺俞治腰強（見胸滿）。束骨治腰如折如結，耳聾，惡風寒，目眩項不可顧，目內眥赤爛。白環俞治腰脊攣痛（見腰脊痛）。

Fēng Chí 風池 (GB 20) treats stooped lower back that induces weakness of the sinews at the nape with loss of use (*Tóng*《銅》).

Fèi Shù 肺俞 (UB 13) treats stiffness of the lower back (see the section on chest fullness).

Shù Gǔ 束骨(UB 65) treats a feeling in the low back as if it is broken or bound up, deafness, aversion to wind-cold, dizzy vision, inability to turn the neck, and redness and erosion on the inner canthus.

Bái Huán Shù 白環俞 (UB 30) treats hypertonicity and pain of the low back and spine (see the section on pain of the lower back and spine).

25. Xu Zhike 許知可 (1079-1154, *Song* 宋 Dynasty), also known as Xu Shuwei 許叔微, was the compiler of *Pǔ Jì Běn Shì Fāng*《普濟本事方》(Skillful Formulas for Universal Salvation).

# 5.29
## *Yāo Jǐ Tòng (Yú Jiàn Bèi Tòng)*
# 腰脊痛（餘見背痛）

## Pain of the lower back and spine
**(for further discussion, see the section on back pain)**

委中主腰痛夾脊至頭幾幾然（《千》）。凡腰腳重痛，於此刺出血，久痼宿疹，亦皆立已。大鐘主腰脊痛。小腸俞、中膂俞、白環俞主腰脊疝痛。次髎、胞肓、承筋主腰脊痛惡寒。合陽主腰脊痛引腹。扶承主腰脊尻臀股陰寒痛。

Wěi Zhōng 委中 (UB 40) governs lower back pain and tightness along the spine all the way up to the head (*Qiān*《千》). For heavy pain of the low back and legs, bleed Wěi Zhōng 委中 (UB 40). It also immediately cures intractable papules.

Dà Zhōng 大鐘 (KI 4) governs pain of the lower back and spine.

Xiǎo Cháng Shù 小腸俞 (UB 27), Zhōng Lǚ Shù 中膂俞 (UB 29), and Bái Huán Shù 白環俞 (UB 30) govern pain of the lower back and spine, as well as *shàn*-mounting pain.

Cì Liáo 次髎 (UB 32), Bāo Huāng 胞肓 (UB 53), and Chéng Jīn 承筋 (UB 56) govern pain of the lower back and spine and aversion to cold.

Hé Yáng 合陽 (UB 55) governs pain of the lower back and spine that radiates to the abdomen.

Fú Chéng 扶承 (UB 36) governs cold pain in low back, spine, sacrum, and coccyx, buttocks, and the inner aspect of the thighs.

涌泉主腰脊相引如解。志室、京門主腰痛脊急（《明下》同）。脾俞、小腸俞、膀胱俞、腰俞、神道、穀中、長強（《明下》同）、大杼、膈關、水分主腰脊急強。腰俞療腰髖疼，腰脊強，不得轉（《明》）。

Yǒng Quán 涌泉 (KI 1) governs [pain] radiating between low back and spine, feeling like they have been dislocated.

淋 222 消渴 195

Zhì Shì 志室 (UB 52) and Jīng Mén 京門 (GB 25) govern lower back pain and tension of the spine (*Míng Xià*《明下》agrees).

Pí Shù 脾俞 (SP 20), Xiǎo Cháng Shù 小腸俞 (UB 27), Páng Guāng Shù 膀胱俞 (UB 28), Yāo Shù 腰俞 (Dū 2), Shén Dào 神道 (Dū 11), Gǔ Zhōng 穀中 (unknown), Cháng Qiáng 長強 (Dū 1) (*Míng Xià* agrees), Dà Zhù 大杼 (UB 11), Gé Guān 膈關 (UB 46), and Shuǐ Fēn 水分 (Rèn 9) govern acute stiffness of the low back and spine.

Yāo Shù 腰俞 (Dū 2) cures pain of the low back and hips, stiffness of the low back and spine, and inability to turn to the sides (*Míng*《明》).

白環俞療腰脊攣痛，大小便不利，百病腰髖疼不遂，腰中冷，不識眠睡。《下》云：療腰脊急強，不能俯仰，起坐難，手足不仁，小便黃，腰尻重不舉。志室、胞肓療腰脊痛急，食不消，腹堅急。膀胱俞療脊急強，腰至足酸重（《下》）。神堂療腰脊急強，逆氣上攻時噎。

Bái Huán Shù 白環俞 (UB 30) cures hypertonicity and pain of the low back and spine, inhibited urination and defecation, paralysis and pain of the low back and hips due to the hundred diseases, cold in the low back, and inability to sleep. *Xià*《下》says: It cures acute stiffness of the low back and spine, inability to bend forward and backward, difficulty getting up and sitting, numbness of the limbs, yellow urine, and heaviness of the low back, sacrum, and coccyx with inability to lift things.

Zhì Shì 志室 (UB 52) and Bāo Huāng 胞肓 (UB 53) cure pain and tension of the low back and spine, non-dispersion of food, and abdominal hardness and tension.

Páng Guāng Shù 膀胱俞 (UB 28) cures acute stiffness of the spine, and aching and heaviness from the low back to the legs (*Xià*).

Shén Táng 神堂 (UB 44) cures acute stiffness of the low back and spine and counterflow qì attacking upward with frequent dysphagia.

大鐘（見淋）治腰脊強痛。志室治腰脊強痛，食飲不消，腹堅急。京骨（見足酸）、中膂俞治腰脊不得俯仰（見消渴）。《明下》云：療腰痛不可俯仰，夾脊膂痛。上下按之應者，從項後至此穴皆灸之，立愈。

Dà Zhōng 大鐘 (KI 4) (see the section on dribbling) treats stiffness and pain of the low back and spine.

Zhì Shì (UB 52) treats stiffness and pain of the low back and spine, inability to digest food, and abdominal hardness and tension.

腸鳴 263
疝 213

Jīng Gǔ 京骨 (UB 64) (see the discussion of aching legs) and Zhōng Lǚ Shù 中膂俞 (UB 29) treat lower back and spine [pain] with inability to bend forward and backward ((see the section on wasting-thirst). *Míng Xià* 《明下》 says: It cures lower back pain, inability to bend forward and backward, and pain of the muscles along the spine. Applying moxibustion to the sites that respond to pressure above and below, from the back of the nape to this point, will cure it immediately.

復溜治腰脊內引痛(《明下》云：腰痛引脊)，不得俯仰起坐，目䀮䀮，善怒多言，舌乾涎自出，足痿不收履，寒不自溫。京骨治筋攣胻酸，髀樞痛，頸項強，腰脊不可俯仰。委中治腰俠脊沉沉然，遺溺，腰重不能舉體，風痹，髀樞痛，可出血，痼疹皆愈。又云：熱病汗不出，足熱厥逆滿，膝不得屈伸，取其經血立愈。

Fù Liū 復溜 (KI 7) treats pain radiating through the medial low back and spine (*Míng Xià* says: Lower back pain radiating to the spine), inability to bend forward or backward, get up or sit, blurred vision, frequent anger, continual talking, dry tongue, uncontrollable drooling, wilting legs with inability to step, and feeling cold with inability to warm oneself.

Jīng Gǔ (UB 64) treats hypertonicity of the sinews, aching lower legs, pain of the thigh pivot, stiffness of the neck and nape, and pain of the lower back and spine with inability to bend forward and backward.

Wěi Zhōng 委中 (UB 40) treats heavy sensation of the low back and along the spine, enuresis, heaviness of the lower back with inability to raise the body, wind *bì*-impediment, and pain of the thigh pivot. It can be bled to cure intractable papules. It is said that bleeding the channel will cure heat disease with absence of sweating, heat reversal of the legs, counterflow fullness, and inability to flex and stretch the knees.

合陽治腰脊強，引腹痛，陰股熱，膝胻酸重，履步難。扶承治腰脊相引如解(《明下》云：療腰脊尻臀腰冷痛)。殷門治腰脊不可俯仰，舉重惡血注之，股外腫。章門(見腸鳴)、次髎治腰脊痛不得轉(見疝)。懸樞治腰脊強(《明》同)，不得屈伸。

Hé Yáng 合陽 (UB 55) treats stiffness of the low back and spine with pain radiating to the abdomen, heat in the inner aspect of the thighs, heavy aching of the knees and legs, and difficulty walking.

Fú Chéng 扶承 (UB 36) treats the low back and spine affecting each other feel as if they are dislocated (*Míng Xià* 《明下》 says: It cures cold pain of the low back, spine, sacrum-coccyx, and buttocks.

Yīn Mén 殷門 (UB 37) treats inability to bend the low back and spine forward and backward, malign blood pooling when lifting a heavy weight, and swelling on the lateral side of the thighs.

Zhāng Mén 章門 (LV 13) (see the section on intestinal rumbling) and Cì Liáo 次髎 (UB 32) treat pain of the lower back and spine, and inability to turn to the sides (see the section on prominent *shàn*-mounting).

Xuán Shū 懸樞 (Dū 5) treats tension and stiffness of the low back and spine (*Míng*《明》agrees) and inability to flex and stretch.

三焦俞治肩背急，腰脊強(《明下》同)，不得俯仰。膀胱俞治腰脊痛。白環俞治腰脊攣痛，大小便不利，腰髖疼，腳膝不遂，溫瘧，腰脊冷疼，不得安臥，勞損風虛。

Sān Jiāo Shù 三焦俞 (UB 22) treats tension of the back and shoulders, stiffness of the low back and spine (*Míng Xià*《明下》agrees), and inability to bend forward and backward.

Páng Guāng Shù 膀胱俞 (UB 28) treats pain of the lower back and spine.

Bái Huán Shù 白環俞 (UB 30) treats hypertonicity and pain of the low back and spine, inhibited urination and defecation, pain of the low back and hips, paralysis of the legs and knees, warm malaria, cold pain of the low back and spine, inability to sleep peacefully, taxation and detriment, and wind vacuity.

《史記》太倉公告宋建曰：君有病，往四五日，君腰脅病不可俯仰，又不得小溲，不亟治，病即入濡腎；及其未舍五臟，急治之。病方今客腎濡，此所謂腎痹也。宋建曰：建故有腰脊痛，往四五日，弄石不能起，即復置之。暮腰脊痛，不得溺，至今不愈。建病得之好持重，即為柔湯使服之，十八日而病愈。然則腰脊傷持重得病而入腎，灸腎俞可也。

*Shǐ Jì*《史記》says: Tài Cāng Gōng told Sòng Jiàn: You have become sick; in four or five days, you will suffer disease of the low back and rib-sides with inability to bend forward and backward as well as inability to urinate. The disease will enter into and immerse the kidneys if you do not quickly treat it. You should get treatment immediately before the disease settles into the five viscera. The disease is now visiting and immersing the kidneys so it is called kidney *bì*-impediment.

Sòng Jiàn said: I have had pain of the low back and spine before. I have not been able to play the stones and raise them [lift weights] in the past four or five days. At dusk, I had pain of the low back and spine with inability to urinate. The disease had never been cured up until now.

Jian's disease was due to liking to lift heavy weights, so I made *Róu Tāng* 柔湯 (Soft Decoction)[26] and asked him to take it. The disease was cured in eighteen days.
If damage to the low back and spine is due to lifting heavy weight and the disease enters the kidneys, it is appropriate to apply moxibustion on Shèn Shù 腎俞 (UB 23).

背痛 483
水腫 459

## 5.30

## *Jǐ Tòng (Yú Jiàn Yāo Jǐ Fēng Jìng Fǎn Zhāng)*

# 脊痛（餘見腰脊風痙反張）

### Pain of the spine

**(for further discussion see the sections on the low back and spine, wind tetany and arched-back rigidity)**

五處、身柱、委中、委陽、崑崙主脊強反折，瘛瘲癲疾（《千》）。膈關等主脊強（見背痛）。崑崙主脊強，背尻骨重。京門、石關主脊痓反折。陰谷主脊內廉痛。至陽療脊急強（《明》）。章門（見水腫）、膈俞（背痛）、胃倉（腹脹）、大腸俞治脊強不得俯仰（《銅》）。

Wǔ Chù 五處 (UB 5), Shēn Zhù 身柱 (Dū 12), Wěi Zhōng 委中 (UB 40), Wěi Yáng 委陽 (UB 39), and Kūn Lún 崑崙 (UB 60) govern arched-back rigidity, and tugging and slackening as well as withdrawal disease (*Qiān* 《千》).

Gé Guān 膈關 (UB 46) governs stiffness of the spine (see the section on back pain).

Kūn Lún 崑崙 (UB 60) governs stiffness of the spine and a heavy sensation of the back and sacrum.

Jīng Mén 京門 (GB 25) and Shí Guān 石關 (KI 18) govern hypertonicity of the spine with arched-back rigidity.

Yīn Gǔ 陰谷 (KI 10) governs pain on the inner aspect of the spine.

Zhì Yáng 至陽 (Dū 9) cures acute stiffness of the spine (*Míng* 《明》).

Zhāng Mén 章門 (LV 13) (see the section on edema), Gé Shù 膈俞 (UB 17) (see the section on back pain), Wèi Cāng 胃倉 (UB 50) (see the section on abdominal fullness), and Dà Cháng Shù

26. *Róu Tāng* 柔湯 (Soft Decoction) is an ancient formula. Its ingredients are unknown.

腰脊 551
寒熱 675
月事 735
消渴 195

大腸俞 (UB 25) treat stiffness of the spine with inability to bend forward and backward (*Tóng*《銅》).

胃俞治脊痛(《銅》見腹脹,《明下》同)。脾俞、大腸俞主腹中氣脹引脊痛,食多身瘦,名曰食晦。先取脾俞,後取季脅(《千》)。膀胱俞療脊急強(見腰脊)。赤白泄洞利,腰脊痛:小腸俞五十壯(見寒熱)。氣穴治賁氣上下,引腰脊痛(見月事)。

Wèi Shù 胃俞 (UB 21) treats pain of the spine (see the section on abdominal fullness in *Tóng*《銅》; *Míng Xià*《明下》agrees).

Pí Shù 脾俞 (UB 20) and Dà Cháng Shù 大腸俞 (UB 25) govern qì distention of the abdomen with pain radiating to the spine and marked emaciation despite eating a lot; this is called *shí huì* 食晦.[27] Treat Pí Shù (UB 20) first, then Jì Xié 季脅 (LV 13) (*Qiān*《千》).

Páng Guāng Shù 膀胱俞 (UB 28) cures acute stiffness of the spine (see the section on [pain of] the low back and spine).

Red and white diarrhea, throughflux diarrhea, and pain of the low back and spine: Apply fifty cones of moxibustion on Xiǎo Cháng Shù 小腸俞 (UB 27) (see the section on [sensations of] cold and heat).

Qì Xué 氣穴 (KI 13) treats rushing qì that moves up and down inducing pain of the low back and spine (see the section on menstruation).

腰俞主月閉,溺赤,脊強互引反折,汗不出。中膂俞治腎虛消渴,腰脊不得俯仰(見消渴)。《明下》云:夾脊膂痛,上下按之應者,從項後至此穴皆灸之,立愈(見腰脊)。

Yāo Shù 腰俞 (Dū 2) governs amenorrhea, reddish urine, stiffness of the spine that induces arched-back rigidity, and absence of sweating.

Zhōng Lǚ Shù 中膂俞 (UB 29) treats kidney vacuity, wasting-thirst, and inability to bend the low back and spine forward and backward (see the section on wasting-thirst). *Míng Xià* says: pain of the muscles along the spine; when a site above or below responds to pressure, from behind the nape to this point, applying moxibustion will cure the disease (see the section on [pain of] the spine).

27. *Shí huì* 食晦: see above footnote on p. 454.

# 5.31
## *Còu Lǐ*

# 腠理

## Interstices

附分治肩背急，風冷客於腠，頸項強痛，不得顧。陽白治背腠寒栗，重衣不得溫（《銅》）。次髎治背腠寒。肝俞療腠中痛（《明下》）。次髎療腰下至足不仁，背腠寒，小便赤淋，心下堅脹（見疝）。

Fù Fēn 附分 (UB 41) treats tension of the back and shoulders, wind-cold visiting the interstices, stiffness and pain of the neck and nape, and inability to turn the neck.

Yáng Bái 陽白 (GB 14) treats cold shivering of the interstices on the back and inability to get warm even when wearing thick clothing (*Tóng*《銅》).

Cì Liáo 次髎 (UB 32) treat cold in the interstices of the back.

Gān Shù 肝俞 (UB 18) cures pain of the interstices (*Míng Xià*《明下》).

Cì Liáo (UB 32) cures numbness from the low back down to the feet, cold in the interstices of the back, dribbling red urine, and hardness and distention below the heart (see the section on prominent *shàn*-mounting).

《史記》扁鵲之言曰：疾居腠理，湯熨之所及也；在血脈，針石之所及也；在腸胃，酒醪之所及也；其在骨髓，雖司命無奈之何也。夫疾之在骨髓，蓋始於居腠理也。使居腠理而能治，雖非聖人之治於無病，亦賢者治將病也。齊元侯乃以醫為好利，欲治不疾以為功，而卒至於不可救。不特齊侯為然，人皆然也。吾故載扁鵲之言於腠理之末以戒人，亦使醫者當治人於將病焉耳。

According to *Shǐ Jì*《史記》, Biǎn Què said: If disease is located in the interstices, decoctions and ironing can reach it; if it is located in the blood vessels, needles and stones can reach it; if it is in the intestines and stomach, liquor and wine can reach it; if it is in the bone and marrow, even the Commander of Fate is helpless.

痰 399
心煩 335
上氣 420
傷寒寒 673
傷寒頭 671
寒熱 675

Disease that is located in the bones and marrow has usually settled in the interstices first. To be able to treat it when it dwells in the interstices - although this is not at the level of the sage who treats what is not sick, it is a person of virtue treating someone who is about to become sick. The Duke Yuàn of Qí thought the doctor [Biǎn Què] was greedy and wanted to take credit for treating someone who was not ill, until [it was too late and] finally the disease could not be treated. It is not just the Duke of Qí; people all think the same way. I recorded Biǎn Què's theory at the end of the section on interstices to warn people, and I also want to let doctors [know] it is appropriate to treat people before disease arises.

## 5.32
## *Gǔ Téng (Gǔ Suǐ)*
# 骨疼（骨髓）
### Pain of the bones
**(Bones and marrow)**

膈俞（見痰）、紫宮、玉堂（並見心煩）療骨疼（《明》）。上關主引骨痛（《千》見瘛瘲）。骨痛：灸絕骨五十壯（見上氣）。商丘主骨痹煩滿。膈俞主皮肉骨痛（見傷寒寒熱）。太白治骨痛（見傷寒頭痛）。復溜治骨寒熱（見寒熱）。骨髓冷痛：上廉七十壯（《千》）。骨會大杼（禁灸），骨病治此；髓會絕骨，髓病治此（《難疏》）。

Gé Shù 膈俞 (UB 17) (see the section on phlegm drool), Zǐ Gōng 紫宮 (Rèn 19), and Yù Táng 玉堂 (Rèn 18) (for all, see the section on vexation of the heart) cure bone pain (*Míng*《明》).

Shàng Guān 上關 (GB 3) governs pain radiating to the bones (see the section on tugging and slackening in *Qiān*《千》).

Bone pain: Apply fifty cones of moxibustion on Jué Gǔ 絕骨 (GB 39) (see the section on qì ascent).

Shāng Qiū 商丘 (SP 5) governs bone *bì*-impediment, vexation and fullness.

Gé Shù (UB 17) governs pain of the skin, flesh, and bones (see the section on cold damage and [sensations of] cold and heat).

Tài Bái 太白 (SP 3) treats bone pain (see the section on cold damage and headaches).

Fù Liū 復溜 (KI 7) treats [sensations of] cold and heat in the bones (see the section on [sensations of] cold and heat).

Cold pain of the bones and marrow: Apply seventy cones of moxibustion on Shàng Lián 上廉 (ST 37) (*Qiān* 《千》).

Dà Zhù 大杼 (UB 11) is the meeting [influential] point of the bones (moxibustion is contraindicated); it treats diseases of the bones; Jué Gǔ 絕骨 (GB 39) is the meeting [influential] point of marrow; it treats diseases of the marrow (*Nán Shū* 《難疏》).

病在骨髓，秦越人以為司命無奈之何。則骨髓有病，病亦憊矣。《八十一難經疏》乃云：骨杼，骨病治此；髓會絕骨，髓病治此。是尚有針灸法矣，可不針灸乎。但《明堂上經》云：大杼禁灸，而《銅人經》云可灸七壯，《明堂下經》云可灸五壯，《素問》亦同。諸經既同，惟《明堂》獨異，灸之可也。況《明堂經》固云禁穴許灸三壯乎，艾炷若小，一、二七壯亦可。更灸上廉、絕骨等穴，尤佳。

When the disease is located in the bones and marrow, Qín Yuèrén thought even the Commander of Fate cannot do anything. When there are diseases of the bones and marrow, the patient is weak. The 81 *Nàn Jīng Shū* 《八十一難經疏》 says: Gǔ Zhù 骨杼 (UB 11) treats diseases of the bones; Jué Gǔ 絕骨 (GB 39) is the meeting [influential] point of marrow; it treats diseases of the marrow. There are still methods of acupuncture and moxibustion, so why can't acupuncture and moxibustion be applied? *Míng Táng Shàng Jīng* 《明堂上經》 says: Moxibustion is contraindicated on Dà Zhù 大杼 (UB 11), while *Tóng Rén Jīng* 《銅人經》 says it is appropriate to apply seven cones of moxibustion on it; and *Míng Táng Xià Jīng* 《明堂下經》 says burning five cones of moxibustion is fine; *Sù Wèn* 《素問》 agrees. All the classics are the same except *Míng Táng* 《明堂》, so moxibustion can be used. And *Míng Táng Jīng* 《明堂經》 also says that three cones of moxibustion can be applied even on those points that are contraindicated for moxibustion. If the size of the cone is small, one or two times seven cones of moxibustion can also be applied. It is even better to apply moxibustion on Shàng Lián 上廉 (ST 37) and Jué Gǔ (GB 39).

# *Zhēn Jiǔ Zī Shēng Jīng*
# 《針灸資生經·第六》

牙緊
605
偏風
396

# 6.01
## *Ěr Míng*
# 耳鳴
## Tinnitus

上關、下關、四白、百會、顱息、翳風、耳門、頷厭、天窗、陽溪、關衝、液門、中渚主耳鳴聾(《千》)。天容、聽會、聽宮、中渚主聾，嘈嘈若蟬鳴。腕骨、陽谷、肩貞、竅陰、俠溪主頷痛引耳，嘈嘈耳鳴無所聞。

Shàng Guān 上關 (GB 3), Xià Guān 下關 (ST 7), Sì Bái 四白 (ST 2), Bǎi Huì 百會 (Dū 20), Lú Xī 顱息 (SJ 19), Yì Fēng 翳風 (SJ 17), Ěr Mén 耳門 (SJ 21), Hàn Yàn 頷厭 (GB 4), Tiān Chuāng 天窗 (SI 16), Yáng Xī 陽溪 (LI 5), Guān Chōng 關衝 (SJ 1), Yè Mén 液門 (SJ 2), and Zhōng Zhǔ 中渚 (SJ 3) govern tinnitus and deafness (*Qiān*《千》).

Tiān Róng 天容 (SI 17), Tīng Huì 聽會 (GB 2), Tīng Gōng 聽宮 (SI 19), and Zhōng Zhǔ (SJ 3) govern deafness and noisy sounds in the ears like the chirping of cicadas.

Wàn Gǔ 腕骨 (SI 4), Yáng Gǔ 陽谷 (SI 5), Jiān Zhēn 肩貞 (SI 9), Qiào Yīn 竅陰 (GB 11 or GB 44), and Xiá Xī 俠溪 (GB 43) govern jaw pain radiating to the ears and noisy sounds in the ears with inability to hear anything.

前谷、後溪主耳鳴，仍取偏歷，大陵。商陽主耳中風聾鳴。刺一分，留一呼；灸三壯，左取右，右取左，如食頃。《明下》云：療耳鳴聾。百會治耳鳴耳聾(《銅》)。絡卻治頭旋耳鳴(《銅》)。浮白治耳鳴嘈嘈無所聞。和髎治耳中眊眊(見牙緊急)。上關治耳中如蟬聲(見偏風)。

Qián Gǔ 前谷 (SI 2) and Hòu Xī 後溪 (SI 3) govern tinnitus; Piān Lì 偏歷 (LI 6) and Dà Líng (PC 7) can also be used.

Shāng Yáng 商陽 (LI 1) governs wind in the ears, deafness, and tinnitus. Needle one fēn deep and retain the needle for one breath; apply three cones of moxibustion; treat on the right side for disease on the left; treat on the left side for disease on the right, [it will be effective in] a short time. *Míng Xià*《明下》says: It cures tinnitus and deafness.

Bǎi Huì (Dū 20) treats tinnitus and deafness (*Tóng*《銅》).

聤耳 567
耳聾 564
無汗 690
頭旋 651
風眩 375
偏頭痛 643

Luò Què 絡卻 (UB 8) treats dizziness and tinnitus (*Tóng*《銅》).

Fú Bái 浮白 (GB 10) treats noisy sounds in the ears with inability to hear anything.

Hé Liáo 和髎 (SJ 22) treats diminished hearing (see the section on clenched jaws).

Shàng Guān 上關 (GB 3) treats ringing in the ears like the sound of cicadas (see the section on hemilateral wind).

耳門治耳鳴如蟬聲（見聤耳）。聽會、聽宮治耳蟬聲（見耳聾）。瘈脈治頭風耳鳴。偏歷、陽溪、商陽（見熱病無汗）、絡卻（見頭旋）、腕骨、前谷治耳鳴。頷厭（見風眩）療耳鳴（《明》）。肩貞主耳鳴無聞（《甲》見傷寒寒熱）。頷厭療耳鳴（見偏頭痛）。

Ěr Mén 耳門 (SJ 21) treats tinnitus like the chirping of cicadas (see the section on purulent ear).

Tīng Huì 聽會 (GB 2) and Tīng Gong 聽宮 (SI 19) treat the chirping of cicadas in the ears (see the section on deafness).

Chì Mài 瘈脈 (SJ 18) treats head wind and tinnitus.

Piān Lì 偏歷 (LI 6), Yáng Xī 陽溪 (LI 5), Shāng Yáng 商陽 (LI 1) (see the section on heat disease with absence of sweating), Luò Què (UB 8) (see the section on dizzy head), Wàn Gǔ 腕骨 (SI 4), and Qián Gǔ 前谷 (SI 2) treat tinnitus.

Hàn Yàn 頷厭 (GB 4) (see the section on wind dizziness) cures tinnitus (*Míng*《明》).

Jiān Zhēn 肩貞 (SI 9) governs tinnitus with inability to hear anything (see the section on cold damage and on [sensations of] cold and heat in *Jiǎ*《甲》).

Hàn Yàn (GB 4) cures tinnitus (see the section on hemilateral headaches).

人之耳鳴，醫者皆以為腎虛所致，是則然矣。然亦有用氣而得者，用心而得者，不可一概論也。若欲無此患，蓋亦不使腎至於虛，且不使氣，不用心可也。或微微耳鳴，只用蔥管置在耳中，令氣透，自不鳴矣。

Doctors all took tinnitus as due to kidney deficiency, which is possible. But it can also be caused by [excessive] use of qì or [excessive] use of the heart-mind. We cannot treat different matters as the same. If we want to prevent this disease, we cannot let the kidneys become deficient, or let qì or the heart be over-used. If there is mild tinnitus, insert the hollow stalk of a green onion into the ear to let qì connect, and the ringing will disappear naturally.

# 6.02
## *Ěr Tòng*
# 耳痛
## Earache

頭風 640
頭痛 643

上關、下關、四白、百會、顱息、翳風、耳門（鳴，《下》同）、曲池、頷厭、天窗、陽溪、關衝、液門、中渚主耳痛。少商主耳前痛。瘈脈、完骨主頭風耳後痛（見頭風，頭痛）。

Shàng Guān 上關 (GB 3), Xià Guān 下關 (ST 7), Sì Bái 四白 (ST 2), Bǎi Huì 百會 (Dū 20), Lú Xī 顱息 (SJ 19), Yì Fēng 翳風 (SJ 17), Ěr Mén 耳門 (SJ 21) (see the section on tinnitus, *Xià* 《下》 agrees), Qū Chí 曲池 (LI 11), Hàn Yàn 頷厭 (GB 4), Tiān Chuāng 天窗 (SI 16), Yáng Xī 陽溪 (LI 5), Guān Chōng 關衝 (SJ 1), Yè Mén 液門 (SJ 2), and Zhōng Zhǔ 中渚 (SJ 3) govern ear pain.

Shào Shāng 少商 (LU 11) governs pain on the anterior aspect of the ear.

Chì Mài 瘈脈 (SJ 18) and Wán Gǔ 完骨 (GB 12) govern head wind with pain on the posterior aspect of the ear (see the sections on head wind and headaches).

耳鳴 561
無汗 690
腰僂 545
勞瘵 188

# 6.03
# *Ěr Lóng*
# 耳聾
## Deafness

天牖（又主耳不聰）、四瀆主耳暴聾（《千》）。外關、會宗主耳渾渾淳淳，聾無所聞。商陽主耳中風聾鳴（見耳鳴）。天牖主耳不聰（《明下》云：療暴聾）。上關等主耳鳴聲（見耳鳴）。商陽（見熱病無汗）、陽谷（《明》同）、百會治耳鳴耳聾（《銅》）。

Tiān Yǒu 天牖 (SJ 16) (also governs hearing loss) and Sì Dú 四瀆 (SJ 9) govern sudden deafness in the ears (*Qiān*《千》).

Wài Guān 外關 (SJ 5) and Huì Zōng 會宗 (SJ 7) govern hearing loss and deafness with inability to hear anything.

Shāng Yáng 商陽 (LI 1) governs deafness and tinnitus due to wind strike (see the section on tinnitus).

Tiān Yǒu (SJ 16) governs hearing loss (*Míng Xià*《明下》says: It cures sudden deafness).

Shàng Guān 上關 (GB 3) and so forth govern tinnitus (see the section on tinnitus).

Shāng Yáng (LI 1) (see the section on heat disease with absence of sweating), Yáng Gǔ 陽谷 (SI 5) (*Míng*《明》agrees), and Bǎi Huì 百會 (Dū 20) treat tinnitus and deafness (*Tóng*《銅》).

束骨（見腰僂）、翳風、上關、後溪、顱囟治耳聾。風池治耳塞。腎俞治耳聾腎虛（見勞瘵）。聽會治耳聾，耳中如蟬聲。聽宮治耳聾如物填塞，無所聞，耳中嘈嘈（《明》云：憹憹嘈嘈蟬鳴）。

Shù Gǔ 束骨 (UB 65) (see the discussion of stooped back), Yì Fēng 翳風 (SJ 17), Shàng Guān 上關 (GB 3), Hòu Xī 後溪 (SI 3), and Lú Xìn 顱囟 (SJ 19) treat deafness.

Fēng Chí 風池 (GB 20) treats stuffed up ears.

Shèn Shù 腎俞 (UB 23) treats deafness and kidney deficiency (see the section on consumption).

Tīng Huì 聽會 (GB 2) treats deafness and ringing in the ears like the sound of cicadas.

Tīng Gōng 聽宮 (SI 19) treats deafness that feels like something is stuffed into the ears, inability to hear, and noisy sounds in the ears (*Míng*《 明 》says: Stuffed up ears with noisy sounds like the chirping of cicadas).

瘧 301
風癇 366
目痛 568
喘 406
中風不 392
心恍惚 322

外關、天窗《明下》同）治耳鳴聾無所聞。竅陰治卒聾，不聞人語。三陽絡、液門治耳暴聾（見瘧）。四瀆治暴氣耳聾。中渚治頭痛耳聾。會宗治耳聾（見風癇）。俠溪治頰頷腫，耳聾，胸痛不可轉，痛無常處。《明下》云：療耳鳴聾。浮白療耳聾（《銅》作鳴）嘈嘈無所聞（《明》）。

Wài Guān 外關 (SJ 5) and Tiān Chuāng 天窗 (SI 16) (*Míng Xià*《 明下 》agrees) treat tinnitus and deafness with inability to hear anything.

Qiào Yīn 竅陰 (GB 11 or GB 44) treats sudden deafness and inability to hear people talking.

Sān Yáng Luò 三陽絡 (SJ 8) and Yè Mén 液門 (SJ 2) treat sudden deafness in the ears (see the section on malaria).

Sì Dú 四瀆 (SJ 9) treats sudden deafness due to qì [diseases].

Zhōng Zhǔ 中渚 (SJ 3) treats headaches and deafness.

Huì Zōng 會宗 (SJ 7) treats deafness (see the section on wind epilepsy).

Xiá Xī 俠溪 (GB 43) treats swollen cheeks and jaw, deafness, and migrating chest pain with inability to turn to the sides. *Míng Xià* says: It cures tinnitus and deafness.

Fú Bái 浮白 (GB 10) cures deafness (*Tóng*《 銅 》says tinnitus) and noisy sounds with inability to hear anything (*Míng*).

玉枕（見目痛）療耳聾。上關療耳聾，狀如蟬聲。《下》云：耳鳴聲。顱息療小兒耳聾（見喘）。耳門、翳風、腦空療耳鳴聾（《下》）。外關、聽會療耳渟渟渾渾，聾無聞。葦筒灸耳病（見中風不語）。肩貞主耳聾（《千》）。耳聾：刺足少陰（見心恍惚）。天牖療暴聾（《明》見瘰癧）。

Yù Zhěn 玉枕 (UB 9) (see the section on eye pain) cures deafness.

Shàng Guān 上關 (GB 3) cures deafness and sounds like the chirping of cicadas. *Xià*《 下 》says: It treats tinnitus.

Lú Xī 顱息 (SJ 19) cures deafness in children (see the section on panting).

Ěr Mén 耳門 (SJ 21), Yì Fēng 翳風 (SJ 17), and Nǎo Kōng 腦空 (GB 19) cure tinnitus and deafness (*Xià*).

Wài Guān 外關 (SJ 5) and Tīng Huì 聽會 (GB 2) cure hearing loss, deafness, and inability to hear.

Apply moxibustion through a reed tube to treat ear diseases (see the section on wind stroke with loss of speech).

Jiān Zhēn 肩貞 (SI 9) governs deafness (*Qiān*《千》).

For deafness, needle Zú Shào Yīn 足少陰 (KI 3) (see the section on heart abstraction).

Tiān Yǒu 天牖 (SJ 16) cures sudden deafness (see the section on scrofula in *Míng*《明》).

**耳聾有用氣得者，氣快則通。傷寒用衣被擁塞得者，病去漸愈。鄉人用札耳草取汁滴，用新羅白草煮粥食，亦驗云。**

If deafness is caused by [excessive] use of qì, it will be cured when qì moves freely. If it caused by covering with clothes during cold damage, it will be cured when the cold damage disappears. People in the countryside make juice from *zhá ěr cǎo* 札耳草, and drop it in the ear; or eat porridge from fresh *luó bái cǎo* 羅白草.[1] They both are effective.

1. *Zhá ěr cǎo* 札耳草 and *luó bái cǎo* 羅白草: The identity of these herbs is unknown.

# 6.04
## *Tíng Ěr (Shēng Chuāng)*
## 聤耳（生瘡）
### Purulent ear
**(Sores)**

下關治聤耳，有膿汁出（《銅》）。耳門治耳有膿汁出，生瘡，聤耳，聤耳（《明》有聾字）如蟬聲，重聽無所聞。風池治耳塞。聽宮治耳如物填塞。聤耳膿出：上關日三壯至二百（《千翼》）。

Xià Guān 下關 (ST 7) treats purulent ear with discharge of pus (*Tóng*《銅》).

Ěr Mén 耳門 (SJ 21) treats discharge of pus from the ears, sores in the ears, hearing loss and purulent ear (*Míng*《明》has deafness) with the chirping of cicadas, hardness of hearing, and inability to hear.

Fēng Chí 風池 (GB 20) treats stuffed up ears.

Tīng Gōng 聽宮 (SI 19) treats ears that feel like something has filled them up.

Purulent ear with discharge of pus: Apply three cones of moxibustion daily up to two hundred on Shàng Guān 上關 (GB 3) (*Qiān Yì*《千翼》).

有二婦人耳久膿出，予以晉礬火煅，候汁乾研細，令挑少許入耳，覺耳漸重而愈。《本事方》紅綿散只用白礬煅用。

There were two ladies who suffered from discharge of pus from the ears. I calcined alum and ground it into fine powder after the liquid was dry. Then I put a little into their ears. They felt their ears getting heavier and then they recovered. *Hòng Mián Săn* 紅綿散 from [*Pŭ Jì*] *Běn Shì Fāng*《本事方》only uses calcined *bái fán* 白礬 [white alum].

頭痛
643

# 6.05
## *Mù Tòng (Mù Míng)*
# 目痛（目瞑）

## Eye pain
**(Heavy eyes)**

陽白主目瞳子痛癢（《千》見不明）。太衝主下眥痛（又云治婦人）。太衝、陽谷、崑崙主目急痛，赤腫。曲泉主目赤、腫痛。陽溪、陽谷主目痛赤。俠溪主外眥赤痛，逆寒泣出，目癢。二間主目眥傷。

Yáng Bái 陽白 (GB 14) governs pain and itching of the pupils (see the section on blindness in *Qiān*《千》).

Tài Chōng 太衝 (LV 3) governs pain of the lower eyelids (another says: It treats female diseases).

Tài Chōng (LV 3), Yáng Gǔ 陽谷 (SI 5), and Kūn Lún 崑崙 (UB 60) govern acute pain of the eyes with redness and swelling.

Qū Quán 曲泉 (LV 8) governs red swollen painful eyes.

Yáng Xī 陽溪 (LI 5) and Yáng Gǔ (SI 5) govern eye pain and redness.

Xiá Xī 俠溪 (GB 43) governs redness and pain of the outer canthus, tearing eyes when cold is counterflowing, and itching eyes.

Èr Jiān 二間 (LI 2) governs damage to the corners of the eyes.

風池、腦戶（《明》同）、玉枕、風府、上星主目痛不能視。先取譩譆，後取天牖、風池、照海主目痛，視如見星。天柱、陶道、崑崙主目如脫。頭維、大陵主目痛如脫（見頭痛）。三間（《明》同）、前谷主目急痛。

Fēng Chí 風池 (GB 20), Nǎo Hù 腦戶 (Dū 17) (*Míng*《明》agrees), Yù Zhěn 玉枕 (UB 9), Fēng Fǔ 風府 (Dū 16), and Shàng Xīng 上星 (Dū 23) govern eye pain and inability to see.

Treat Yī Xī 譩譆 (UB 45) first, then Tiān Yǒu 天牖 (SJ 16), Fēng Chí (GB 20), and Zhào Hǎi 照海 (KI 6) to govern eye pain and seeing stars.

Tiān Zhù 天柱 (UB 10), Táo Dào 陶道 (Dū 13), and Kūn Lún 崑崙 (UB 60) govern a feeling in the eyes as if they are about to burst from their sockets.

Tóu Wéi 頭維 (ST 8) and Dà Líng 大陵 (PC 7) govern eye pain as if they are about to burst from their sockets (see the section on headaches).

Sān Jiān 三間 (LI 3) (*Míng* 《明》 agrees) and Qián Gǔ 前谷 (SI 2) govern acute pain of the eyes.

陽白治頭目痛目眵(《銅》)。目窗治頭面浮腫，痛引目外眥上赤痛，忽頭旋，目䀮䀮遠視不明。上星、腦戶治目睛痛，不能遠視。玉枕治目痛不能視。《明下》云：目痛如脫。天柱療頭風，目如脫(《明》)。

Yáng Bái 陽白 (GB 14) treats headaches and eye pain with discharge from the eyes (*Tóng* 《銅》).

Mù Chuāng 目窗 (GB 16) treats puffy swelling of the head and face with pain, pain radiating to above the outer canthus with redness, sudden dizziness, blurred vision, and seeing dimly afar.

Shàng Xīng 上星 (Dū 23) and Nǎo Hù 腦戶 (Dū 17) treat painful eyeballs and inability to see distant objects.

Yù Zhěn 玉枕 (UB 9) treats eye pain with inability to see. *Míng Xià* 《明下》 says: Eye pain as if about to burst out of their sockets.

Tiān Zhù 天柱 (UB 10) cures head wind and eyes that feel as if they are about to burst from their sockets (*Míng*).

心俞、陰蹻療目痛。飛揚、陽谷療頭眩眼痛。玉枕療目內攣，系急痛，失枕，頭重項痛，風眩目痛，頭寒多汗，耳聾鼻塞。小兒三五歲，兩眼每至春秋生白翳遮瞳子，痛不可忍：灸九椎節上一壯。小兒熱毒風盛，眼睛痛：灸手中指本節頭三壯，名拳尖。

Xīn Shù 心俞 (UB 15) and Yīn Qiāo 陰蹻 (KI 6 or KI 8) cure eye pain.

Fēi Yáng 飛揚 (UB 58) and Yáng Gǔ 陽谷 (SI 5) cure dizzy head and eye pain.

Yù Zhěn (UB 9) cures hypertonicity of the eyes, acute pain of the eye tie, crick in the neck, heaviness of the head, pain of the nape, wind dizziness, eye pain, coldness of the head, profuse sweating, deafness, and nasal congestion.

For 3 or 5 year old children with white screens covering the pupils during the spring and fall, and unbearable pain, apply one cone of moxibustion on the 9th vertebra.

目淚 573
頭痛 643
面腫 655
傷寒 661

Heat toxins and wind excess in children with eye pain: Apply three cones of moxibustion on the base joint of the middle finger. The name of this point is Quán Jiān 拳尖.

四白主目痛，僻戾，目不明（《千》）。齦交主目痛不明。下廉主眼痛。眼急痛，不可遠視：灸當陽隨年壯。前谷主目痛（見目淚）。風癢赤痛：人中近鼻柱灸二壯。通里，百會，後頂療頭目痛（並見頭痛）。崑崙主目如拔（《千》見瘧）。

Sì Bái 四白 (ST 2) governs eye pain, deviation, and dim vision (*Qiān*《千》).

Yín Jiāo 齦交 (Dū 28) governs eye pain with dim vision.

Xià Lián 下廉 (LI 8) governs eye pain.

For acute eye pain and inability to see distant objects, apply same number of cones as the age of the patient on Dāng Yáng 當陽 (non-channel).[2]

Qián Gŭ 前谷 (SI 2) governs eye pain (see tearing of the eyes).

Wind itchiness with redness and pain: Apply two cones of moxibustion on the philtrum, near the nose pillar.

Tōng Lĭ 通里 (HT 5), Băi Huì 百會 (Dū 20), and Hòu Dĭng 後頂 (Dū 19) cure pain of the head and eyes (for all, see the section on headaches).

Kūn Lún 崑崙 (UB 60) governs a feeling in the eyes like they are being pulled out (see the section on malaria in *Qiān*).

陶道治頭重目瞑（《銅》與《明》同）。大迎治目不得閉（見面腫）。風門治傷寒目瞑（見傷寒雜病）。天柱治目瞑視。腦空療頭風目瞑（《明》）。《銅》云：腦風頭痛。天府療頭眩目瞑，遠視䀮䀮。目窗主目瞑，遠視䀮䀮（《千》）。承漿主目瞑，身汗出。

Táo Dào 陶道 (Dū 13) treats heaviness of the head and eyes (*Tóng*《銅》and *Míng*《明》agree).

Dà Yíng 大迎 (ST 5) treats inability to close the eyes (see the section on facial swelling).

Fēng Mén 風門 (UB 12) treats cold damage and heavy eyes (see the section on cold damage and miscellaneous diseases).

Tiān Zhù 天柱 (UB 10) treats heavy eyes.

2. Dāng Yáng 當陽 is located one cùn into the anterior hairline, directly above the pupils.

Nǎo Kōng 腦空 (GB 19) cures head wind and heavy eyes (*Míng*《明》). *Tóng*《銅》says: It treats head wind and headaches. 風癇 366 驚癇 363

Tiān Fǔ 天府 (LU 3) cures dizzy head, heavy eyes, and seeing dimly afar.

Mù Chuāng 目窗 (GB 16) governs heavy eyes and seeing dimly afar (*Qiān*《千》).

Chéng Jiāng 承漿 (Rèn 24) governs heavy eyes and sweating.

目微澀痛，或兩旁生小米珠，頻去其睫自愈，不必針灸。

For mild pain and dryness of the eyes or small rice-size bumps growing to the sides, removing the eye lashes frequently cures the disease. Acupuncture is not necessary.

## 6.06
## *Mù Shàng Shì (Mù Shùn Dòng)*
# 目上視（目瞤動）
## Upward staring eyes
**(Twitching of the eyelids)**

申脈主目反上視，若赤痛從內眥始（《千》）。陽白、上星、本神、大都、曲泉、俠溪、三間、前谷、攢竹、玉枕主目系急，目上插。絲竹空、前頂主目上插，憎風寒。神庭（見風癇）、囟會（見驚癇）治目上不識人。

Shēn Mài 申脈 (UB 62) governs upward staring eyes with redness and pain starting from the inner canthus (*Qiān*).

Yáng Bái 陽白 (GB 14), Shàng Xīng 上星 (Dū 23), Běn Shén 本神 (GB 13), Dà Dū 大都 (SP 2), Qū Quán 曲泉 (LV 8), Xiá Xī 俠溪 (GB 43), Sān Jiān 三間 (LI 3), Qián Gǔ 前谷 (SI 2), Zǎn Zhú 攢竹 (UB 2), and Yù Zhěn 玉枕 (UB 9) govern tension of eye tie and upturned eyes.

Sī Zhú Kōng 絲竹空 (SJ 23) and Qián Dǐng 前頂 (Dū 21) govern upturned eyes and aversion to wind and cold.

Shén Tíng 神庭 (Dū 24) (see the section on wind epilepsy) and Xìn Huì 囟會 (Dū 22) (see the section on fright epilepsy) treat upturned eyes and loss of consciousness.

咳逆 417 肝俞治目上視（見咳逆）。筋縮療目轉上及目瞪（《明下》見驚癇）。臨泣
中風 379 主兒癇反視（《千》見驚癇）。肝俞療目上視（《明下》見目不明）。筋縮
目不明 579 治目轉上垂（《銅》見驚癇）》。治眼戴睛上插，眼反戴眼（並見中風）。

Gān Shù 肝俞 (UB 18) treats upward staring eyes (see the section on coughing counterflow).

Jīn Suō 筋縮 (Dū 8) cures upturned staring eyes (see the section on fright epilepsy in *Míng Xià*《明下》).

Lín Qì 臨泣 (GB 15 or GB 41) governs epilepsy in children with upturned eyes (see fright epilepsy in *Qiān*《千》).

Gān Shù (UB 18) cures upward staring eyes (see the section on blurred vision in *Míng Xià*).

Jīn Suō (Dū 8) treats spinning of the eyes, and drooping upper [eyelids] (see the section on fright epilepsy in *Tóng*《銅》). It also treats upturned and upcast eyes (for all of these, see the section on wind stroke).

承泣（《銅》見目淚）主目瞤動，與項口相引。《甲乙》云：目瞤動，與頭口參相引，喎僻口不能言。顴髎治口喎，面赤目黃，眼瞤動不止，䪼腫齒痛。地倉治眼瞤動不止，目不得閉（見口喎）。攢竹治眼瞼瞤動（見目不明）。目不明，淚出，目眩瞢，瞳子癢，遠視䀮䀮，昏夜無見，目瞤動（餘同上承泣）刺承泣。

Chéng Qì 承泣 (ST 1) (see the section on tearing eyes in *Tóng*《銅》) governs twitching eyelids that pull the nape and mouth. *Jiǎ Yǐ*《甲乙》says: It treats twitching eyelids that pull the head and mouth, deviation of the mouth, and inability to speak.

Quán Liáo 顴髎 (SI 18) treats deviation of the mouth, red face and yellow eyes, incessant twitching of the eyes, swollen cheeks, and toothache.

Dì Cāng 地倉 (ST 4) treats incessant twitching of the eyes and inability to close the eyes (see the section on deviation of the mouth).

Zǎn Zhú 攢竹 (UB 2) treats twitching eyelids (see the section on blurred vision).

Blurred vision, tearing eyes, dizzy vision, itching pupils, seeing dimly afar, inability to see at dusk and in the evening, and twitching eyelids (the rest [of the symptoms] treated by Chéng Qì (ST 1) are the same as above): needle Chéng Qì (ST 1).

# 6.07
## *Mù Lèi Chū*
## 目淚出
## Tearing eyes

目翳 584
目痛 568
口喎 591
目瞤 571

液門（《明下》云：目澀䀮䀮，頭痛泣出）、前谷、後溪、腕骨、神庭、百會、天柱、風池、天牖主目泣出。肝俞等主目淚出，多眵，矆（見目翳）。俠溪主泣出目癢（見目痛）。承泣主目淚出。

Yè Mén 液門 (SJ 2) (*Míng Xià*《明下》says: Dry eyes with blurred vision, headaches, and tearing), Qián Gŭ 前谷(SI 2), Hòu Xī 後溪 (SI 3), Wàn Gŭ 腕骨 (SI 4), Shén Tíng 神庭 (Dū 24), Băi Huì 百會 (Dū 20), Tiān Zhù 天柱 (UB 10), Fēng Chí 風池 (GB 20), and Tiān Yŏu 天牖 (SJ 16) govern tearing eyes.

Gān Shù 肝俞 (UB 18) and so forth govern tearing eyes with a lot of discharge from the eyes, as well as poor vision (see the section on eye screens).

Xiá Xī 俠溪 (GB 43) governs tearing itchy eyes (see the section on eye pain).

Chéng Qì 承泣 (ST 1) governs tearing eyes.

行間（見口喎）、神庭治目淚出（《銅》見鼻涕）。臨泣治多淚（見翳）。齦交治目淚眵汁，內眥赤癢痛，生白翳。風池治目淚出，欠氣多。睛明治氣眼冷淚（見眼翳）。承泣治目瞤冷淚。頭維治風淚出（見目瞤）。腕骨治目冷淚生翳。

Xíng Jiān 行間 (LV 2) (see the section on deviation of the mouth) and Shén Tíng 神庭 (Dū 24) treat tearing eyes (see the section on sniveling in *Tóng*《銅》).

Lín Qì 臨泣 (GB 15 or GB 41) treats profuse tearing (see the section on [eye] screens).

Yín Jiāo 齦交 (Dū 28) treats tearing eyes with discharge and red, itching, painful inner canthus with white screens.

Fēng Chí (GB 20) treats tearing eyes and frequent yawning.

口喎 591 目瞤 571

Jīng Míng 睛明 (UB 1) treats qì disorders of the eyes[3] with cold tears (see the section on eye screens).

Chéng Qì 承泣 (ST 1) treats twitching eyelids with cold tears (see the section on deviation of the mouth).

Tóu Wéi 頭維 (ST 8) treats tearing due to wind (see the section on twitching of the eyelids).

Wàn Gǔ 腕骨 (SI 4) treats cold tears in the eyes with screens.

行間（口喎）、魚際療目泣出（《明》）。心俞療目𥆧𥆧淚出（《千》）。睛明主目遠視，惡風目淚出，憎寒頭痛，目眩瞢，內眥赤痛，遠視𥆧𥆧無見，眥癢痛淫膚白翳（《千》）。目淚出：刺承泣（見目瞤）。前谷主目痛泣出，甚者如脫。行間治目淚出（見口喎）。

Xíng Jiān 行間 (LV 2) (see the section on deviation of the mouth) and Yú Jì 魚際 (LU 10) cure tearing eyes (*Míng*《明》).

Xīn Shù 心俞 (UB 15) cures blurred vision and tearing eyes (*Qiān*《千》).

Jīng Míng 睛明 (UB 1) governs farsightedness, aversion to wind, tearing eyes, aversion to cold, headaches, dizzy vision, redness and pain of the inner canthus, seeing dimly afar, inability to see, itching and pain of the canthus, and *yín fū* 淫膚[4] with white screens (*Qiān*).

Tearing eyes: Prick Chéng Qì (ST 1) (see the section on twitching of the eyelids).

Qián Gǔ 前谷 (SI 2) governs eye pain with tearing, as if about to burst from the sockets when the pain is severe.

Xíng Jiān (LV 2) treats tearing eyes (see the section on deviation of the mouth).

予用真熊膽治人目疾（赤瞤翳淚皆除，神效）。

I use bear gall bladder to treat eye diseases.[5] (It can remove redness, twitching, screens, and tearing of the eyes. It is divinely effective.)

3. Qì disorders of the eyes are usually caused by liver qì constraint due to anger. The symptoms include blurred vision, tearing eyes, swollen eyelids, and dryness of the eyes.

4. *Yín fū* 淫膚 is a type of polyp growing over the eyes, or pterygium, usually due to heat.

5. Today this is ethically questionable and prohibitively expensive.

# 6.08

## *Mù Xuàn*

# 目眩

## Dizzy vision

鼻涕 616
瘛瘲 354
肩背痛 486
腰傴 545
腹滿 445
歷節風 707
胸滿 470
咳逆 417

通谷治頭重目眩，善驚引鼽衄，頸項痛，目䀮䀮（《銅》）。神庭（見鼻涕）、上關（見瘛瘲）、涌泉、譩譆（見肩背痛）、束骨（見腰傴）、魚際、大都（見腹滿）治目眩。

Tōng Gǔ 通谷 (UB 66) treats heaviness of the head, dizzy vision, susceptibility to fright leading to nosebleeds and sniveling, pain of the neck and nape, and blurred vision (*Tóng*《銅》).

Shén Tíng 神庭 (Dū 24) (see the section on sniveling), Shàng Guān 上關 (GB 3) (see the section on tugging and slackening), Yǒng Quán 涌泉 (KI 1), Yī Xī 譩譆 (UB 45) (see the section on shoulder and back pain), Shù Gǔ 束骨 (UB 65) (see the discussion of stooped lower back), Yú Jì 魚際 (LU 10), and Dà Dū 大都 (SP 2) (see the section on abdominal fullness) treat dizzy vision.

本神治目眩，頸項強急痛，胸脅相引，不得轉側。飛揚（見歷節風）、肺俞治頭目眩（見胸滿）。肝俞治目眩循眉痛（見咳逆）。絲竹空治目眩頭痛目赤，視物䀮䀮，風癇目戴上不識人，眼睫毛倒，發狂，吐涎沫，發即無時。

Běn Shén 本神 (GB 13) treats dizzy vision, acute pain and stiffness of the neck and nape, pulling sensation between the chest and rib-sides, and inability to turn to the sides.

Fēi Yáng 飛揚 (UB 58) (see the section on joint-running wind) and Fèi Shù 肺俞 (UB 13) treat dizziness in the head and eyes (see the section on chest fullness.)

Gān Shù 肝俞 (UB 18) treats dizzy vision and pain along the eyebrows (see the section on coughing counterflow).

Sī Zhú Kōng 絲竹空 (SJ 23) treats randomly occurring dizzy vision, headaches, red eyes, blurred

腹脹 449 傷寒無 690 風勞 371 瘛瘲 354

vision, wind epilepsy, upcast eyes,[6] loss of consciousness, ingrown eye lashes, mania, and vomiting of drool and foam.

天府治目眩遠視𥆨𥆨。支正、三焦俞治目眩頭痛（見腹脹）。風池治目眩若（見傷寒無汗）。風門治身熱目眩（見風勞）。臨泣治目眩，枕骨合顱痛，惡寒。風府治頭痛頸項急，目眩。神庭治頭風目眩，淚出。

Tiān Fǔ 天府 (LU 3) treats dizzy vision and seeing dimly afar.

Zhī Zhèng 支正 (SI 7) and Sān Jiāo Shù 三焦俞 (UB 22) treat dizzy vision and headaches (see the section on abdominal fullness).

Fēng Chí 風池 (GB 20) treats dizzy vision (see the section on cold damage with absence of sweating).

Fēng Mén 風門 (UB 12) treats generalized heat and dizzy vision (see the section on wind taxation).

Lín Qì 臨泣 (GB 15 or GB 41) treats dizzy vision, pain at Hé Lú 合顱 (Dū 17) on the occiput, and aversion to cold.

Fēng Fǔ 風府 (Dū 16) treats headache, tension of the neck and nape, and dizzy vision.

Shén Tíng 神庭 (Dū 24) treats head wind, dizzy vision, and tearing eyes.

上星治目眩（《明下》同）睛痛，不能遠視。前頂、五處治頭風目眩，目戴上（見瘛瘲）。臨泣治目眩鼻塞，目生白翳。四白治頭痛目眩（《明》同），眼白翳，微風，目動不息。前關療風赤眼，頭痛目眩目澀（《明》）。

Shàng Xīng 上星 (Dū 23) treats dizzy vision (*Míng Xià*《明下》agrees) with eye pain and inability to see distant objects.

Qián Dǐng 前頂 (Dū 21) and Wǔ Chù 五處 (UB 5) treat head wind, dizzy vision, and upcast eyes (see the section on tugging and slackening).

Lín Qì (GB 15 or GB 41) treats dizzy eyes, nasal congestion, and white screens in the eyes.

Sì Bái 四白 (ST 2) treats headaches, dizzy vision (*Míng*《明》agrees), white screens in the eyes, and incessant eye movement caused by mild wind.

6. Volume 45 of *Jǐng Yuè Quán Shū*《景岳全書·卷之四十五》(Jǐngyuè's Complete Compendium) states: The symptom of upcast eyes occurs after suppuration of pox or after severe sweating and diarrhea. It is usually characterized by upturned eyes, or the white of eyes (sclera) showing.

Qián Guān 前關 (GB 1 or Tài Yáng) cures *fēng chì yǎn* 風赤眼 wind redness of the eyes,[7] headaches, dizzy vision and dry eyes (*Míng*《明》).

四白(《銅》同)、涌泉、大杼療頭痛目眩。束骨療頭痛目眩(《下》又云：療風赤胎赤，兩目眥爛)、身熱，肌肉動。前谷療目眩淫淫。攢竹療頭目風眩，眉頭痛，鼽衄，目䀮䀮無遠見(《下》)。囟會療頭目眩。

Sì Bái 四白 (ST 2) (*Tóng*《銅》agrees), Yǒng Quán 涌泉 (KI 1), and Dà Zhù 大杼 (UB 11) cure headaches and dizzy vision.

Shù Gǔ 束骨 (UB 65) cures headaches, dizzy vision (*Xià*《下》says: It cures *fēng chì* 風赤 wind redness, *tāi chì* 胎赤 fetal redness,[8] and erosion of both canthi), generalized heat, and muscle twitching.

Qián Gǔ 前谷 (SI 2) cures progressively worsening dizzy vision.

Zǎn Zhú 攢竹 (UB 2) cures wind dizziness of the head and eyes, pain at the medial end of the eyebrows, sniveling, nosebleeds, blurred vision, and inability to see distant objects (*Xià*).

Xìn Huì 囟會 (Dū 22) cures dizziness of the head and eyes.

岐伯灸頭旋目眩，及偏頭痛不可忍，牽眼䀮䀮遠視：灸兩眼小眥上髮際各一壯，立瘥。率谷主醉酒風熱發，兩目眩痛(《千》)。大都主目眩。承漿、前頂、天柱、腦空、目窗主目眩瞑。天柱、陶道(《明下》同)、崑崙主目眩，目如脫。又云：瘧多汗，目如脫，項如拔，崑崙主之。

Qí Bó's moxibustion prescription for spinning head, dizzy vision, and unbearable hemilateral headaches that induce blurred vision with inability to see distant objects: Apply one cone each on the sites within the hairline above the smaller [outer] canthus. This will cure the disease immediately.

Shuài Gǔ 率谷 (GB 8) governs drunkenness with onset of wind heat and dizzy vision with painful eyes (*Qiān*《千》).

Dà Dū 大都 (SP 2) governs dizzy vision.

Chéng Jiāng 承漿 (Rèn 24), Qián Dǐng 前頂 (Dū 21), Tiān Zhù 天柱 (UB 10), Nǎo Kōng 腦空 (GB 19), and Mù Chuāng 目窗 (GB 16) govern dizzy heavy eyes.

7. *Fēng chì yǎn* 風赤眼 (wind redness of the eyes) may indicate *fēng huǒ yǎn* 風火眼 (wind fire eyes), which is due to attack of wind heat. The symptoms include red painful swollen eyes, blurred vision, and tearing eyes. It is similar to the diagnosis of conjunctivitis in Western medicine.

8. *Tāi chì* 胎赤 or fetal redness is redness and erosion of the canthus of the eyes in newborns. It is due to insufficient cleaning of the eyes after birth.

目不明
579 Tiān Zhù 天柱 (UB 10), Táo Dào 陶道 (Dū 13) (*Míng Xià*《明下》agrees), and Kūn Lún 崑崙 (UB 60) govern dizzy vision and eyes that feel as if they are about to burst from their sockets. It also says: For malaria with profuse sweating, eyes that feel as if they are about to burst from their sockets, and the nape feels like it is being pulled: Kūn Lún (UB 60) can govern this.

大敦主目不欲視，太息。神庭、水溝主頭痛，目不可視。承泣主目眩（見目不明）。通里、百會療頭目眩疼（《明》）。後頂療目眩痛（《下》目不明）。臨泣、中渚治目眩（《銅》並見目翳）。頷厭主目眩（《千》見偏頭[痛]）。

Dà Dūn 大敦 (LV 1) governs no desire to look and sighing.

Shén Tíng 神庭 (Dū 24) and Shuǐ Gōu 水溝 (Dū 26) govern headaches and inability to see.

Chéng Qì 承泣 (ST 1) governs dizzy vision (see the section on blurred vision).

Tōng Lǐ 通里 (HT 5) and Bǎi Huì 百會 (Dū 20) cure dizziness of head and eyes with pain (*Míng*《明》).

Hòu Dǐng 後頂 (Dū 19) cures dizzy vision and eye pain (see the section on blurred vision in *Xià*《下》).

Lín Qì 臨泣 (GB 15 or GB 41) and Zhōng Zhǔ 中渚 (SJ 3) treat dizzy vision (for all, see the section on eye screens in *Tóng*《銅》).

Hàn Yàn 頷厭 (GB 4) governs dizzy vision (see the section on hemilateral head[aches] in *Qiān*《千》).

## 6.09
## *Mù Bù Míng (Mù Máng Máng, Mù Àn, Mù Miǎo)*
## 目不明 （目䀮䀮　目暗　目眇）

目痛 568
脊 555
咳逆 417
頭風 640

### Blurred vision
**(Blurred vision, diminished vision, blindness)**

腎俞、偏歷、後頂治目䀮䀮（《銅》）。攢竹治目䀮䀮，視物不明，眼中赤（明作熱）痛，及瞼瞤動。又云：三度以細棱針刺之，目大明。養老、合谷、曲差（《明》同）治目視不明。肩中俞治寒熱目視不明。

Shèn Shù 腎俞 (UB 23), Piān Lì 偏歷 (LI 6), and Hòu Dǐng 後頂 (Dū 19) treat blurred vision (*Tóng*《銅》).

Zǎn Zhú 攢竹 (Dū 2) treats blurred vision, inability to see clearly, redness (*Míng*《明》says heat) and pain of the eyes, and facial twitching. It also says: Vision will be bright when you prick it with a thin three-edged needle three times.

Yǎng Lǎo 養老 (SI 6), Hé Gǔ 合谷 (LI 4), and Qū Chā 曲差 (UB 4) (*Míng* agrees) treat blurred vision.

Jiān Zhōng Shù 肩中俞 (SI 15) treats [sensations of] cold and heat as well as blurred vision.

風池（見目痛）、五處治目不明。目窗治忽頭旋目䀮䀮，遠視不明。又云：三度刺目大明。復溜（見脊），肝俞治起則目䀮䀮（見咳逆）。頭維治偏痛，目視物不明。三里治目不明。人年三十以上，不灸三里，令氣上衝目。《明下》云：令氣上眼暗，所以三里下氣也。水泉治婦人目䀮䀮，不能遠視。頷厭療目無所見（《明》見風眩）。攢竹（見頭風）、腎俞（《下》見勞）、崑崙療目䀮䀮。

Fēng Chí 風池 (GB 20) (see the section on eye pain) and Wǔ Chù 五處 (UB 5) treat blurred vision.

Mù Chuāng 目窗 (GB 16) treats sudden dizziness, blurred vision, and seeing dimly afar. It also says: Pricking it three times will brighten vision.

Fù Liū 復溜 (KI 7) (see the section on [pain of the lower back and] spine) and Gān Shù 肝俞 (UB 18) treat blurred vision when getting up (see the section on coughing counterflow).

Tóu Wéi 頭維 (ST 8) treats hemilateral headaches and blurred vision.

Sān Lǐ 三里 (ST 36) treats blurred vision. When someone over 30 does not apply moxibustion on Sān Lǐ (ST 36), it lets qì run upward into the eyes. *Míng Xià*《明下》says: When qì is allowed to run upward and causes blurred vision, Sān Lǐ (ST 36) descends the qì.

Shuǐ Quán 水泉 (KI 5) treats blurred vision in women and inability to see distant objects.

Hàn Yàn 頷厭 (GB 4) cures inability to see (see the section on wind dizziness in *Míng*《明》).

Zǎn Zhú 攢竹 (UB 2) (see the section on head wind), Shèn Shù 腎俞 (UB 23) (see taxation in *Xià*《下》), and Kūn Lún 崑崙 (UB 60) cure blurred vision.

後頂療目不明，惡風寒，頭目眩痛（《下》）。肝俞療目生白翳（解溪同），氣短唾血，目上視，多怒狂衄，目䀮䀮。脅堂療目黃遠視䀮䀮。天牖主目不明（《千》）。天柱、陶道、崑崙主目不明，目如脫。

Hòu Dǐng 後頂 (Dū 19) cures blurred vision, aversion to cold, and dizziness of the head and eyes with pain (*Xià*).

Gān Shù (UB 18) cures white screens in the eyes (same as Jiě Xī 解溪 (ST 41)), shortness of qì, spitting of blood, upward staring eyes, frequent anger, mania and nosebleeds, and blurred vision.

Xié Táng 脅堂 (LV 14) cures yellow eyes and blurred vision when look afar.

Tiān Yǒu 天牖 (SJ 16) governs blurred vision (*Qiān*《千》).

Tiān Zhù 天柱 (UB 10), Táo Dào 陶道 (Dū 13), and Kūn Lún (UB 60) govern blurred vison and eyes that feel as if they are about to burst from their sockets.

承泣主目不明，淚出，目眩瞢，瞳子癢，遠視䀮䀮，昏夜無見（《甲乙》）。陽白主目瞳子痛癢，遠視䀮䀮，昏夜無見。腎俞、胃俞、心俞、百會、內關、復溜、太泉、腕骨、中渚（《明下》同）、攢竹、睛明、委中、崑崙、天柱、本神、大杼、頷厭、通谷、曲泉、後頂、絲竹空主目䀮䀮不明，惡風寒（《千》）。

Chéng Qì 承泣 (ST 1) governs blurred vision, tearing eyes, dizziness, blurred vision, itchiness of the pupils, seeing dimly afar, and night blindness (*Jiǎ Yǐ*《甲乙》).

Yáng Bái 陽白 (GB 14) governs itching painful pupils, seeing dimly afar, and inability to see at dusk and in the evening.

Shèn Shù 腎俞 (UB 23), Wèi Shù 胃俞 (UB 21), Xīn Shù 心俞 (UB 15), Bǎi Huì 百會 (Dū 20), Nèi Guān 內關 (PC 6), Fù Liū 復溜 (KI 7), Tài Quán 太泉 (KI 3), Wàn Gǔ 腕骨 (SI 4), Zhōng Zhǔ 中渚 (SJ 3) (*Míng Xià* (《明下》agrees), Zǎn Zhú 攢竹 (UB 2), Jīng Míng 睛明 (UB 1), Wěi Zhōng 委中 (UB 40), Kūn Lún 崑崙 (UB 60), Tiān Zhù 天柱 (UB 10), Běn Shén 本神 (GB 13), Dà Zhù 大杼 (UB 11), Hàn Yàn 頷厭 (GB 4), Tōng Gǔ 通谷 (UB 66), Qū Quán 曲泉 (LV 8), Hòu Dǐng 後頂 (Dū 19), and Sī Zhú Kōng 絲竹空 (SJ 23) govern blurred vision and aversion to cold (*Qiān*《千》).

風池等主目痛不能視(見目痛)。肝虛目不明:灸肝俞二百壯,小兒斟酌可灸一二七壯。小兒奶澼目不明:灸肩中俞各二十壯(《明》)。

Fēng Chí 風池 (GB 20) and so forth govern eye pain and inability to see (see the section on eye pain).

Blurred vision due to liver deficiency: Apply two hundred cones of moxibustion on Gān Shù 肝俞 (UB 18); apply seven or two time seven cones of moxibustion on children.

Blurred vision in children due to breast milk afflux: Apply twenty cones of moxibustion on Jiān Zhōng Shù 肩中俞 (SI 15) (*Míng*《明》).

《千金方》戒人喪明之由云:生食五辛,接熱食飲,刺頭出血過多,極目遠視,夜讀注書,久處煙火,博弈不休,日沒後讀書,飲酒不已,熱餐面食,抄寫多年,雕鏤細作,泣淚過多,房室不節,數向日月輪看,月下讀書,夜視星月,極目瞻視山川草木(十八件)。又有馳騁田獵,冒涉風霜,迎風追獸,日夜不息者,並是傷目之由也。其讀書博弈等過度患目者,名肝勞。若欲治之,非三年閉目不視,不可得瘥。徒自瀉肝,及作諸治,終是無效。

The *Qiān Jīn Fāng*《千金方》warns people about the causes of blindness: eating the five acrid foods together with hot food; excessive pricking to bleed on the head; looking as far as the eye can see; concentrated reading at night; staying in smoke for a long time; playing chess constantly; reading after sunset; incessant drinking of liquor; eating hot food and noodles; copying and writing for many years; carving tiny things; crying too much; unregulated sexual activity; looking at the sun and moon frequently; reading under the moonlight; looking at the moon and stars at night; looking at mountains, trees, and bushes as far as eye can see (a total of eighteen reasons). Also riding and hunting when there is wind and frost, chasing animals against the wind, doing these things day and night without rest are causes for damage to the eyes.

When excessive reading and playing chess harm the eyes, it is called liver taxation. If we want to treat it, ask the person to close his eyes and not look at anything for three years; otherwise, it won't be cured. It is not effective to drain the liver and treat other things.

《本事方》云：讀書之苦傷肝損目。誠然。晉范寧嘗苦目痛，就張湛求方。湛戲之曰云云：用損讀書一，減思慮二，專內視三，簡外觀四，旦早起五，夜早眠六。凡六物，熬以神火，下以氣簁，蘊於胸中。七日，然後納諸方寸，修之一時，近能數其目睫，遠視尺棰之餘。長服不已，動見牆壁之外，非但明目，乃亦延年。審如是而行之，非可謂之嘲戲，亦奇方也，以其勸戒人有理。姑備載之，以示後人。

[*Pǔ Jì*] *Běn Shì Fāng*《本事方》says: Too much reading damages the liver and the eyes. This is true. Fàn Níng of *Jìn* suffered eye pain and went to Zhāng Zhàn for treatment. Zhàn joked: First, reduce reading; second, cut down on thought and anxiety; third, focus on looking inward; fourth, reduce watching outward; fifth, get up early; sixth, sleep early. All six things boil the spirit fire, filtrate it through a qì sieve, and store it in the chest. In seven days, after it has been collected and concentrated into one square cùn and cultivated for a while, [the practitioner] can count his own eyelashes close up or see past the end of a ruler far off. If he takes this[9] for a long time, he can see things beyond a wall. It does not just brighten the eyes, but it also extends a person's years. If we follow this, it is not a joke, but a miraculous method. This is reasonable so I record it here to instruct people.

眼暗：灸大椎數節第十，當脊中安灸二百壯，以多為佳，最驗（《千》）。《明堂》云：人年三十以上，若不灸三里，令氣上衝目。《明下》云眼暗。

For blurred vision, apply two hundred cones of moxibustion on the tenth vertebra, counting from the big vertebrae, and right on the spine. The more cones, the better. It is most effective (*Qiān*《千》). *Míng Táng*《明堂》says: After thirty years of age, if moxibustion is not applied on Sān Lǐ 三里 (ST 36), qì rushes up into the eyes (*Míng Xià*《明下》says: [This causes] blurred vision).

《千金方》云：讀書博弈等過度患目者，名肝勞，若欲治之，非三年閉目不視，不可得瘥。徒自瀉肝，及作諸治，終是無效。則是目者，不可使之勞也。古人蓋有養之之法。如彭真人龜年常患目疾，不計晝夜，瞪目注視，以去昏暗，閉之少頃，依法再行，積功而視秋毫。

The *Qiān Jīn Fāng*《千金方》says: Reading and playing chess harm the eyes. This is called liver taxation. If we want to treat it, the person should close his eyes for three years and the disease can be cured. Only draining the liver or treating in other ways are not effective. So we cannot exhaust the eyes. It seems that ancient people had other methods of taking care of the eyes. For example, a Daoist holy man named Péng suffered from eye disease when he was old. He stared at things no matter day or night to remove the blurriness. He would close the eyes for a while and then repeat it again. Eventually, he could see the tip of an autumn hair [very small things].

9. 'Takes this' as in taking a dose of medicine.

徐真人甲常患目疾，暗室正坐，運睛旋還八十一數，閉目集神，再運不數，而神光自現，狀如金輪，永除昏暗。

A Daoist holy man named Xú Jiǎ frequently suffered eye disease. He would sit in a dark room and rotate his eyes 81 times, closing his eyes and concentrating his spirit. Then he would rotate them again countless times. Then a spirit light spontaneously appeared like a gold wheel and the blurriness disappeared forever.

施真人自記歌亦云運睛除目暗（此見《抱朴子》），皆養之之法也。若用藥，則地黃丸、羊肝丸等，與用當歸、芍藥、黃連等分為末，以雪水煎濃汁，乘熱頻洗者，最佳云（見《既效方》）。

*Zì Jì Gē* 自記歌 (Self-Recorded Songs) of the Daoist holy man Shī also says: Rotate the eyes to remove blurred vision (see *Bào Pǔ Zǐ*《抱朴子》). These are all methods of nourishing oneself. As for herbs, take *Dì Huáng Wán* 地黃丸 (Rehmannia Pill) or *Yáng Gān Wán* 羊肝丸 (Goat's Liver Pill). Or make a powder of equal portions of *dāng guī* 當歸 (Angelicae Radix), *sháo yào* 芍藥 (Paeoniae Radix), and *huáng lián* 黃連 (Coptidis Rhizoma); boil it in snow water to make a concentrated liquid; wash the eyes with it while it is hot. This works the best (see *Jì Xiào Fāng*《既效方》).

腦空治癲風引目眇（見腦痛）。

Nǎo Kōng 腦空 (GB 19) treats epilepsy that induces blindness (see the section on brain pain).

# 6.10

## *Mù Yì Mó (Bái Yì, Juàn Mù, Wèi Mù)*

# 目翳膜（白翳　睊目　膭目）

## Eye screens

**(White screens, strabismus, painful eyes)**

至陰主目翳（《千》）。丘墟主目翳，瞳子不見。後溪主眥爛有翳，又主目赤有翳。前谷、京骨主目中白翳。京骨主目反白，白翳從內眥始。肝俞、上星、風池、睛明、齦交、承泣、四白、巨髎、瞳子髎主目淚出多眵矇，內眥赤痛癢，生白膚翳。

Zhì Yīn 至陰 (UB 67) governs screens in the eyes (*Qiān*《千》).

Qiū Xū 丘墟 (GB 40) governs screens in the eyes so the pupil cannot be seen.

Hòu Xī 後溪 (SI 3) governs erosion of the canthus and screens in the eyes. It also governs red eyes with screens.

Qián Gǔ 前谷 (SI 2) and Jīng Gǔ 京骨 (UB 64) govern white screens in the eyes.

Jīng Gǔ 京骨 (UB 64) governs pathological white in the eyes and white screens that start at the inner canthus.

Gān Shù 肝俞 (UB 18), Shàng Xīng 上星 (Dū 23), Fēng Chí 風池 (GB 20), Jīng Míng 睛明 (UB 1), Yín Jiāo 齦交 (Dū 28), Chéng Qì 承泣 (ST 1), Sì Bái 四白 (ST 2), Jù Liáo 巨髎 (ST 3), and Tóng Zǐ Liáo 瞳子髎 (GB 1) govern tearing and profuse discharge from the eyes; red, painful, and itching inner canthus; and white screens in the eyes.

承光治目生白膜（《銅》）。臨泣治目生白膜，多淚，又治目眩，生白翳。睛明治攀睛翳膜覆瞳子，惡風淚出，目內眥癢痛，小兒雀目疳眼，大人氣眼冷淚，目視物不明，大眥努肉侵睛。《明》云：膚翳白膜覆瞳子，眼暗，雀目冷淚。

Chéng Guāng 承光 (UB 6) treats white screens (*Tóng*《銅》).

Lín Qì 臨泣 (GB 15 or GB 41) treats white screens in the eyes and profuse tearing. It also treats dizzy vision and white screens in the eyes.

Jīng Míng 睛明 (UB 1) treats screens in the eyes that creep over the pupils, aversion to wind, tearing eyes, itching and pain of the inner canthus, sparrow eyes in children, *gān* eyes, qì eyes with cold tears in adults, *yí* eyes,[10] blurred vision, and outcropping creeping over the eyes[11] from the big [inner] canthus. *Míng*《 明 》says: It treats screens covering the pupils, blurred vision, sparrow eyes, and cold tears.

青盲 589
腋腫 496
目淚 573
咳逆 417
目眩 575

巨髎治白翳覆瞳子（ 見青盲 ）。少澤治目上膚翳覆瞳子 。丘墟（ 見腋腫 ）、瞳子髎治目中翳膜（ 見青盲 ）。中渚治目眩生翳膜 。臨泣 、腕骨 、齦交（ 並見目淚 ）、肝俞（ 見咳逆 ）、四白（ 見目眩 ）、關衝 、前谷治目生白翳 。至陰治目生翳 。

Jù Liáo 巨髎 (ST 3) treats white screens covering the pupils (see the section on clear-eye blindness).[12]

Shào Zé 少澤 (SI 1) treats screens covering the pupils.

Qiū Xū 丘墟 (GB 40) (see the section on swelling of the axilla) and Tóng Zǐ Liáo 瞳子髎 (GB 1) treat screens in the eyes (see the section on clear-eye blindness).

Zhōng Zhǔ 中渚 (SJ 3) treats dizzy vision with screens in the eyes.

Lín Qì (GB 15 or GB 41), Wàn Gǔ 腕骨 (SI 4), Yín Jiāo 齦交 (Dū 28) (for all, see the section on tearing eyes), Gān Shù 肝俞 (UB 18) (see the section on coughing counterflow), Sì Bái 四白 (ST 2) (see the section on dizzy vision), Guān Chōng 關衝 (SJ 1), and Qián Gǔ 前谷 (SI 2) treat white screens in the eyes.

Zhì Yīn 至陰 (UB 67) treats screens in the eyes.

太淵治目生白翳（《 明下 》同 ），眼眥赤筋，缺盆中引痛 。陽溪治目風赤爛有翳 。角孫治目生膚翳 。至陰療目翳睆睆 。合谷療目不明，生白翳（《 下 》）。張仲文療風眼，卒生翳膜，兩目痛不可忍：灸手中指本節頭節間尖上三壯，炷如麥，左灸右，右灸左 。

Tài Yuān 太淵 (LU 9) treats white screens in the eyes (*Míng Xià*《 明下 》agrees), red sinews in the canthus, and pain radiating to the empty basin.

10. This character indicates some type of eye disease, but the specific symptoms are unknown.

11. An outcropping is a gray-white fleshy growth over the eye. In Western medicine, it is called pterygium.

12. Clear-eye blindness is caused by liver and kidney deficiency, combined with spleen deficiency. This results in insufficient blood supply to the eyes. In the beginning, symptoms include blurred vision and objects appear to have a green or yellow tint; later they may go blind.

青盲 589

Yáng Xī 陽溪 (LI 5) treats eye wind, redness and erosion with screens in the eyes.

Jiǎo Sūn 角孫 (SJ 20) treats screens in the eyes.

Zhì Yīn 至陰 (UB 67) cures blurred vision with screens.

Hé Gǔ 合谷 (LI 4) cures blurred vision and white screes in the eyes (*Xià*《 下 》).

Zhāng Zhòngwén's treatment for wind eye[13] with sudden onset of screens, and unbearable eye pain: Apply three cones of moxibustion on the tip of the base joint of the middle finger; use grain-of-wheat size cones. Apply moxibustion on the left side when the disease is on the right side; apply moxibustion on the right side when the disease is on the left side.

前溪主目中白翳( 《 千 》 )。解溪主白幕覆珠子無所見 。目卒生翳：灸大指節横文三壯，左灸右，右灸左良 。肝俞 、解溪療目生白翳( 《 明下 》見目不明 )。水溝主睊目 。上關( 見青肓 )、偏歷主臆目䀮䀮 。

Qián Xī 前溪 governs white screens in the eyes (*Qiān*《 千 》).

Jiě Xī 解溪 (ST 41) governs white screens covering the pupil, and inability to see.

Sudden onset of screens in the eyes: Apply three cones of moxibustion on the transverse crease of the thumb. It is good to apply moxibustion on the left side when the disease is on the right; or to apply moxibustion on the right when the disease is on the left.

Gān Shù 肝俞 (UB 18) and Jiě Xī (ST 41) cure white screens in the eyes (see the section on blurred vision in *Míng Xià*).

Shuǐ Gōu 水溝 (Dū 26) governs strabismus.

Shàng Guān 上關 (GB 3) (see the section on clear-eye blindness) and Piān Lì 偏歷 (LI 6) govern painful eyes with blurred vision.

予游學會稽，絕早觀書，辰牌方食，久之患目澀。倦游而歸，同舍遺以鹽精，數次揩目而疾除。鹽精且爾，則青鹽之能治目固也。古方蓋用青鹽揩牙，因掬在手洗目而目明云（鹽精乃鹽倉地下之精英）。

I traveled to study in Kuài Jī 會稽; [while there] I read books as early in the day as possible and ate in the *chén* 辰 double-hour [7-9 am]. After a long time, I had dry eyes. I came back [each day] when I was tired of studying. My roommate left some salt essence which I used to rub the eyes frequently and the disease disappeared. Salt essence can do it; green salt [lake salt] can also certainly treat the

13. Wind eye is caused by wind heat. The symptoms include itchy eyes, erosion of the canthus, and tearing eyes. All the symptoms get worse when exposed to wind.

目不明 579
翳 584
目痛 568
傷寒無 690

eyes. An ancient method is to use green salt to rub the teeth, then hold it in the hands to wash the eyes and brighten the vision (Salt essence is the essence under a salt warehouse).

## 6.11

## *Mù Chì (Mù Huáng, Mù Qīng)*

## 目赤 (目黃 目青)

### Red eyes

**(Yellow eyes, green eyes)**

懸厘治目兌眥赤痛(《銅》)。攢竹治眼赤痛(見目不明)。風池治目內眥赤痛，氣發耳塞，目不明。崑崙、太淵，陽溪治目赤(見翳)。俠溪治目外眥赤，目眩。液門治目赤澀。《千》云：主目澀暴變。內關治目赤支滿。目窗(見目痛)、大陵治目赤(見傷寒無汗)。

Xuán Lí 懸厘 (GB 6) treats red painful canthii (*Tóng*《銅》).

Zǎn Zhú 攢竹 (UB 2) treats red painful eyes (see the section on blurred vision).

Fēng Chí 風池 (GB 20) treats red painful inner canthus, plugged ears due to qì effusion, and blurred vision.

Kūn Lún 崑崙 (UB 60), Tài Yuān 太淵 (LU 9), and Yáng Xī 陽溪 (LI 5) treat red eyes (see the section on [eye] screens).

Xiá Xī 俠溪 (GB 43) treats redness in the outer canthus, and dizzy vision.

Yè Mén 液門 (SJ 2) treats red dry eyes. *Qiān*《千》says: It governs dry eyes with sudden changes.

Nèi Guān 內關 (PC 6) treats red eyes and propping fullness.

Mù Chuāng 目窗 (GB 16) (see the section on eye pain) and Dà Líng 大陵 (PC 7) treat red eyes (see the section on cold damage with absence of sweating).

上星、肝俞主內眥赤痛癢(《千》)。支溝主女人脊急目赤。申脈(見目痛)、太衝等、曲泉、陽溪(並見目痛)主赤痛腫。束骨(《千》同)、京

淚 573
翳 584
目痛 568
腹脹 449

骨治內眥赤爛（《銅》）。前關療風赤眼（《明》見目眩）。小兒二三歲，忽兩眼大小眥俱赤：灸手大指次指間後寸半口陷中，各三壯。

Shàng Xīng 上星 (Dū 23) and Gān Shù 肝俞 (UB 18) govern redness, pain, and itching of the inner canthus (*Qiān*《千》).

Zhī Gōu 支溝 (SJ 6) governs tension of the spine and red eyes in women.

Shēn Mài 申脈 (UB 62) (see the section on eye pain), Tài Chōng 太衝 (LV 3) and so forth, Qū Quán 曲泉 (LV 8), and Yáng Xī 陽溪 (LI 5) (for all, see the section on eye pain) govern red painful swollen eyes.

Shù Gǔ 束骨 (UB 65) (*Qiān* agrees) and Jīng Gǔ 京骨 (UB 64) treat redness and erosion on the inner canthus (*Tóng*《銅》).

Qián Guān 前關 (GB 1) cures wind redness of the eyes (see the section on dizzy vision in *Míng*《明》).

Two or three year old children with sudden onset of redness in both canthii of the eyes: Apply three cones of moxibustion each in the depression a half cùn proximal to the space between the thumb and index finger.

目赤痛從目眥始：取陰蹻（《千》）。睛明（見淚）、後溪、目窗（目痛）、瞳子髎（見翳）主目赤。肝勞邪氣眼赤：當陽百壯。風癢赤：灸人中（見目痛）。腦戶、膽俞、意舍、陽綱（並見腹脹）治目黃（《銅》）。中管、大陵主目黃振寒（《千》）。勞宮（《銅》同）主黃膽目黃。青靈治目黃。期門治目青而嘔（《千》同）。太泉主目中白睛青（《千》）。

Red painful eyes starting from the corner of the eyes: treat Yīn Qiāo 陰蹻 (KI 6 or KI 8) (*Qiān*).

Jīng Míng 睛明 (UB 1) (see the section on tearing [eyes]), Hòu Xī 後溪 (SI 3), Mù Chuāng 目窗 (GB 16) (see the section on eye pain), and Tóng Zǐ Liáo 瞳子髎 (GB 1) (see the section on [eye] screens) govern red eyes.

Red eyes due to liver taxation and evil qì: Apply a hundred cones of moxibustion on Dāng Yáng 當陽 [see the footnote above].

Red itching [eyes] due to wind: Apply moxibustion on Rén Zhōng 人中 (Dū 26) (see the section on eye pain).

Nǎo Hù 腦戶 (Dū 17), Dǎn Shù 膽俞 (UB 19), Yì Shě 意舍 (UB 49), and Yáng Gāng 陽綱 (UB 48) (for all, see the section on abdominal fullness) treat yellowing of the eyes (*Tóng*).
Zhōng Guǎn 中管 (Rèn 12) and Dà Líng 大陵 (PC 7) govern yellowing of the eyes and quivering with cold (*Qiān*《千》).

Láo Gōng 勞宮 (PC 8) (*Tóng*《 銅 》agrees) governs jaundice and yellowing of the eyes.

Qīng Líng 青靈 (PC 2) treats yellowing of the eyes.

Qī Mén 期門 (LV 14) treats green eyes and vomiting (*Qiān*《 千 》agrees).

Tài Quán 太泉 (LU 9) governs blue whites of the eyes (*Qiān*).

## 6.12
## *Qīng Huāng (Què Mù, Gān Yǎn)*
# 青肓（雀目　疳眼）

## Clear-eye blindness
**(Sparrow eye, eye *gān*)**

商陽、巨髎、上關、承光、瞳子髎、絡卻主青肓無所見。期門、太泉主目青（見目痛）。絡卻治青風內障，目無所見（《銅》）。巨髎治青肓目無見，遠視䀮䀮，白翳覆瞳子。瞳子髎治青肓目無見，遠視䀮䀮，目中翳膜，頭痛，目外眥赤痛。

Shāng Yáng 商陽 (LI 1), Jù Liáo 巨髎 (ST 3), Shàng Guān 上關 (GB 3), Chéng Guāng 承光 (UB 6), Tóng Zǐ Liáo 瞳子髎 (GB 1), and Luò Què 絡卻 (UB 8) govern clear-eye blindness.

Qī Mén (LV 14) and Tài Quán (LU 9) govern green eyes (see the section on eye pain).

Luò Què 絡卻 (UB 8) treats green-blue wind with internal obstruction and blindness (*Tóng*).

Jù Liáo (ST 3) treats clear-eye blindness, inability to see, seeing dimly afar, and white screens covering the pupils.

Tóng Zǐ Liáo (GB 1) treats clear-eye blindness, seeing dimly afar, screens in the eyes, headaches, and red painful outer canthus.

商陽治青肓，右取左，左取右（見頷腫）。小兒目澀怕明，狀如青肓：灸中渚各一壯（《明》）。小兒疳眼：合谷各一壯。睛明治疳眼（《銅》）。睛明治小兒雀目疳眼。《明》云：療眼暗，雀目冷淚。肝俞主熱病瘥後食五辛，多患眼暗如雀目（《千》）。小兒雀目，夜不見物：灸手大指甲後一寸內廉橫文頭白肉際，各一壯。（《單方》云：雀腦血點效）。

Shāng Yáng 商陽 (LI 1) treats clear-eye blindness. Treat the left side when the disease is on the right or treat the right side when the disease in on the left (see the section on swelling [in the lower cheeks and] under the chin).

Dry eyes in children with aversion to light appearing like clear-eye blindness: Apply one cone of moxibustion on Zhōng Zhǔ 中渚 (SJ 3) (*Míng*《 明 》).

Eye *gān* 疳[14] in children: Apply one cone of moxibustion on Hé Gǔ 合谷 (LI 4).

Jīng Míng 睛明 (UB 1) treats eye *gān* (*Tóng*《 銅 》).

Jīng Míng 睛明 (UB 1) treats sparrow eye and eye *gān* in children. *Míng* says: It cures blurred vision and sparrow eyes with cold tears.

Gān Shù 肝俞 (UB 18) governs blurred vision like sparrow eyes that often arises when someone eats the five acrid foods after recovering from heat disease (*Qiān*《 千 》).

Sparrow eyes in children and night blindness: Apply one cone of moxibustion each on the border of white flesh at the inner end of the transverse crease, one cùn proximal to the thumb nail. (*Dān Fāng*《 單方 》(Single Formulas) says: Marking it with blood from the brain of a sparrow is effective).

14. Eye *gān* 疳 is caused by spleen deficiency with liver constraint, as well as steaming of damp-heat. The symptoms include dry eyes with aversion to light, screens in iris, dryness in sclera, sores in the eyes, thirst, diarrhea, and a swollen belly.

偏風 396

## 6.13
## *Kǒu Yǎn Wāi (Yú Jiàn Zhòng Fēng, Piān Fēng Bù Yǔ)*

# 口眼喎（餘見中風　偏風不語）

## Deviation of the mouth and eyes
**(for further discussion see the sections on wind stroke and hemilateral wind with loss of speech)**

承泣、四白、巨髎、上關、大迎(《銅》同)、顴骨、強間、風池、迎香、水溝主口喎僻不能言(《千》)。頰車、顴髎主口僻痛，惡風寒，不可嚼。水溝、齦交主口不能禁水漿，喎僻。風頭耳後痛，煩心，足不收，失履，口喎僻：完骨主之(《甲》)。

Chéng Qì 承泣 (ST 1), Sì Bái 四白 (ST 2), Jù Liáo 巨髎 (ST 3), Shàng Guān 上關 (GB 3), Dà Yíng 大迎 (ST 5) (*Tóng*《銅》agrees), Quán Gǔ 顴骨 (Cheek Bone, non-channel), Qiáng Jiān 強間 (Dū 18), Fēng Chí 風池 (GB 20), Yíng Xiāng 迎香 (LI 20), and Shuǐ Gōu 水溝 (Dū 26) govern deviation of the mouth and inability to speak (*Qiān*《千》).

Jiá Chē 頰車 (ST 6) and Quán Liáo 顴髎 (SI 18) govern deviation and pain of the mouth, aversion to cold, and inability to chew.

Shuǐ Gōu (Dū 26) and Yín Jiāo 齦交 (Dū 28) govern inability to hold water or liquid in the mouth due to deviation.

Wind in the head and pain behind the ears, vexation of the heart, loss of use of the feet, inability to walk, and deviation of the mouth: Wán Gǔ 完骨 (GB 12) can treat this (*Jiǎ*《甲》).

上關、下關治偏風(並見偏風)。承光治口喎，鼻多清涕，風眩頭痛(《銅》)。通天治口喎，鼻多清涕，衄血，頭重。列缺、完骨治口面喎(並見偏風)。翳風治口眼(《明下》作吻)喎斜，失欠脫頷，口噤不開，吃不能言，頰腫牙車痛。

Shàng Guān (GB 3) and Xià Guān 下關 (ST 7) treat hemilateral wind (for all, see the section on hemilateral wind).

Chéng Guāng 承光 (UB 6) treats deviation of the mouth, copious clear snivel, wind dizziness, and headache (*Tóng*《銅》).

眼瞤 571
心痛 312

Tōng Tiān 通天 (UB 7) treats deviation of the mouth, copious clear snivel, nosebleeds, and heaviness of the head.

Liè Quē 列缺 (LU 7) and Wán Gǔ 完骨 (GB 12) treat deviation of the mouth and face (see the section on hemilateral wind).

Yì Fēng 翳風 (SJ 17) treats deviation of the mouth and eyes (*Míng Xià*《 明下 》says lips), dislocated chin when yawning, clenched jaws, loss of speech, and swelling of the cheeks and jaws.

承漿治偏風口喎(《明下》同)。巨髎治瘛瘲口喎。顴髎治口喎眼瞤動(見眼瞤)。承泣治口眼喎斜，目瞤面葉葉動牽口眼，目視䀮䀮，冷淚眼眥赤痛(《明》同)。地倉治偏風口喎，目不得閉，失音不語，飲食不收，水漿漏落，眼瞤動不止，病左治右，右治左；艾如粗釵腳大。若大口轉喎，卻灸承漿七七壯愈。

Chéng Jiāng 承漿 (Rèn 24) treats hemilateral wind and deviation of the mouth (*Míng Xià* agrees).

Jù Liáo 巨髎 (ST 3) treats tugging and slackening and deviation of the mouth.

Quán Liáo 顴髎 (SI 18) treats deviation of the mouth and twitching eyelids (see the section on twitching of the eyelids).

Chéng Qì 承泣 (ST 1) treats deviation of the mouth and eyes, twitching eyelids and face with a pulling sensation of the mouth and eyes, blurred vision, cold tears, and red painful corners of the eyes (*Míng*《 明 》agrees).

Dì Cāng 地倉 (ST 4) treats hemilateral wind and deviation of the mouth, inability to close the eyes, loss of speech, inability to hold food with leakage of liquid [due to deviation of the mouth], and incessant twitching of the eyes. Treat the left side for the disease of the right; treat the right side for the disease of the left; burn cones the size of the leg of a thick hairpin.

Apply seven times seven cones of moxibustion on Chéng Jiāng 承漿 (Rèn 24) to cure deviation of the mouth.

行間治口喎，四肢逆冷，嗌乾煩渴，瞋不欲視，目淚出，太息。通谷治失欠口喎，食飲善嘔，暴啞不能言(《明下》同)。太淵治口僻(見心痛)。溫溜、偏歷、二間(《明下》云：口眼斜)、內庭治口喎。衝陽治偏風，口眼喎，胕腫，齒齲痛，發寒熱。

Xíng Jiān 行間 (LV 2) treats deviation of the mouth, cold limb reversal, dry throat, vexing thirst, staring but with no desire to see,[15] tearing eyes, and sighing.

15. This is due to facial paralysis; the eyes cannot close so it appears that the person is staring; but they are not consciously looking at anything.

鼻涕
616
偏風
396

Tōng Gǔ 通谷 (UB 66) treats yawning, deviation of the mouth, frequent retching when eating, and sudden loss of speech (*Míng Xià*《明下》agrees).

Tài Yuān 太淵 (LU 9) treats deviation of the mouth (see the section on heart pain).

Wēn Liū 溫溜 (LI 7), Piān Lì 偏歷 (LI 6), Èr Jiān 二間 (LI 2) (*Míng Xià* says: deviation of the mouth and eyes), and Nèi Tíng 內庭 (ST 44) treat deviation of the mouth.

Chōng Yáng 衝陽 (ST 42) treats hemilateral wind, deviation of the mouth and eyes, swollen elbows, pain from tooth decay, and [sensations of] cold and heat.

和髎（見鼻涕）療口噼（《明》）。列缺（《下》同）、地倉（見偏風）療口喎。巨窌療面風寒，鼻準上腫，癰痛，招搖視瞻，瘛瘲，口噼。地倉療偏風口喎，失音不言，不得飲水，食漏落，脈瞤動。

Hé Liáo 和髎 (LI 19) (see the section on sniveling) cures deviation of the mouth (*Míng*《明》).

Liè Quē 列缺 (LU 7) (*Xià*《下》agrees) and Dì Cāng 地倉 (ST 4) (see the section on hemilateral wind) cure deviation of the mouth.

Jù Liáo 巨窌 (ST 3) cures wind-cold in the face, swollen tip of the nose, pain due to welling-abscess, shaking of the head that affects vision, tugging and slackening, and deviation of the mouth.

Dì Cāng 地倉 (ST 4) cures hemilateral wind, deviation of the mouth leading to loss of speech and inability to drink water with leakage of food, and twitching vessels.

灸風中脈，口眼喎斜，其狀喎向右者，謂左邊脈中風而緩，宜灸左；喎左灸右，炷如麥粒，各二七壯，頻灸取盡風氣。聽會、頰車、地倉二穴。

Moxibustion for wind striking the vessels, with deviation of the eyes and mouth to the right, which is due to wind striking the vessels of the left side and inducing weakness: It is approriate to apply moxibustion on the left side. Apply moxibustion on the right side if the mouth and eyes deviate to the left. Burn cones the size of a grain of wheat. Frequently burn two times seven cones of moxibustion to remove all the wind qì. Apply moxibustion bilaterally on Tīng Huì 聽會 (GB 2), Jiá Chē 頰車 (ST 6), and Dì Cāng (ST 4).

口喎 591
瘛瘲 354
口噤 605
狂 345

## 6.14

## *Kǒu Yīn Yǎ (Shé Bù Néng Yán, Yú Jiàn Zhòng Fēng Shī Yīn)*

# 口喑啞（舌不能言　餘見中風失音）

## Loss of voice

**(Loss of speech; for further discussion, see the sections on wind stroke and loss of voice)**

合谷、水溝主喑（《千》見口噤）。承泣等（見口喎）、地倉（《明》同）、大迎、魚際、通里（見風痙）主不能言。腦戶等主喑不能言（見瘛瘲）。孔最、暗門療失音（《明》見下）。風府（《下》同）、承漿（《下》）療喑不能言。

Hé Gǔ 合谷 (LI 4) and Shuǐ Gōu 水溝 (Dū 26) govern loss of voice (see the section on clenched jaws in *Qiān*《千》).

Chéng Qì 承泣 (ST 1) and so forth (see the section on deviation of the mouth), Dì Cāng 地倉 (ST 4) (*Míng*《明》agrees), Dà Yíng 大迎 (ST 5), Yú Jì 魚際 (LU 10), and Tōng Lǐ 通里 (HT 5) (see the section on wind tetany) govern inability to speak.

Nǎo Hù 腦戶 (Dū 17) and so forth govern loss of voice (see the section on tugging and slackening).

Kǒng Zuì 孔最 (LU 6) and Yīn Mén 暗門 (Dū 15) cure loss of voice (*Míng*, see *Xià*《下》).

Fēng Fǔ 風府 (Dū 16) (*Xià* agrees) and Chéng Jiāng 承漿 (Rèn 24) (*Xià*) cure loss of voice.

翳風、通里療暴喑不能言（《下》）。聽宮（《明》同）治失聲（《銅》）。頰車治失音（見口噤）。陰郄治失音不能言。間使（見狂）、合谷主喑不能言（《千》見口噤）。天鼎治暴喑氣哽。《明下》云：暴喑咽腫，食不下，喉鳴（《銅》）。

Yì Fēng 翳風 (SJ 17) and Tōng Lǐ 通里 (HT 5) cure sudden loss of voice and inability to speak (*Xià*).

Tīng Gōng 聽宮 (SI 19) (*Míng*《明》agrees) treats loss of voice (*Tóng*《銅》).

Jiá Chē 頰車 (ST 6) treats loss of voice (see the section on clenched jaws).

心痛 312
頰腫 632
口噤 605
口喎 591
悲 331

Yīn Xī 陰郄 (HT 6) treats loss of voice and inability to speak.

Jiān Shǐ 間使 (PC 5) (see the section on mania) and Hé Gǔ 合谷 (LI 4) govern loss of voice and inability to speak (see the section on clenched jaws in *Qiān* 《千》).

Tiān Dǐng 天鼎 (LI 17) treats sudden loss of voice and qì choking. *Míng Xià* 《明下》 says: It treats sudden loss of voice, swollen throat, difficulty getting food down, and throat rales (*Tóng* 《銅》).

靈道（見心痛）、天突（《明下》）、天窗（《明下》同）治暴暗不能言，口噤（見頰腫）。支溝（見口噤）、通谷（見口喎）、三陽絡治暴啞（《明下》同）。頰車治牙關不開，口噤不語（《明下》同），失音，牙關痛，頷頰腫（《明》同）。

Líng Dào 靈道 (HT 4) (see the section on heart pain), Tiān Tū 天突 (Rèn 22) (*Míng Xià*), and Tiān Chuāng 天窗 (SI 16) (*Míng Xià* agrees) treat sudden loss of voice, inability to speak, and clenched jaws (see the section on swelling [and pain] around [lips] and cheek).

Zhī Gōu 支溝 (SJ 6) (see the section on clenched jaws), Tōng Gǔ 通谷 (UB 66) (see the section on deviation of the mouth), and Sān Yáng Luò 三陽絡 (SJ 8) treat sudden loss of voice (*Míng Xià* agrees).

Jiá Chē 頰車 (ST 6) treats clenched jaws with loss of speech (*Míng Xià* agrees), loss of voice, painful jaws, and swollen chin and cheeks (*Míng* 《明》 agrees).

日月治言語不正（見悲）。小兒五六歲不語者，心氣不足，舌本無力，發轉難：心俞三壯；或足兩踝各三壯（《千》）。廉泉（《明》同）、然谷（《甲乙》作通谷）、陰谷主舌下腫，難言，舌縱涎出（《千》）。風府主舌緩，瘖（《明下》同），不能言，舌急語難。

Rì Yuè 日月 (GB 24) treats abnormal speech (see the section on [anxiety and] sorrow [of the heart]).

5 or 6 year old children with loss of speech, insufficient heart qì, weak root of the tongue with difficulty moving it freely: Apply three cones of moxibustion on Xīn Shù 心俞 (UB 15); or on the inner and outer malleolus of the foot (*Qiān*).

Lián Quán 廉泉 (Rèn 23) (*Míng* agrees), Rán Gǔ 然谷 (KI 2) (*Jiǎ Yǐ* 《甲乙》 says Tōng Gǔ (UB 66)), and Yīn Gǔ 陰谷 (KI 10) govern swelling beneath the tongue, difficulty speaking, protracted tongue, and drooling (*Qiān*).

Fēng Fǔ 風府 (Dū 16) governs slack tongue, loss of voice (*Míng Xià*《明下》agrees), inability to speak, and hypertonicity of the tongue with difficulty speaking.

支溝、天窗、扶突、曲鬢、靈道主暴喑不能言。復溜主舌卷不能言。通里主不能言。魚際主痙上氣，失喑不能言。啞門治頸項強，舌緩不能言（《銅》）。《明》云：失音不能言，舌急。

Zhī Gōu 支溝 (SJ 6), Tiān Chuāng 天窗 (SI 16), Fú Tū 扶突 (LI 18), Qū Bìn 曲鬢 (GB 7), and Líng Dào 靈道 (HT 4) govern sudden loss of voice and inability to speak.

Fù Liū 復溜 (KI 7) governs curled tongue with inability to speak.

Tōng Lǐ 通里 (HT 5) governs inability to speak.

Yú Jì 魚際 (LU 10) governs tetany with qì ascent and loss of voice.

Yǎ Mén 啞門 (Dū 15) treats stiffness of the neck and nape, slack tongue with loss of speech (*Tóng*《銅》). *Míng*《明》says: It treats loss of voice with inability to speak and hypertonicity of the tongue.

啞門，一名舌橫，一名舌厭。督脈陽維之會，入繫舌本，則是穴也。其舌本所繫歟，凡舌緩不能言者，宜治此。

Yǎ Mén (Dū 15) is also named Shé Héng 舌橫, or Shé Yàn 舌厭. This point is where the Dū vessel and the yángwéi [mài] meet and connect to the root of the tongue. So if there is weakness of the tongue with inability to speak, it is appropriate to treat this point.

廉泉治舌下腫，難言，舌縱涎出，咳嗽上氣，喘息，嘔沫，口噤，舌根急縮，下食難（《銅》）。

Lián Quán 廉泉 (Rèn 23) treats swelling beneath the tongue, difficulty speaking, protracted tongue and drooling, cough with qì ascent, panting, vomiting foam, clenched jaws, acute contraction of the root of the tongue, and difficulty getting food down (*Tóng*).

廉泉，一名舌本，蓋舌之根本也。故能治舌下腫難言，舌縱涎出，舌根急縮諸病。與《千金方》所療略同。凡有此等疾者，宜針灸此。

Lián Quán (Rèn 23) is also named as Shé Běn 舌本; it is the root of the tongue. It can treat various disorders such as swelling beneath the tongue, protracted tongue and drooling, acute contraction of the root of the tongue, and so forth. This is similar to the treatment in the *Qiān Jīn Fāng*《千金方》. It is appropriate to needle or apply moxibustion on this point for the various disorders.

唾血 402

大迎治舌強不能言。翳風主不能言（《千》瘛瘲）。

Dà Yíng 大迎 (ST 5) treats stiffness of the tongue with inability to speak.

Yì Fēng 翳風 (SJ 17) governs loss of speech (see the section on tugging and slackening in *Qiān*《千》).

## 6.15
## *Shé Jiàng (Tǔ Shé, Zhòng Shé)*
# 舌強（吐舌 重舌）
## Stiffness of the tongue
**(Protrusion of the tongue; double tongue[16])**

中衝治舌強（《銅》見心痛）。陰谷治舌縱涎下，煩逆，溺難，小腹急，引陰痛，股內廉痛。天突治舌下急（見唾血）。然谷治舌縱（《千》作瘲）。解溪主口痛囓舌（《千》）。天突主俠舌縫脈青。魚際主舌上黃，身熱。

Zhōng Chōng 中衝 (PC 9) treats stiffness of the tongue (see heart pain in *Tóng*《銅》).

Yīn Gǔ 陰谷 (KI 10) treats protracted tongue and drooling, vexation and counterflow, difficulty urinating, tension of the smaller abdomen that induces pain of the genital area and on the medial aspect of the thigh.

Tiān Tū 天突 (Rèn 22) treats tension beneath the tongue (see the section on spitting of blood).

Rán Gǔ 然谷 (KI 2) treats protracted tongue (*Qiān* says slackening).

Jiě Xī 解溪 (ST 41) governs painful mouth and biting the tongue (*Qiān*).

Tiān Tū 天突 (Rèn 22) governs green vessels alongside the tongue seam (frenulum).

Yú Jì 魚際 (LU 10) governs yellow [coating] on the tongue and generalized heat.

16. Double tongue is the name of a disorder. Symptoms include: swelling beneath the tongue that is shaped like another tongue. It is caused by heat accumulation of the heart and spleen.

喉痹 629
不能言 392
風癇 366
狂 345
癲癇 357
驚 323
口啞 594

魚際治舌上黃(《銅》見寒熱)。竅陰治舌強(見喉痹)。廉泉治舌根急縮(見不能言)。陽谷療吐舌戾頸(《明》見狂言),小兒吐舌(並見風癇),治小兒舌強,嘲奶不得(《下》見口噤)。治小兒重舌:灸行間隨年壯,又灸兩足外踝上三壯。

Yú Jì 魚際 (LU 10) treats yellow [coating] on the tongue (see the section on [sensations of] cold and heat in *Tóng*《銅》).

Qiào Yīn 竅陰 (GB 44 or GB 11) treats stiffness of the tongue (see the section on throat *bì*-impediment).

Lián Quán 廉泉 (Rèn 23) treats acute contraction of the root of the tongue (see the section on loss of speech).

Yáng Gǔ 陽谷 (SI 5) cures protrusion of the tongue, perverse neck [torticollis or wryneck] (see the section on manic raving in *Míng*《明》), protrusion of the tongue in children (for all, see the section on wind epilepsy); it treats stiffness of the tongue in children and inability to suck breast milk (see the section on clenched jaws in *Xià*《下》).

To treat double tongue in children: Apply the same number of cones as the patient's age on Xíng Jiān 行間 (LV 2) or apply three cones of moxibustion on lateral malleolus.

滑肉門(見狂)、少海(癲癇)、溫溜療吐舌(見狂)。大迎治舌強(《銅》見啞)。築賓(見狂言)、太乙治吐舌(見癲狂)。關衝主舌卷(《千》見心煩)。陽溪等(見癲狂)、二間等(見驚)、飛揚等、溫溜等(並見癲狂)主吐舌。啞門主舌強。風府主舌急。陰谷主舌瘲。廉泉治舌縱,舌根急縮(並見口啞)。

Huá Ròu Mén 滑肉門 (ST 24) (see the section on mania), Shào Hǎi 少海 (HT 3) (see the section on withdrawal and epilepsy), and Wēn Liū 溫溜 (LI 7) cure protrusion of the tongue (see the section on mania).

Dà Yíng 大迎 (ST 5) treats stiffness of the tongue (see the section on muteness in *Tóng*).

Zhù Bīn 築賓 (KI 9) (see the section on manic raving) and Tài Yǐ 太乙 (ST 23) treat protrusion of the tongue (see the section on withdrawal and mania).

Guān Chōng 關衝 (SJ 1) governs curled tongue (see the section on vexation of the heart in *Qiān*《千》).

Yáng Xī 陽溪 (LI 5) and so forth (see the section on withdrawal and mania), Èr Jiān 二間 (LI 2) and so forth (see the section on fright), Fēi Yáng 飛揚 (UB 58), Wēn Liū 溫溜 (LI 7) (for all, see the section on withdrawal and mania) and so forth govern protrusion of the tongue.

口噤 605
心痛 312
腸鳴 263
風痙 373
咳逆 417

Yǎ Mén 啞門 (Dū 15) governs stiffness of the tongue.

Fēng Fǔ 風府 (Dū 16) governs hypertonicity of the tongue.

Yīn Gǔ 陰谷 (KI 10) governs slackening of the tongue.

Lián Quán 廉泉 (Rèn 23) treats protraction of the tongue and acute contraction of the root of the tongue (for all, see the section on muteness).

## 6.16

## *Kǒu Huǎn (Qiàn Shēn, Shī Qiàn)*

# 口緩（欠伸　失欠）

## Slack mouth

**(Yawning and stretching, yawning)**

地倉、大迎主口緩不收，不能言（《千》）。合谷、水溝主唇吻不收（見口噤）。失欠，頰車蹉：灸背第五椎，一日二七壯。滿三日未瘥：灸氣衝二百壯。胸前喉下甲骨中是，亦名氣堂，又灸三陰交百壯，三報之。

Dì Cāng 地倉 (ST 4) and Dà Yíng 大迎 (ST 5) govern slack mouth and loss of speech (*Qiān*《千》).

Hé Gǔ 合谷 (LI 4) and Shuǐ Gōu 水溝 (Dū 26) govern inability to contract the lips (see the section on clenched jaws).

After yawning the jaw cannot close: Apply two times seven cones of moxibustion daily on the fifth vertebra. If the disease is not cured in three days, apply two hundred cones of moxibustion on Qì Chōng 氣衝 (ST 30). [Or] the point below the throat in front of the chest on the cartilage is named Qì Táng 氣堂; a hundred cones of moxibustion can also be applied on Sān Yīn Jiāo 三陰交 (SP 6); give three sessions.

通里主數欠頻伸（見心痛）。下關、大迎、翳風主口失欠，下牙齒痛。內庭主喜頻伸數欠，惡聞人音（《銅》同）。漏谷主強欠（見腸鳴）。太淵治數欠不得息（見風痙）。經渠治數欠（見咳逆）。風池治目淚出，欠氣多。

口喎 591 口啞 594 風癇 366

Tōng Lǐ 通里 (HT 5) governs frequent yawning and stretching (see the section on heart pain).

Xià Guān 下關 (ST 7), Dà Yíng 大迎 (ST 5), and Yì Fēng 翳風 (SJ 17) govern yawning and pain of the lower teeth.

Nèi Tíng 内庭 (ST 44) governs frequent yawning and dislike for hearing people talk (*Tóng*《銅》agrees).

Lòu Gǔ 漏谷 (SP 7) governs belching (see the section on intestinal rumbling).

Tài Yuān 太淵 (LU 9) treats frequent yawning and inability to breathe (see the discussion of arched-back rigidity).

Jīng Qú 經渠 (LU 8) treats frequent yawning (see the section on coughing counterflow).

Fēng Chí 風池 (GB 20) treats tearing eyes and frequent yawning.

脾俞治黄疸喜欠，不嗜食(《千》同)。衝陽主傷寒病，振寒而欠。翳風(見口喎，《下》同)、通谷治失欠(見口喎)。風府主舌緩(《千》見口啞)。啞門治舌緩(見口啞)。崑崙主口閉。翳風主不能言(《千》並見瘈瘲)。小兒喜欠(風癇)：上關(見上關門)。

Pí Shù 脾俞 (UB 20) treats jaundice, frequent yawning, and no desire to eat (*Qiān*《千》agrees).

Chōng Yáng 衝陽 (ST 42) governs cold damage, quivering with cold, and yawning.

Yì Fēng (SJ 17) (see the section on deviation of the mouth; *Xià*《下》agrees) and Tōng Gǔ 通谷 (UB 66) treat yawning (see the section on deviation of the mouth).

Fēng Fǔ 風府 (Dū 16) governs slack tongue (see the section on muteness in *Qiān*).

Yǎ Mén 啞門 (Dū 15) treats slack tongue (see the section on muteness).

Kūn Lún 崑崙 (UB 60) governs clenched jaws.

Yì Fēng (SJ 17) governs loss of speech (*Qiān*; also see the section on tugging and slackening).

Frequent yawning in children (see the section on wind epilepsy): Shàng Guān 上關 (GB 3) (See the section on Shàng Guān (GB 3)).

有婦人臟燥悲泣數欠，《金匱》有大棗湯，謾合服愈（方見《本事》）。

A woman had visceral agitation with sorrow, crying, and frequent yawning; she slowly drank one *gě* of *Dà Zǎo Tāng* 大棗湯 (Jujube Decoction) from *Jīn Guì* 《金匱》(Golden Cabinet) and the disease was cured (for the formula, see *Běn Shì* 《本事》).

## 6.17
## *Chǐ Qǔ*
## 齒齲
## Tooth decay

角孫療齒牙不嚼物，齲痛腫(《明》)。耳門療齒齲。三間、陽谷、衝陽(見口喎)、內庭、厲兌、四瀆、液門、陽谷、上關(《下》同)治齒齲痛(《銅》)。少海治齒齲痛，又治齒寒，腦風頭痛。合谷、偏歷、三陽絡(《明下》云：療齒痛)、耳門治齒齲。

Jiǎo Sūn 角孫 (SJ 20) cures inability to chew with pain and swelling from tooth decay (*Míng* 《明》).

Ěr Mén 耳門 (SJ 21) cures tooth decay.

Sān Jiān 三間 (LI 3), Yáng Gǔ 陽谷 (SI 5), Chōng Yáng 衝陽 (ST 42) (see the section on deviation of the mouth), Nèi Tíng 內庭 (ST 44), Lì Duì 厲兌 (ST 45), Sì Dú 四瀆 (SJ 9), Yè Mén 液門 (SJ 2), Yáng Gǔ 陽谷 (SI 5), and Shàng Guān 上關 (GB 3) (*Xià* 《下》 agrees) treat pain from tooth decay (*Tóng* 《銅》).

Shào Hǎi 少海 (HT 3) treats pain from tooth decay, cold teeth, brain wind, and headaches.

Hé Gǔ 合谷 (LI 4), Piān Lì 偏歷 (LI 6), Sān Yáng Luò 三陽絡 (SJ 8) (*Míng Xià* 《明下》 says: They cure toothache), and Ěr Mén (SJ 21) treat tooth decay.

三間、大迎、正營治齒齲痛。完骨治齒齲(見癲疾)。兌端、目窗、正營、耳門治唇吻強，上齒齲痛(《千》)。厲兌、三間、衝陽、偏歷、小海、合谷、內庭、復溜主齲齒。曲鬢主齒齲。下關、大迎、翳風、完骨主牙齒齲痛。

Sān Jiān (LI 3), Dà Yíng 大迎 (ST 5), and Zhèng Yíng 正營 (GB 17) treat pain from tooth decay.

Wán Gǔ 完骨 (GB 12) treats tooth decay (see the section on withdrawal and epilepsy).

Duì Duān 兌端 (Dū 27), Mù Chuāng 目窗 (GB 16), Zhèng Yíng 正營 (GB 17), and Ěr Mén (SJ 21) treat stiff lips and pain from decay of the upper teeth (*Qiān*《 千 》).

Lì Duì 厲兌 (ST 45), Sān Jiān 三間 (LI 3), Chōng Yáng 衝陽 (ST 42), Piān Lì 偏歷 (LI 6), Xiǎo Hǎi 小海 (SI 8), Hé Gǔ 合谷 (LI 4), Nèi Tíng 內庭 (ST 44), and Fù Liū 復溜 (KI 7) govern tooth decay.

Qū Bìn 曲鬢 (GB 7) governs tooth decay.

Xià Guān 下關 (ST 7), Dà Yíng 大迎 (ST 5), Yì Fēng 翳風 (SJ 17), and Wán Gǔ 完骨 (GB 12) govern pain from tooth decay.

《傳》曰：唇亡齒寒，謂前齒非牙也。《說文》云：齲，齒蠹也，謂齒蠹而痛也。其不因齲蠹而痛者，謂齒囊也，蓋風寒入腦髓爾。《素問》謂大寒至骨髓，故頭痛齒亦痛。當以此治之。

*Zhuàn*《 傳 》says: 'dead lips and cold teeth.' This indicates the anterior teeth. *Shuō Wén*《 說文 》says: Tooth decay is [caused by] tooth worms and when there are tooth worms, there is pain. If the pain is not due to tooth worms, it is called tooth sacks, which are due to wind-cold entering the brain. *Sù Wèn*《 素問 》says: When severe cold enters the bone marrow, there are headaches and toothache. We should follow this theory when giving treatment.

# 6.18
## *Kǒu Shé Gān Kǔ (Rè Chòu)*
# 口舌乾苦（熱臭）
## Dry tongue and mouth with bitterness
**(Hot odor)**

心煩 335
喉痹 629
瘧 301
勞瘵 188
痃癖 433
腸鳴 263
腹脹 449

膽俞、商陽、小腸俞主口舌乾，食飲不下。勞宮、少澤、三間、太衝主口熱，口乾，口爛。太溪、少澤主咽乾，口熱，唾如膠。曲澤、章門主口乾。少陰主舌卷口乾。陽陵泉主口苦，嗌仲介介然。

Dǎn Shù 膽俞 (UB 19), Shāng Yáng 商陽 (LI 1), and Xiǎo Cháng Shù 小腸俞 (UB 27) govern dry tongue and mouth with difficulty getting food and drink down.

Láo Gōng 勞宮 (PC 8), Shào Zé 少澤 (SI 1), Sān Jiān 三間 (LI 3), and Tài Chōng 太衝 (LV 3) govern heat in the mouth, dry mouth, and erosion of the mouth.

Tài Xī 太溪 (KI 3) and Shào Zé (SI 1) govern dry throat, heat in the mouth, and glue-like spittle.

Qū Zé 曲澤 (PC 3) and Zhāng Mén 章門 (LV 13) govern dry mouth.

Shào Yīn 少陰 (HT 6) governs curled tongue and dry mouth.

Yáng Líng Quán 陽陵泉 (GB 34) govern bitter taste in the mouth and a scratchy feeling in the throat.

關衝（又見心煩）等主舌卷口乾（見喉痹）。曲澤治身熱煩渴口乾（《銅》）。三間（見瘧）、肺俞（見勞瘵）、不容（見痃癖）、章門（見腸鳴）、商陽（見瘧）、竅陰（見喉痹）、兌端治口乾（《銅》）。膽俞治口苦舌乾（見腹脹）。《明下》云：口舌乾，食不下。

Guān Chōng 關衝 (SJ 1) (also see the section on vexation of the heart) and so forth govern curled tongue and dry mouth (see the section on throat *bi*-impediment).

Qū Zé (PC 3) treats generalized heat, vexation, thirst, and dry mouth (*Tóng*《銅》).

脊 555
淋 222
喉痹 629
飧泄 246
傷寒 661
唾血 402
口疳 605

Sān Jiān 三間 (LI 3) (see the section on malaria), Fèi Shù 肺俞 (UB 13) (see the section on consumption), Bù Róng 不容 (ST 19) (see the section on strings and aggregations), Zhāng Mén 章門 (LV 13) (see the section on intestinal rumbling), Shāng Yáng 商陽 (LI 1) (see the section on malaria), Qiào Yīn 竅陰 (GB 11 or GB 44) (see the section on throat *bì*-impediment), and Duì Duān 兌端 (Dū 27) treat dry mouth (*Tóng*《銅》).

Dǎn Shù 膽俞 (UB 19) treats bitter taste in the mouth and dry tongue (see the section on abdominal fullness). *Míng Xià*《明下》says: It treats dry tongue and mouth and difficulty getting food down.

復溜（見脊）、大鐘（見淋）、尺澤治舌乾（見喉痹）。下廉治唇乾，涎出不覺（見飧泄）。少衝（見傷寒）、大鐘（見淋）治口中熱。肝俞、曲澤（見唾血）、少澤療口乾（《明》）。曲澤療口乾（見傷寒）。

Fù Liū 復溜 (KI 7) (see the section on [pain of the lower back and] spine), Dà Zhōng 大鐘 (KI 4) (see the section on dribbling), and Chǐ Zé 尺澤 (LU 5) treat dry tongue (see the section on throat *bì*-impediment).

Xià Lián 下廉 (LI 8 or ST 39) treats dry lips and uncontrollable drooling (see the section on swill diarrhea).

Shào Chōng 少衝 (HT 9) (see the section on cold damage) and Dà Zhōng 大鐘 (KI 4) (see the section on dribbling) treat heat in the mouth.

Gān Shù 肝俞 (UB 18), Qū Zé 曲澤 (PC 3) (see the section on spitting of blood), and Shào Zé 少澤 (SI 1) cure dry mouth (*Míng*《明》).

Qū Zé 曲澤 (PC 3) cures dry mouth (see the section on cold damage).

勞宮治大小人口中腥臭，胸脅支滿（《銅》）。《千》云：主老小口中腫腥臭。《明下》云：療小兒齦爛臭（見口疳）。少衝治口熱咽酸（見傷寒）。

Láo Gōng 勞宮 (PC 8) treats fishy-smelling mouth in children and adults and propping fullness of the chest and rib-sides (*Tóng*); *Qiān*《千》says: It governs swelling, fishy-smelling mouth in young and old; *Míng Xià* says: It cures erosion and fishy-smelling gums in children (see the section on *gān* of the mouth).

Shào Chōng (HT 9) treats heat in the mouth and a sour taste in the throat (see the section on cold damage).

## 6.19
## *Kǒu Chǐ Gān Chuāng (Yá Yín Zhǒng, Yá Guān Jí)*

# 口齒疳瘡（牙齦腫　牙關急）

### *Gān* sores of the mouth and teeth
**(Swollen gums, clenched jaws)**

承漿治口齒疳蝕生瘡（《銅》）。承漿療口中生瘡（《明》）。小兒口有瘡蝕，齦爛臭穢衝人：灸勞宮各一壯（《下》）。天衝治牙齦腫（《銅》）。角孫治齒齦腫，小兒疳濕瘡（見瘡）。

Chéng Jiāng 承漿 (Rèn 24) treats *gān* erosion and sores in the mouth and teeth (*Tóng*《銅》).

Chéng Jiāng (Rèn 24) cures sores in the mouth (*Míng*《明》).

Eroding sores in the mouth of children, erosion of the gums, foul breath assaulting people: Apply one cone of moxibustion on Láo Gōng 勞宮 (PC 8) (*Xià*《下》).

Tiān Chōng 天衝 (GB 9) treats gum swelling (*Tóng*).

Jiǎo Sūn 角孫 (SJ 20) treats gum swelling, *gān*, and damp sores in children (see the discussion of sores).

《史記》：齊大夫病齲齒，太倉公灸其左太陽明脈。即為苦參湯，日漱三升，出入五六日，病已。得之風，及臥開口，食而不漱。餘見"齒齲。"

*Shǐ Jì*《史記》says: A senior official of Qí suffered tooth decay. Master Tài Cāng applied moxibustion on the tàiyáng and yángmíng vessels[17] on the left side. He made *Kǔ Shēn Tāng* 苦參湯 (Flavescent Sophora Decoction), [asked him to] drink three *shēng* each day for five or six days, and the disease was cured. This disease is caused by wind, or opening the mouth while sleeping, or not rinsing the mouth after eating. For further discussion, see tooth decay.

17. One character (yáng 陽) appears to be missing here.

中風 379
口喎 591
偏風 396
癲疾 360
牙疼 609
口噤 605

完骨主牙車急（中風）。翳風治牙車痛（見口喎）。下關治牙車脫（見偏風）。水溝（見癲疾）、上關（見牙疼）、頰車（見口噤）治牙關不開（《銅》）。和髎治牙車引急，頭重痛，耳中嘈嘈，頷頰腫。聽會治牙車脫臼，相離三寸。《明》云：牙車急痛，不得嚼食（餘見中風偏風）。

Wán Gǔ 完骨 (GB 12) governs tension of the jaws (see the section on wind stroke).

Yì Fēng 翳風 (SJ 17) treats painful jaws (see the section on deviation of the mouth).

Xià Guān 下關 (ST 7) treats dislocation of the jaws (see the section on hemilateral wind).

Shuǐ Gōu 水溝 (Dū 26) (see the section on withdrawal and epilepsy), Shàng Guān 上關（ GB 3) (see the section on toothache), and Jiá Chē 頰車 (ST 6) (see the section on clenched jaws) treat clenched jaws (*Tóng*《銅》).

Hé Liáo 和髎 (SJ 22 or LI 19) treats tension of the jaws, painful heavy head, noisy sounds in the ears, and swollen chin and cheeks.

Tīng Huì 聽會 (GB 2) treats dislocation of the jaws, separating by 3 cùn. *Míng*《明》says: It treats acute pain of the jaws and inability to chew (for further discussion, see the section on wind stroke and hemilateral wind).

# 6.20

## *Chǐ Jìn (Kǒu Jìn, Yú Jiàn Zhòng Fēng)*

# 齒噤（口噤　餘見中風）

## Clenched jaws

**(Clenched jaws; for further discussion, see the section of wind stroke)**

頰頷 632
頰腫 632
口喎 591
舌腫 597
唇頰 632
偏風 396
口啞 594
風痙 373

天容、廉泉、魄戶、氣舍、扶突主咳逆，上氣喘息，嘔沫，齒噤（《千》）。然谷治初生兒臍風口噤，痿厥洞泄（《銅》）。曲鬢（《明下》見頸項）治口噤不能言（見頰頷）。天窗（見頰腫）、翳風治口噤（見口喎）。廉泉治口噤，舌根縮（見舌腫）。

Tiān Róng 天容 (SI 17), Lián Quán 廉泉 (Rèn 23), Pò Hù 魄戶 (UB 42), Qì Shě 氣舍 (ST 11), and Fú Tū 扶突 (LI 18) govern coughing counterflow, qì ascent and panting, vomiting of foam, and clenched jaws (*Qiān* 《千》).

Rán Gǔ 然谷 (KI 2) treats umbilical wind with clenched jaws in newborns, wilting reversal, and throughflux diarrhea (*Tóng* 《銅》).

Qū Bìn 曲鬢 (GB 7) (see the section on [stiffness of] the neck and nape in *Míng Xià* 《明下》) treats clenched jaws with loss of speech (see the discussion of the cheeks and under the chin).

Tiān Chuāng 天窗 (SI 16) (see the section on swelling [and pain around lips and] cheeks) and Yì Fēng 翳風 (SJ 17) treat clenched jaws (see the section on deviation of the mouth).

Lián Quán 廉泉 (Rèn 23) treats clenched jaws and contraction of the root of the tongue (see the discussion of swollen tongue).

合谷（見唇頰）、列缺（見偏風）、頰車（見口啞）、禾髎治口噤不開。大迎治風痙口噤（見風痙）。支溝治口噤不開，暴啞不能言。外關、內庭、三里、商丘、大泉主僻噤（《甲》云：口僻刺太泉，引而下之）。齦交、上關、大迎、翳風主口噤不開，引鼻中。

Hé Gǔ 合谷 (LI 4) (see the discussion of lips and cheeks), Liè Quē 列缺 (LU 7) (see the section on hemilateral wind), Jiá Chē 頰車 (ST 6) (see the section on muteness), and Hé Liáo 禾髎 (LI 19) treat clenched jaws.

少氣
426

Dà Yíng 大迎 (ST 5) treats wind tetany and clenched jaws (see the section on wind tetany).

Zhī Gōu 支溝 (SJ 6) treats clenched jaws, sudden loss of speech.

Wài Guān 外關 (SJ 5), Nèi Tíng 內庭 (ST 44), Sān Lǐ 三里 (ST 36), Shāng Qiū 商丘 (SP 5), and Dà Quán 大泉 (KI 3) govern deviated clenched mouth (*Jiǎ*《甲》says: Needle Tài Quán 太泉 (KI 3) for deviation of the mouth, to bring [the evil qì] down and drain it).

Yín Jiāo 齦交 (Dū 28), Shàng Guān 上關 (GB 3), Dà Yíng (ST 5), and Yì Fēng 翳風 (SJ 17) govern clenched jaws with a pulling sensation in the nose.

合谷、水溝(《明下》同)主唇吻不收，喑不能言，口噤。商丘、曲鬢主口噤(並《千》)。承漿療面風口不開，口生瘡。《明下》云：療口噤。廉泉療齦噤(見少氣)。兌端療口噤鼓頷(《下》)。

Hé Gǔ 合谷 (LI 4) and Shuǐ Gōu 水溝 (Dū 26) (*Míng Xià*《明下》agrees) govern inability to contract the lips, loss of voice, and clenched jaws.

Shāng Qiū (SP 5) and Qū Bìn 曲鬢 (GB 7) govern clenched jaws (both in *Qiān*《千》).

Chéng Jiāng 承漿 (Rèn 24) cures facial wind, inability to open the mouth, and sores in the mouth. *Míng Xià* says: It cures clenched jaws.

Lián Quán 廉泉 (Rèn 23) cures clenched gums (see the section on qì shortage).

Duì Duān 兌端 (Dū 27) cures clenched jaws and chattering of the jaws (Xià《下》).[18]

翳風療口噤不開。禾髎療口不可開，及尸厥。小兒生二七日內著噤，不吮奶多啼者，是客風中於臍，循流至心脾二臟之經，使舌強唇痙，嘲奶不得。此疾新，施方藥，不望十全。大抵以去客風無過，灸承漿七壯，次灸頰車各二壯。

Yì Fēng 翳風 (SJ 17) cures clenched jaws.

Hé Liáo 禾髎 (LI 19) cures inability to open the mouth and deathlike reversal.

When a newborn baby, which is two times seven days old, suffers clenched jaws, inability to suck milk, and cries a lot, it is due to visiting wind striking the umbilicus. It then flows to the heart and spleen channels causing stiffness of the tongue, tetany of the lips, and inability to suck milk. This is a modern disease; we can treat it with herbs, but cannot expect it to be one hundred percent effective. Removing the visiting wind is not wrong; apply seven cones of moxibustion on Chéng Jiāng 承漿 (Rèn 23) and apply two cones of moxibustion on Jiá Chē 頰車 (ST 6).

18. Chattering jaws is due to coldness. In English we say chattering teeth.

# 6.21
## *Yá Téng*
## 牙疼
## Toothache

大迎、顴髎、聽會、曲池主齒痛惡寒(《千》)。浮白主牙齒痛，不能言。陽谷、正營主上牙齒痛。陽谷、液門、商陽、二間、四瀆主下牙齒痛。角孫、頰車主牙齒不能嚼(《明》同)。風齒疼痛：灸外踝上高骨前交脈二壯；又以線量手中指至掌後横文，折為四分，量横文後當臂中。灸二壯，愈。隨左右。

Dà Yíng 大迎 (ST 5), Quán Liáo 顴髎 (SI 18), Tīng Huì 聽會 (GB 2), and Qū Chí 曲池 (LI 11) govern toothache and aversion to cold (*Qiān*《千》).

Fú Bái 浮白 (GB 10) governs toothache and inability to speak.

Yáng Gǔ 陽谷 (SI 5) and Zhèng Yíng 正營 (GB 17) govern aching of the upper teeth.

Yáng Gǔ 陽谷 (SI 5), Yè Mén 液門 (SJ 2), Shāng Yáng 商陽 (LI 1), Èr Jiān 二間 (LI 2), and Sì Dú 四瀆 (SJ 9) govern aching of the lower teeth.

Jiǎo Sūn 角孫 (SJ 20) and Jiá Chē 頰車 (ST 6) govern inability to chew (*Míng*《明》agrees).

Pain due to wind teeth[19]: apply two cones of moxibustion on the site at the crossing vessel anterior to the high bone above the lateral malleolus;[20] or use string to measure the distance between [the tip of] the middle finger to the transverse crease proximal to the palms, fold the string into quarters, then use it to measure from the transverse crease up the arm. Apply two cones of moxibustion [on the site at the end of the string]. This will cure the disease. Follow left or right [based on the affected site].

有老婦人舊患牙疼，人教將兩手掌交叉，以中指頭盡處為穴。灸七壯，永不疼。恐是外關也。穴在手少陽去腕後二寸陷中。泉司梢子妻

19. Wind teeth is caused by wind attacking the teeth when there is vacuity in the yángmíng 陽明 channels. The symptoms include swollen gums and loose teeth.

20. This is probably in the vicinity of Jué Gǔ 絕骨 (GB 39) but the exact location is not clear.

風痙 373 頰頷 632 頰腫 632 咳逆 417

舊亦苦牙疼，人為灸手外踝穴近前些子，遂永不疼。但不知《千金》所謂外踝上者，指足外踝耶？手外踝耶？識者當辨之。

An old lady suffered from toothache. Someone asked her to cross her hands, then located the point at the tip of the middle finger. She applied seven cones of moxibustion on the point and the toothache never came back again. This might be Wài Guān 外關 (SJ 5). It is located in the depression two cùn proximal to the wrist, on the hand shàoyáng channel.

The wife of a boatman also suffered toothache, so someone applied moxibustion on the site slightly anterior to the styloid process of the ulna, and the pain was gone forever. However, when *Qiān Jīn*《千金》says 'above the lateral malleolus,'[21] I do not know if it means the lateral malleolus of the foot, or the styloid process of the ulna on hand. The knowledgeable should differentiate this.

翳風治牙車痛（《銅》見口喎）。大迎治牙疼，頰頷腫（見風痙）。曲鬢治頰頷腫，引牙車不得開（詳見頰頷）。正營治牙齒痛，唇吻急強，齒齲痛。陽溪、懸顱、手三里治齒痛（見頭）。商陽治齒痛惡寒（見頷腫）。

Yì Fēng 翳風 (SJ 17) treats painful jaws (see deviation of the mouth in *Tóng*《銅》).

Dà Yíng 大迎 (ST 5) treats toothache and swollen cheeks and jaw (see the section on wind tetany).

Qū Bìn 曲鬢 (GB 7) treats swollen cheeks and jaw causing inability to open the jaws (for the details, see the discussion of swelling [and pain around] the cheek and under the chin).

Zhèng Yíng 正營 (GB 17) treats toothache, acute stiffness of the lips, and pain from tooth decay.

Yáng Xī 陽溪 (LI 5), Xuán Lú 懸顱 (GB 5), and Shǒu Sān Lǐ 手三里 (LI 10) treat toothache (see the section on the headaches).

Shāng Yáng 商陽 (LI 1) treats toothache and aversion to cold (see the section on swelling under the chin).

兌端治齒齦痛。小海治寒熱齒齦腫，風眩，頸項痛。上關（《銅》同）療風牙疼，牙車不開，口噤，嚼物鳴（《明》）。厥陰俞療牙痛（見咳逆）。

Duì Duān 兌端 (Dū 27) treats painful gums.

Xiǎo Hǎi 小海 (SI 8) treats [sensations of] cold and heat, swollen gums, wind dizziness, and pain of the neck and nape.

21. *Wài huái* 外踝 can mean the lateral malleolus or the styloid process of the ulna. Without adding the word for hand or foot, it is hard to tell which is meant.

Shàng Guān 上關 (GB 3) (*Tóng*《 銅 》agrees) cures pain from wind teeth, inability to open the jaws, clenched jaws, and sounds [from the jaws] when chewing food (*Míng*《 明 》).

Jué Yīn Shù 厥陰俞 (UB 14) cures toothache (see the section on coughing counterflow).

《良方》灸牙疼法：隨左右所患肩尖，微近後骨縫中，小舉臂取之，當骨解陷中，灸五壯。予親灸數人皆愈。灸畢，項大痛，良久乃定，永不發。

*Liáng Fāng*《 良方 》has a moxibustion treatment for toothache: Use the same side as the affected site. Lift the arm a little, and locate the point slightly posterior to the tip of the shoulder in the seam of the joint, in the depression between the bones. Apply five cones of moxibustion.

I applied moxibustion on several people here, and they were all cured. After the moxibusiton is complete, there will be neck pain that will disappear after a long time. But the toothache will never come back.

予親病齒痛，百方治不驗，用此法瘥。

My relative suffered toothache, and was not cured even after treatment with a hundred formulas. It was cured after using this method.

辛帥舊患傷寒，方愈，食青梅，既而牙疼甚。有道人為之灸，屈手大指本節後陷中，灸三壯。初灸覺病牙癢，再灸覺牙有聲，三壯痛止。今二十年矣。恐陽溪穴也（《銅》云：治齒痛，手陽明脈入齒縫中。左痛灸右，右痛灸左）。

Commander Xīn suffered cold damage. He ate green plums right after the disease was cured, and then he had a toothache. A Daoist applied three cones of moxibustion on the depression proximal to the base joint of the thumb when flexing the finger. After the first moxibustion session, his teeth itched. In the next moxibustion session, he perceived a sound in his teeth. The toothache stopped after three cones. It has been twenty years since then. This might be Yáng Xī 陽溪 (LI 5) (*Tóng* says: It treats toothache, because the hand yángmíng channel enters the teeth. Apply moxibustion on right side when the pain is on the left; apply moxibustion on the left side when the pain is on the right).

鼻衄 620
息肉 614
目痛 568
風癇 366
鼻涕 616
風眩 375
頭重 653

## 6.22
## *Bí Sāi Bù Lì (Bù Wén Xiāng Chòu)*
# 鼻塞不利（不聞香臭）

### Nasal congestion
**(Loss of sense of smell)**

曲差、上星、迎香、素髎、水溝、齦交、通天、禾髎、風府主鼻塞，喘息不利，鼻涕，鼽衄有瘡。承靈等主鼻窒，喘息不通（見鼻衄）。厲兌、京骨、前谷主鼻不利涕黃。齦交主息肉不利（見息肉）。天柱主不知香臭。

Qū Chā 曲差 (UB 4), Shàng Xīng 上星 (Dū 23), Yíng Xiāng 迎香 (LI 20), Sù Liáo 素髎 (Dū 25), Shuǐ Gōu 水溝 (Dū 26), Yín Jiāo 齦交 (Dū 28), Tōng Tiān 通天 (UB 7), Hé Liáo 禾髎 (LI 19), and Fēng Fǔ 風府 (Dū 16) govern nasal congestion, inability to breathe, runny nose, sniveling, and nosebleeds, as well as nasal sores.

Chéng Líng 承靈 (GB 18) and so forth govern nasal congestion and difficulty breathing (see the section on nosebleeds).

Lì Duì 厲兌 (ST 45), Jīng Gǔ 京骨 (UB 64), and Qián Gǔ 前谷 (SI 2) govern blockage of the nose with yellow snivel.

Yín Jiāo (Dū 28) governs polyps inhibiting [the nasal passages] (see the discussion of polyps).

Tiān Zhù 天柱 (UB 10) governs loss of sense of smell.

中管主鼻間焦臭。眉衝療頭痛鼻塞（《明》）。玉枕（見目痛）、百會（見風癇）、明堂（見鼻涕）、當陽、臨泣（見風眩）療鼻塞。迎香療鼻息不聞香臭。風府療鼻不得息。天牖療鼻塞不聞香臭（《下》）。至陰（見頭重）治鼻塞。

Zhōng Guǎn 中管 (Rèn 12) governs smelling a burnt odor.

Méi Chōng 眉衝 (UB 3) cures headaches and nasal congestion (*Míng*《明》).

Yù Zhěn 玉枕 (UB 9) (see the section on eye pain), Bǎi Huì 百會 (Dū 20) (see the section on wind epilepsy), Míng Táng 明堂 (see the section on sniveling), Dāng Yáng 當陽 (non-channel), and Lín Qì 臨泣 (GB 15 or GB 41) (see the section on wind dizziness) cure nasal congestion.

Yíng Xiāng 迎香 (LI 20) cures loss of sense of smell when breathing.

Fēng Fǔ 風府 (Dū 16) cures inability to breathe.

Tiān Yǒu 天牖 (SJ 16) cures nasal congestion and loss of sense of smell (*Xià*《下》).

Zhì Yīn 至陰 (UB 67) (see the section on heaviness of the head) treats nasal congestion.

上星（《明下》同）、百會、囟會（《明》同）、承光治鼻塞不聞香臭。若是鼻塞：灸囟會，日七壯，至四日漸退，五日頓愈（《銅》）。臨泣（見風眩，《明》同）、通天治鼻塞悶。步郎治鼻塞不通（《明》同）。臨泣治目眩鼻塞。前谷、齦交治鼻塞不利。承靈治鼽衄息不利。素髎治鼻塞息肉不消，多涕生瘡（《千》）。

Shàng Xīng 上星 (Dū 23) (*Míng Xià*《明下》agrees), Bǎi Huì 百會 (Dū 20), Xìn Huì 囟會 (Dū 22) (*Míng*《明》agrees), and Chéng Guāng 承光 (UB 6) treat nasal congestion and loss of sense of smell.

For nasal congestion: Apply seven cones of moxibustion daily on Xìn Huì (Dū 22). The congestion will gradually be relieved over the next four days, and will be cured in five days (*Tóng*《銅》).

Lín Qì 臨泣 (GB 15 or GB 41) (see wind dizziness; *Míng* agrees) and Tōng Tiān 通天 (UB 7) treat nasal congestion with stuffiness.

Bù Láng 步郎 (KI 22) treats nasal blockage (*Míng* agrees).

Lín Qì 臨泣 (GB 15 or GB 41) treats dizzy vision and nasal congestion.

Qián Gǔ 前谷 (SI 2) and Yín Jiāo 齦交 (Dū 28) treat inhibited nasal orifices.

Chéng Líng 承靈 (GB 18) treats sniveling and nosebleeds, as well as difficulty breathing.

Sù Liáo 素髎 (Dū 25) treats nasal congestion, polyps that do not disperse, profuse snivel, and sores (*Qiān*《千》).

按《銅人》云：素髎穴諸方闕治療法，《千金》治鼻塞息肉不消，多涕生瘡。而今之《千金》只云：主鼻喎僻多涕，鼽衄有瘡。又云：主鼻窒喘息不利。與此文稍異，豈古今本不同耶。

The treatment method for Sù Liáo (Dū 25) according to *Tóng Rén*《銅人》: "*Qiān Jīn*《千金》says it treats nasal congestion, polyps that do not disperse, profuse snivel, and sores." But today *Qiān Jīn* only says: "It governs deviation of the nose, profuse snivel, runny nose, nosebleeds, and sores." It also says: "It treats nasal congestion and difficulty breathing." There is a little discrepancy between these passages; it may be due to a different version of the text in ancient times and nowadays.

厲兌治惡風鼻不利 。水溝等主不知香臭(《千》見鼻涕 )。

Lì Duì 厲兌 (ST 45) treats aversion to wind and blockage of the nose.

Shuĭ Gōu 水溝 (Dū 26) and so forth govern loss of sense of smell (see the section on sniveling in *Qiān*《千》).

## 6.23

## *Bí Yŏu Xī Ròu (Shēng Chuāng)*

# 鼻有息肉（生瘡）

## Polyps in the nose

**(Sores)**

齦交主鼻中息肉不利，鼻頭額頞中痛，鼻中有蝕瘡(《千》)。曲差等主鼽衄有瘡( 見鼻塞 )。腦空主癘鼻( 見鼻痛 )。鼻中息肉：灸上星二百壯，又灸俠上星兩傍，相去三寸，各百壯 。迎香治鼻有息肉，不聞香臭，衄血(《銅》)。

Yín Jiāo 齦交 (Dū 28) governs polyps in the nose that inhibit [breathing], pain of the tip and bridge of the nose, as well as the forehead, and sores eroding the nose (*Qiān*).

Qū Chā 曲差 (UB 4) and so forth govern sniveling and nosebleeds, as well as sores (see the section on nasal congestion).

Năo Kōng 腦空 (GB 19) governs leprosy of the nose (see the section on pain of the nose).

Polyps in the nose: Apply two hundred cones of moxibustion on Shàng Xīng 上星 (Dū 23) and a hundred cones of moxibustion on the sites three cùn lateral to Shàng Xīng (Dū 23).

Yíng Xiāng 迎香 (LI 20) treats polyps in the nose, loss of sense of smell, and nosebleeds (*Tóng*《銅》).

齦交治鼻中息肉，蝕瘡。素髎治息肉不消，多涕生瘡。禾髎（見鼻涕）療衄衄有瘡（《明》）。巨窌療鼻準上腫癰痛（見口喎）。

鼻涕 616
口喎 591

Yín Jiāo 齦交 (Dū 28) treats polyps in the nose and eroding sores.

Sù Liáo 素髎 (Dū 25) treats polyps that do not disperse, profuse snivel, and nasal sores.

Hé Liáo 禾髎 (LI 19) (see the section on sniveling) cures runny nose, nosebleeds, and nasal sores (*Míng*《明》).

Jù Liáo 巨窌 (ST 3) cures swelling of the tip of the nose and pain due to welling-abscesses (see the section on deviation of the mouth).

《單方歌》云：狗頭灰方寸，丁香半錢匕，細研吹鼻中，息肉化為水。

*Dān Fāng Gē*《單方歌》says: Grind a square-cùn size [spoonful][22] of *gǒu tóu huī* 狗頭灰 [an alternate name for *mǎ bó* 馬勃 (Lasiosphaera seu Calvatia)] and a half-qián size spoonful of *dīng xiāng* 丁香 (Caryophylli flos) into fine powder and blow it into the nose. The polyps will dissolve into water.

22. *Fāng cùn bǐ* 方寸匕 (square-inch sized spoon) is an ancient type of measuring spoon for herbs. Its bowl is one cùn by one cùn in dimension. The volume of a square-inch spoon is 2.74 milliliter of liquid, or about 1 gram of powdered herbs.

口喎
591
癇
354

# 6.24

## Bí Tì Chū (Bí Gān, Bí Tì)

# 鼻涕出（鼻乾　鼻嚏）

## Sniveling

**(Dry nose; sneezing)**

小兒多涕，是腦門被冷風拍著及肺寒也：灸囟會三壯（《明》）。《明堂》：療頭風，多鼻涕，鼻塞。禾髎療鼻窒口喎僻，鼻多清涕出，不可止，鼽衄有瘡（《下》同）。崑崙療鼻衄多涕。風門療鼻衄不止，鼻垂清涕（《下》）

Frequent sniveling in children is caused by cold wind attacking the forehead and cold in the lungs: Apply three cones of moxibustion on Xìn Huì 囟會 (Dū 22) (*Míng*《明》). *Míng Táng*《明堂》says: It cures head wind, profuse snivel, and nasal congestion.

Hé Liáo 禾髎 (LI 19) cures nasal congestion, deviation of the mouth, frequent incessant runny nose with clear discharge, sniveling, nosebleeds, and sores (*Xià*《下》agrees).

Kūn Lún 崑崙 (UB 60) cures nosebleeds and frequent sniveling.

Fēng Mén 風門 (UB 12) cures incessant nosebleeds and runny nose with clear snivel (*Xià*).

禾髎治鼻洞涕，生瘡（《銅》）。風門治鼻鼽出清涕（見傷寒雜病）。通天、承光治口喎，鼻多清涕（並見口喎）。前頂治小兒鼻多清涕（見癇）。神庭治頭風目眩，鼻出清涕不止，目淚出。神庭、攢竹、迎香、風門、合谷、至陰、通谷主鼻鼽清涕出（《千》）。

Hé Liáo (LI 19) treats throughflux sniveling and nasal sores (*Tóng*《銅》).

Fēng Mén (UB 12) treats runny nose with clear snivel (see the section on cold damage and miscellaneous diseases).

Tōng Tiān 通天 (UB 7) and Chéng Guāng 承光 (UB 6) treat deviation of the mouth and copious clear snivel (for all, see the section on deviation of the mouth).

Qián Dǐng 前頂 (Dū 21) treats frequent runny nose with clear snivel in children (see the section on withdrawal and epilepsy).

Shén Tíng 神庭 (Dū 24) treats head wind, dizzy vision, incessant runny nose with clear snivel, and tearing eyes. 鼻塞 612

Shén Tíng (Dū 24), Zǎn Zhú 攢竹 (UB 2), Yíng Xiāng 迎香 (LI 20), Fēng Mén 風門 (UB 12), Hé Gǔ 合谷 (LI 4), Zhì Yīn 至陰 (UB 67), and Tōng Gǔ 通谷 (UB 66) govern runny nose with clear snivel (*Qiān*《千》). 上氣 420

曲差等主鼻喎僻多涕（見鼻塞）。復溜主涎出鼻痛。水溝、天牖主鼻不收涕，不知香臭。厲兌、京骨、前谷主涕黃（《千》見鼻塞）。鼻中乾，鼻衄等凡二十二病，皆灸絕骨五十壯（見上氣）。

Qū Chā 曲差 (UB 4) and so forth govern deviation of the nose and frequent sniveling (see the section on nasal congestion).

Fù Liū 復溜 (KI 7) governs drooling and pain of the nose.

Shuǐ Gōu 水溝 (Dū 26) and Tiān Yǒu 天牖 (SJ 16) govern sniveling and loss of sense of smell.

Lì Duì 厲兌 (ST 45), Jīng Gǔ 京骨 (UB 64), and Qián Gǔ 前谷 (SI 2) govern yellow snivel (see the section on nasal congestion).

For the 22 diseases, such as dry nose, nosebleeds, and so forth: Apply fifty cones of moxibustion on Jué Gǔ 絕骨 (GB 39) (see the section on qì ascent).

執中母氏久病鼻乾，有冷氣。問諸醫者，醫者亦不曉。但云病去自愈。即而病去，亦不愈也，後因灸絕骨而漸愈。執中亦嘗患此，偶絕骨微痛而著艾，鼻乾亦失去。初不知是灸絕骨之力，後閱《千金方》有此證，始知鼻乾之去因絕骨也。若鼻涕多：宜灸囟會、前頂。大人小兒之病，初無以異焉耳。

My mother was sick for a long time and suffered dry nose with cold qì. She asked various doctors, but they did not know why. They said the symptoms will disappear after the disease goes away, but it did not happen like that. The symptoms gradually got better after applying moxibustion on Jué Gǔ (GB 39).

I, Zhízhōng 執中, also suffered these symptoms. I felt slight pain at Jué Gǔ (GB 39) so I applied moxibustion on it, and the dryness of the nose was gone. Initially I did not know that applying moxibustion on Jué Gǔ (GB 39) was so powerful until I read the records in *Qiān Jīn Fāng*《千金方》; then I knew that dryness of the nose disappeared because of Jué Gǔ (GB 39).

Profuse snivel: Apply moxibustion on Xìn Huì 囟會 (Dū 22) and Qián Dǐng 前頂 (Dū 21). In the early stage of disease, there is no big difference between children and adults.

風門、五處主時時嚏不已(《千》)。頷厭療好嚏(《明》)。風門治多涕(《銅》見傷寒)。《本事方》許知可自停飲，食已必嚏，服棗膏丸愈(時暫嚏添衣項上愈)。

Fēng Mén 風門 (UB 12) and Wǔ Chù 五處 (UB 5) govern frequent sneezing (*Qiān*《千》).

Hàn Yàn 頷厭 (GB 4) cures frequent sneezing (*Míng*《明》).

Fēng Mén (UB 12) treats profuse snivel (see the section on cold damage in *Tóng*《銅》).

[*Pǔ Jì*] *Běn Shì Fāng*《本事方》says Xǔ Zhīkě[23] sneezed after eating and drinking. This was cured by taking *Zǎo Gāo Wán* 棗膏丸 [Jujube Paste Pill] (wearing more clothing on the nape cures occasional sneezing).

23. Xǔ Zhīkě 許知可 was the compiler of [*Pǔ Jì*] *Běn Shì Fāng*《本事方》.

# 6.25
## *Bí Tòng (Yú Jiàn Bí Chuāng)*
# 鼻痛（餘見鼻瘡）

息肉 614
口喎 591
鬼擊 343

### Pain of the nose
**(for further discussion, see nasal sores)**

腦空、竅陰主鼻管疽發為癘鼻（《千》）。復溜主涎出，鼻中痛。巨髎治面風寒，鼻頔上腫，壅痛（《銅》）。肝俞主鼻中酸（《千》）。齦交主額頞中痛（見息肉）。巨窌療鼻準上腫癰痛（見口喎）。鬼擊鼻出血：灸人中並水分、陰交（見鬼擊）。

Nǎo Kōng 腦空 (GB 19) and Qiào Yīn 竅陰 (GB 11 or GB 44) govern flat-abscesses in the nose that become leprosy of the nose (*Qiān*).

Fù Liū 復溜 (KI 7) governs drooling and pain of the nose.

Jù Liáo 巨髎 (ST 3) treats wind-cold in the face, swelling at the root of the nose, congestion, and pain (*Tóng*).

Gān Shù 肝俞 (UB 18) governs achiness of the nose (*Qiān*).

Yín Jiāo 齦交 (Dū 28) governs pain of the forehead and the bridge of the nose (see the section on polyps [in the nose]).

Jù Liáo 巨窌 (ST 3) cures swelling, welling-abscesses, and pain at the tip of the nose (see the section on deviation of the mouth).

Nosebleeds due to ghost strike: Apply moxibustion on Rén Zhōng 人中 (Dū 26), Shuǐ Fēn 水分 (Rèn 9) and Yīn Jiāo 陰交 (Rèn 7) (see the section on ghost strikes).

鼻塞
612

## 6.26
## *Bí Nǜ*
# 鼻衄
## Nosebleeds

神庭等主鼻鼽（《千》見鼻涕）。曲差等主鼽衄有瘡（見鼻塞）。承靈（《銅》同）、風池、風門、譩譆、後溪主鼻衄窒喘息不通。中管、三間、偏歷、厲兌、承筋（銅同）、京骨、崑崙、承山、飛揚、隱白主頭熱鼽衄。

Shén Tíng 神庭 (Dū 24) and so forth govern nosebleeds (see the section on sniveling in *Qiān*《千》).

Qū Chā 曲差 (UB 4) and so forth govern sniveling and nosebleeds, as well as nasal sores (see the section on nasal congestion).

Chéng Líng 承靈 (GB 18) (*Tóng*《銅》agrees), Fēng Chí 風池 (GB 20), Fēng Mén 風門 (UB 12), Yī Xī 譩譆 (UB 45), and Hòu Xī 後溪 (SI 3) govern nosebleeds, nasal congestion, and inability to breathe.

Zhōng Guǎn 中管 (Rèn 12), Sān Jiān 三間 (LI 3), Piān Lì 偏歷 (LI 6), Lì Duì 厲兌 (ST 45), Chéng Jīn 承筋 (UB 56) (*Tóng* agrees), Jīng Gǔ 京骨 (UB 64), Kūn Lún 崑崙 (UB 60), Chéng Shān 承山 (UB 57), Fēi Yáng 飛揚 (UB 58), and Yǐn Bái 隱白 (SP 1) govern heat in the head, sniveling, and nosebleeds.

京骨（《銅》同）、申脈主衄不止，淫濼。郄門主衄血嘔血。隱白、委中主衄血劇不止。涌泉主衄不止。水溝、天牖主鼻鼽不得息，及衄不止（《甲乙》）。天府治衄血不止，針四分（《銅》）。上髎、後溪、風府、啞門治諸陽熱氣盛，衄血不止。

Jīng Gǔ (UB 64) (*Tóng* agrees) and Shēn Mài 申脈 (UB 62) govern incessant nosebleeds and weakness.

Xī Mén 郄門 (PC 4) governs nosebleeds and vomiting of blood.

Yǐn Bái 隱白 (SP 1) and Wěi Zhōng 委中 (UB 40) govern severe incessant nosebleeds.

肩背痛 486
息肉 614
目眩 575
唾血 402
腹脹 211
涕出 616
口喎 591

Yǒng Quán 涌泉 (KI 1) governs incessant nosebleeds.

Shuǐ Gōu 水溝 (Dū 26) and Tiān Yǒu 天牖 (SJ 16) govern runny nose, inability to breathe, and incessant nosebleeds (*Jiǎ Yǐ*《甲乙》).

Tiān Fǔ 天府 (LU 3) treats incessant nosebleeds; needle 4 fēn deep (*Tóng*《銅》).

Shàng Liáo 上髎 (UB 31), Hòu Xī 後溪 (SI 3), Fēng Fǔ 風府 (Dū 16), and Yǎ Mén 啞門 (Dū 15) treat excessive heat qì in all the yáng [channels] and incessant nosebleeds.

通天治衄血頭重。禾髎、兌端、勞宮治衄血不止。曲泉、隱白、譩譆（見肩背痛）、陰郄、迎香治衄血（見息肉）。偏歷、合谷、二間（《明下》同）、崑崙、通谷（見目眩）治鼽衄。曲泉治衄血喘呼，小腹痛攻咽喉。

Tōng Tiān 通天 (UB 7) treats nosebleeds and heaviness of the head.

Hé Liáo 禾髎 (LI 19), Duì Duān 兌端 (Dū 27), and Láo Gōng 勞宮 (PC 8) treat incessant nosebleeds.

Qū Quán 曲泉 (LV 8), Yǐn Bái 隱白 (SP 1), Yī Xī 譩譆 (UB 45) (see the section on [aching] pain of the shoulder and back), Yīn Xī 陰郄 (HT 6), and Yíng Xiāng 迎香 (LI 20) treat nosebleeds (see the section on polyps [in the nose]).

Piān Lì 偏歷 (LI 6), Hé Gǔ 合谷 (LI 4), Èr Jiān 二間 (LI 2) (*Míng Xià*《明下》agrees), Kūn Lún 崑崙 (UB 60), and Tōng Gǔ 通谷 (UB 66) (see the section on dizzy vision) treat sniveling and nosebleeds.

Qū Quán (LV 8) treats nosebleeds, panting, and pain of the smaller abdomen that attacks the throat.

太溪（見唾血）、隱白（見腹脹）、風門（見涕出）、兌端、腦空療衄血不止。禾髎（見鼻涕）療鼽衄有瘡（《明》）。攢竹療鼽衄（《下》見頭風）。巨髎療鼻準上腫癰痛（見口喎）。

Tài Xī 太溪 (KI 3) (see the section on spitting of blood), Yǐn Bái (SP 1) (see the section on abdominal fullness), Fēng Mén 風門 (UB 12) (see the section on sniveling), Duì Duān (Dū 27), and Nǎo Kōng 腦空 (GB 19) cures incessant nosebleeds.

Hé Liáo 禾髎 (LI 19) (see the section on sniveling) cures sniveling and nosebleeds as well as nasal sores (*Míng*《明》).

Zǎn Zhú 攢竹 (UB 2) cures sniveling and nosebleeds (see the section on head wind in *Xià*《下》).

Jù Liáo 巨髎 (ST 3) cures swelling of the tip of the nose and pain due to welling-abscess (see the section on deviation of the mouth).

治口喎鼻出血不止，名腦衄：灸上星五十壯（《集效》）。徐德占教衄者急灸項後髮際兩筋間宛宛中三壯，立定。蓋血自此入腦注鼻中，常人以綿勒頸後，尚可止衄，此灸決效無疑（《良》）。腦衄：灸上星五十壯（《千》見唾血）。

Treatment for deviation of the mouth with incessant nosebleeds, which is called spontaneous bleeding of the brain: Apply fifty cones of moxibustion on Shàng Xīng 上星 (Dū 23) (*Jí Xiào*《集效》).

Xú Dézhàn taught that people with nosebleeds should quickly apply three cones of moxibustion in the depression between the two sinews of the nape, within the posterior hairline. It stops the bleeding right away. This might because blood enters the brain and pours into the nose from this site. People often tie the back of the neck with silk string, which can also stop the bleeding. This moxibustion is effective without a doubt (*Liáng*《良》).

Spontaneous bleeding of the brain: Apply fifty cones of moxibustion on Shàng Xīng (Dū 23) (see the section on spitting of blood in *Qiān*《千》).

執中母氏忽患鼻衄，急取藥服，凡平昔與人服有效者皆不效。因閱《集效方》（本出《千金》）云：口喎鼻出血不止，名腦衄，灸上星五十壯。尚疑頭上不宜多灸，只灸七壯而止，次日復作，再灸十四壯而愈。有人鼻常出膿血，予教灸囟會亦愈。則知囟會、上星皆治鼻衄云。

My mother suffered sudden nosebleeds and took herbs right away. But those herbs, which usually are effective on other people, were not effective for her. So I read *Jí Xiào Fāng*《集效方》(The version from *Qiān Jīn*《千金》) says: Deviation of the mouth and incessant nosebleeds is called spontaneous bleeding of the brain. Apply fifty cones of moxibustion on Shàng Xīng (Dū 23). I doubted that it is appropriate to use so much moxibustion on the head, so I only burned seven cones and [the nosebleed] stopped but came back the next day. I applied fourteen cones of moxibustion again and cured the disease. Someone else had pus and blood coming from the nose. I taught him to apply moxibustion on Xìn Huì 囟會 (Dū 22) and it was also effective. So I know both Xìn Huì (Dū 22) and Shàng Xīng (Dū 23) can be used to treat nosebleeds.

鼻衄等：灸絕骨（《千》見上氣）。前谷治衄血（《銅》見咳）。譩譆治溫瘧，肩背痛，目眩鼻衄，喘逆腹脹，肩髆內廉痛，不得俯仰。

Nosebleeds and so forth: Apply moxibustion on Jué Gǔ 絕骨 (GB 39) (see the section on qì ascent in *Qiān*《千》).

Qián Gǔ 前谷 (SI 2) treats nosebleeds (see the section on cough in *Tóng*《銅》).

Yī Xī 譩譆 (UB 45) treats warm malaria, pain of the shoulders and back, dizzy vision, nosebleeds, panting counterflow, abdominal distention, pain of the medial aspect of the shoulders and arms, and inability to bend forward and backward.

風門治鼻鼽（見傷寒）。衄時癢癢：便灸足大指節橫理三毛中十壯，劇者百壯。衄不止灸之，並治陰卵腫（《千》）；又灸風府一穴四壯，不止又灸；或灸涌泉各百壯。

Fēng Mén 風門 (UB 12) treats nasal congestion (see the section on cold damage).

Itching during nosebleeds: Apply ten cones of moxibustion in the three-hair region proximal to the transverse crease of the big toe; burn a hundred cones for severe cases or incessant bleeding. This also treats swollen testicles (*Qiān*). Or apply four cones of moxibustion on Fēng Fǔ 風府 (Dū 16); continue if the bleeding does not stop. Or apply a hundred cones of moxibustion on Yǒng Quán 涌泉 (KI 1).

腹脹
211
陰痿縮
198

## 6.27
## Yān Hóu Zhǒng Tòng (Shēng Chuāng)

# 咽喉腫痛（生瘡）

### Sore swollen throat
**(Sores)**

風府治咽喉痛（《銅》）。膽俞治咽痛，食不下（見腹脹）。風府（《明》同）、天窗、勞宮主喉嗌痛（《千》）。中渚、支溝、內庭（《千》云：咽中引痛）主嗌痛。涌泉、大鐘主咽中痛，不可內食。間使（《甲》作行間）主嗌中如扼（《銅》云如哽）。

Fēng Fǔ 風府 (Dū 16) treats sore throat (*Tóng*《銅》).

Dǎn Shù 膽俞 (UB 19) treats sore throat with difficulty getting food down (see the section on abdominal fullness).

Fēng Fǔ (Dū 16) (*Míng*《明》agrees), Tiān Chuāng 天窗 (SI 16), and Láo Gōng 勞宮 (PC 8) govern sore throat (*Qiān*《千》).

Zhōng Zhǔ 中渚 (SJ 3), Zhī Gōu 支溝 (SJ 6), and Nèi Tíng 內庭 (ST 44) (*Qiān* says: pain of the throat) govern sore throat.

Yǒng Quán 涌泉 (KI 1) and Dà Zhōng 大鐘 (KI 4) govern sore pharynx with inability to eat.

Jiān Shǐ 間使 (PC 5) (*Jiǎ*《甲》says: Xíng Jiān 行間 (LV 2)) governs a feeling in the throat as if being strangled (*Tóng* says: It feels like choking on something).

膝關治喉咽痛（《銅》見風痹）。天窗（《明下》同）治喉痛。水突主喉咽腫。前谷、照海、中封主嗌偏腫，不可咽（《千》）。中封等主喉腫（見陰痿縮）。然谷、太溪主嗌內腫，氣走咽喉，不能言。

Xī Guān 膝關 (LV 7) treats sore throat (see the section on wind *bì*-impediment in *Tóng*).

Tiān Chuāng (SI 16) (*Míng Xià*《明下》agrees) treats sore throat.

Shuǐ Tū 水突 (ST 10) governs swollen throat.

Qián Gǔ 前谷 (SI 2), Zhào Hǎi 照海 (KI 6), and Zhōng Fēng 中封 (LV 4) govern swollen throat with inability to swallow (*Qiān*《千》). 咳逆 417

Zhōng Fēng (LV 4) and so forth governs swollen throat (see the section on wilted and retracted genitals). 唾血 402

Rán Gǔ 然谷 (KI 2) and Tài Xī 太溪 (KI 3) govern swelling of the throat, qì running through the throat, and inability to speak.

喉腫，胸脅支滿：灸尺澤百壯。人迎治咽喉癰腫（見咳逆上氣）。太溪（見唾血）、中渚治咽腫。璇璣治喉痹咽腫，水漿不下。液門治咽外腫，寒厥臂痛，不能上下。然谷治咽內腫。水突、氣舍治咽腫（上氣）。天突治喉中生瘡不得下食（《銅》、《明》云：療喉中熱瘡）。璇璣療喉痹咽癰，水漿不下。

Swollen throat and propping fullness of the chest and rib-sides: Apply a hundred cones of moxibustion on Chǐ Zé 尺澤 (LU 5).

Rén Yíng 人迎 (ST 9) treats swollen welling-abscesses in the throat (see the section on coughing counterflow and qì ascent).

Tài Xī (KI 3) (see the section on spitting of blood) and Zhōng Zhǔ 中渚 (SJ 3) treat swollen throat.

Xuán Jī 璇璣 (Rèn 21) treats throat *bì*-impediment, swollen pharynx, and inability to get water down.

Yè Mén 液門 (SJ 2) treats swelling of the outer aspect of the throat, cold reversal, and arm pain with inability to move it up and down.

Rán Gǔ (KI 2) treats swelling of the throat.

Shuǐ Tū 水突 (ST 10) and Qì Shě 氣舍 (ST 11) treat swollen throat (see the section on qì ascent).

Tiān Tū 天突 (Rèn 22) treats sores in the throat and inability to eat (*Tóng*《銅》and *Míng*《明》say: It cures hot sores in the throat).

Xuán Jī 璇璣 (Rèn 21) cures throat *bì*-impediment, welling-abscesses in the throat, and inability to get water down.

上氣 420
胸痛 469
淋 222
膈痛 481
頸腫 636

# 6.28
## *Hóu Yàn Míng (Zá Bìng)*
## 喉咽鳴（雜病）
### Throat rales
**(Miscellaneous diseases)**

扶突、天突、太溪主喉鳴，暴忤氣哽（《千》）。少商、太衝、經渠主喉中鳴。魚際主喉中焦乾。咽冷聲破，灸天瞿五十壯（見上氣）。天突、扶突治喉中如水雞聲（《銅》）。天溪治喉中作聲（見胸痛）。

Fú Tū 扶突 (LI 18), Tiān Tū 天突 (Rèn 22), and Tài Xī 太溪 (KI 3) govern throat rales and sudden qì choking (*Qiān*《千》).

Shào Shāng 少商 (LU 11), Tài Chōng 大衝 (LV 3), and Jīng Qú 經渠 (LU 8) govern throat rales.

Yú Jì 魚際 (LU 10) governs dry throat.

Cold in the throat and loss of voice: Apply fifty cones of moxibustion on Tiān Qú 天瞿 (Rèn 22) (see the section on qì ascent).

Tiān Tū (Rèn 22) and Fú Tū (LI 18) treat croaking of frogs in the throat (*Tóng*《銅》).

Tiān Xī 天溪 (SP 18) treats sounds in the throat (see the section on chest pain).

大鐘（見淋）、大包主喉鳴（見膈痛）。天突治喉內如水雞聲（《明》見嗽）。《下》云：喉中鳴翕翕（見頸腫）。陽陵泉、天池（見上氣）、膻中療喉鳴（《明下》見膈痛）。

Dà Zhōng 大鐘 (KI 4) (see the section on dribbling) and Dà Bāo 大包 (SP 21) (see the section on pain of the diaphragm) govern throat rales.

Tiān Tū (Rèn 22) treats croaking of frogs in the throat (see the section on cough in *Míng*《明》). *Xià*《下》 says: vigorous throat rales (see the section on acute swelling [of the neck]).

Yáng Líng Quán 陽陵泉 (GB 34), Tiān Chí 天池 (PC 1) (see the section on qì ascent), and Dàn Zhōng 膻中 (Rèn 17) cure throat rales (see the section on pain of the diaphragm in *Míng Xià*《明下》).

小兒喉中鳴，咽乳不利：灸璇璣三壯。液門、四瀆主呼吸短氣，咽中如息肉狀。少府、蠡溝主嗌中有氣，如息肉狀（《銅》同）。然谷、太溪主嗌內腫，氣走咽喉。風池主喉咽僂引，項攣不收。

Throat rales in children and inhibited swallowing of milk: Apply three cones of moxibustion on Xuán Jī 璇璣 (Rèn 21).

Yè Mén 液門 (SJ 2) and Sì Dú 四瀆 (SJ 9) govern shortness of breath and a feeling like polyps in the throat.

Shào Fǔ 少府 (HT 8) and Lí Gōu 蠡溝 (LV 5) govern qì in the throat and a feeling like polyps (*Tóng*《銅》agrees).

Rán Gǔ 然谷 (KI 2) and Tài Xī 太溪 (KI 3) govern swelling of the throat and qì running through the throat.

Fēng Chí 風池 (GB 20) governs constriction of the throat, hypertonicity of the nape and loss of use.

心痛 312
喉痹 629
疝 220
口喎 591
煩心 335
傷寒 661

# 6.29
## *Yān Hóu Gān*
## 咽喉乾
## Dry throat

極泉、太淵（見心痛）、偏歷（見喉痹）、太衝（見疝）、天突治咽乾（《銅》見唾血）。魚際治喉乾燥，寒栗鼓頷，咳引尻痛溺出，嘔血。行間治咽乾煩渴（見口喎）。神門治咽乾不嗜食（見煩心）。

Jí Quán 極泉 (HT 1), Tài Yuān 太淵 (LU 9) (see the section on heart pain), Piān Lì 偏歷 (LI 6) (see the section on throat *bì*-impediment), Tài Chōng 太衝 (LV 3) (see the section on prominent *shàn*-mounting), and Tiān Tū 天突 (Rèn 22) treat dry throat (see the section on spitting of blood in *Tóng*《銅》).

Yú Jì 魚際 (LU 10) treats dry throat, shivering and chattering of the jaws,[24] cough induced sacral and coccyx pain, as well as urinary incontinence, and vomiting blood.

Xíng Jiān 行間 (LV 2) treats dry throat, and vexation thirst (see the section on deviation of the mouth).

Shén Mén 神門 (HT 7) treats dry throat and no desire to eat (see the section on vexation of the heart).

照海治嗌乾（《明》同），四肢惰，善悲不樂。少衝治咽酸（見傷寒，《千》同）。魚際療喉焦乾（《明》見肘痛）。太溪、少澤主咽乾（《千》見口喎乾）。復溜、照海、太衝、中封主嗌乾。

Zhào Hǎi 照海 (KI 6) treats dry throat (*Míng*《明》agrees), lazy limbs, and frequent sorrow and unhappiness.

Shào Chōng (HT 9) treats aching throat (see the section on cold damage; *Qiān*《千》agrees).

Yú Jì (LU 10) cures scorched dry throat (see the section on elbow pain in *Míng*).

24. Chattering of the jaws: is usually called chattering teeth in English and is due to cold.

Tài Xī 太溪 (KI 3) and Shào Zé 少澤 (SI 1) govern dry throat (see the sections on deviation of the mouth and dry mouth in *Qiān*).

Fù Liū 復溜 (KI 7), Zhào Hǎi 照海 (KI 6), Tài Chōng 太衝 (LV 3), and Zhōng Fēng 中封 (LV 4) govern dry throat.

## 6.30
## *Hóu Bì*
## 喉痹
## Throat *bì*-impediment

凡喉痹，脅中暴逆：先取衝脈，後取三里、雲門，各瀉之，又刺手小指端出血，立已（《千》）。三里、溫溜（《明下》同）、曲池、中渚、豐隆（《銅》同）主喉痹不能言。神門、合谷、風池主喉痹。

Throat *bì*-impediment with sudden counterflow in the rib-sides: drain the *chōng mài* first, then Sān Lǐ 三里 (ST 36) and Yún Mén 雲門 (LU 2); also bleed the end of the little finger. The disease will be cured immediately (*Qiān*《千》).

Sān Lǐ (ST 36), Wēn Liū 溫溜 (LI 7) (*Míng Xià*《明下》agrees), Qū Chí 曲池 (LI 11), Zhōng Zhǔ 中渚 (SJ 3), and Fēng Lóng 豐隆 (ST 40) (*Tóng*《銅》agrees) govern throat *bì*-impediment and inability to speak.

Shén Mén 神門 (HT 7), Hé Gǔ 合谷 (LI 4), and Fēng Chí 風池 (GB 20) govern throat *bì*-impediment.

完骨、天牖、前谷主喉痹，頸項腫，不可俯仰，頰腫引耳後。璇璣、鳩尾主喉痹咽腫，水漿不下。天鼎、氣舍、膈俞主喉痹哽噎，咽腫不得消，食飲不下。涌泉（《明》同）、然谷主喉痹，哽咽寒熱。

Wán Gǔ 完骨 (GB 12), Tiān Yǒu 天牖 (SJ 16), Qián Gǔ 前谷 (SI 2) govern throat *bì*-impediment, swollen neck and nape, inability to bend forward and backward, and swelling of the cheeks that radiates to behind the ears.

Xuán Jī 璇璣 (Rèn 21) and Jiū Wěi 鳩尾 (Rèn 15) govern throat *bì*-impediment, swollen throat, and inability to get water down.

膝痛 536
咳逆 417
胸滿 470

Tiān Dǐng 天鼎 (LI 17), Qì Shě 氣舍 (ST 11), and Gé Shù 膈俞 (UB 17) govern throat *bì*-impediment, choking and dysphagia, swollen throat that does not disperse, and difficulty getting food and drink down.

Yǒng Quán 涌泉 (KI 1) (*Míng*《明》agrees) and Rán Gǔ 然谷 (KI 2) govern throat *bì*-impediment and choking in the throat with [sensations of] cold and heat.

中府、陽交主喉痹，胸滿塞，寒熱。天容、缺盆(《明》同)、大杼、膈俞、雲門、尺澤、二間、厲兌、涌泉、然谷主喉痹哽咽，寒熱。三間(《明》同，《銅》同)、陽溪主喉痹，咽如哽。

Zhōng Fǔ 中府 (LU 1) and Yáng Jiāo 陽交 (GB 35) govern throat *bì*-impediment, stuffy chest, and [sensations of] cold and heat.

Tiān Róng 天容 (SI 17), Quē Pén 缺盆 (ST 12) (*Míng* agrees), Dà Zhù 大杼 (UB 11), Gé Shù (UB 17), Yún Mén 雲門 (LU 2), Chǐ Zé 尺澤 (LU 5), Èr Jiān 二間 (LI 2), Lì Duì 厲兌 (ST 45), Yǒng Quán 涌泉 (KI 1), and Rán Gǔ (KI 2) govern throat *bì*-impediment, choking, and [sensations of] cold and heat.

Sān Jiān 三間 (LI 3) (*Míng* and *Tóng*《銅》agree) and Yáng Xī 陽溪 (LI 5) govern throat *bì*-impediment, and a feeling in the throat as if choking on something.

天突主喉痹，咽乾急。大陵、偏歷主喉痹嗌乾。關衝(《銅》同)、竅陰、少澤主喉痹。舌卷，口喎乾，喉痹，氣逆咳嗽，口中涎唾：灸肺俞七壯，亦可隨年壯，至百壯。陽輔、陽交(並見膝痛)、厲兌、下廉、然谷、經渠、完骨、膈俞、缺盆、氣舍(見咳逆)、雲門(見胸滿)、陽溪、合谷、溫溜、中府、浮白治喉痹(《銅》)。

Tiān Tū 天突 (Rèn 22) governs throat *bì*-impediment and acute dry throat.

Dà Líng 大陵 (PC 7) and Piān Lì 偏歷 (LI 6) govern throat *bì*-impediment and dry throat.

Guān Chōng 關衝 (SJ 1) (*Tóng* agrees), Qiào Yīn 竅陰 (GB 44), and Shào Zé 少澤 (SI 1) govern throat *bì*-impediment.

For curled tongue, deviation of the mouth with dryness, throat *bì*-impediment, qì counterflow and cough, and drool and spittle in the mouth: Apply seven cones of moxibustion on Fèi Shù 肺俞 (UB 13), or burn the same number of cones as the age of the patient up to a hundred.

Yáng Fǔ 陽輔 (GB 38), Yáng Jiāo 陽交 (GB 35) (for all, see the section on knee pain), Lì Duì (ST 45), Xià Lián 下廉 (ST 37), Rán Gǔ (KI 2), Jīng Qú 經渠 (LU 8), Wán Gǔ 完骨 (GB 12), Gé Shù (UB 17), Quē Pén (ST 12), Qì Shě 氣舍 (ST 11) (see the section on coughing counterflow), Yún Mén (LU 2) (see the section on chest fullness), Yáng Xī (LI 5), Hé Gǔ 合谷 (LI 4), Wēn Liū

溫溜 (LI 7), Zhōng Fǔ 中府 (LU 1), and Fú Bái 浮白 (GB 10) treat throat *bì*-impediment (*Tóng*《銅》).

大杼治喉痹煩滿。天容治喉痹寒熱，咽中如鯁。天鼎治喉痹咽腫，不得食飲，食不下，喉鳴。前谷治頷腫喉痹。二間治喉痹，頷腫，肩背痛，振寒。曲池治喉痹不能言。竅陰治喉痹，舌強，口乾，肘不舉。少澤治喉痹，舌強，口乾，心煩。

Dà Zhù 大杼 (UB 11) treats throat *bì*-impediment with vexation and fullness.

Tiān Róng 天容 (SI 17) treats throat *bì*-impediment, [sensations of] cold and heat, and a feeling like a fish bone is stuck in the throat.

Tiān Dǐng 天鼎 (LI 17) treats throat *bì*-impediment, swollen throat, inability to eat or difficulty getting food down, and throat rales.

Qián Gǔ 前谷 (SI 2) treats swelling under the chin and throat *bì*-impediment.

Èr Jiān 二間 (LI 2) treats throat *bì*-impediment, swelling under the chin, pain of the shoulders and back, and quivering with cold.

Qū Chí 曲池 (LI 11) treats throat *bì*-impediment and inability to speak.

Qiào Yīn 竅陰 (GB 44) treats throat *bì*-impediment, stiff tongue, dry mouth, and inability to raise the elbows.

Shào Zé 少澤 (SI 1) treats throat *bì*-impediment, stiff tongue, dry mouth, and vexation of the heart.

大陵治喉痹，口乾，身熱頭痛，短氣，胸脅痛。浮白療寒熱喉痹(《明》)。膈俞、經渠療喉痹。二間療喉痹，咽如有物傷，忽振寒。《下》云：喉痹咽腫，多臥善睡。小兒急喉痹：灸天突一壯(《下》)。(有醫者說藥不下喉，當以曲竹管灌藥，效。)

Dà Líng 大陵 (PC 7) treats throat *bì*-impediment, dry mouth, generalized heat, headaches, shortness of breath, and pain of the chest and rib-sides.

Fú Bái (GB 10) cures [sensations of] cold and heat and throat *bì*-impediment (*Míng*《明》).

Gé Shù 膈俞 (UB 17) and Jīng Qú 經渠 (LU 8) cure throat *bì*-impediment.

Èr Jiān (LI 2) cures throat *bì*-impediment, a feeling in the throat like it has been damaged by something, and sudden quivering with cold. *Xià*《下》says: It treats throat *bì*-impediment, swollen throat, and somnolence.

耳鳴 561 Acute throat *bì*-impediment in children: Apply one cone of moxibustion on Tiān Tū 天突 (Rèn
面腫 655 22) (*Xià*《下》). (Some doctors say: If unable to swallow herbs, pour in the herbs with a curved bamboo tube. This is effective).

## 6.31

## *Chún Jiá Zhǒng Tòng (Yí Hàn Zhǒng)*

# 唇頰腫痛（頤頷腫）

### Swelling and pain around the lips

**(Swelling of the lower cheeks and under the chin)**

合谷主唇吻不收（《千》見口緩）。緊唇：灸虎口，男左女右。又灸承漿三壯。三間療唇口乾（《明》見瘧）。下廉治唇乾涎出（《銅》見飧泄）。光明（《銅》同）、足臨泣（《明下》同）主喜嚙頰。

Hé Gǔ 合谷 (LI 4) governs inability to contract the lips (see the discussion of slack mouth in *Qiān*《千》).

Tightness of the lips: Apply moxibustion on the tiger's mouth (Hǔ Kǒu 虎口); apply it on the left side for males and the right side for females; in addition apply three cones of moxibustion on Chéng Jiāng 承漿 (Rèn 24).

Sān Jiān 三間 (LI 3) cures dry mouth and lips (see the section on malaria in *Míng*《明》).

Xià Lián 下廉 (LI 8) treats dry lips and drooling (see the section on swill diarrhea in *Tóng*《銅》).

Guāng Míng 光明 (GB 37) (*Tóng* agrees) and Zú Lín Qì 足臨泣 (GB 41) (*Míng Xià*《明下》agrees) govern frequent biting of one's own cheeks.

巨窌、天窗主頰腫痛（《明》同）。京骨、陽谷主自嚙唇。腕骨等主頷痛（見耳鳴）。迎香治唇腫痛（《銅》治偏風）。正營治牙痛，唇吻急強。上關（《明下》同）、兌端治唇吻強。大迎治唇吻瞤動（見面腫）。

Jù Liáo 巨窌 (ST 3) and Tiān Chuāng 天窗 (SI 16) govern swelling and pain of the cheeks (*Míng* agrees).

Jīng Gǔ 京骨 (UB 64) and Yáng Gǔ 陽谷 (SI 5) govern biting one's own lips. 耳聾 564

Wàn Gǔ 腕骨 (SI 4) and so forth govern pain under the chin (see the section on tinnitus). 牙關 605

Yíng Xiāng 迎香 (LI 20) treats painful swollen lips (see the section on hemilateral wind in *Tóng* 《銅》). 風痓 371 口喎 591

Zhèng Yíng 正營 (GB 17) treats toothache and acute stiffness of the lips.

Shàng Guān 上關 (GB 3) (*Míng Xià*《明下》agrees) and Duì Duān 兌端 (Dū 27) treats stiffness of the lips.

Dà Yíng 大迎 (ST 5) treats twitching lips (see the section on facial swelling).

膺窗、太衝治唇腫。俠溪（見耳聾）、和髎（見牙關）、頰車治頷頰腫（見口噤）。曲鬢治頰頷腫，引牙車不得開，急痛，口噤不能言。完骨治頰腫。大迎治頰頷腫（見風痓）。翳風治脫頷頰腫（見口喎）。

Yīng Chuāng 膺窗 (ST 16) and Tài Chōng 太衝 (LV 3) treat swollen lips.

Xiá Xī 俠溪 (GB 43) (see the section on deafness), Hé Liáo 和髎 (SJ 22) (see the section on the [clenched] jaws), and Jiá Chē 頰車 (ST 6) treat swelling of the cheeks and under the chin (see the section on clenched jaws).

Qū Bìn 曲鬢 (GB 7) treats swelling of the cheeks and under the chin, inability to open the jaws, acute pain, and clenched jaws with inability to speak.

Wán Gǔ 完骨 (GB 12) treats swollen cheeks.

Dà Yíng (ST 5) treats swelling of the cheeks and under the chin (see the section on wind tetany).

Yì Fēng 翳風 (SJ 17) treats dislocated mandible and swollen cheeks (see the section on deviation of the mouth).

腕骨、陽谷治頸項腫寒熱。支正治頷腫。手三里治頰頷腫，瘰歷。少商治腮頷腫。成君綽忽腮頷腫大如升，甄權針此立愈。商陽治頤頷腫，齒痛，惡寒，肩背急相引缺盆痛，目青盲：灸三壯，右取左，左取右，食頃立已。

Wàn Gǔ (SI 4) and Yáng Gǔ (SI 5) treat swollen neck and nape and [sensations of] cold and heat.

Zhī Zhèng 支正 (SI 7) treats swelling under the chin.

Shǒu Sān Lǐ 手三里 (LI 10) treats swelling of the cheeks and under the chin and scrofula.

面痛 658 齒齲 601

Shào Shāng 少商 (LU 11) treats swelling of the cheeks and under the chin. Chéng Jūnzhuō suffered sudden swelling of his cheeks and under his chin. [The swelling] was as big as a *shēng*.[25] Zhēn Quán needled this point and cured the disease immediately.

Shāng Yáng 商陽 (LI 1) treats swelling of the cheeks and under the chin, toothache, aversion to cold, tension of the shoulders and back that radiates painfully into the empty basin [supraclavicular fossa], and clear-eye blindness: Apply three cones of moxibustion on the left side for diseases on the right; or on the right for diseases on the left. This will cure it soon.

完骨等主頰腫（《千》見喉痹）。攢竹等主頰痛（見面痛）。角孫主頸頷柱滿。兌端等主唇吻強（見齒齲）。足臨泣療胸膈滿悶，腋下腫，善噛頰（《明下》）。水溝療面腫唇動葉葉，肺風，狀如蟲行。

Wán Gǔ 完骨 (GB 12) and so forth govern swollen cheeks (see the section on throat *bì*-impediment in *Qiān*《千》).

Zǎn Zhú 攢竹 (UB 2) and so forth govern cheek pain (see the section on facial pain).

Jiǎo Sūn 角孫 (SJ 20) governs stiffness and distention of the neck and under the chin.

Duì Duān 兌端 (Dū 27) and so forth govern stiff lips (see the section on tooth decay).

Zú Lín Qì 足臨泣 (GB 41) cures fullness and oppression of the chest and diaphragm, swelling under the axilla, and frequently biting one's own cheeks (*Míng Xià*《明下》).

Shuǐ Gōu 水溝 (Dū 26) cures facial swelling, twitching lips that look like worms crawling, and lung wind.

李襲興稱武德中出鎮潞州，甄權以新撰《明堂》示予：有刺史成君綽忽頸腫如數升，喉中閉塞，水粒不下三日矣。余屈權救之，針其右手次指之端，如食頃，氣息即通。明日，飲啖如故（《千金翼》）。按《銅人》云：少商穴在手大指端內側去爪甲角如韭葉。成君綽腮頷腫大如升（云云同上），甄權針之立愈。病狀少異，功效實同。但李云次指端，《銅人》云大指端，未知其孰是。果針少商，當在大指端也。姑兩存之，以俟識者。

Lǐ Xíxìng was a guard in Lùzhōu during the Wǔ Dé 武德 period,[26] Zhēn Quán showed me [Sūn Sīmiǎo] the newly written *Míng Táng*《明堂》: Provincial governor Chéng Jūnzhuō suffered

25. *Shēng* 升 is a unit of dry measurement for grain, approximately equal to 1 deciliter. Here it indicates the size of the swelling.

26. The *Wǔ Dé* 武德 period indicates the time between 618 and 626 CE.

sudden swelling on his neck. [The swelling] was as big as several shēng. He also had a blockage of the throat and inability to get water and food down for three days. I [Sūn] deferred to Zhēn Quán to treat him. He needled the tip of his right index finger, and the patient could breathe after a while and eat normally the next day (*Qiān Jīn Yì* 《千金翼》).

Note that *Tóng Rén* 《銅人》 says: Shào Shāng 少商 (LU 11) is located at the medial aspect of the thumb, the distance of a leek leaf from the nail. Chéng Jūnzhuō suffered sudden swelling of his cheeks and under his chin; [the swelling] was as big as a shēng (same as above). Zhēn Quán needled him and cured the disease immediately.

The symptoms are little different, but the results are the same. However Lǐ said the tip of the index finger, while *Tóng Rén* says the tip of the thumb. I do not know which is correct. If Shào Shāng (LU 11) was needled, it must be located on the tip of the thumb. I put these passages together here to wait for someone who might know.

腋腫 496
風痹 377
癰疽 694
足麻 509
勞瘵 188
肩痛 486
偏風 396
目眩 575
咳逆 417

# 6.32
## *Jǐng Xiàng Jiàng (Jí Zhǒng)*
## 頸項強（急腫）
## Stiffness of the neck and nape
**(Acute swelling)**

腕骨、陽谷治頸項腫，寒熱（《銅》）。丘墟治頸腫（見腋腫）。大迎治寒熱頸痛，瘰歷。消濼（見風痹）、竅陰治項痛（見癰疽）。風門治傷寒頸項強（見傷寒雜病）。京骨（見足麻）、大杼治頸項強，不可俯仰（見瘧，《明》同）。

Wàn Gǔ 腕骨 (SI 4) and Yáng Gǔ 陽谷 (SI 5) treat swollen neck and nape and [sensations of] cold and heat (*Tóng*《銅》).

Qiū Xū 丘墟 (GB 40) treats neck swelling (see the section on swelling of the axilla).

Dà Yíng 大迎 (ST 5) treats [sensations of] cold and heat, neck pain, and scrofula.

Xiāo Luò 消濼 (SJ 12) (see the section on wind *bì*-impediment) and Qiào Yīn 竅陰 (GB 44) treat neck pain (see the section on welling and flat-abscesses).

Fēng Mén 風門 (UB 12) treats cold damage and stiffness of the neck and nape (see the section on cold damage and miscellaneous diseases).

Jīng Gǔ 京骨 (UB 64) (see the section on numbness of the legs) and Dà Zhù 大杼 (UB 11) treat stiffness of the neck and nape with inability to bend forward and backward (see the section on malaria; *Míng*《明》agrees).

魄戶（見勞瘵）、肩井治頸項不得顧（見肩痛）。天牖、後溪治項強不得顧。完骨（見偏風）、頷厭治頸項痛。本神治頸項強痛（見目眩）。風池治痎瘧，頸項痛，不得顧。通天治頸項轉側難。頰車、大椎、氣舍（見咳逆）、腦空治頸項強，不得顧。

Pò Hù 魄戶 (UB 42) (see the section on consumption) and Jiān Jǐng 肩井 (GB 21) treat inability of the neck and nape to turn (see the section on [aching] pain of the shoulders [and back]).

目眩 575
瘰癧 702
頭痛 643
腦痛 649

Tiān Yǒu 天牖 (SJ 16) and Hòu Xī 後溪 (SI 3) treat stiff neck with inability to turn.

Wán Gǔ 完骨 (GB 12) (see the section on hemilateral wind) and Hàn Yàn 頷厭 (GB 4) treat pain of the neck and nape.

Běn Shén 本神 (GB 13) treats stiffness and pain of the neck and nape (see the section on dizzy vision).

Fēng Chí 風池 (GB 20) treats malaria, neck and nape pain, and inability to turn.

Tōng Tiān 通天 (UB 7) treats difficulty turning the neck and nape to the sides.

Jiá Chē 頰車 (ST 6), Dà Zhuī 大椎 (Dū 14), Qì Shě 氣舍 (ST 11) (see the section on coughing counterflow), and Nǎo Kōng 腦空 (GB 19) treat neck and nape stiffness with inability to turn.

天柱治頸項筋急不得顧。人迎治項氣悶腫，食不下。後頂、外丘治頸項痛，惡風寒。齦交、風府治頸項急不得顧（見目眩）。臂臑（見瘰癧）、強間治頸項強（見頭痛）。少澤（《明》同）、前谷、後溪、陽谷、完骨、崑崙、小海、攢竹主項強急痛，不可顧（《千》）。

Tiān Zhù 天柱 (UB 10) treats sinew tension of the neck and nape with inability to turn.

Rén Yíng 人迎 (ST 9) treats neck qì[27] with oppression and swelling and difficulty getting food down.

Hòu Dǐng 後頂 (Dū 19) and Wài Qiū 外丘 (GB 36) treat neck and nape pain and aversion to wind-cold.

Yín Jiāo 齦交 (Dū 28) and Fēng Fǔ 風府 (Dū 16) treat neck and nape tension with inability to turn (see the section on dizzy vision).

Bì Nào 臂臑 (LI 14) (see the section on scrofula) and Qiáng Jiān 強間 (Dū 18) treat stiffness of the neck and nape (see the section on headaches).

Shào Zé 少澤 (SI 1) (*Míng*《明》agrees), Qián Gǔ 前谷 (SI 2), Hòu Xī 後溪 (SI 3), Yáng Gǔ 陽谷 (SI 5), Wán Gǔ 完骨 (GB 12), Kūn Lún 崑崙 (UB 60), Xiǎo Hǎi 小海 (SI 8), and Zǎn Zhú 攢竹 (UB 2) govern neck stiffness with acute pain and inability to turn (*Qiān*《千》).

消濼、本神、通天、強間、風府、瘖門、天柱、風池、齦交、天衝、陶道、外丘、通谷、玉枕主項如拔，不可左右顧。《明》云：天柱（見目眩）、強間（見頭痛）療項如拔。《下》云：天柱療項如拔（見腦痛）。

27. Neck qì seems to be the name of a disease, but no further information has so far been found. Perhaps it is goiter.

目痛 568 風眩 375

Xiāo Luò 消濼 (SJ 12), Běn Shén 本神 (GB 13), Tōng Tiān 通天 (UB 7), Qiáng Jiān 強間 (Dū 18), Fēng Fǔ 風府 (Dū 16), Yīn Mén 瘖門 (Dū 15), Tiān Zhù 天柱 (UB 10), Fēng Chí 風池 (GB 20), Yín Jiāo 齦交 (Dū 28), Tiān Chōng 天衝 (GB 9), Táo Dào 陶道 (Dū 13), Wài Qiū 外丘 (GB 36), Tōng Gǔ 通谷 (UB 66), and Yù Zhěn 玉枕 (UB 9) govern a pulling sensation in the nape and inability to turn sides.

*Míng* says: Tiān Zhù 天柱 (UB 10) (see the section on dizzy vision) and Qiáng Jiān 強間 (Dū 18) (see the section on headaches) cure a pulling sensation in the nape.

*Xià*《下》says: Tiān Zhù (UB 10) cures a pulling sensation in the nape (see the section on brain pain).

天容、前谷、角孫、腕骨、支正主頸項腫痛，不可顧。天容主頸項癰，不能言。飛揚、涌泉、頷厭、後頂主頸項疼，歷節汗出。角孫主頸項柱滿。浮白療頸項癰腫(《銅》同)，不能言及癭，肩不舉(《明》)。

Tiān Róng 天容 (SI 17), Qián Gǔ (SI 2), Jiǎo Sūn 角孫 (SJ 20), Wàn Gǔ 腕骨 (SI 4), and Zhī Zhèng 支正 (SI 7) govern swelling and pain of the neck and nape with inability to turn.

Tiān Róng (SI 17) governs welling-abscess on the neck and nape and inability to speak.

Fēi Yáng 飛揚 (UB 58), Yǒng Quán 涌泉 (KI 1), Hàn Yàn 頷厭 (GB 4), and Hòu Dǐng (Dū 19) govern neck and nape pain and joint-running[28] with sweating.

Jiǎo Sūn 角孫 (SJ 20) governs blockage and fullness of the neck and nape.

Fú Bái 浮白 (GB 10) cures swollen welling-abscesses on the neck and nape (*Tóng*《銅》agrees), inability to speak, goiter, and inability to raise the shoulders (*Míng*《明》).

曲差療心煩滿，汗不出，頭項痛，身熱，目視不明。通天療項痛重，暫起僵仆。瘖門療項強不得顧。玉枕(見目痛)、完骨(見風眩)療項痛。風府療頭(《明》有痛)項急，不可傾側。陽谷療脅痛頸腫，寒熱。

Qū Chā 曲差 (UB 4) cures vexation and fullness of the heart, absence of sweating, headaches, nape pain, generalized fever, and blurred vision.

Tōng Tiān 通天 (UB 7) cures pain and heaviness of the nape and collapse when attempting to stand up.

Yīn Mén 瘖門 (Dū 15) cures neck stiffness with inability to turn.

28. Joint-running is short for joint-running wind. This is a condition with joint pain all over the body.

Yù Zhěn 玉枕 (UB 9) (see the section on eye pain) and Wán Gǔ 完骨 (GB 12) (see the section on wind dizziness) cure nape pain.

Fēng Fǔ 風府 (Dū 16) cures tension of the head and nape (*Míng* says headache) and inability to lean to the sides.

Yáng Gǔ 陽谷 (SI 5) cures pain of the rib-sides, swollen neck, and [sensations of] cold and heat.

天突療身寒熱，頸腫，喉中鳴翕翕，胸中氣鯁鯁（《下》）。天井療頸項及肩背痛（見肘痛）。曲鬢療頸項強，不得顧，引牙齒痛，口噤不能言。

Tiān Tū 天突 (Rèn 22) cures generalized [sensations of] cold and heat, neck swelling, throat rales, and qì choking in the chest (*Xià*《下》).

Tiān Jǐng 天井 (SJ 10) cures pain of the neck, nape, shoulders and back (see the section on elbow pain).

Qū Bìn 曲鬢 (GB 7) cures stiffness of the neck and nape with inability to turn, pain radiating in the teeth, clenched jaws, and inability to speak.

癇
357
腦痛
649
目眩
575
鼻涕
616

# 6.33

## *Tóu Fēng (Tóu Xuàn, Yòu Jiàn Tóu Xuán)*

## 頭風（頭眩　又見頭旋）

### Head wind

**(Dizzy head; also see the section on spinning head)**

五處療頭眩風悶（《明》）。百會（見癇）、腦空（見目眩）、天柱（見腦痛）療頭風。神聰療頭風目眩，狂亂風癇。左主如花，右主如果。前頂療頭風熱痛，頭腫風癇。後頂療風眩目䀮䀮，額顱上痛。上星療頭風目眩（《下》）。

Wǔ Chù 五處 (UB 5) cures dizzy head and oppression due to wind (*Míng*《明》).

Bǎi Huì 百會 (Dū 20) (see the section on withdrawal and epilepsy), Nǎo Kōng 腦空 (GB 19) (see the section on dizzy vision), and Tiān Zhù 天柱 (UB 10) (see the section on brain pain) cure head wind.

Shén Cōng 神聰 (non-channel) cures head wind and dizzy vision, mania, and wind epilepsy. The [point on the] left governs like a flower; the [point on the] right governs like a fruit.[29]

Qián Dǐng 前頂 (Dū 21) cures head wind with hot pain, swelling of the head, and wind epilepsy.

Hòu Dǐng 後頂 (Dū 19) cures wind dizziness, blurred vision, and pain of the forehead and skull.

Shàng Xīng 上星 (Dū 23) cures head wind and dizzy vision (*Xià*《下》).

前頂治頭風目眩，面赤（《明下》作皮）腫（《銅》）。下廉、五處（見目眩）、神庭（見鼻涕）治頭風。神庭主風頭眩，善嘔煩滿（《千》）。天牖、風門（《明下》同）、崑崙、關元、關衝主風眩頭痛。

Qián Dǐng (Dū 21) treats head wind, dizzy vision, and red swollen face (*Míng Xià*《明下》 says: skin) (*Tóng*《銅》).

Xià Lián 下廉 (LI 8), Wǔ Chù (UB 5) (see the section on dizzy vision), and Shén Tíng 神庭 (Dū 24) (see the section on sniveling) treat head wind.

29. This means the results of the point on the right are better than those of left.

Shén Tíng 神庭 (Dū 24) governs dizzy head due to wind, frequent retching, vexation, and fullness (*Qiān*《千》).

Tiān Yǒu 天牖 (SJ 16), Fēng Mén 天牖 (UB 12) (*Míng Xià*《明下》agrees), Kūn Lún 崑崙 (UB 60), Guān Yuán 關元 (Rèn 4), and Guān Chōng 關衝 (SJ 1) govern wind dizziness and headaches.

前頂、後頂、頷厭主風眩偏頭痛。上星主風頭眩，顏清。囟會主風頭眩，頭痛顏清。完骨主風頭耳後痛（瘈脈同），煩心（《銅》同）。跗陽主痿厥，風頭重痛。俠溪主胸中寒如風狀，頭眩，兩頰痛。腎俞、攢竹、承光、絲竹空、瘈脈、和髎主風頭痛。

Qián Dǐng 前頂 (Dū 21), Hòu Dǐng 後頂 (Dū 19), and Hàn Yàn 頷厭 (GB 4) govern wind dizziness and hemilateral headaches.

Shàng Xīng 上星 (Dū 23) governs dizzy head due to wind and clean [pale] face.

Xìn Huì 囟會 (Dū 22) governs dizzy head due to wind, headaches, and clear [pale] face.

Wán Gǔ 完骨 (GB 12) governs head wind, pain behind the ears (same as Chì Mài 瘈脈 (SJ 18)), and vexation of the heart (*Tóng*《銅》agrees).

Fū Yáng 跗陽 (UB 59) governs wilting reversal and head wind with heaviness and pain.

Xiá Xī 俠溪 (GB 43) governs cold in the chest that feels like wind [blowing], dizzy head, and cheek pain.

Shèn Shù 腎俞 (UB 23), Zǎn Zhú 攢竹 (UB 2), Chéng Guāng 承光 (UB 6), Sī Zhú Kōng 絲竹空 (SJ 23), Chì Mài 瘈脈 (SJ 18) and Hé Liáo 和髎 (LI 19) govern the pain of head wind.

上星主風頭引頷痛。合谷、五處主風頭熱。天牖療頭風面腫（《下》作目眩），項強不得轉（《明》）。囟會治頭風生白屑，多睡（《明》同）。針佳。以油鹽揩發根，頭風永除（《銅》）。頭風腫癢：針眉衝（許）。通里、百會療頭目眩痛（《明》）。陽谷療頭眩（見狂）。

Shàng Xīng (Dū 23) governs head wind with pain radiating under the chin.

Hé Gǔ 合谷 (LI 4) and Wǔ Chù 五處 (UB 5) govern heat in the head due to wind.

Tiān Yǒu (SJ 16) cures head wind, facial swelling (*Xià*《下》says dizzy eyes), and stiff neck with inability to turn (*Míng*《明》).

Xìn Huì 囟會 (Dū 22) treats head wind with white scales and sleepiness (*Míng*《 明 》agrees). Acupuncture is best. Rub the hair roots with oily salt; this will remove the head wind forever (*Tóng*《 銅 》).

Head wind with swelling and itching: needle Méi Chōng 眉衝 (UB 3) (*Xǔ* 許).[30]

Tōng Lǐ 通里 (HT 5) and Bǎi Huì 百會 (Dū 20) cure dizziness and pain of the head and eyes (*Míng*).

Yáng Gǔ 陽谷 (SI 5) cures dizzy head (see the section on mania).

**《素問》論頭痛，本於大寒內至骨髓；則頭風者亦本於風寒入腦髓耶。《本事方》論婦人患頭風者十居其半，或者婦人無巾以御風寒鄒？男子間有患之者，非頭上少髮，必其囟會前頂之髮禿也。欲灸頭風，宜先囟會、百會、前頂等穴。其頭風連目痛者，當灸上星、神聰、後頂等穴。予嘗自灸驗，教人灸亦驗云。**

*Sù Wèn*《 素問 》discusses headaches: Severe cold entering the bone marrow is the root; so head wind is due to wind-cold entering the brain marrow.

[*Pǔ Jì*] *Běn Shì Fāng*《 本事方 》discusses head wind: Half of women suffer head wind; is this because they do not have scarves to prevent wind-cold? Men also suffer head wind occasionally; either because they have less hair on their heads, or because they have hair loss on the area of Xìn Huì (Dū 22) and Qián Dǐng 前頂 (Dū 21).

To apply moxibustion for head wind, it is appropriate to first apply it on Xìn Huì (Dū 22), Bǎi Huì (Dū 20), Qián Dǐng (Dū 21) and so forth. Or apply it on Shàng Xīng 上星 (Dū 23), Shén Cōng 神聰 (non-channel), Hòu Dǐng 後頂 (Dū 19) and so forth if the head wind is associated with eye pain.

I tried moxibustion on myself, and it is effective; I taught other people, and it also worked well.

**《本事》云：下虛者，腎虛也，腎厥則頭痛（宜玉真丸。上虛者，肝虛也；肝厥則頭暈，宜鉤藤散）。**

*Běn Shì*《 本事 》says: Vacuity of the lower body is kidney vacuity. Kidney reversal causes headaches (It is appropriate to take *Yù Zhēn Wán* 玉真丸 (True Jade Pill). Vacuity of the upper body is liver vacuity. Liver reversal causes dizziness, it is appropriate to take *Gōu Téng Sǎn* 鉤藤散 (Uncaria Powder)).

30. Xǔ 許 refers to Xǔ Shūwēi 許叔微, the compiler of *Pǔ Jì Běn Shì Fāng*《 普濟本事方 》(Skillful Formulas for Universal Salvation). See the book appendix.

# 6.34

## *Tóu Tòng (Piān Tóu Tòng, Yú Jiàn Shāng Hán Tóu Tòng)*

## 頭痛（偏頭痛　餘見傷寒頭痛）

## Headaches

**(Hemilateral headaches; for further discussion, see the section on cold damage and headaches)**

中風 379
瘧 301
膈 481
目眩 575
寒熱 675
腹脹 211
傷寒無 690

解溪（見中風）、承光（《明》同）治風眩頭痛，嘔吐心煩（《銅》）。膽俞治頭痛振寒，汗不出。大杼治頭痛振寒（見瘧）。啞門治頭痛風汗不出。合谷、天池（見膈）、絲竹空（見目眩）、魚際（見寒熱）、四白（見目眩）、天衝、三焦俞（見腹脹）、風池（見傷寒無汗）治頭痛。

Jiě Xī 解溪 (ST 41) (see the section on wind stroke) and Chéng Guāng 承光 (UB 6) (*Míng*《明》agrees) treat wind dizziness, headaches, vomiting, and vexation of the heart (*Tóng*《銅》).

Dǎn Shù 膽俞 (UB 19) treats headaches, quivering with cold, and absence of sweating.

Dà Zhù 大杼 (UB 11) treats headaches and quivering with cold (see the section on malaria).

Yǎ Mén 啞門 (Dū 15) treats headaches and absence of sweating due to wind.

Hé Gǔ 合谷 (LI 4), Tiān Chí 天池 (PC 1) (see the section on [pain in] the diaphragm), Sī Zhú Kōng 絲竹空 (SJ 23) (see the section on dizzy vision), Yú Jì 魚際 (LU 10) (see the section on [sensations of] cold and heat), Sì Bái 四白 (ST 2) (see the section on dizzy vision), Tiān Chōng 天衝 (GB 9), Sān Jiāo Shù 三焦俞 (UB 22) (see the section on abdominal fullness), and Fēng Chí 風池 (GB 20) (see the section on cold damage with absence of sweating) treat headaches.

神道治寒（《明下》作身）熱，頭痛，進退痎瘧，恍惚悲愁（《明》同），健忘驚悸。陽溪治厥逆頭痛，胸滿不得息。豐隆治厥頭痛，面浮腫，風逆，四肢腫，身濕。至陰治鼻塞頭重，風寒從足小指起，脈痹上下帶胸脅痛無常，轉筋，寒熱汗不出，煩心。

Shén Dào 神道 (Dū 11) treats cold (*Míng Xià*《明下》says body) and heat, headaches, malaria, abstraction and sorrow (*Míng* agrees), forgetfulness, and fright palpitations.

Yáng Xī 陽溪 (LI 5) treats reverse counterflow, headaches, chest fullness, and inability to breathe.

面腫 655 傷寒 661

Fēng Lóng 豐隆 (ST 40) treats reversal headaches, puffy facial swelling, wind counterflow, swollen extremities and generalized dampness.

Zhì Yīn 至陰 (UB 67) treats nasal congestion, heaviness of the head, wind-cold starting from the little toes, vessel *bì*-impediment moving up and down with migrating pain of the chest and rib-sides, cramping, [sensations of] cold and heat, absence of sweating, and vexation of the heart.

青靈治頭痛振寒，目黃脅痛。強間治腦旋目運，頭痛不可忍，煩心，嘔吐涎沫，發無時，項強不可顧。崑崙治頭痛，肩背急。風府治頭痛頸項急，不得顧，目眩。曲差治頭項痛。顱息療身熱頭痛，不可反側(《明》)。

Qīng Líng 青靈 (HT 2) treats headaches, quivering with cold, yellow eyes, and rib-side pain.

Qiáng Jiān 強間 (Dū 18) treats spinning head, dizzy vision, insufferable headaches, vexation of the heart, vomiting of drool and foam at random times, and stiff neck with inability to turn.

Kūn Lún 崑崙 (UB 60) treats headaches and tension of the shoulders and back.

Fēng Fǔ 風府 (Dū 16) treats headaches, tension of the neck and nape, inability to turn, and dizzy vision.

Qū Chā 曲差 (UB 4) treats head and nape pain.

Lú Xī 顱息 (SJ 19) cures generalized heat, headaches, and inability to turn to the sides (*Míng*《明》).

魚際療頭痛甚，汗不出。腦戶(見面腫)療頭痛。百會、通里療頭目眩痛(《下》)。中衝(見傷寒)、命門(《上》同)療身熱如火，頭痛如破(《明下》)。溫溜療寒熱頭痛，善噦，衄，肩不舉。

Yú Jì 魚際 (LU 10) cures severe headaches and absence of sweaing.

Nǎo Hù 腦戶 (Dū 17) (see the section on facial swelling) cures headaches.

Bǎi Huì 百會 (Dū 20) and Tōng Lǐ 通里 (HT 5) cure dizziness and pain of the head and eyes (*Xià*《下》).

Zhōng Chōng 中衝 (PC 9) (see the section on cold damage) and Mìng Mén 命門 (Dū 4) (*Shàng*《上》agrees) cure generalized heat that feels like fire burning inside and headache that feel like the head is broken (*Míng Xià*《明下》).

Wēn Liū 溫溜 (LI 7) cures [sensations of] cold and heat, headaches, frequent hiccups, nosebleeds, and inability to raise the shoulders.

率谷療醉後酒風發，頭重，皮膚腫，兩角眩痛。小兒食時頭痛（《千》同）及五心熱：灸譩譆各一壯。天柱、陶道、大杼（一作本神）、孔最、後溪主頭痛。腦戶、腦空、通天主頭重痛。頭維、大陵主頭痛如破，目痛如脫（《甲》云：喘逆煩痛，嘔吐汗流）。

Shuài Gǔ 率谷 (GB 8) cures episodes of liquor wind[31] when drunk, heaviness of the head, swollen skin, dizziness, and pain of the corners of the head.

Headaches in children while eating (*Qiān* 《千》 agrees) with five heart heat: Apply one cone of moxibustion on Yī Xī 譩譆 (UB 45).

Tiān Zhù 天柱 (UB 10), Táo Dào 陶道 (Dū 13), Dà Zhù 大杼 (UB 11) (some say Běn Shén 本神 (GB 13)), Kǒng Zuì 孔最 (LU 6), and Hòu Xī 後溪 (SI 3) govern headaches.

Nǎo Hù 腦戶 (Dū 17), Nǎo Kōng 腦空 (GB 19), and Tōng Tiān 通天 (UB 7) govern headaches and heaviness of the head.

Tóu Wéi 頭維 (ST 8) and Dà Líng 大陵 (PC 7) govern headache that feel like the head is broken, eye pain with a feeling that they are about to burst from their sockets (*Jiǎ* 《甲》 says: They treat panting counterflow, vexation, pain, vomiting, and sweating).

竅陰、強間（《明》同）主頭痛如椎刺，不可動。目窗、中渚、完骨、命門、豐隆、外丘、通谷、京骨、臨泣、小海、承筋、陽陵泉主頭痛寒熱，汗出不惡寒。神庭、水溝主寒熱頭痛，喘渴，目不可視。消濼主寒熱痹，頭痛。五處等主頭痛（見癒瘲）。崑崙、解溪、曲泉、飛揚、前谷、少澤、通里主頭眩痛。

Qiào Yīn 竅陰 (GB 11 or GB 44) and Qiáng Jiān 強間 (Dū 18) (*Míng* 《明》 agrees) govern headaches that feel like the piercing of an awl and inability to move.

Mù Chuāng 目窗 (GB 16), Zhōng Zhǔ 中渚 (SJ 3), Wán Gǔ 完骨 (GB 12), Mìng Mén 命門 (Dū 4), Fēng Lóng 豐隆 (ST 40), Wài Qiū 外丘 (GB 36), Tōng Gǔ 通谷 (UB 66), Jīng Gǔ 京骨 (UB 64), Lín Qì 臨泣 (GB 15 or GB 41), Xiǎo Hǎi 小海 (SI 8), Chéng Jīn 承筋 (UB 56), and Yáng Líng Quán 陽陵泉 (GB 34) govern headaches, [sensations of] cold and heat, and sweating without aversion to cold.

Shén Tíng 神庭 (Dū 24), Shuǐ Gōu 水溝 (Dū 26) govern [sensations of] cold and heat, headaches, panting, thirst, and inability to see.

Xiāo Luò 消濼 (SJ 12) governs cold or heat *bì*-impediment and headaches.

31. Liquor wind is wind attack that occurs after getting drunk. The symptoms include generalized heat, fatigue, profuse sweating, aversion to wind, and shortness of breath.

齒齲 601 Wǔ Chù 五處 (UB 5) and so forth govern headaches (see the section on tugging and slackening).

Kūn Lún 崑崙 (UB 60), Jiě Xī 解溪 (ST 41), Qū Quán 曲泉 (LV 8), Fēi Yáng 飛揚 (UB 58), Qián Gǔ 前谷 (SI 2), and Tōng Lǐ 通里 (HT 5) govern dizziness and headaches.

若頭痛，筋攣骨重，少氣，噦噫，滿，時驚，不嗜臥，咳嗽煩冤，其脈舉之則弦，按之石堅，由腎氣不足而內著，其氣逆而上行，謂之腎厥。宜灸關元百壯，服玉真丸（《指》）。若頭痛連齒，時發時止，連年不已，此由風寒留於骨髓，髓以腦為主，腦逆故頭痛，齒亦痛。宜白附子散，灸曲鬢七壯，左痛灸左，右痛灸右。

Headaches, hypertonicity of the sinews, heavy bones, qì shortage, hiccups, belching, fullness, frequent fright, no desire to sleep, cough, vexation and low spirits; wiry pulse as hard as a stone when pressed. This is caused by kidney qì insufficiency internally and qì counterflowing upward. It is called kidney reversal. It is appropriate to apply a hundred cones of moxibustion on Guān Yuán 關元 (Rèn 4) and take *Yù Zhēn Wán* 玉真丸 (True Jade Pill) (*Zhǐ*《指》).

Headaches with pain radiating to the teeth, on and off but lasting for years. It is caused by wind-cold staying in the bone marrow; the marrow dominates the brain, so brain counterflow results in headaches and toothache. It is appropriate to try *Bái Fù Zǐ Sǎn* 白附子散 (Typhonium Powder) and apply seven cones of moxibustion on Qū Bìn 曲鬢 (GB 7). Burn moxa on the left for pain on the left; burn moxa on the right for pain on the right.

少海（見齒齲）、完骨治頭痛（《銅》見心煩）。《千》云：主風頭耳後痛。腦空等，天衝主癲疾頭痛（《千》見癲）。

Shào Hǎi 少海 (HT 3) (see the section on tooth decay) and Wán Gǔ 完骨 (GB 12) treat headaches (see the section on vexation of the heart in *Tóng*《銅》). *Qiān*《千》says: They govern head wind with pain behind the ears.

Nǎo Kōng 腦空 (GB 19) and so forth and Tiān Chōng 天衝 (GB 9) govern epilepsy diseases and headaches (see the section on withdrawal and epilepsy in *Qiān*).

《素問》嘗論有數歲頭痛不已者，大寒內至骨髓，髓以腦為主，腦逆故頭痛齒亦痛，名曰厥逆頭痛。亦有腎厥、肝厥頭痛者，如《本事方》所謂下虛者，腎虛也，腎厥則頭痛；上虛者，肝虛也，肝厥則頭暈是也，皆可隨證治之。若真頭疼，則朝發夕死，夕發朝死矣（詳見《難經疏》）。人而患此，亦未如之何。要之，亦有所自，其在根本不固耶。若欲蓄艾，須先百會、囟會等穴，而丹田、氣海等穴，尤所當灸，以補養之，毋使至於此極可也。

傷寒寒 673
傷寒頭 671
目眩 575

*Sù Wèn*《素問》once discussed constant headaches that lasted several years; this is caused by severe cold entering the bone marrow. Marrow governs the brain; the brain counterflows resulting in headaches and toothaches. This is called reverse counterflow with headaches. There are also headaches due to kidney reversal and liver reversal, for example what was said in [*Pǔ Jì*] *Běn Shì Fāng*《本事方》: Vacuity of the lower body is kidney vacuity; kidney reversal causes headaches. Vacuity of upper body is liver vacuity; liver reversal causes dizziness. They can all be treated according to their pattern.

True headaches come on in the morning and expire in the evening, or come on in the evening and expire in the morning (see the details in *Nàn Jīng Shū*《難經疏》). People who suffer this don't know what to do for themselves. To summarize, [each headache] has its own reason, and is due to instability of the root. If we want to apply moxibustion, we should apply it on Bǎi Huì 百會 (Dū 20), Xìn Huì 囟會 (Dū 22) and so forth first; we also need to burn moxibustion on Dān Tián 丹田 (cinnabar field), Qì Hǎi 氣海 (Rèn 6), and so forth to supplement. This will prevent [the unstable root] from reaching its extremity.

前頂等主風眩偏頭痛（《千》見頭風）。懸厘治頭偏痛（見傷寒寒熱）。懸厘主偏頭痛，引目外眥（見傷寒頭痛）。頷厭療風（《銅》云：頭風）眩目無見，偏頭痛引目外眥急，耳鳴好嚏，頸痛（《明》）。岐伯灸偏頭痛（見目眩）。

Qián Dǐng 前頂 (Dū 21) and so forth govern wind dizziness and hemilateral headaches (see the section on head wind in *Qiān*《千》).

Xuán Lí 懸厘 (GB 6) treats hemilateral headaches (see the section on cold damage with [sensations of] cold and heat).

Xuán Lí (GB 6) governs hemilateral headaches that radiate to the outer canthus (see the section on cold damage and headaches).

Hàn Yàn 頷厭 (GB 4) cures wind (*Tóng*《銅》says: head wind) dizziness, inability to see, hemilateral headaches with tension radiating to the outer canthus, tinnitus, frequent sneezing, and neck pain (*Míng*《明》). Qí Bó applied moxibustion for hemilateral headaches (see the section on dizzy vision).

後頂治頭偏痛（《銅》）。玉枕主頭半寒痛（《千》）。《甲》云：頭眩目痛，頭半寒。正營治頭項偏痛。懸顱治熱病煩滿，汗不出，頭偏痛，引目外眥赤，身熱齒痛（《明》同）。懸厘治頭偏痛，煩心不欲食（並《銅》）。

Hòu Dǐng 後頂 (Dū 19) treats hemilateral headaches (*Tóng*《銅》).

Yù Zhěn 玉枕 (UB 9) governs cold pain of half of the head (*Qiān*《千》). *Jiă*《甲》said: It treats dizzy head, eye pain, and coldness of half of the head.

Zhèng Yíng 正營 (GB 17) treats hemilateral pain of the head and nape.

Xuán Lú 懸顱 (GB 5) treats heat disease, vexation, fullness, absence of sweating, hemilateral headaches that induce redness in the outer canthus, generalized heat, and toothaches (*Míng*《明》agrees).

Xuán Lí 懸厘 (GB 6) treats hemilateral headaches, vexation of the heart, and no desire to eat (all in *Tóng*).

# 6.35
## *Nǎo Tòng (Nǎo Fēng)*
# 腦痛 （腦風）

痰 399
面腫 655

## Brain pain
### (Brain wind)

強間治腦旋（《銅》見頭痛）。天柱治頭旋腦痛。《明下》云：療頭風腦重，目如脫，項如拔，項強痛不顧。玉枕治腦風，疼不可忍。承靈治腦風，頭痛，惡風寒。腦空治腦風頭痛不可忍，目瞑，心悸，發即為癲，風引目眇。

Qiáng Jiān 強間 (Dū 18) treats spinning brain (see the section on headaches in *Tóng*).

Tiān Zhù 天柱 (UB 10) treats dizziness and brain pain. *Míng Xià*《明下》says: It cures head wind and heaviness of the brain, the eyes feel as if they are about to burst out of their sockets, the nape feels dislocated, and stiffness and pain of the nape with inability to turn it.

Yù Zhěn (UB 9) treats brain wind with unbearable pain.

Chéng Líng 承靈 (GB 18) treats brain wind, headaches, and aversion to wind-cold.

Nǎo Kōng 腦空 (GB 19) treats brain wind, unbearable headaches, blurred vision, palpitations, withdrawal disease when [these symptoms] occur, and blurred vision due to wind.

上廉治腦風，頭痛。率谷治腦兩角強痛（見痰）。喑門療頭風，腦疼。風池（見面腫）療腦痛。小兒囟開不合：灸臍上下各五分二穴，各三壯。灸瘡未合，囟先合矣（《下》）。少海治腦風（《銅》見齒齲）。凡口鼻出血不止，名腦衄：上星五十壯（《千》）。

Shàng Lián 上廉 (LI 9) treats brain wind and headaches.

Shuài Gǔ 率谷 (GB 8) treats stiffness and pain of the corners of the head (see the section on phlegm drool).

Yīn Mén 喑門 (Dū 15) cures head wind and brain pain.

Fēng Chí 風池 (GB 20) (see the section on facial swelling) cures brain pain.

Fontanels not closing up in children: Apply three cones of moxibustion on the two points that are located five fēn above and below the umbilicus. The fontanels will close before the moxa sores heal (*Xià*《下》).

Shào Hǎi 少海 (HT 3) treats brain wind (see the section on tooth decay in *Tóng*《銅》).

Incessant bleeding from the mouth and nose is called spontaneous bleeding of the brain: Apply fifty cones of moxibustion on Shàng Xīng 上星 (Dū 23) (*Qiān*《千》).

有士人患腦熱疼，甚則自床投下，以腦拄地，或得冷水粗得，而疼終不已，服諸藥不效。人教炙囟會而愈。熱疼且可炙，況冷疼乎。凡腦痛、腦旋、腦瀉，先宜炙囟會，而強間等穴，蓋其次也。

A scholar suffered from hot pain of the brain; he would throw himself from his bed and press his head on the ground when it was severe; or pour cold water [on himself] for temporary relief, but the pain would never go away. No herbs were effective. Someone instructed him to apply moxibustion on Xìn Huì 囟會 (Dū 22) and he recovered. Even hot pain can be treated with moxibustion, as well as cold pain.

Brain pain, dizziness, and brain leakage[32]: It is appropriate to apply moxibustion on Xìn Huì (Dū 22) first; then Qiáng Jiān 強間 (Dū 18) and so forth.

32. Brain leakage indicates acute or chronic sinusitis.

腦痛 649
目眩 575
目痛 568
風癇 366

# 6.36
## *Tóu Xuán (Tóu Zhòng)*
## 頭旋（頭重）
## Spinning head [dizziness]
**(Heaviness of the head)**

目窗治忽頭旋（《銅》見目痛）。絡卻治頭旋耳鳴。天柱治頭旋（見腦痛）。岐伯灸頭旋（見目眩）。申脈治坐如在舟車中（《銅》見腰腳）。

Mù Chuāng 目窗 (GB 16) treats sudden onset of spinning head (see the section on eye pain in *Tóng*《銅》).

Luò Què 絡卻 (UB 8) treats spinning head and tinnitus.

Tiān Zhù 天柱 (UB 10) treats spinning head (see the section on brain pain).

Qí Bó applied moxibustion for spinning head (see the section on dizzy vision).

Shēn Mài 申脈 (UB 62) treats a sensation as if sitting in a boat or wagon (see the section on the lower back and legs in *Tóng*).

母氏隨執中赴任，為江風所吹，自覺頭動搖如在舟車上，如是半年，乃大吐痰，遍服痰藥，並灸頭風諸穴，方愈。

My mother followed me to my working place. The wind blew in from the river and she felt like her head was moving as if sitting in a boat or wagon. This lasted about half a year and she was spitting up a lot of phlegm. It was cured after taking herbs to treat phlegm and applying moxibustion on the various points for head wind.

治頭風搖動，灸腦後玉枕中間七壯（《千翼》）。玉枕療失枕頭重（《明》見目痛）。《下》云：療頭重如石。百會療頭重（見風癇）。百會療腦重鼻塞，頭目眩痛（《下》）。陶道療頭重目眩。

To treat head wind and dizziness: Apply seven cones of moxibustion on Yù Zhěn 玉枕 (UB 9) which is on the back of the head (*Qiān Yì*《千翼》).

頭痛 643 頭風 640 癲 343 鼻衄 620 風痹 377 勞 188

Yù Zhěn 玉枕 (UB 9) cures heaviness of the head and crick in the neck (see the section on eye pain in *Míng*《明》). *Xià*《下》says: It cures heaviness of the head that feels like a stone.

Bǎi Huì 百會 (Dū 20) cures heaviness of the head (see the section on wind epilepsy).

Bǎi Huì (Dū 20) cures brain heaviness, nasal congestion, dizziness of the head and eyes with pain (*Xià*).

Táo Dào 陶道 (Dū 13) cures heaviness of the head and dizzy vision.

率谷（見頭痛）療頭重。跗陽（見頭風）、腦戶等主頭重痛（《千》見頭痛）。至陰治頭重（《銅》見頭痛）。天柱療腦重（《明下》見腦）。啞門（見癲）、通天（見鼻衄）、跗陽（見風痹）治頭重（《銅》）。腎俞治頭重（見勞）。頭重風勞，腦戶五壯。頭重不能勝，灸腦戶下寸半（《千翼》）。

Shuài Gǔ 率谷 (GB 8) (see the section on headaches) cures heaviness of the head.

Fū Yáng 跗陽 (UB 59) (see the section on head wind), Nǎo Hù 腦戶 (Dū 17), and so forth govern heaviness and pain of the head (see the section on headaches in *Qiān*《千》).

Zhì Yīn 至陰 (UB 67) treats heaviness of the head (see the section on headaches in *Tóng*《銅》).

Tiān Zhù 天柱 (UB 10) cures heaviness of the brain (see the section on the brain [pain] in *Míng Xià*《明下》).

Yǎ Mén 啞門 (Dū 15) (see the section on withdrawal, [epilepsy, tugging and slackening]), Tōng Tiān 通天 (UB 7) (see the section on nosebleeds), and Fù Yáng (UB 59) (see the section on wind *bì*-impediment) treat heaviness of the head (*Tóng*).

Shèn Shù 腎俞 (UB 23) treats heaviness of the head (see the section on taxation).

Heaviness of the head and wind taxation: Apply five cones of moxibustion on Nǎo Hù (Dū 17).

Heaviness of the head with inability to hold it up: Apply moxibustion on the site 1.5 cùn below Nǎo Hù (Dū 17) (*Qiān Yì*《千翼》).

# 6.37
# *Tóu Zhǒng*

水腫
459

# 頭腫

## Swelling of the head

腦戶治頭腫（《銅》）。前頂療頭風熱痛，頭腫大。腫極，即以三棱針刺之，繞寸以下，其頭痛腫立瘥（《明》）。上星療頭風頭腫，皮腫面虛，鼻塞頭痛。囟會療頭皮腫，生白屑。完骨治頭面腫（《銅》見癲）。腦戶治頭腫。公孫主頭面腫。完骨等主頭面氣腫（並見水腫）。

Nǎo Hù 腦戶 (Dū 17) treats swelling of the head (*Tóng*《銅》).

Qián Dǐng 前頂 (Dū 21) cures head wind, hot pain, and swelling of the head. For extreme swelling, bleed it with a three-edged needle or bleed 1 cùn around it; the headache and swelling will be cured immediately (*Míng*《明》).

Shàng Xīng 上星 (Dū 23) cures head wind with swelling, swelling of the skin and puffy face, nasal congestion, and headaches.

Xìn Huì 囟會 (Dū 22) cures swollen scalp with white flakes.

Wán Gǔ 完骨 (GB 12) treats head and facial swelling (see the discussion of withdrawal in *Tóng*).

Nǎo Hù (Dū 17) treats swelling of the head.

Gōng Sūn 公孫 (SP 4) governs head and facial swelling.

Wán Gǔ (GB 12) governs qì swelling of the head and face (for all, see the section on edema).

驚癎
363

# 6.38
## *Dǐng Zhǒng Tòng*

# 頂腫痛

## Painful swelling of the vertex

曲差治頂痛(《銅》)。前頂治小兒驚癎頂腫(見驚癎)。

Qū Chā 曲差 (UB 4) treats pain of the vertex (*Tóng*《銅》).

Qián Dǐng 前頂 (Dū 21) treats fright epilepsy and swollen vertex in children (see the section on fright epilepsy).

澧陽有士人之子驚風後頂腫，醫以半夏、南星為細末，新水調敷而愈。若灸則宜灸前頂等穴云。

The son of a scholar in Lǐ Yáng suffered swelling of the vertex after fright wind. The doctor ground *bàn xià* 半夏 (Pinelliae Rhizoma) and *nán xīng* 南星 (Arisaematis Rhizoma) into a fine powder, mixed it with newly-drawn water and applied it topically. The disease was cured. It is appropriate to apply moxibustion on Qián Dǐng (Dū 21) and so forth.

## 6.39
## *Miàn Zhǒng (Yú Jiàn Shuǐ Zhǒng)*
## 面腫（餘見水腫）

偏風 396
頭痛 643
膝痛 536

### Facial swelling
**(for further discussion, see the section on edema)**

巨窌主面惡見寒，頰腫痛（《千》）。上星、天牖治頭風面虛腫（《銅》）。囟會治目眩（《明下》云：面赤暴腫）。前頂治面赤腫。目窗治頭面浮腫痛，引目外眥上赤痛。完骨治頭面浮腫。水溝治面腫唇動，狀如蟲行。又云：風水面腫，針此穴出水盡，頓愈。

Jù Liáo 巨窌 (ST 3) governs aversion to cold in the face and swelling and pain of the cheeks (*Qiān*《千》).

Shàng Xīng 上星 (Dū 23) and Tiān Yǒu 天牖 (SJ 16) treat head wind and puffy swelling of the face (*Tóng*《銅》).

Xìn Huì 囟會 (Dū 22) treats dizzy vision (*Míng Xià*《明下》says: facial redness with sudden onset of swelling).

Qián Dǐng 前頂 (Dū 21) treats red swollen face.

Mù Chuāng 目窗 (GB 16) treats puffy swelling and pain of the head and face with pain and redness radiating to the outer canthus.

Wán Gǔ 完骨 (GB 12) treats puffy swelling of the head and face.

Shuǐ Gōu 水溝 (Dū 26) treats facial swelling and twitching lips that look like worms crawling. It also says: For wind-water with facial swelling, needle this point to drain out the water. It will cure the disease immediately.

迎香治面癢腫（見偏風）。大迎治風壅面浮腫，目不得閉，唇吻瞤動不止，針之頓愈。合谷治面腫，唇吻不收，喑不能言，口噤不開。溫溜治面虛腫。豐隆（見頭痛）、承漿、陽交（見膝痛）治面腫。

Yíng Xiāng 迎香 (LI 20) treats itchy swollen face (see the section on hemilateral wind).

水腫 459 腦風 649

Dà Yíng 大迎 (ST 5) treats puffy swelling of the face due to wind congestion, inability to close the eyes, and incessant twitching of the lips. The disease will be cured immediately after needling this point.

Hé Gǔ 合谷 (LI 4) treats facial swelling, inability to contract the lips, loss of voice, and clenched jaws.

Wēn Liū 溫溜 (LI 7) treats vacuity swelling of the face.

Fēng Lóng 豐隆 (ST 40) (see the section on headaches), Chéng Jiāng 承漿 (Rèn 24), and Yáng Jiāo 陽交 (GB 35) (see the section on knee pain) treat facial swelling.

厲兌治寒瘧，面腫，足胻寒。陷谷（見水腫）治面目浮腫。百會治飲酒面赤（《明》見風癇）。解溪治頭風面赤。腦戶療面赤腫，頭痛（《明》）。厲兌療面浮腫。水溝（見腦風）、天牖療面腫。陷谷療頭面虛腫。

Lì Duì 厲兌 (ST 45) treats cold malaria, facial swelling, and coldness of the lower legs.

Xiàn Gǔ 陷谷 (ST 43) (see the section on edema) treats puffy swelling of the face and eyes.

Bǎi Huì 百會 (Dū 20) treats facial redness after drinking liquor (see the section on wind epilepsy in *Míng*《明》).

Jiě Xī 解溪 (ST 41) treats head wind and facial redness.

Nǎo Hù 腦戶 (Dū 17) cures red swollen face and headaches (*Míng*).

Lì Duì (ST 45) cures puffy facial swelling.

Shuǐ Gōu 水溝 (Dū 26) (see the section on brain wind) and Tiān Yǒu 天牖 (SJ 16) cure facial swelling.

Xiàn Gǔ (ST 43) cures facial swelling due to vacuity.

風池療肺風面赤，目視䀮䀮，項強不得顧，面腫皮軟，腦疼。上星、囟會、前頂、腦戶、風池主面赤腫（《千》）。陷谷、上星、囟會、前頂（並見水腫）、公孫治卒面腫（《銅》見狂言）。陷谷等、陽陵泉等、天樞等、中府等、解溪主面腫（並見水腫）。

Fēng Chí 風池 (GB 20) cures lung wind,[33] facial redness, blurred vision, stiff neck with inability to turn, facial swelling with soft skin, and brain pain.

33. Lung wind is caused by wind toxins attacking the lungs. The symptoms include itchy sores on the skin, facial sores, and redness and erosion of the tip of the nose.

Shàng Xīng 上星 (Dū 23), Xìn Huì 囟會 (Dū 22), Qián Dǐng 前頂 (Dū 21), Nǎo Hù 腦戶 (Dū 17), and Fēng Chí 風池 (GB 20) govern red swollen face (*Qiān* 《千》).

Xiàn Gǔ 陷谷 (ST 43), Shàng Xīng (Dū 23), Xìn Huì (Dū 22), Qián Dǐng (Dū 21) (for all, see the section on edema), and Gōng Sūn 公孫 (SP 4) treat sudden facial swelling (see the section on manic raving in *Tóng* 《銅》).

Xiàn Gǔ (ST 43), Yáng Líng Quán 陽陵泉 (GB 34), Tiān Shū 天樞 (ST 25), Zhōng Fǔ 中府 (LU 1) and so forth, and Jiě Xī 解溪 (ST 41) govern facial swelling (for all, see the section on edema).

有人因入水得水腫，四肢皆腫，面亦腫。人為灸水分並氣海，翌朝，視其面如削矣。恐面腫亦可灸水分云。

Someone suffered edema because he entered the water. He had swelling of the limbs and face.

Someone applied moxibustion on Shuǐ Fēn 水分 (Rèn 9) and Qì Hǎi 氣海 (Rèn 6). The next morning, people saw that his face looked slender. So it is approriate to apply moxibustion on Shuǐ Fēn (Rèn 9) for facial swelling.

咳 414 狂 345 驚 323 勞 188

# 6.40
## *Miàn Tòng (Miàn Chì, Miàn Hēi)*
## 面痛（面赤　面黑）

## Facial pain
**(Red face; black [dark] face)**

攢竹、齦交、玉枕主面赤，頰中痛(《千》)。中渚主顳顬痛，頷顱熱痛，面赤。懸厘主面皮赤痛。腎俞、內關主面赤熱。天窗、天突主面皮熱。腦戶治面赤目黃(《銅》)。懸顱治面膚赤痛。

Zǎn Zhú 攢竹 (UB 2), Yín Jiāo 齦交 (Dū 28), and Yù Zhěn 玉枕 (UB 9) govern facial redness and painful cheeks (*Qiān*《千》).

Zhōng Zhǔ 中渚 (SJ 3) governs pain of the temples, hot pain of the chin and skull, as well as facial redness.

Xuán Lí 懸厘 (GB 6) governs red painful facial skin.

Shèn Shù 腎俞 (UB 23) and Nèi Guān 內關 (PC 6) govern red hot face.

Tiān Chuāng 天窗 (SI 16) and Tiān Tū 天突 (Rèn 22) govern hot facial skin.

Nǎo Hù 腦戶 (Dū 17) treats facial redness and yellow eyes (*Tóng*《銅》).

Xuán Lú 懸顱 (GB 5) treats red painful facial skin.

行間主面蒼黑(《千》)。太衝主面塵黑。支溝(見咳)、間使(見狂)、液門(見驚)主面赤。解溪主面赤(見風)。氣海療冷病面黑(《明下》)。腎俞療面黃黑(並見勞)。關衝主面黑(見風)。

Xíng Jiān 行間 (LV 2) governs grayish black [dark] face (*Qiān*).

Tài Chōng 太衝 (LV 3) governs black [dark] face.

Zhī Gōu 支溝 (SJ 6) (see the section on cough), Jiān Shǐ 間使 (PC 5) (see the section on mania), and Yè Mén 液門 (SJ 2) (see the section on fright) govern red face.

Jiě Xī 解溪 (ST 41) governs red face (see the discussion of wind).

Qì Hǎi 氣海 (Rèn 6) cures cold diseases with a dark facial complexion (*Míng Xià* 《明下》).

Shèn Shù 腎俞 (UB 23) cures yellow and dark facial complexion (for all, see the section on taxation).

Guān Chōng 關衝 (SJ 1) governs dark facial complexion (see the discussion of wind).

# *Zhēn Jiǔ Zī Shēng Jīng*
# 《針灸資生經·第七》

# 7.01
## *Shāng Hán (Rè Bìng, Yīn Zhèng, Yáng Zhèng)*
## 傷寒（熱病　陰證　陽證）

## Cold damage
**(Heat disease; yīn disease; yáng disease)**

凡熱病刺陷谷，足先寒，寒上至膝，乃出針。身痹洗淅振寒，季脅支滿痛，熱病先腰脛酸，喜渴數飲，身清，清則項痛而寒且酸，足熱不欲言，頭痛顛顛然，先取涌泉，及太陽井滎。

For heat disease, prick Xiàn Gǔ 陷谷 (ST 43). First the feet will feel cold; when the coldness ascends up to the knees, remove the needles.

Generalized *bì*-impediment, quivering with cold as if soaked with water, propping fullness and pain of the rib-sides, heat disease first with aching low back and lower legs, thirst with desire to drink, chilly body, pain of the nape with cold aching, heat in the legs, no desire to talk, and headache with anxiety: treat Yǒng Quán 涌泉 (KI 1) first, then the *jǐng*-well and *yíng*-spring points of the tàiyáng [channels].

熱中少氣厥寒，灸之熱去：灸涌泉三壯。煩心不嗜食，灸涌泉熱去。四逆喘氣，偏風，身汗出而清：皆取俠溪。凡溫病身熱五日以上，汗不出：刺太泉留針一時取針。若未滿五日者，禁針。凡好太息，不嗜食，多寒熱汗出，病至則喜嘔，嘔已乃衰：即取公孫及井俞。

Heat strike with qì shortage and cold reversal: Apply moxibustion to remove the heat, apply three cones of moxibustion on Yǒng Quán (KI 1).

Vexation of the heart with no desire to eat: Apply moxibustion on Yǒng Quán (KI 1) to remove heat.

Limb reversal, panting, hemilateral wind, and generalized sweating with chilliness: treat Xiá Xī 俠溪 (GB 43).

Warm disease with generalized heat for five days or more and absence of sweating: needle Tài Quán 太泉 (LU 9); retain the needle for a while then remove it. If the disease has been less than five days, needling is contraindicated.

黃膽
668

Tendency to sigh, no desire to eat, frequent bouts of [sensations of] cold and heat with sweating; frequent retching at the onset of the disease but the symptoms wane after retching: treat Gōng Sūn 公孫 (SP 4) and the *jǐng*-well points.

實則腸中切痛，厥，頭面腫起，煩心狂，多飲，不嗜臥。虛則鼓脹，腹中氣大滿熱痛，不嗜食，霍亂：公孫主之。凡熱病煩心，足寒清多汗：先取然谷，後取太溪，大指間動脈，皆先補之。凡溫病可針刺五十九穴，又身之穴六百五十有五，其三十六穴，灸之有害，七十九穴，刺之為災。

In repletion, there is cutting pain of the intestines, reversal, swelling of the head and face, vexation of the heart, mania, drinking frequently, and no desire to sleep. In vacuity, there is drum distention, severe qì fullness of the abdomen with hot pain, no desire to eat, and sudden turmoil [cholera]: Gōng Sūn (SP 4) can govern this.

Heat disease with vexation of the heart, cold chilly legs, and profuse sweating: treat Rán Gǔ 然谷 (KI 2) first, then Tài Xī 太溪 (KI 3) and the vessel in the big toe. Supplement first.

In warm disease, needle the 59 points. There are 655 points in the body, but 36 points of them will do harm when moxibustion is applied and 79 points will bring disaster when needled.

江南諸師秘仲景要方不傳。顳顬穴，針灸治溫病（見黃膽）。《指迷方》灸陰毒傷寒法：其狀不躁不渴，唇青腰背重，咽喉及目睛痛，心腹煩痛，舌縮面青，吃噫氣喘，嘔逆冷汗，向暗不語。以生蔥約十餘莖，去根，粗皮，顛倒紙卷徑闊二寸，勿令緊，欲通氣；以快刀切，每一餅子高半寸，安在臍心，用熨斗火熨，蔥軟易之，不過十餘次，患人即蘇，後服正氣藥。

The doctors south of the Yángzǐ river keep [Zhāng] Zhòngjǐng's formulas secret and won't release them.

Niè Rú 顳顬 (GB 19) treats warm disease (see the section on jaundice).

*Zhǐ Mí Fāng*《指迷方》has a method of applying moxibustion for yīn toxins and cold damage: the symptoms include absence of irritability and thirst, but with green lips, heaviness of the lower and upper back, sore throat, eye pain, vexation and pain of the heart and abdomen, contracted tongue, green face, vomiting and panting, retching counterflow with cold sweats, and loss of speech. Get ten stalks of raw green onions, remove the roots and the rough peel, wrap them upside down with paper into a roll 2 cùn in diameter. Do not make it too tight so that air can flow through it; cut it with sharp knife into half cùn high cakes. Put it on the umbilicus, and iron it with an iron, change the green onions when they become soft. The patient will recover in not more than ten treatments. Then take herbs to correct the qì.

灸結胸傷寒法：其狀胸滿短氣，按之即痛，或吐逆滿悶，或大便不通，諸藥不能救者，巴豆七粒和皮，肥黃連七寸去須，同搗爛作一丸，安在臍心上，以手按下稍實緊，捻艾皂子大，於藥上灸，甚者不過三五壯，立愈。續用補藥一二日，若病半月微有氣，皆瘳。

A method of applying moxibustion for chest binds and cold damage: The symptoms include chest fullness, shortness of breath, pain upon pressure; vomiting counterflow, fullness and oppression; and constipation. For those people who cannot be saved by the various herbs. Use seven pieces of *bā dòu* 巴豆 (Crotonis Fructus) with the skin and a thick piece of *huáng lián* 黃連 (Coptidis Rhizoma) seven cùn long with the fine roots removed; grind these together into a paste and make pellets. Put one in the center of umbilicus and press it with the hands to make it firm. Roll moxa cones the size of a *zào zǐ* 皂子 (seed of Gleditsiae Fructus) and place one on the top of the herbs. If the case is serious burn no more than three or five cones and it will cure the disease immediately. The patient should take supplementing herbs for one or two days. This will cure the disease for patients who are still breathing, even if they have been sick for half a month.

治氣虛陽脫，體冷無脈，氣息欲絕，不省人事，及傷寒陰厥，百藥不效，蔥熨法：蔥以索纏如盞許大，切去根及葉，惟存白長二寸許，如大餅餤，先以火脅一面令通熱，艾勿令灼人；及以熱處搭病人臍連臍下，其上以熨斗滿貯火熨之，令蔥餅中熱氣熨入肌肉中。須預作三四餅，一餅壞不可熨，又易一餅，良久，病患當漸醒，手足溫，有汗則瘥，更服四逆湯輩溫其內，萬萬無憂。

Qì vacuity with collapse of yáng, generalized coldness with an absence of a pulse, the breath is about to expire, unconsciousness, as well as cold damage and yīn reversal: the hundred herbs are ineffective. Use the green onion ironing method: Tie a bundle of green onions together with string. Make it about the diameter of a bowl; cut off the roots and leaves, only retaining about two cùn lengths of the white stem. It will look like a big pastry. Burn mugwort on one side of it to make it hot; do not burn the mugwort on the patient. Apply the hot side to the patient's umbilicus and the area below it; put an iron full of fire on the top to iron it and let the hot qì flow from inside the green onion pastry into the flesh. Make three or four pastries in advance; change pastries when one cannot be ironed anymore. The patient will gradually wake up after a long time; the disease will recover when his limbs get warm and he sweats. In addition he should take *Sì Nì Tāng* 四逆湯 (Counterflow Cold Decoction) and similar formulas to warm the body, so he will not worry any more.

予伯兄病傷寒，冥冥不知人八日，四體堅冷如石，藥不復可入，用此遂瘥。集賢[院]校理胡全夫用此拯人之危，不可勝數（《良》）。

My cousin suffered cold damage and had been unconscious for eight days. His limbs were stiff and cold as stone, and he could not take any herbs. After applying this method, he recovered. An editor in the Jíxían [Yuàn][1] named Hú Quánfū used it to rescue people in urgent conditions; [effective] cases are countless (*Liáng*《良》)

初得病，或先頭痛身寒熱，或澀澀欲守火，或腰背強直，面目如飲酒狀，此傷寒初得一二日。但列火灸心下三處：第一處去心下一寸，名巨闕；第二處去心下二寸，名上管；第三處去心下三寸，名胃管；各灸五十壯，大人可五十壯，小兒可三壯，亦隨其年灸之，大小以意斟量（《千》）。

At the beginning of disease, people have headaches with generalized [sensations of] cold and heat; or shivering with desire to stay close to the fire; or stiff lower and upper back, and a [red] face that looks like they have just drank liquor. This is first or second day after contacting cold damage. Apply moxibustion on three sites below the heart: the first site is located one cùn below the heart, it is called Jù Quē 巨闕 (Rèn 14); the second site is located two cùn below the heart, it is called Shàng Guǎn 上管 (Rèn 13); the third site is located three cùn below the heart, it is called Wèi Guǎn 胃管 (Rèn 12).[2] Apply fifty cones of moxibustion on each site; burn fifty cones of moxibustion on adults, and three cones on children. Or apply the same number of cones as the patient's age, determining the measure of cones based on whether an adult or child (*Qiān*《千》).

若病者三四日以上，宜先灸胸上二十壯：以繩度鼻正上盡髮際，中屈繩斷去半，便從髮際入髮中灸繩頭，名曰天聰。又灸兩顳顬，又灸兩風池，又灸肝俞百壯，餘處各二十壯。又灸太衝三十壯，神驗。

If someone suffers the disease for more than three or four days, it is appropriate to apply twenty cones of moxibustion on the chest: Measure from the tip of the nose to the hairline with a string, cut the string into half, and then measure with it from the hairline. Apply moxibustion at the end of the string. It is called Tiān Cōng 天聰. Or apply twenty cones of moxibustion on the bilateral points of Niè Rú 顳顬 (GB 19) and Fēng Chí 風池 (GB 20). Burn a hundred cones on Gān Shù 肝俞 (UB 18) and twenty cones on the rest of the points. Also apply thirty cones of moxibustion on Tài Chōng 太衝 (LV 3). It is divinely effective.

凡治傷寒，惟陰證可灸，餘皆當針。故《千金方》惟云刺取，而《素問》亦云病甚者為五十九刺，所以瀉諸陽、胸中、胃中、四肢、五臟之熱也（見《熱論篇》）。若溫病身熱五日以上，汗不出，可刺太泉；未滿五日，禁針爾（《千金》）。而《千金》於頭痛，身寒，熱病，乃灸巨闕、上管，中管三處，豈亦是陰證耶？其狀蓋云或澀澀欲守火是也。醫者當辨之，

1. A bureau started in the *Táng* (唐) Dynasty. The editor who works there is called the *jí xián xiào lǐ* 集賢校理.

2. Wèi Guǎn 胃管 can refer to Rèn 12 or Rèn 13, but according to the earlier text, Shàng Guǎn 上管 (Rèn 13) is already mentioned, so here it should indicate Rèn 12.

To treat cold damage, moxibustion can only be applied on yīn patterns; acupuncture should be applied on other patterns. So *Qiān Jīn Fāng*《千金方》says to apply acupuncture [on cold damage with fevers] only and *Sù Wèn*《素問》also says to needle 59 points for serious disease, and drain heat from all the yáng channels, chest, stomach, limbs and five viscera (see the chapter called *Rè Lùn Piān*《熱論篇》(Treatise on Heat)).

For warm disease with generalized heat that has lasted for more than five days and absence of sweating, needle Tài Quán 太泉 (KI 3); if less than five days, needling is contraindicated (*Qiān Jīn*《千金》). But *Qiān Jīn* says to apply moxibustion on Jù Quē 巨闕 (Rèn 14), Shàng Guǎn 上管 (Rèn 13), and Zhōng Guǎn 中管 (Rèn 12) for headaches, cold body, and heat disease. These are not yīn patterns. The symptoms might include shivering with desire to stay close to the fire. Doctors should differentiate this.

通里治熱病，卒心中懊憹，數欠頻伸，悲恐，目眩頭痛，面赤而熱，心悸，肘臂臑痛，實則肢腫，虛則不能言，苦嘔，喉痹，少氣遺溺(《銅》)。期門治婦人傷寒。過經不解，當針期門，使經不傳。

Tōng Lǐ 通里 (HT 5) treats heat disease, sudden anguish in the heart, frequent yawning and stretching, sorrow and fear, dizzy vision, headaches, hot red face, palpitations, and pain of the elbows and arms. In repletion, there are swollen limbs; in vacuity, there is inability to speak, vomiting, throat *bì*-impediment, qì shortage, and enuresis (*Tóng*《銅》).

Qī Mén 期門 (LV 14) treats cold damage in women.

Channel passage but still unresolved[3]: it is appropriate to needle Qī Mén (LV 14); then there will be no transmission along the channels.

中管療天行傷寒(《明》)。曲澤療傷寒病溫濕，身熱口乾。膈俞主傷寒嗜臥，怠惰不欲動搖，身常濕，不能食(《千》)。少衝治熱病煩滿，上氣心痛，痰冷少氣，悲恐善(《明》作喜)驚，掌熱胸痛，口熱咽酸，乍寒乍熱，手攣不伸，引腋痛(《銅》)。

Zhōng Guǎn (Rèn 12) cures epidemic cold damage (*Míng*《明》).

Qū Zé 曲澤 (PC 3) cures cold damage with warm dampness, generalized heat, and dry mouth.

Gé Shù 膈俞 (UB 17) governs cold damage with somnolence, fatigue, no desire to move, frequent generalized dampness, and inability to eat (*Qiān*《千》).

3. Channel passage but still unresolved: This refers to a complication occurring after mistakenly using purgative treatment when evil qì has transferred from tàiyáng to shàoyáng channels; or after using vomiting and purgative treatment when an exterior pattern has already been resolved from the tàiyáng channels.

Shào Chōng 少衝 (HT 9) treats heat disease, vexation and fullness, qì ascent, heart pain, cold phlegm, qì shortage, sorrow, fear and frequent (*Míng*《明》says susceptibility to) fright, hot palms, chest pain, heat in the mouth, sour taste in the throat, sudden bouts of cold and heat, and hypertonicity of the arms with inability to stretch and pain radiating to the axilla (*Tóng*《銅》).

曲池治傷寒餘疾，皮膚乾燥。通里主熱病，先不樂數日(《千》)。魚際、陽谷主熱病，振栗鼓頷，腹滿陰痿，色不變。尺澤主氣膈喜嘔，鼓頷，不得汗。腎俞主頭身熱赤，振栗，腰中四肢淫濼，欲嘔。

Qū Chí 曲池 (LI 11) treats cold damage and other diseases, and dry skin.

Tōng Lǐ 通里 (HT 5) governs heat disease and unhappiness for several days (*Qiān*).

Yú Jì 魚際 (LU 10) and Yáng Gǔ 陽谷 (SI 5) govern heat disease, shivering, chattering of the jaws, abdominal fullness, and yīn wilting (impotence) without changes in the complexion.

Chǐ Zé 尺澤 (LU 5) governs dysphagia-occlusion, frequent retching, chattering of the jaws, and absence of sweating.

Shèn Shù 腎俞 (UB 23) governs heat and redness of the head and body, shivering, soreness and weakness of the low back and four limbs, and frequent retching.

三間主氣熱，身熱喘(《甲》云：寒熱口乾，身熱喘息，目急痛，善驚)。魚際治熱病寒栗鼓頷，腹滿陰痿，色不變。中衝、少衝、關衝、勞宮、大陵、陽溪、天窌主熱病煩心，心悶汗不出，掌中熱，心痛身熱如火，舌本痛。

Sān Jiān 三間 (LI 3) governs qì-type heat, generalized heat and panting (*Jiǎ*《甲》says: [sensations of] cold and heat, dry mouth, generalized heat, panting, acute pain of the eyes, and frequent fright).

Yú Jì (LU 10) treats heat disease with shivering and chattering of the jaws, abdominal fullness, and yīn wilting without changes in the complexion.

Zhōng Chōng 中衝 (PC 9), Shào Chōng (HT 9), Guān Chōng 關衝 (SJ 1), Láo Gōng 勞宮 (PC 8), Dà Líng 大陵 (PC 7), Yáng Xī 陽溪 (LI 5), and Tiān Liáo 天窌 (SJ 15) govern heat disease, vexation and oppression of the heart, absence of sweating, heat in the palms, heart pain, generalized heat that feels like there is fire inside, and pain at the root of the tongue.

間使主熱病煩心，喜噦，胸中澹澹，喜動而熱。巨闕主煩心喜嘔。曲澤主傷寒溫病，身熱煩心，口乾。支正、少海主熱病先腰脛酸，喜渴數飲食，身熱項強痛。天井主振寒頸項痛。委中主熱病夾脊痛。風門治傷寒頸項強，目瞑（《明》有鼻塞字），多嚏鼻鼽，出清涕（《銅》）。

Jiān Shǐ 間使 (PC 5) governs heat disease, vexation of the heart, frequent hiccups, a rolling sensation in the chest, tendency to move a lot, and heat.

Jù Quē 巨闕 (Rèn 14) governs vexation of the heart and frequent retching.

Qū Zé 曲澤 (PC 3) governs cold damage, warm disease, generalized heat, vexation of the heart, and dry mouth.

Zhī Zhèng 支正 (SI 7) and Shào Hǎi 少海 (HT 3) govern heat disease first with aching low back and lower legs, susceptibility to thirst, frequent eating and drinking, and generalized heat with stiffness and pain of the nape.

Tiān Jǐng 天井 (SJ 10) governs quivering with cold and pain of the neck and nape.

Wěi Zhōng 委中 (UB 40) governs heat disease with pain along the spine.

Fēng Mén 風門 (UB 12) treats cold damage, stiffness of the neck and nape, blurred vision (*Míng* 《明》 has nasal congestion), frequent sneezing, and running nose with clear snivel (*Tóng* 《銅》).

陰毒沉困，藥餌難為工，但灸臍中三百壯，艾如半棗。手足不暖，不可治也（見《本事方》）。或心迷耳聾叫不應，因食冷得疾者，予以理中湯救數人矣。若復渴則煎五苓散與服，或煎人參湯服，皆效。（《千金》云：傷寒多從風寒得之，始表中風寒，入裡則不消矣。未有溫覆而不消也。）

For deep oppression of yīn toxins when herbal medicine has difficulty doing its work: Apply three hundred cones of moxibustion on Qí Zhōng 臍中 (Rèn 8); burn cones the size of half of a date. It is not treatable if the limbs are cold (see [*Pǔ Jì*] *Běn Shì Fāng* 《本事方》).

If someone has confusion, deafness, and does not respond when called, and they got this condition from eating cold food, I have used *Lǐ Zhōng Tāng* 理中湯 (Center Rectifying Decoction) to rescue several such people. If the patient is thirsty, cook *Wǔ Líng Sǎn* 五苓散 (Poria Five Powder) or *Rén Shēn Tāng* 人參湯 (Ginseng Decoction) and have him drink it. They are both effective. (*Qiān Jīn* 《千金》 says: Cold damage is usually caused by wind-cold. In the beginning, the exterior is stuck by wind-cold; it will not dissipate once it enters the interior unless warm application [of herbal medicine] is used.)

# 7.02
## *Huáng Dǎn*
# 黃膽
## Jaundice

脾俞、胃管、太溪主黃膽(《千》)。然谷主黃膽，一足寒一足熱，喜渴。太衝主黃膽熱中，喜渴。中封、五里主身黃，時有微熱(《甲乙》云：不嗜食，少氣，身體重)。脊中主黃膽腹滿不能食。脾俞主黃膽喜欠，不下食，脅下滿欲吐，身重不欲動。

Pí Shù 脾俞 (UB 20), Wèi Guǎn 胃管 (Rèn 12 or Rèn 13), and Tài Xī 太溪 (KI 3) govern jaundice (*Qiān*《千》).

Rán Gǔ 然谷 (KI 2) governs jaundice, a cold sensation on one foot and a hot sensation on the other, and susceptibility to thirst.

Tài Chōng 太衝 (LV 3) governs jaundice, heat stroke, and susceptibility to thirst.

Zhōng Fēng 中封 (LV 4) and Wǔ Lǐ 五里 (LV 10) govern yellow body and frequent mild heat (*Jiǎ Yǐ*《甲乙》says: no desire to eat, qì shortage, and heavy body).

Jǐ Zhōng 脊中 (Dū 6) governs jaundice, abdominal fullness, and inability to eat.

Pí Shù (UB 20) governs jaundice, frequent yawning, inability to get food down, fullness below the rib-sides, desire to vomit, and generalized heaviness with no desire to move.

勞宮主黃膽目黃。中管、大陵主目黃振寒。脾俞治黃膽(《銅》見腹脹)。脾俞療腰身黃脹滿，腹肚泄痢，身重，四肢不收，黃膽邪氣積聚，腹痛寒熱(《明》)。章門療身黃羸瘦(《明下》見鼓脹)。

Láo Gōng 勞宮 (PC 8) governs jaundice and yellow eyes.

Zhōng Guǎn 中管 (Rèn 12) and Dà Líng 大陵 (PC 7) govern yellow eyes and quivering with cold.

Pí Shù (UB 20) treats jaundice (see the section on abdominal fullness in *Tóng*《銅》).

Pí Shù 脾俞 (UB 20) cures yellowing of the lower back with distention and fullness, diarrhea, dysentery, generalized heaviness, loss of use of the limbs, jaundice, accumulation of evil qì, abdominal pain, and [sensations of] cold and heat (*Míng* 《 明 》).

Zhāng Mén 章門 (LV 13) cures yellowing of the body and marked emaciation (see the section on drum distention in *Míng Xià* 《 明下 》).

寅門穴治馬黃黃膽。上齦里穴針三鋥，治馬黃黃膽。上腭穴針三鋥，治馬黃黃膽，四時等病。舌下穴俠舌兩邊，針治黃膽。唇裡穴針三鋥，治馬黃黃膽，寒暑溫疫。顳顬穴，針灸治四時寒暑所苦，疸氣溫病。夾人中穴，火針治馬黃黃膽疫，通身並黃，語音已不轉者。

Yín Mén 寅門 (non-channel)[4] treats horse yellow jaundice.[5]

Needle Shàng Yín Lǐ 上齦里 (non-channel)[6] three times to treat horse yellow jaundice.

Needle Shàng È 上腭 (non-channel)[7] three times to treat horse yellow jaundice and seasonal epidemic diseases.

Shé Xià 舌下 (non-channel) is located bilaterally alongside the tongue; needle it to treat jaundice.

Needle Chún Lǐ 唇裡 (non-channel)[8] three times to treat horse yellow jaundice and warm epidemics due to cold and summerheat.

Needle Niè Rú 顳顬 (GB 19) to treat people suffering from cold and summerheat all year around, jaundice qì, and warm disease.

Use a fire needle on the sides of Rén Zhōng 人中 (Dū 26) to treat horse yellow jaundice, yellow color all over the body, and slurred speech.

俠承漿穴治馬黃急疫。巨闕七壯，治馬黃黃膽急疫等病。上管灸七壯，治馬黃黃膽。男陰縫穴扳陰反向上灸，治馬黃黃膽。風府針之，治頭中百病，馬

4. Yín Mén 寅門 is located on the midline approximately 1.8 cùn posterior to the anterior hairline. According to *Qiān Jīn Yào Fāng* 《 千金要方 》: Measure from the tip of the nose to anterior hairline with a string, fold it into thirds, then measure with one third back from the anterior hairline. The point is located at the end of the string.

5. Horse yellow jaundice is a type of jaundice, but the specific details are unknown.

6. Shàng Yín Lǐ 上齦里 is located on the inner aspect of the mouth, level with Rén Zhōng 人中 (Dū 26).

7. Shàng È 上腭 is located on the upper palate, at the end of the cleft of the palate, right above the gums.

8. Chún Lǐ 唇裡 is located on the inner aspect of the lower lip, level with Chéng Jiāng 承漿 (Rèn 24).

黃黃膽。熱府針灸治馬黃黃膽。肺俞灸主黃膽，通治百毒。心俞、肝俞、脾俞、腎俞、腳後跟針灸，治馬黃黃膽，寒暑諸毒。耳中穴灸，治馬黃黃膽，寒暑疫毒。頰裡穴針，主治馬黃黃膽，寒暑溫疫，頰兩邊同法。手太陽灸隨年壯，治黃膽。臂石子頭穴，灸七壯，治馬黃黃膽。錢孔穴，灸百壯，治黃膽。太衝穴針灸，治馬黃溫疫(《千》)。

Jiá Chéng Jiāng 俠承漿 (non-channel) treats horse yellow [jaundice] and acute epidemics.

Apply seven cones of moxibustion on Jù Quē 巨闕 (Rèn 14) to treat horse yellow jaundice and other acute epidemics.

Apply seven cones of moxibustion on Shàng Guǎn 上管 (Rèn 13) to treat horse yellow jaundice.

To treat horse yellow jaundice in males, apply moxibustion on Yīn Fèng 陰縫 (non-channel) while pushing the testes out of the way.

Needle Fēng Fǔ 風府 (Dū 16) to treat the hundred diseases of the head and horse yellow jaundice.

Needle and apply moxibustion on Rè Fǔ 熱府 (GB 20 or UB 12) to treat horse yellow jaundice.

Apply moxibustion on Fèi Shù 肺俞 (UB 13) to govern jaundice and treat the hundred toxins in general.

Needle and apply moxibustion on Xīn Shù 心俞 (UB 15), Gān Shù 肝俞 (UB 18), Pí Shù 脾俞 (UB 20), Shèn Shù 腎俞 (UB 23) as well as on the heel to treat horse yellow jaundice, and all toxins due to cold and summerheat.

Needle Ěr Zhōng 耳中 (non-channel)[9] to treat horse yellow jaundice, cold, summer heat, and epidemic toxins.

Needle Jiá Lǐ 頰裡 (non-channel)[10] to treat horse yellow jaundice and warm epidemics due to [sensations of] cold and heat. Use the same method on both sides.

Apply the same number of cones as the age of patient on Shǒu Tài Yáng 手太陽[11] to treat jaundice.

Apply seven cones of moxibustion on Pì Shí Zǐ Tóu 臂石子頭 (non-channel)[12] to treat horse yellow jaundice.

---

9. Ěr Zhōng 耳中 is located on the crux of the helix, directly above auditory meatus.

10. Jiá Lǐ 頰裡 is located on the inner aspect of the mouth, level with and 1 cùn lateral (posterior) to the corners of the mouth.

11. Shǒu Tài Yáng 手太陽: The location of this point is unknown.

12. Pì Shí Zǐ Tóu 臂石子頭 should be written Bì Shí Zǐ Tóu 臂石子頭. It is located 3 cùn above Tài Yuān 太淵 (LU 9).

Apply a hundred cones of moxibustion on Qián Kǒng 錢孔 (non-channel)[13] to treat jaundice.

Needle and apply moxibustion on Tài Chōng 太衝 (LV 3) to treat horse yellow and warm epidemics (*Qiān*《千》).

五苓散治疸病發渴立效。瘀熱在裡，身黃腫，煎茵陳下（服此不效，方可針灸）。

*Wǔ Líng Sǎn* 五苓散 (Poria Five Powder) treats the onset of jaundice with thirst. It is effective immediately.

For stasis and heat inside with a yellow swollen body: Drink boiled *yīn chén* 茵陳 (Artemisiae Scopariae Herba) (needle or apply moxibustion only if this is ineffective).

# 7.03

## *Shāng Hán Tóu Tòng (Yú Jiàn Tóu Tòng)*

## 傷寒頭痛（餘見頭痛）

## Cold damage with headaches

**(for further discussion, see the section on headaches)**

溫溜主傷寒寒熱，頭痛噦衄，肩不舉（《千》）。懸顱主熱病頭痛身熱。懸厘、鳩尾主熱病偏頭痛，引目外眥。少澤主振寒，小指不用，頭痛。神道、關元主身熱頭痛，進退往來。三焦俞主頭痛，食不下。

Wēn Liū 溫溜 (LI 7) governs cold damage, [sensations of] cold and heat, headaches, belching, nosebleeds, and inability to raise the shoulders (*Qiān*).

Xuán Lú 懸顱 (GB 5) governs heat disease with headaches and generalized heat.

Xuán Lí 懸厘 (GB 6) and Jiū Wěi 鳩尾 (Rèn 15) govern heat disease with hemilateral headaches and pain radiating to the outer canthus.

Shào Zé 少澤 (SI 1) governs quivering with cold, loss of use of the little finger, and headaches.

13. Qián Kǒng 錢孔 is located on the line between the nipples and umbilicus, at the junction of this line and the lower border of the rib cage.

傷寒 661 傷寒寒 673 寒熱 675

Shén Dào 神道 (Dū 11) and Guān Yuán 關元 (Rèn 4) govern generalized heat that comes and goes with headaches.

Sān Jiāo Shù 三焦俞 (UB 22) governs headaches and difficulty getting food down.

太白主熱病，先頭重顏痛，煩悶心身熱，熱爭則腰痛不可俯仰，又熱病滿悶不得臥，身重骨痛不相知。溫溜治傷寒身熱，頭痛噦逆，肩不得舉（《銅》）。風池治頭痛。魚際、液門、中渚、通里主頭痛（《千》）。

Tài Bái 太白 (SP 3) governs heat disease that first has heaviness of the head and facial pain, vexation and oppression of the heart, and heat in the body; when the heat contends, there is inability to bend the lower back forward and backward; or heat disease with fullness and oppression, inability to sleep, generalized heaviness, painful bones, and unconsciousness.

Wēn Liū 溫溜 (LI 7) treats cold damage with generalized heat, headaches, belching counterflow, and inability to lift the shoulders (*Tóng*《銅》).

Fēng Chí 風池 (GB 20) treats headaches.

Yú Jì 魚際 (LU 10), Yè Mén 液門 (SJ 2), Zhōng Zhǔ 中渚 (SJ 3), and Tōng Lǐ 通里 (HT 5) govern headaches (*Qiān*《千》).

天池療頭痛（此見寒熱）。支正等主頭眩痛（見傷寒寒熱）。頭痛顛顛然，先取涌泉云云（見傷寒）。魚際療頭痛汗不出（見寒熱）。

Tiān Chí 天池 (PC 1) cures headaches (for this, see the section on [sensations of] cold and heat).

Zhī Zhèng 支正 (SI 7) and so forth govern dizziness and headaches (see the section on cold damage and [sensations of] cold and heat).

Headaches with anxiety: Treat Yǒng Quán 涌泉 (KI 1) first (see the section on cold damage).

Yú Jì (LU 10) cures headaches with absence of sweating (see the section on [sensations of] cold and heat).

治傷寒頭痛藥多矣，惟濃煎五苓散服，必效，不必針灸。予屢施與人皆效故也。

There are a lot of herbs to treat cold damage with headaches, but only a concentrated decoction of *Wǔ Líng Sǎn* 五苓散 (Poria Five Powder) is absolutely effective. Acupuncture is not necessary. I use it to treat patients and it always effective.

# 7.04

## *Shāng Hán Hán Rè (Yú Jiàn Zì Hàn, Shāng Hán Wú Hàn)*

## 傷寒寒熱（餘見自汗　傷寒無汗）

## Cold damage, [sensations of] cold and heat

**(for further discussion, see the sections on spontaneous sweating, and cold damage with absence of sweating)**

支正、少海主熱病，先腰脛酸，喜渴，身熱項強，振寒寒熱。《甲》云：主振寒寒熱，頸項腫，實則肘攣頭眩痛，虛則生疣痂（《千》）。曲澤主傷寒溫病，身熱煩心，口乾。《甲》云：主心澹善驚，身熱煩心，口乾手清，逆氣嘔唾，肘瘛，善搖頭顏青，汗出不過眉。

Zhī Zhèng 支正 (SI 7) and Shào Hǎi 少海 (HT 3) govern heat disease, first with aching low back and lower legs, frequent thirst, generalized heat, neck stiffness, quivering with cold, and [sensations of] cold and heat. *Jiǎ*《甲》says: They govern shivering with cold, [sensations of] cold and heat, and swollen neck and nape. In repletion, there is hypertonicity of the elbows, dizziness, and headaches; in vacuity, there are warts and scabs (*Qiān*《千》).

Qū Zé 曲澤 (PC 3) governs cold damage, warm disease, generalized heat, vexation of the heart, and dry mouth. *Jiǎ* says: It governs a rolling sensation in the heart, susceptibility to fright, generalized heat, vexation of the heart, dry mouth, cool hands, qì counterflow, vomiting and spitting, slack elbows, frequent shaking of the head, green-blue facial complexion, and sweating that does not go past the eyebrows.

三間主氣熱身熱喘。《甲》云：寒熱口乾，身熱喘息，口急痛，善驚。肩貞主寒熱項適歷。《甲》云：耳鳴無聞，引缺盆、肩中熱痛，麻小不舉。溫溜主傷寒寒熱頭痛。商丘主寒熱好嘔。

Sān Jiān 三間 (LI 3) governs qì-type heat, generalized heat, and panting. *Jiǎ* says: It treats [sensations of] cold and heat, dry mouth, generalized heat, panting, acute pain of the mouth, and susceptibility to fright.

Jiān Zhēn 肩貞 (SI 9) governs [sensations of] cold and heat and scrofula of the neck. *Jiǎ* says: It treats tinnitus, inability to hear, hot pain radiating between the empty basin and the shoulders, numbness, and mild inability to lift [the shoulders].

Wēn Liū 溫溜 (LI 7) governs cold damage, [sensations of] cold and heat, and headaches.

Shāng Qiū 商丘 (SP 5) governs [sensations of] cold and heat and frequent vomiting.

大椎主傷寒熱盛煩嘔。膈俞、中府主寒熱，皮肉骨痛，少氣不得臥，支滿。肩井、關衝主寒熱淒索，氣上不得臥。列缺主寒熱掌中熱。曲池主傷寒餘熱不盡。天井主傷寒振寒，頸項痛。衝陽主振寒而欠。後溪主身熱惡寒。

Dà Zhuī 大椎 (Dū 14) governs [sensations of] cold and heat, vexation, and vomiting with exuberant heat.

Gé Shù 膈俞 (UB 17) and Zhōng Fǔ 中府 (LU 1) govern [sensations of] cold and heat, pain of the skin, flesh, and bones, qì shortage with inability to lie down, and propping fullness.

Jiān Jǐng 肩井 (GB 21) and Guān Chōng 關衝 (SJ 1) govern [sensations of] cold and heat, qì ascent, and inability to lie down.

Liè Quē 列缺 (LU 7) governs [sensations of] cold and heat and heat in the palms.

Qū Chí 曲池 (LI 11) governs [sensations of] cold and heat with residual heat.

Tiān Jǐng 天井 (SJ 10) governs [sensations of] cold and heat, quivering with cold, and pain of the neck and nape.

Chōng Yáng 衝陽 (ST 42) governs quivering with cold and yawning.

Hòu Xī 後溪 (SI 3) governs generalized heat and aversion to cold.

肩痛 486
勞瘵 188

# 7.05

## *Hán Rè (Yòu Jiàn shāng Hán Hán Rè, Zhòng Fēng Hán Rè)*

# 寒熱（又見傷寒寒熱　中風寒熱）

## [Sensations of] cold and heat

**(also see the sections on cold damage with [sensations of] cold and heat, and wind stroke with [sensations of] cold and heat)**

復溜治骨寒熱汗注不止（《銅》）。至陽治寒熱解散，淫濼脛酸，四肢重痛，少氣難言（《明》同）。光明治身解寒，淫濼脛酸，不能久立。啞門治寒熱風痙，脊強反折（《銅》）。

Fù Liū 復溜 (KI 7) treats [sensations of] cold and heat in the bones and incessant pouring of sweat (*Tóng*《銅》).

Zhì Yáng 至陽 (Dū 9) treats [sensations of] cold and heat, sluggishness, weak and aching lower legs, heavy painful limbs, qì shortage, and difficulty speaking (*Míng*《明》agrees).

Guāng Míng 光明 (GB 37) treats sluggish body with a cold sensation, weak aching lower legs, and inability to stand for long.

Yǎ Mén 啞門 (Dū 15) treats [sensations of] cold and heat, wind tetany, and arched-back rigidity (*Tóng*).

陶道、神堂（見肩痛）、風池治灑淅寒熱。陰郄治灑淅畏寒，厥逆。魚際治灑淅惡風寒，虛熱，舌黃身熱，頭痛咳嗽，汗不出，痹走胸背痛，不得息。浮白治發寒熱。腎俞治頭重身熱（見勞瘵）。顱囟治身熱頭重，脅痛不得轉側。

Táo Dào 陶道 (Dū 13), Shén Táng 神堂 (UB 44) (see the section on [aching] pain of the shoulders [and back]), and Fēng Chí 風池 (GB 20) treat [sensations of] cold and heat with aversion to cold as if after soaking in the rain.

Yīn Xī 陰郄 (HT 6) treats aversion to cold as if after soaking in the rain and reverse counterflow.

Yú Jì 魚際 (LU 10) treats aversion to wind-cold as if after soaking in the rain, vacuity heat, yellow tongue, generalized heat, headaches, cough, absence of sweating, *bì*-impediment with pain of the chest and back, and inability to breathe.

腹脹 211
勞瘵 188
傷寒 661
頭痛 643
腋腫 496
痰 399

Fú Bái 浮白 (GB 10) treats onset of [sensations of] cold and heat.

Shèn Shù 腎俞 (UB 23) treats heaviness of the head and generalized heat (see the section on consumption).

Lú Xìn 顱囟 (SJ 19) treats generalized heat, heaviness of the head, pain of the rib-sides, and inability to turn to the sides.

太白、陽綱治身熱（並見腹脹）。曲差治身體煩熱。腦空治勞疾羸瘦，體熱。肺俞治寒熱喘滿（見勞瘵）。天池治寒熱胸膈滿（見膈滿）。少衝治乍寒乍熱（見傷寒）。神道（見頭痛）、少海治寒熱。

Tài Bái 太白 (SP 3) and Yáng Gāng 陽綱 (UB 48) treat generalized heat (see the section on abdominal fullness).

Qū Chà 曲差 (UB 4) treats vexation and heat in the body.

Nǎo Kōng 腦空 (GB 19) treats taxation, marked emaciation, and generalized heat.

Fèi Shù 肺俞 (UB 13) treats [sensations of] cold and heat and panting fullness (see the section on consumption).

Tiān Chí 天池 (PC 1) treats [sensations of] cold and heat and fullness of the chest and diaphragm (see the discussion of fullness of the diaphragm).

Shào Chōng 少衝 (HT 9) treats sudden bouts of cold and heat (see the section on [sensations of] cold and heat).

Shén Dào 神道 (Dū 11) (see the section on headaches) and Shào Hǎi 少海 (HT 3) treat [sensations of] cold and heat.

膽俞治振寒（見頭痛）。臨泣治灑淅振寒（見腋腫）。魚際療虛熱灑灑毛豎，惡風寒，舌上黃，身熱咳嗽喘，痹走胸背不得息，頭痛甚，汗不出，熱煩心，少氣不足（《明》）。膈俞療寒熱骨痛（見痰）。

Dǎn Shù 膽俞 (UB 19) treats quivering with cold (see the section on headaches).

Lín Qì 臨泣 (GB 15 or GB 41) treats quivering with cold as if after soaking in the rain (see the section on swelling of the axilla).

Yú Jì 魚際 (LU 10) cures vacuity heat, [aversion to cold] as if after soaking in the rain with the body-hair raised, aversion to wind-cold, yellow tongue, generalized heat, cough and panting, *bì*-impediment of the chest and back, inability to breathe, severe headaches, absence of sweating, heat vexation, and qì shortage (*Míng*《明》).

Gé Shù 膈俞 (UB 17) cures [sensations of] cold and heat and pain of the bones (see the section on phlegm [drool]).

頸腫 636
勞 188
虛損 174

天突（見頸腫）療身寒熱（《下》）。腦空療身寒熱，引項強急。飛揚、光明主寒熱（《千》見傷寒無汗）。臟腑積聚，心腹滿，腰背痛，飲食不消，吐逆，寒熱往來，小便不利，羸瘦少氣，三焦俞隨年（又見勞）；又胃管百壯（至千壯佳）。

Tiān Tū 天突 (Rèn 22) (see the section on [acute] swelling of the neck) cures generalized [sensations of] cold and heat (*Xià*《下》).

Nǎo Kōng 腦空 (GB 19) cures generalized [sensations of] cold and heat that induces stiffness and tension of the nape.

Fēi Yáng 飛揚 (UB 58) and Guāng Míng 光明 (GB 37) govern [sensations of] cold and heat (see the section on cold damage with absence of sweating in *Qiān*《千》).

Accumulations and binds in the organs, fullness of the heart and abdomen, lower and upper back pain, non-dispersion of food, vomiting counterflow, alternating [sensations of] cold and heat, inhibited urination, marked emaciation, and qì shortage: Apply same number of cones as the age of the patient on Sānjiāo Shù 三焦俞 (UB 22) (also see the section on taxation); or burn a hundred cones on Wèi Guǎn 胃管 (Rèn 12 or Rèn 13) (it is good to burn up to a thousand cones).

小腸俞主三焦寒熱（如灸腎法），隨年。又膀胱、三焦津液下，大小腸寒熱，赤泄洞痢，腰脊痛。又小便不利，婦人帶下，五十壯。四肢寒熱，腰疼不得俯仰，身黃腹滿，食嘔，舌根直：灸脾俞並椎三穴，各七壯。盜汗，寒熱惡寒：肺俞隨年壯，針五分；又陰都百壯。多汗寒熱，玉枕五十（《千翼》）。涌泉主身體腰脊如解（見虛損）。

Xiǎo Cháng Shù 小腸俞 (UB 27) governs [sensations of] cold and heat in the sānjiāo (the same indications as the kidney moxibustion); burn the same number of cones as the patient's age. It also governs the descent of fluids from the urinary bladder and sānjiāo, cold and heat in the large and small intestines, red diarrhea, throughflux diarrhea, pain of the lower back and spine, inhibited urination, and abnormal vaginal discharge: Apply fifty cones of moxibusiton.

[Sensations of] cold and heat of the limbs, lower back pain with inability to bend forward and backward, yellow body, abdominal fullness, vomiting after eating, and stiff root of the tongue: Apply seven cones of moxibustion on the three points of Pí Shù 脾俞 (UB 20) and the vertebra [the point below the spinous process at the same level].

腹痛 209 Night sweating, [sensations of] cold and heat, and aversion to cold: Apply the same number of cones as the patient's age on Fèi Shù 肺俞 (UB 13); needle five fēn deep. Or apply a hundred cones of moxibustion on Yīn Dū 陰都 (KI 19).

Profuse sweating with [sensations of] cold and heat: Apply fifty cones of moxibustion on Yù Zhěn 玉枕 (UB 9) (*Qiān Yì*《千翼》).

Yǒng Quán 涌泉 (KI 1) governs a feeling in the body as if the lower back and spine were separated (see the section on vacuity detriment).

## 7.06

## *Fù Hán Rè Qì (Lěng Qì, Yòu Jiàn Láo)*

# 腹寒熱氣（冷氣　又見勞）

### Cold and hot qì in the abdomen

**(Cold qì; also see the section on taxation)**

行間主腹痛而熱（《千》）。中極主腹中熱（並見腹痛）。五臟熱，及身體熱，脈弦急：著灸第十四椎，與臍相當，五十壯。老小增損之。若虛寒至百壯，橫三間寸灸之。氣衝主身熱（腹痛）。

Xíng Jiān 行間 (LV 2) governs abdominal pain with heat (*Qiān*《千》).

Zhōng Jí 中極 (Rèn 3) governs heat in the abdomen (for all, see the section on abdominal pain).

Heat in five viscera, generalized heat, and a wiry tense pulse: Apply fifty cones of moxibustion on the fourteenth vertebra, which is level with the umbilicus. Adjust the number of the cones according to the age of the person. Apply a hundred cones of moxibustion for vacuity cold, following [the technique of] *héng sān jiān cùn* (Transverse Three Cùn Method).[14]

Qì Chōng 氣衝 (ST 30) governs generalized heat (see the section on abdominal pain).

凡腹中熱，喜渴涎出，是蛔也。手持之，勿令得移，以針刺中管（亦不可容易針）。氣衝主腹中大熱不安（見腹脹）。關元主寒氣入腹。久冷：灸天樞

14. *Héng Sān Jiān Cùn* 橫三間寸 (Transverse Three Cùn Method) is a moxibustion technique. It is usually used as suppurating moxibustion. It is further discussed in Volume 2.

百壯（見癥瘕）。陰陵泉（見水腫）、三陰交（見痃癖）治腹寒。隱白療腹中寒熱（《明》見腹脹）。

癥瘕 435
水腫 459
痃癖 433
瘛瘲 354
傷寒 661
積聚 437

Heat in the abdomen and frequent thirst with drooling is due to round worms. Hold [the the mass of worms] with your hand and do not let them move; then needle Zhōng Guǎn 中管 (Rèn 12) (This cannot be needled carelessly).

Qì Chōng 氣衝 (ST 30) governs severe heat in the abdomen with restlessness (see the section on abdominal fullness).

Guān Yuán 關元 (Rèn 4) governs cold qì entering the abdomen.

Enduring cold: Apply a hundred cones of moxibustion on Tiān Shū 天樞 (ST 25) (see the section on concretions and conglomerations).

Yīn Líng Quán 陰陵泉 (SP 9) (see the section on edema) and Sān Yīn Jiāo 三陰交 (SP 6) (see the section on strings and aggregations) treat cold in the abdomen.

Yǐn Bái 隱白 (SP 1) cures [sensations of] cold and heat in the abdomen (see the section on abdominal fullness in *Míng*《明》).

下廉療熱風冷痹。上關等主寒熱（《千》見瘛瘲癲）。飛揚等治寒熱（《銅》各見癲疾）。啞門等治寒熱（見瘛瘲）。少衝治乍寒乍熱（見傷寒）。岐伯云：但是積冷虛乏病，皆宜灸關元（《明下》）。

Xià Lián 下廉 (LI 8) cures heat, wind, and cold *bì*-impediment.

Shàng Guān 上關 (GB 3) and so forth govern [sensations of] cold and heat (see the sections on tugging and slackening as well as withdrawal in *Qiān*《千》).

Fēi Yáng 飛揚 (UB 58) and so forth treat [sensations of] cold and heat (see the section on withdrawal and epilepsy in *Tóng*《銅》).

Yǎ Mén 啞門 (Dū 15) and so forth treat [sensations of] cold and heat (see the section on tugging and slackening).

Shào Chōng 少衝 (HT 9) treats sudden bouts of cold and heat (see the section on cold damage). Qí Bó said: It is appropriate to apply moxibustion on Guān Yuán (Rèn 4) to treat cold accumulations and fatigue (*Míng Xià*《明下》).

三里療臟腑久積冷氣，心腹脹滿。天樞療久積冷氣，繞臍切痛，時上衝心（《銅》同）。中極療冷氣（見積聚）。漏谷（見痃癖）、會陽治冷氣（《銅》見泄瀉）。下管治六腑氣寒，不嗜食。氣海治冷氣上衝心。

上氣 420
結氣 426
腹滿 445
心痛 312

Sān Lǐ 三里 (ST 36) cures enduring accumulations of cold qì in the viscera and bowels and distention and fullness of the heart and abdomen.

Tiān Shū 天樞 (ST 25) cures enduring accumulations of cold qì and cutting pain around umbilicus that frequently rushes upward to the heart (*Tóng*《銅》agrees).

Zhōng Jí 中極 (Rèn 3) cures cold qì (see the section on accumulations and binds).

Lòu Gǔ 漏谷 (SP 7) (see the section on strings and aggregations) and Huì Yáng 會陽 (UB 35) treat cold qì (see the section on diarrhea in *Tóng*).

Xià Guǎn 下管 (Rèn 10) treats cold qì in the six bowels with no desire to eat.

Qì Hǎi 氣海 (Rèn 6) treats cold qì rushing upward to the heart.

隱白主腹中寒冷氣，脹滿（《千》）。太衝主上氣冷發，腹中雷鳴（見上氣）。結氣寒冷：灸太倉百壯（見結氣）。凡臍下絞痛，流入陰中，發作無時，此冷氣：灸關元百壯。商丘主心下寒（見腹滿）。鳩尾、少衝、商丘主心寒，冷氣上：灸龍頷百壯（並心痛）。陽交主寒厥驚狂。衝門治腹寒氣滿（《銅》見積聚）。

Yǐn Bái 隱白 (SP 1) governs cold in the abdomen due to cold qì, distention, and fullness (*Qiān*《千》).

Tài Chōng 太衝 (LV 3) governs qì ascent due to cold and thunderous rumbling in the abdomen (see the section on qì ascent).

Qì binds and coldness: Apply a hundred cones of moxibustion on Tài Cāng 太倉 (Rèn 12) (see the section on bound up qì).

Colicky pain below the umbilicus radiating into the genitals, occurring randomly, this is cold qì: Apply a hundred cones of moxibustion on Guān Yuán 關元 (Rèn 4).

Shāng Qiū 商丘 (SP 5) governs cold below the heart (see the section on abdominal fullness).

Jiū Wěi 鳩尾 (Rèn 15), Shào Chōng 少衝 (HT 9), and Shāng Qiū (SP 5) govern cold in the heart. Cold qì running upward: Apply a hundred cones of moxibustion on Lóng Hàn 龍頷 (non-channel)[15] (together with heart pain).

Yáng Jiāo 陽交 (GB 35) governs cold reversal, fright, and mania.

Chōng Mén 衝門 (SP 12) treats abdominal coldness and qì fullness (see the section on accumulations and binds in *Tóng*).

15. Lóng Hàn 龍頷 is located approximately 1.5 cùn above Jiū Wěi 鳩尾 (Rèn 15).

《千金翼》云：五勞六極，復生七傷，變生七氣。積聚堅牢如杯，留在腹內，心痛煩冤，不食，時來時去，發作無常。寒氣為病，則吐逆心滿；熱氣為病，則恍惚悶亂，長如眩冒，又復失精云云。宜服局方七氣湯。若冷氣忽作，藥灸不及，只用火針微刺諸穴與疼處，須臾即定，神效。

*Qiān Jīn Yì*《千金翼》says: The five taxations and six extremes generate the seven damages, and then transform into the seven qì. Accumulations and binds are as hard as a cup and stay inside the abdomen, [with additional symptoms of] heart pain and vexation, inability to eat, and [these symptoms] come and go without regular timing.

In diseases caused by cold qì, [the patient has] vomiting counterflow and fullness of the heart; in diseases caused by hot qì, [the patient has] abstraction, oppression and confusion, dizziness, and seminal loss. It is appropriate to take *Qī Qì Tāng* 七氣湯 (Seven Qì Decoction) from *Jú Fāng* 局方. For sudden onset of cold qì which cannot be reached by herbs and moxibustion, just use a fire needle to prick the various points and the painful area. This will settle the problem immediately. It has divine effects.

## 7.07
## Shēn Hán Bì (Shī Bì Bù Rén, Yòu Jiàn Shǒu Zú Bì Bù Rén)

# 身寒痹（濕痹不仁　又見手足痹不仁）

### Generalized cold *bì*-impediment
**(Damp *bì*-impediment with numbness;**
**also see the section on *bì*-impediment of the limbs with numbness)**

膈俞（《明》同）治身常濕（《銅》見痃癖）。豐隆主身濕（《千》）。曲池、列缺主身濕搖，時時寒。中封主痿厥，身體不仁，少氣濕重。合陽主膝股重。漏谷主久濕痹不能行。《銅》云：不能久立。

Gé Shù 膈俞 (UB 17) (*Míng*《明》agrees) treats frequent generalized dampness (see the section on strings and aggregations in *Tóng*《銅》).

Fēng Lóng 豐隆 (ST 40) governs generalized dampness (*Qiān*《千》).

Qū Chí 曲池 (LI 11) and Liè Quē 列缺 (LU 7) govern generalized dampness with shaking, and frequent cold in the body.

Zhōng Fēng 中封 (LV 4) governs wilting reversal, generalized numbness, qì shortage, and severe dampness.

Hé Yáng 合陽 (UB 55) governs heavy knees and thighs.

Lòu Gǔ 漏谷 (SP 7) governs damp *bì*-impediment and inability to walk. *Tóng* says: It treats inability to stand for long.

懸鐘主濕痹不腫，髀筋急瘛脛痛。絕骨主髀軀痛，膝脛骨搖，酸痹不仁，筋縮，諸節酸折。臨泣主身痹，洗淅振寒。商丘主骨痹煩滿。凡身體不仁，先取京骨，後取中封、絕骨，皆瀉之。中封主痿厥，身體不仁，少氣濕重，膝腫。

Xuán Zhōng 懸鐘 (GB 39) governs damp *bì*-impediment without swelling, tugging, and tension of the sinews of the thighs with lower leg pain.

膝痛 536
月事 735

Jué Gǔ 絕骨 (GB 39)[16] governs pain of the hips and body, shaking of the knees and lower leg bones, aching *bì*-impediment and numbness, sinew contraction, and aching joints that feel as if they are broken.

Lín Qì 臨泣 (GB 41) governs generalized *bì*-impediment and quivering with cold as if after soaking in the rain.

Shāng Qiū 商丘 (SP 5) governs bone *bì*-impediment, vexation and fullness.

Numbness of the body: Drain Jīng Gǔ 京骨 (UB 64) first, then Zhōng Fēng 中封 (LV 4) and Jué Gǔ (GB 39).

Zhōng Fēng (LV 4) governs wilting reversal, numbness of the body, qì shortage, severe dampness, and swelling of the knees.

風市主緩縱痿痹，腨腸疼冷不仁。中瀆主寒氣在分肉間痛，苦痹不仁。陽關主膝外廉痛，不可屈伸，脛痹不仁。絕骨主痠痹不仁，又主身重（見《上》）。環跳治冷風濕痹（《銅》見腰痛）。條口（見膝痛）治濕痹。

Fēng Shì 風市 (GB 31) governs weakness, slackening, wilting, *bì*-impediment, and calf pain with coldness and numbness.

Zhōng Dú 中瀆 (GB 32) governs cold qì in the flesh with pain, *bì*-impediment, and numbness.

Yáng Guān 陽關 (GB 33) governs pain of the outer aspect of the knees, inability to flex and stretch, and numbness of the lower legs.

Jué Gǔ (GB 39) governs aching *bì*-impediment with numbness and generalized heaviness (see *Shàng* 《上》).

Huán Tiào 環跳 (GB 30) treats cold, wind, and damp *bì*-impediment (see lower back pain in *Tóng* 《銅》).

Tiáo Kǒu 條口 (ST 38) (see the section on knee pain) treats damp *bì*-impediment.

下髎治寒濕內傷（見月事）。委中療風濕痹（《明》見腳弱）。下廉療偏風熱風，冷痹不遂，風濕痹，灸瘡瘥，冷痹即已。魚際療痹走胸背（《明》見寒熱，《銅》同）。

Xià Liáo 下髎 (UB 34) treats cold-damp internal damage (see the section on menstruation).

16. According to *Qiān Jīn Yào Fāng* 《千金要方》, Volume 30, Jué Gǔ 絕骨 (GB 39) should be Yáng Fǔ 陽輔 (GB 38).

Wěi Zhōng 委中 (UB 40) cures wind-damp *bì*-impediment (see the section on weak legs in *Míng*《明》).

Xià Lián 下廉 (ST 39) cures hemilateral wind and hot wind, cold *bì*-impediment and paralysis, and wind-damp *bì*-impediment; cold *bì*-impediment will be cured after the moxa sores heal.

Yú Jì 魚際 (LU 10) cures *bì*-impediment running through the chest and back (see the section on [sensations of] cold and heat in *Míng*; *Tóng*《銅》agrees).

治冷痹脛膝疼，腰腳攣急，足冷氣上，不能久立，有時厭厭嗜臥，手足沉重，日覺羸瘦，名復連病。令人極無情地，常愁不樂，健忘嗔喜。有如此候，即當灸懸鐘、絕骨隨年，一灸即愈，不得再灸也。若年月久更發，依法更灸。若意便欲多者，七日外更七壯。《千翼·虛損論》曰：疾之所起，生自五勞，五勞既用，二臟先損，心腎受邪，即生六極。一曰氣極，氣極令內虛。五臟不足，外受邪氣，多寒濕痹云云。又曰：五勞六極七傷，七氣積聚，變為病者。甚則令人得大風緩急，濕痹不仁，偏枯筋縮，四肢拘攣，令人無子云云。

Cold *bì*-impediment with knee and lower leg pain, hypertonicity of the lower back and legs, cold legs with qì ascent, inability to stand for long, frequent feeling of sleepiness, heavy limbs, and gradually becoming markedly emaciated: This is called *fù lián* 復連 disease. It usually makes people apathetic, constantly worried, unhappy, and forgetful, [or] with alternating anger and joy. If someone has these symptoms, apply moxibustion on Xuán Zhōng 懸鐘 (GB 39) [also known as] Jué Gǔ 絕骨 (GB 39). Burn the same number of cones as the patient's age. Once the disease is cured, no more moxibustion should be applied.

If the disease returns years later, follow this method and apply moxibustion again. If someone wants to do more, apply seven cones of moxibustion after seven days. *Qiān Yì · Xū Sǔn Lùn*《千翼·虛損論》says: Disease arises from five taxations. The five taxations first damage the heart and kidneys, then generate the six extremes. One of them is called qì extreme and can lead to internal vacuity. Insufficiency of the five viscera inside and attack of evil qì outside with cold-damp *bì*-impediment will arise. It also says: The five taxations, six extremes, and seven damages, as well as accumulations of the seven qì, can induce disease. In severe cases, this makes people suffer severe acute wind, damp *bì*-impediment with numbness, hemilateral paralysis and contraction of the sinews, hypertonicity of the limbs, and infertility.

# 7.08

## *Zì Hàn (Shāng Hán Zì Hàn, Dào Hàn)*

# 自汗（傷寒自汗　盜汗）

## Spontaneous sweating

**(Cold damage, spontaneous sweating, night sweating)**

玉枕（見目痛）療多汗（《明》）。膈俞（見痰）療汗出。陰蹻療女人汗出（見月事）。陰蹻等（見腹痛）主汗出（《千》）。飛揚、涌泉、頷厭、後頂主頸項疼，歷節汗出。崑崙主瘧多汗（《千》）。然谷主溫瘧汗出。

目痛 568
月事 735
腹痛 441
卒疝 213
瘰歷 702
肺氣 412
喜噫 281
瘧 301
勞 188

Yù Zhěn 玉枕 (UB 9) (see the section on eye pain) cures profuse sweating (*Míng*《明》).

Gé Shù 膈俞 (UB 17) (see the section on phlegm [drool]) cures sweating.

Yīn Qiāo 陰蹻 (KI 6 or KI 8) cures sweating in women (see the section on menstruation).

Yīn Qiāo (KI 6 or KI 8) and so forth (see the section on abdominal pain) govern sweating (*Qiān*《千》).

Fēi Yáng 飛揚 (UB 58), Yǒng Quán 涌泉 (KI 1), Hàn Yàn 頷厭 (GB 4), and Hòu Dǐng 後頂 (Dū 19) govern pain of the neck and nape and joint-running with sweating.

Kūn Lún 崑崙 (UB 60) governs malaria with profuse sweating (*Qiān*).

Rán Gǔ 然谷 (KI 2) governs warm malaria with sweating.

復溜治骨寒熱，汗注不止（《銅》）。大敦治心痛汗出（見卒疝）。缺盆治汗出（見瘰歷）。中府治風汗出（見肺氣）。少商治汗出而寒（見喜噫）。衝陽主汗出（見瘧），灸手足心熱盜汗（見勞）。

Fù Liū 復溜 (KI 7) treats [sensations of] cold and heat in the bones with incessant pouring of sweat (*Tóng*《銅》).

Dà Dūn 大敦 (LV 1) treats heart pain and sweating (see the discussion of sudden *shàn*-mounting).

Quē Péng 缺盆 (ST 12) treats sweating (see the section on scrofula).

Zhōng Fǔ 中府 (LU 1) treats sweating during wind attack (see the section on lung qì).

Shào Shāng 少商 (LU 11) treats sweating while feeling cold (see the section on [frequent] belching).

Chōng Yáng 衝陽 (ST 42) governs sweating (see the section on malaria). For heat in the palms and soles with night sweating: Apply moxibustion (see the section on taxation).

牡蠣散治臥即盜汗，風虛頭痛。牡蠣熬黃、白朮、防風各三兩，酒服方寸匕，日二。止汗之驗，無出此方。一切泄汗服之，三日皆愈。此《千金方》所載也。《本事方》云：如惡風加防風一倍，氣虛加朮，面腫加牡蠣，蓋增益之也。亦有牡蠣散治虛勞盜汗不止，牡蠣煅、麻黃根、黃耆等分為末。每二錢，水一盞煎七分，溫服。予皆用之驗，故附此（《本事》又有二方）。

*Mŭ Lì Săn* 牡蠣散 (Oyster Shell Powder) treats night sweating while asleep, wind vacuity, and headaches. Take three liǎng each of *mŭ lì* 牡蠣 (Ostreae Cocha) that has been fried until yellow, *bái zhú* 白朮 (Atractylodis Macrocephalae Rhizoma), and *fáng féng* 防風 (Saphshnikoviae Gruel), and drink a square-inch spoonful with liquor twice a day. Nothing else can stop sweating as effectively as this. Taking this formula for three days can treat all leakage of sweat. This is what was recorded in *Qiān Jīn Fāng*《千金方》.

[*Pŭ Jì*] *Běn Shì Fāng*《本事方》says: Double the dosage of *fáng féng* (Saposhnikoviae Radix Gruel), for aversion to cold, increase the dosage of *bái zhú* (Atractylodis Macrocephalae Rhizoma) for qì vacuity, and increase the dosage of *mŭ lì* (Ostreae Cocha) for facial swelling. *Mŭ Lì Săn* (Oyster Shell Powder) can also be used to treat vacuity taxation with incessant sweating. Make a powder of equal portions of calcined *mŭ lì* (Ostreae Cocha), *má huáng gēn* 麻黃根 (Ephedrae Radix), and *huáng qí* 黃耆 (Astragali Radix). Cook two qián of powder in one bowl of water, down to seventy percent of the volume, and drink it while it is warm. It has been effective whenever I use it, so I attached it here. (There are two more formulas in *Běn Shì Fāng*).

列缺、曲池主熱病煩心心悶，先手臂身熱瘛瘲，脣口聚，鼻張，目下汗出如珠（《千》）。五處、攢竹、正營、上管、缺盆、中府主汗出寒熱。承漿主汗出衄血不止。百會主汗出而嘔、痙。

Liè Quē 列缺 (LU 7) and Qū Chí 曲池 (LI 11) govern heat disease, vexation and oppression of the heart, heat in the arms and body with tugging and slackening, twitching lips, flaring nostrils, and sweat that appears like pearls under the eyes (*Qiān*《千》).

Wǔ Chù 五處 (UB 5), Zǎn Zhú 攢竹 (UB 2), Zhèng Yíng 正營 (GB 17), Shàng Guǎn 上管 (Rèn 13), Quē Péng 缺盆 (ST 12), and Zhōng Fǔ 中府 (LU 1) govern sweating with [sensations of] cold and heat.

Chéng Jiāng 承漿 (Rèn 24) governs sweating and incessant nosebleed.

Bǎi Huì 百會 (Dū 20) governs sweating, vomiting, and tetany.

大都主熱病汗出，且厥足清。《外臺》乃云：汗不出，厥，手足清。復溜主寒熱無所安，汗出不止，風逆四肢腫。凡熱病煩心，足寒清，多汗：先取然谷，後取太溪，大指間動脈，皆先補之。列缺（水腫）、肺俞、心俞主汗出（中風）。

Dà Dū 大都 (SP 2) governs heat disease, sweating, and reversal with cold legs. *Wài Tái*《外臺》says: absence of sweating, reversal, and cold limbs.

Fù Liū 復溜 (KI 7) governs [sensations of] cold and heat, irritability, incessant sweating, wind counterflow, and swollen extremities.

Heat disease, vexation of the heart, cold chilly legs, and profuse sweating: Supplement Rán Gǔ 然谷 (KI 2) first, then Tài Xī 太溪 (KI 3), as well as the vessel in the big toe [and the second toe].

Liè Quē 列缺 (LU 7) (see the section on edema), Fèi Shù 肺俞 (UB 13), and Xīn Shù 心俞 (UB 15) govern sweating (see the section on wind stroke).

傷寒自汗，蓋陰證也。惟理中湯最佳。予屢教人服驗。若只額上有微汗，與夫上一節有汗者，最宜煎五苓散服之（見《既效方》）。《單方歌》云：疫病汗如水，《論》中號濕溫，燒故竹扇灰，湯調效莫論。其論頗有理，藥必可用也。（多汗亦有用心得者，宜灸心俞，服鎮心丹皆效）。

Cold damage with spontaneous sweating is a yīn pattern. *Lǐ Zhōng Tāng* 理中湯 (Center Rectifying Decoction) is the best formula for it. I ask people to drink it and it is always effective. If someone has only slight sweating on the forehead, or sweats on the upper section [unknown meaning], it is more appropriate to cook *Wǔ Líng Sǎn* 五苓散 (Poria Five Powder) (see *Jì Xiào Fāng*《既效方》).

*Dān Fāng Gē*《單方歌》says: The Discussion calls epidemic disease with watery sweat 'damp-warmth.' Burn an old bamboo fan into ash and mix it with a decoction;[17] this is effective. The discussion is reasonable, so the herbs can be used. (Profuse sweating can also be caused by con-

17. It is unclear if this refers to one of the above decoctions or something else.

寒熱
675

sumption of the heart. It is appropriate to apply moxibustion on Xīn Shù (UB 15); taking *Zhèn Xīn Dān* 鎮心丹 (Heart Settling Elixir) is also effective).

多汗瘧病：譩譆（五十）。多汗，四肢不舉，少力：橫文五十，長平五十。多汗盜汗（並見寒熱）。

Profuse sweating with malarial disease: Yī Xī 譩譆 (UB 45) (apply fifty cones of moxibustion).

Profuse sweating, inability to lift the four limbs, and weakness: Apply fifty cones of moxibustion on Héng Wén 橫文 (SP 15) and Cháng Píng 長平 (LV 13).

Profuse sweating (for all, see the section on [sensations of] cold and heat).

## 7.09
## *Hàn Bù Chū*
# 汗不出
## Absence of sweating

凡胸滿短氣不得汗，皆針補手太陰以出汗（《千》）。少澤、復溜、崑崙主瘧寒汗不出。偏歷主風瘧汗不出。少澤治瘧寒熱汗不出（《銅》）。上星治痎瘧振寒，熱汗不出。啞門治頭痛風汗不出。心俞（見狂，《明》同）、曲差治心中煩滿，汗不出（《明》同）。

Chest fullness, shortness of breath, and absence of sweating: Needle with supplementation Shǒu Tàiyīn手太陰 (LU 3) to induce sweating (*Qiān*《千》).

Shào Zé 少澤 (SI 1), Fù Liū 復溜 (KI 7), and Kūn Lún 崑崙 (UB 60) govern malaria, coldness, and absence of sweating.

Piān Lì 偏歷 (LI 6) governs wind, malaria, and absence of sweating.

Shào Zé (SI 1) treats malaria, [sensations of] cold and heat, and absence of sweating (*Tóng*《銅》).

Shàng Xīng 上星 (Dū 23) treats malaria, quivering with cold, and fever with absence of sweating.

Yǎ Mén 啞門 (Dū 15) treats headaches, wind, and absence of sweating.

Xīn Shù 心俞 (UB 15) (see the section on mania; *Míng* 《明》 agrees) and Qū Chà 曲差 (UB 4) treat vexation and absence of sweating (*Míng* agrees).

陶道治灑淅寒熱，脊強汗不出（《明》同）。膽俞治振寒汗不出（見頭痛）。命門治頭痛如破，身熱如火，汗不出。上脘治身熱汗不出（見霍亂）。至陰（見頭痛）、魚際（見寒熱）、曲泉（見疝）、俠溪（見胸脅滿）、中膂俞治汗不出（見消渴）。

頭痛 643
霍亂 271
寒熱 675
疝 213
胸脅滿 470
消渴 195
唾血 402
寒熱 675

Táo Dào 陶道 (Dū 13) treats aversion to cold as if after soaking in the rain, [sensations of] cold and heat, stiffness of the spine, and absence of sweating (*Míng* 《明》 agrees).

Dǎn Shù 膽俞 (UB 19) treats quivering with cold and absence of sweating (see the section on headaches).

Mìng Mén 命門 (Dū 4) treats headache that feel like the head is broken, generalized heat that feels like there is fire inside, and absence of sweating.

Shàng Wǎn 上脘 (Rèn 13) treats generalized heat and absence of sweating (see the section on sudden turmoil).

Zhì Yīn 至陰 (UB 67) (see the section on headaches), Yú Jì 魚際 (LU 10) (see the section on [sensations of] cold and heat), Qū Quán 曲泉 (LV 8) (see the section on prominent *shàn*-mounting), Xiá Xī 俠溪 (GB 43) (see the section on fullness of the chest and rib-sides), and Zhōng Lǚ Shù 中膂俞 (UB 29) treat absence of sweating (see the section on wasting-thirst).

偏歷治風汗不出。竅陰治手足煩熱，汗不出，轉筋。命門（見頭痛）、肺俞（見汗）療汗不出（《明》）。曲澤療汗出不過肩（見唾血）。曲澤主汗出不過肩（《甲》見傷寒寒熱）。魚際療汗不出（見寒熱）。

Piān Lì 偏歷 (LI 6) treats wind and absence of sweating.

Qiào Yīn 竅陰 (GB 11 or GB 44) treats vexation, heat in the limbs, absence of sweating, and cramping.

Mìng Mén (Dū 4) (see the section on headaches) and Fèi Shù 肺俞 (UB 13) (see the section on sweating) cure absence of sweating (*Míng*).

Qū Zé 曲澤 (PC 3) cures sweating that does not pass the shoulders (see the section on spitting of blood).

Qū Zé (PC 3) governs sweating that does not pass the shoulders (see the section on cold damage with [sensations of] cold and heat in *Jiǎ* 《甲》).

Yú Jì 魚際 (LU 10) cures absence of sweating (see the section on [sensations of] cold and heat).

## 7.10
## *Shāng Hán Wú Hàn*
# 傷寒無汗
## Cold damage with absence of sweating

大都療熱病汗不出，手足逆冷，腹滿善嘔，目眩煩心，四肢腫（《明下》）。凡溫病身熱五日以上，汗不出，刺太泉留針一時取針。若未滿五日，禁刺。勞宮主熱病三日以往，不得汗，怵惕。《甲乙》亦云：主熱病煩滿欲嘔噦，三日以往不得汗，怵惕，胸脅不可反側，咳滿，溺赤小便血，衄不止，嘔吐血，氣逆噫不止，嗌中痛，食不下，善渴，口中爛，掌中熱，欲嘔（《千》）。

Dà Dū 大都 (SP 2) cures heat disease, absence of sweating, cold counterflow of the limbs, abdominal fullness, frequent retching, dizzy vision, vexation of the heart, and swollen limbs (*Míng Xià*《明下》).

Warm disease with generalized heat for more than five days with absence of sweating: Needle Tài Quán 太泉 (LU 9); retain the needle for one two-hour period and remove it. If it is less than five days, acupuncture is contraindicated.

Láo Gōng 勞宮 (PC 8) governs heat disease of more than three days with absence of sweating and apprehensiveness. *Jiǎ Yǐ*《甲乙》says: It treats heat disease with vexation, fullness, and desire to retch, absence of sweating after three days with apprehensiveness, inability to turn the chest and rib-sides, cough, fullness, reddish urine and blood in the urine, incessant nosebleeds, vomiting of blood, qì counterflow with incessant belching, throat pain, difficulty getting food down, frequent thirst, sores in the mouth, heat in the palms, and frequent retching (*Qiān*《千》).

孔最主臂厥熱痛，汗不出（《明》云：熱病汗不出），皆灸刺之，此穴可出汗。經渠、陽池、陽谷、合谷（《明下》同）、前谷、內庭、後溪、腕骨、支溝（《明下》同）、厲兌、衝陽、解溪主熱病汗不出。

Kǒng Zuì 孔最 (LU 6) governs arm reversal with hot pain and absence of sweating (*Míng*《明》says: For heat disease with absence of sweating), apply moxibustion and needling. This point can induce sweating.

Jīng Qú 經渠 (LU 8), Yáng Chí 陽池 (SJ 4), Yáng Gǔ 陽谷 (SI 5), Hé Gǔ 合谷 (LI 4) (*Míng Xià*《明下》agrees), Qián Gǔ 前谷 (SI 2), Nèi Tíng 內庭 (ST 44), Hòu Xī 後溪 (SI 3), Wán Gǔ 腕骨 (SI 4), Zhī Gōu 支溝 (SJ 6) (*Míng Xià* agrees), Lì Duì 厲兌 (ST 45), Chōng Yáng 衝陽 (ST 42), and Jiě Xī 解溪 (ST 41) govern heat disease with absence of sweating.

中衝等主熱病汗不出（見傷寒諸病）。命門、膀胱俞、上管、曲差、上星、陶道、天柱、上窌、懸厘、風池主煩滿汗不出。飛揚主下部寒熱，汗不出，體重。玉枕、大杼、肝俞、心俞、膈俞、陶道主汗不出，淒厥惡寒。光明主腹足清，寒熱汗不出。

Zhōng Chōng 中衝 (PC 9) and so forth govern heat disease with absence of sweating (see the sections on the various cold damage diseases).

Mìng Mén 命門 (Dū 4), Páng Guāng Shù 膀胱俞 (UB 28), Shàng Guǎn 上關 (Rèn 13), Qū Chà 曲差 (UB 4), Shàng Xīng 上星 (Dū 23), Táo Dào 陶道 (Dū 13), Tiān Zhù 天柱 (UB 10), Shàng Liáo 上窌 (UB 31), Xuán Lí 懸厘 (GB 6), and Fēng Chí 風池 (GB 20) govern vexation, fullness, and absence of sweating.

Fēi Yáng 飛揚 (UB 58) governs [sensations of] cold and heat of the lower body, absence of sweating, and heaviness of the body.

Yù Zhěn 玉枕 (UB 9), Dà Zhù 大杼 (UB 11), Gān Shù 肝俞 (UB 18), Xīn Shù 心俞 (UB 15), Gé Shù 膈俞 (UB 17), and Táo Dào (Dū 13) govern absence of sweating, cold reversal, and aversion to cold.

Guāng Míng 光明 (GB 37) governs cold abdomen and legs, [sensations of] cold and heat, and absence of sweating.

曲泉主身熱頭痛，汗不出。魚際主頭痛不甚汗出。尺澤主氣膈喜嘔，鼓頷，不得汗，煩心身痛。液門、中渚、通里主熱病先不樂，頭痛面熱無汗。傷寒溫病，善搖頭，顏清，汗出不過肩，曲澤主之（《甲》）。委中治熱病汗不出云云，取其經血立愈（《銅》）。

Qū Quán 曲泉 (LV 8) governs generalized heat, headaches, and absence of sweating.

Yú Jì 魚際 (LU 10) governs headaches with less sweating.

Chǐ Zé 尺澤 (LU 5) governs dysphagia-occlusion, frequent retching, chattering of the jaws, absence of sweating, vexation of the heart, and generalized pain.

Yè Mén 液門 (SJ 2), Zhōng Zhǔ 中渚 (SJ 3), and Tōng Lǐ 通里 (HT 5) govern heat disease with unhappiness first, then headaches, hot face, and absence of sweating.

腹滿 445 Cold damage and warm disease with frequent head shaking, chilly face, and sweating that does not pass the shoulders: Qū Zé 曲澤 (PC 3) can govern it (*Jiǎ*《甲》).

Wěi Zhōng 委中 (UB 40) treats heat disease with absence of sweating. Bleeding the channel will cure the disease immediately (*Tóng*《銅》).

孔最治熱病汗不出，此穴可灸三壯，即汗出(《明下》同)。

Kǒng Zuì 孔最 (LU 6) treats heat disease with absence of sweating. Applying three cones of moxibustion on this point will induce sweating (*Míng Xià*《明下》agrees).

陷谷、厲兌、膈俞、中渚、大都(見腹滿)、支溝、陽谷(《明》同)、腕骨、前谷治熱病汗不出。懸顱治熱病煩滿，汗不出(《明》同)。懸厘治熱病汗不出，頭偏痛，煩心不欲食。譩譆治熱病汗不出。大杼治傷寒汗不出，脊強。

Xiàn Gǔ 陷谷 (ST 43), Lì Duì 厲兌 (ST 45), Gé Shù 膈俞 (UB 17), Zhōng Zhǔ 中渚 (SJ 3), Dà Dū 大都 (SP 2) (see the section on abdominal fullness), Zhī Gōu 支溝 (SJ 6), Yáng Gǔ 陽谷 (SI 5) (*Míng*《明》agrees), Wán Gǔ 腕骨 (SI 4), and Qián Gǔ 前谷 (SI 2) treat heat disease with absence of sweating.

Xuán Lú 懸顱 (GB 5) treats heat disease, vexation, and absence of sweating (*Míng*《明》agrees).

Xuán Lí 懸厘 (GB 6) treats heat disease, absence of sweating, hemilateral headaches, vexation of the heart, and no desire to eat.

Yī Xī 譩譆 (UB 45) treats heat disease and absence of sweating.

Dà Zhù 大杼 (UB 11) treats cold damage, absence of sweating, and stiffness of the spine.

經渠治熱病汗不出，暴痹喘，足(《明》作逆)心痛，嘔吐。商陽治熱病汗不出(《明下》同)。中衝治熱病汗不出，掌熱，身如火，心痛煩滿，舌強。太溪治熱病汗不出，默默嗜臥，溺黃，消癉，大便難。

Jīng Qú 經渠 (LU 8) treats heat disease, absence of sweating, severe *bì*-impediment, panting, leg (*Míng* says: counterflow) and heart pain, and vomiting.

Shāng Yáng 商陽 (LI 1) treats heat disease with absence of sweating (*Míng Xià* agrees).

Zhōng Chōng 中衝 (PC 9) treats heat disease, absence of sweating, heat in the palms, the body feels like it is on fire, and heart pain with vexation and fullness, as well as stiffness of the tongue.

Tài Xī 太溪 (KI 3) treats heat disease, absence of sweating, quiet and somnolence, yellowish urine, pure heat wasting-thirst, and constipation.

風池治溫病汗不出，目眩、苦頭痛。太陵治熱病汗不出，臂攣腋腫，善笑不休，心懸若飢，喜悲泣驚恐，目赤，小便如血，嘔逆，狂言不樂。勞宮治熱病三日汗不出，怵惕，胸脅痛不可轉，大小便血，衄血不止，氣逆嘔噦，煩渴，食飲不下。

Fēng Chí 風池 (GB 20) treats warm disease, absence of sweating, dizzy vision, and headaches.

Tài Líng 太陵 (PC 7) treats heat disease, absence of sweating, hypertonicity of the arms, swelling of the axilla, frequent incessant laughter, the heart is suspended as if hungry, frequent sorrow, crying, fright, and fear, red eyes, bloody urine, retching counterflow, manic raving, and unhappiness.

Láo Gōng 勞宮 (PC 8) treats heat disease for three days with absence of sweating, apprehensiveness, pain of the chest and rib-sides with inability to turn to the sides, bloody urine and stool, incessant nosebleeds, qì counterflow, retching, vexation, thirst, and difficulty getting food and drink down.

光明治熱病汗不出，卒狂，虛則痿痹坐不能起，實則足胻熱膝痛，身體不仁，善嚙頰。中衝治熱病煩悶，汗不出，掌熱，身如火，心痛舌強（《明下》云：身熱如火，頭痛如破）。

Guāng Míng 光明 (GB 37) treats heat disease, absence of sweating, and sudden mania. In vacuity, there is wilting and *bì*-impediment with inability to get up from sitting; in repletion, there is hot pain of the legs and knees, numbness of the body, and frequently biting of one's own cheeks.

Zhōng Chōng (PC 9) treats heat disease, vexation and oppression, absence of sweating, heat in the palms, the body feels like it is on fire, heart pain, and stiffness of the tongue (*Míng Xià*《明下》 says: the body feels like it is on fire with headaches that feel like the head is broken).

天池療熱病汗不出，胸滿頸痛，四肢不舉，腋下腫，上氣胸中有聲，喉喝（《明下》）。相識患陰證傷寒，四肢厥冷不省，予與理中湯服，至第二服，汗出如雨矣，神哉。

Tiān Chí 天池 (PC 1) cures heat disease, absence of sweating, chest fullness, neck pain, inability to lift the limbs, swelling of the axilla, qì ascent with sounds in the chest, and a rattling sound in the throat (*Míng Xià*).

Someone I knew suffered a yīn pattern of cold damage, with cold reversal in the limbs, and unconsciousness. I gave him *Lǐ Zhōng Tāng* 理中湯 (Center-Rectifying Decoction). After taking the second dose, he sweated profusely like rain. It was a miracle.

## 7.11

## *Fā Bēi (Yōng Jū, Yáng, Yú Jiàn Zhì Lòu)*

# 發背（癰疽　瘍　餘見痔漏）

### Sores on the back

**(Welling and flat-abscesses; sores; for further discussion, see the section on hemorrhoids and fistulas)**

頻刺風門，泄諸陽熱氣，背永不發癰疽（《銅》）。灸發背法：或不見瘡頭，以濕紙敷，先乾者是。以大蒜去皮生切錢子，先安一蒜錢在上，次艾灸三壯。換蒜復三灸，如此易無數。痛灸至不痛，不痛灸至痛，方住。

Needle Fēng Mén 風門 (UB 12) frequently to drain hot qì from all the yáng channels; welling- and flat-abscesses will never erupt on the back (*Tóng*《銅》).

Method of applying moxibustion for sores on the back: If the head of the sore cannot be seen, apply the wet paper on the sores; the place that dries out first is the head. Peel the skin off of fresh garlic and cut it into slices the size of a coin. First place a coin-size slice of garlic on [the head of the sore], then apply three cones of moxibustion. Change the garlic and burn three more cones; keep changing the slices without counting. If the sore was painful, apply moxibustion until the pain goes away; if the sore was not painful, apply moxibustion until the person feels pain; then stop.

若第一日急灸減九分，二日灸減八分，至第七日尚可。自此以往，灸已後時。灸訖，以石上生者龍鱗薜荔洗研，取汁湯溫呷，即瀉出惡物去根。凡疔瘡，頭瘡，魚臍等瘡，一切無名者悉治（《集效》）。

If the sore is reduced by ninety percent immediately after applying moxibustion in the first day and eighty percent in the second day, [moxibustion] can still be applied until the seventh day. After that, moxibustion is not necessary. After the moxibustion is complete, rinse and grind *lóng lín bì lì* 龍鱗薜荔 (Hederae Cauli et Folium) that grew on a stone; decoct the juice and sip it while is warm. This can drain malign things and remove the root [of the sores]. It can treat all boils, sores, head sores, fish umbilicus sores, and so forth; as well as sores that have no name (*Jí Xiào*《集效》).

凡發腫至堅有根者，名曰石癰。治法當上灸之百壯，石子當碎出。如不出，益壯乃佳(《千》)。論曰：凡發背皆因服五石寒食更生散所致，亦有單服鐘乳而發者，又有生平不服而自發背者。其候率多於背兩胛間起，初如粟米大，或痛或癢，仍作赤色。

Swelling from sores on the back that becomes hard and have a root, are called stone welling-abscess. The treatment method is to apply a hundred cones of moxibustion on them. The stone should break through and come out. If it does not come out, burning more cones is good (*Qiān*《千》).

The discussion says: Generally sores erupting on the back are caused by taking *Wǔ Shí* [*Sǎn*] 五石散 (Five Stones Powder) or *Hán Shí* [*Sǎn*] 寒食散 (Take Cold Powder), and *Gēng Shēng* Sǎn 更生散 (Change Life Powder).[18] It can also occur after taking only *zhōng rǔ* [*shí*] 鐘乳石 (Stalactitum) or occur spontaneously without taking any of these things. The symptoms usually start on the back between the two scapulae. In the beginning, the [sores] are the size of millet with itching or pain and redness.

人皆初不以為事，日漸長大，不過十日，遂至於死。臨困之時，以闊三寸高一寸瘡有數十孔，以手按之，諸孔中皆膿出，尋時失音。所以養生者，小覺背上癢痛有異，即火急取淨土水和為泥，捻作餅子，厚二分、闊一寸半，以粗艾大作炷灸泥上，帖著瘡上灸之，一炷一易餅子。

People ignore this in the beginning, but it grows gradually day by day, and the patient will die in ten days. By the time the person is about to die, each sore is one cùn high and three cùn wide with tens of holes, and pus comes out when pressed. The patient loses his voice in very short time. So to nourish life, when someone begins to feel something wrong on the back with itching and pain, they should quickly mix clean soil and water into mud, then twist it into the cakes two fēn high and 1.5 cùn wide. Place the mud directly on the sores, then burn big moxa cones made from coarse mugwort on it. Change the cake after each cone.

若粟米大時，可灸七餅子即瘥。如榆莢大，灸七七餅炷即瘥。如錢大，可日夜灸，不限炷數。仍服五香連翹湯，及鐵漿諸藥攻之，乃愈。凡腫起背胛中，頭白如黍粟，四邊相連腫赤黑，令人悶亂，即名發背，禁房室酒肉蒜面。若不灸治，即入內殺人。若灸當瘡上七八百壯。有人不識，多作雜腫治者，皆死。

18. *Wǔ Shí Sǎn* 五石散 (Five Stones Powder), and *Hán Shí* [*Sǎn*] 寒食散 (Take Cold Powder) are different names for the same formula. It contains *zhōng rǔ* [*shí*] 鐘乳石 (Stalactitum) and four other minerals and is used to treat weakness and taxation. The formula is hot, so the patient needs to eat cold foods to reduce the heat *Gēng Shēng Sǎn* 更生散 (Change Life Powder) is also named *Wǔ Shí Gēng Shēng Sǎn* 五石更生散 (Five Stones Change Life Powder). Its functions are similar to *Wǔ Shí Sǎn* 五石散 (Five Stones Powder) but with even more hot herbs.

If the sores are the size of millet, it will be cured after applying moxibustion on seven cakes. If the sores are the size of elm seeds, it will heal after applying moxibustion on seven times seven cakes. If the sores are as big as a coin, moxibustion can be applied day and night without limit. Also ask the patient to take *Wǔ Xiāng Lián Qiào Tāng* 五香連翹湯 (Five Fragrances with Forsythia Decoction), *tiě jiāng* 鐵漿 (Ferri Aqua) and so forth to attack it. The sores will be cured.

If the swelling arises on the back and [between] the scapulae, with white heads that look like millet, connected with each other on all sides, and the color of the swelling is dark red, making the person feel oppressed and confused: This is called sores on the back. Sexual activities, liquor, meat, garlic and wheat-flour should be avoided.

If moxibustion is not applied, [the sores] enter inwardly and kill people. When applying moxibustion, it is appropriate to burn seven or eight hundred cones of moxibustion on the sores. There are doctors who do not know this and treat it as a miscellaneous swelling. Their patients all die.

郭戶為予言，鄉裡有善治發背癰疽者，皆於瘡上灸之，多至三二百壯，無有不愈。但艾炷小作之，炷小則人不畏灸，灸多則作效矣。蓋得此法也，然亦不必泥此。近有一醫以治外科得名，有人發背瘡大如碗，有數孔，醫亦無藥可治，只以艾遍敷在瘡上，灸之久而方疼。則以瘡上皆死肉，故初不覺疼也。旋以藥調治之愈。蓋出於意表也。

The Guō family told me that someone in their village was good at treating sores on the back, welling-abscesses, and flat-abscesses. He always applied moxibustion on the sores, and burned as many as two or three hundred cones. All the diseases were cured. But the cones should be small in size so people won't be afraid of moxibustion, and can stand more cones, which is effective. We do not have to limit ourselves to these methods.

Recently, there was a doctor who was famous for treating external diseases. Someone suffered sores on his back; the sore was as big as a bowl and had several holes in it. The doctor was unable to treat him with herbs, so he applied moxa cones all over the sores and burned them for a long time. The patient began to feel pain. It must be because there was dead flesh in the sores, so the patient did not feel the pain at first. He gave the patient herbs to recuperate afterwards and the patient recovered. This goes beyond my expectations.

王蘧疽發於背，張生以艾火加瘡上，自旦及暮，凡一百五十壯，知痛乃已。明日鑷去黑痂，膿血盡潰，膚理皆紅，亦不復痛。始別以藥附之，日一易焉。易時旋剪去黑爛惡肉，月許瘡乃平。是歲秋夏間，京師士大夫病疽者七人，余獨生。此雖司命事，然固有料理，不知其方，遂至不幸者（見王蘧發背方序）。

腰腳痛 542
膝痛 536
腋腫 496

A flat-abscess erupted on Wáng Qú's back; Scholar Zhāng applied a total of one hundred and fifty cones of moxibustion on the sores from dawn till dusk, until [Wáng Qú] felt pain. The next day, [Scholar Zhāng] removed the black crust [on the sores] with tweezers; both pus and blood drained out and the skin was red. There was no pain anymore. [Scholar Zhāng] then begin to apply herbs on the sores, and changed the herbs every day. He cut out the black eroded malign flesh at the same time. It took more than one month to heal the sores.

Between fall and summer one year, seven scholars in capital suffered flat-abscesses and I was the only one to survive. Although this is destiny, there is certainly taking care of the situation as well. If one doesn't know the formulas he will arrive at misfortune (see the preface of *Fā Bèi Fāng* 發背方 (Formulas for Sores on the back) by Wáng Qú).

陽輔治腋腫疽馬刀（見腰腳痛）。犢鼻治膝臏癰腫（見膝痛）。竅陰主營（《明》作骨）疽發厲，項痛引頭（《明》同），目痛（《銅》云：治癰疽頭痛心煩）。凡疽卒著五指，筋急不得屈伸者：灸踝骨中央數十壯，或至百壯。

Yáng Fǔ 陽輔 (GB 38) treats swelling of the axilla, flat-abscesses, and saber lumps (see the section on low back and leg pain).

Dú Bí 犢鼻 (ST 35) treats welling-abscesses and swelling of the patellae (see the section on knee pain).

Qiào Yīn 竅陰 (GB 44) governs severe eruptions of flat-abscesses in the *yíng*-construction (*Míng* 《明》 says bones), nape pain radiating to the head (*Míng* agrees), and eye pain. *Tóng* 《銅》 says: It treats welling and flat-abscesses, headaches, and vexation of the heart.)

Flat-abscesses suddenly appearing on the fingers and sinew tension with inability to flex and stretch: Apply several tens or a hundred cones of moxibustion in the center of the ankle bone.

附骨疽，灸間使後一寸，隨年壯，立瘥。天突療肺癰，唾膿血，氣壅不通（《明》）。膻中療肺癰，咳嗽上氣，唾膿，不下食，胸中氣滿如塞。小海治瘍腫振寒。太衝、臨泣（見腋腫）治馬刀瘍瘻。《單方歌》云：惡患是石癰，不針可藥取，當上灸百壯，石子出如雨。

Bone flat-abscesses (suppurative osteomyelitis): Apply moxibustion on the site one cùn proximal to Jiān Shǐ 間使 (PC 5). Burn the same number of cones as the patient's age. This will cure the disease immediately.

Tiān Tū 天突 (Rèn 22) cures lung abscesses with spitting of blood and pus and qì blockage (*Míng*).

Dàn Zhōng 膻中 (Rèn 17) cures lung abscesses, cough with qì ascent, spitting pus, inability to get food down, and qì fullness of the chest that feels like it is plugged up.

Xiǎo Hǎi 小海 (SI 8) treats swollen sores and quivering with cold.

Tài Chōng 太衝 (LV 3), Lín Qì 臨泣 (GB 41) (see the section on swelling of the axilla) treat saber lumps, sores, and fistulas. *Dān Fāng Gē*《 單方歌 》(Single Formula Songs) says: Stone welling-abscess is a malign disease; do not needle it but you can use herbs. It is appropriate to apply a hundred cones of moxibustion on it; the stones will come out like rain.

余嘗為劉和叔序《 灸癰疽方 》云：必以毒藥攻於內，伐其根也 。又以火艾灼其外，宣其毒也 。法盡于此矣 。癰疽始作，灼艾服大黃等藥，無不愈者（ 大黃宜隨人虛實服 ）。王子高病背疽，京師外醫以為不可治 。得一徐人教以灼艾如棗大，近千壯 。魯直數患背瘡，亦灼艾而愈 。灸為第一法也（ 《 必 》 ）。

I wrote a preface for *Jīu Yōng Jū Fāng*《 灸癰疽方 》(Applying Moxibustion for Welling- and Flat-Abscesses) by Líu Héshū, saying that we must use toxic herbs to attack internally so that the root is cut and burn moxibustion externally to disperse the toxins. All methods are within this principle. At the beginning stage of welling and flat-abscesses, apply moxibustion and take *dà huáng* 大黄 (Rhei Radix et Rhizoma) and so forth. This will cure the disease (*dà huáng* according to whether the person is vacuous or replete). When Wáng Zǐgāo[19] suffered a flat abscess on his back, external doctors[20] in capital thought it was not treatable. Someone from Xú said to apply close to a thousand cones of moxibustion the size of date kernels on it. Lǔzhí[21] frequently suffered sores on his back and was also cured by applying moxibustion. So moxibustion is the first method (*Bì*《 必 》).

19. Based on the previous text, Wáng Zǐgāo 王子高 may be another name for Wáng Qú 王蘧.

20. In ancient times, there were internal and external doctors. Internal doctors are the predecessor of modern doctors of internal medicine; external doctors were in charge of expelling evils and this category does not exist anymore.

21. Lǔzhí 魯直 may refer to Huáng Tíngjiān 黃庭堅 who was an artist, scholar, government official, and poet during the *Sòng* Dynasty. He was predominantly known as a calligrapher, but was also admired for his painting and poetry. He was one of the Four Masters of the *Sòng* Dynasty.

# 7.12
## *Yǐng Liú (Ròu Liú)*

# 瘿瘤（肉瘤）

## Goiter
**(Fleshy tumors)**

咳逆上
420

天府（《甲乙》作天窗）、臑會、氣舍主瘤癭氣咽腫。通天主癭，久五十壯。胸堂、羊矢灸百壯。腦戶、通天、消濼、天突主頸有大氣。臑會治項癭氣瘤（《明》）。《下》云：療癭及臂氣腫。氣舍治瘤癭（見咳逆上氣）。

Tiān Fǔ 天府 (LU 3) (*Jiǎ Yǐ*《甲乙》says Tiān Chuāng 天窗 (SI 16)), Nào Huì 臑會 (SJ 13), and Qì Shě 氣舍 (ST 11) govern tumors, goiter, and swollen throat.

Tōng Tiān 通天 (UB 7) governs goiter; apply fifty or a hundred cones of moxibustion on Xiōng Táng 胸堂 (Rèn 17) and Yáng Shǐ 羊矢 (LV 12).

Nǎo Hù 腦戶 (Dū 17), Tōng Tiān (UB 7), Xiāo Luò 消濼 (SJ 12), and Tiān Tū 天突 (Rèn 22) govern great qì of the neck.

Nào Huì 臑會 (SJ 13) treats goiter on the neck (*Míng*《明》). *Xià*《下》says: It cures goiter and qì swelling of the arms.

Qì Shě (ST 11) treats goiter (see the section on coughing counterflow and qì ascent ).

浮白療癭，肩不舉（《銅》云：治癭氣）。肺俞療癭氣。癭上氣短氣，灸肺俞百壯。癭上氣胸滿，雲門五十壯。癭惡氣：天府五十壯（《千金翼》云：又胸堂百壯）。癭，勞氣：衝陽，隨年壯。癭：灸天瞿三百，橫三間寸灸之。

Fú Bái 浮白 (GB 10) cures goiter and inability to raise the shoulders (*Tóng*《銅》says: It treats goiter).

Fèi Shù 肺俞 (UB 13) cures goiter.

Goiter with qì ascent and shortness of breath: Apply a hundred cones of moxibustion on Fèi Shù (UB 13).

Goiter with qì ascent and chest fullness: Apply fifty cones of moxibustion on Yún Mén 雲門 (LU 2).

Goiter with malign qì: Apply fifty cones of moxibustion on Tiān Fǔ 天府 (LU 3) (*Qiān Jīn Yì*《千金翼》says: Apply a hundred cones of moxibustion on Xiōng Táng 胸堂 (Rèn 17).

Goiter and taxation qì: Apply the same number of cones as the patient's age on Chōng Yáng 衝陽 (ST 42).

Goiter: Apply three hundred cones of moxibustion on Tiān Qú 天瞿 (Rèn 22), following the Transverse Three Cùn Method.

癭氣面腫：通天五十壯。癭：灸中封隨年壯。諸癭：灸肩髃左右相對宛宛處，男左十八壯，右十七壯，女右十八壯，左十七壯；或再三取，瘥止。又風池百壯，又兩耳後髮際百壯，又頭衝（一作頸衝）灸之，各隨年壯（《千金翼》云：一名臂臑）。

Goiter with facial swelling: Apply fifty cones of moxibustion on Tōng Tiān 通天 (UB 7).

Goiter: Apply the same number of cones as the patient's age on Zhōng Fēng 中封 (LV 4).

All goiters: Apply moxibustion on the depression at Jiān Yú 肩髃 (LI 15) on the left and right sides. Burn eighteen cones of moxibustion on the left and seventeen cones on the right side of males; burn eighteen cones of moxibustion on the right and seventeen cones on the left side of females; keep doing this until the disease is cured. Or apply a hundred cones of moxibustion on Fēng Chí 風池 (GB 20); or within the hairline behind the ear; or burn the same number of cones as the patient's age on Tóu Chōng 頭衝 (one version says Jǐng Chōng 頸衝) (LI 14) (*Qiān Jīn Yì* says: It is also named as Bì Nào 臂臑 (LI 14)).

癭，惡氣：大椎橫三間寸灸之；風池，耳上髮際、大椎各百壯；大椎兩邊各寸半，小垂下各三十；又臂臑隨年壯，凡五處，共九穴；又垂兩手兩腋上文頭各三百壯，針亦良（《千翼》）。

Goiter and malign qì: Apply moxibustion on Dà Zhuī 大椎 (Dū 14), following the Transverse Three Cùn Method; or burn a hundred cones of moxibustion on Fēng Chí (GB 20), the site in the hairline above the ears, and Dà Zhuī (Dū 14); or burn thirty cones of moxibustion on the sites 1.5 cùn lateral and slightly below Dà Zhuī (Dū 14); or apply the same number of cones as the patient's age on Bì Nào (LI 14). All the nine points listed above are located in five places.[22] Also apply three hundred cones of moxibustion at the end of the fold above the two axillae when the arm drops down. Needling is also good (*Qiān Yì*《千翼》).

22. In other words, there are five points. Four are bilateral, making nine sites.

大智禪師云：皮膚頭面生瘤，大如拳，小如栗，或軟或硬，不痛，不可輒針灸。天南星生乾皆得，滴少醋研膏；先將小針刺病處令氣透，以藥膏攤紙上貼，三五易瘥。此亦一說也，故並存之。

Monk Master Dà Zhì said: tumors arise on the skin, head, and face; the size may be as big as a fist or as small as chestnut; hard or soft, but without pain. Acupuncture and moxibustion are not always applicable. Obtain raw or dried *tiān nán xīng* 天南星 (Arisaematis Rhizoma), mix it with a few drops of vinegar, and grind it into a paste. First needle with a fine needle to let qì penetrate, then place the paste on paper and apply it on [the tumor]. When you have changed the paste three or five times, the disease will be cured. This also is another theory, so I put it here.

治腦瘻諸節諸癰腫牢堅治之方：削附子令如棋子厚，正著腫上，以少唾濕附子，艾灸附子令熱徹；附子欲乾，輒更唾濕之，常令附子熱徹 。附子欲乾，輒更氣入腫中，無不愈 。此法絕妙不傳（《千翼》）。凡肉瘤勿治，治則殺人 。（《肘後方》云：不得針灸 。）

The method to treat brain fistulas, swelling and hardness of all the joints, and welling-abscesses: Cut a piece of *fù zǐ* 附子 (Aconiti Radix Lateralis) as thick as a chess piece, place it on the swollen area, moisten the *fù zǐ* with a little spittle, and apply moxibustion on it to heat it thoroughly. Once the *fù zǐ* dries out, moisten it again with spittle, and keep warming it thoroughly. When the *fù zǐ* dries out, it sends qì into the swelling, thus curing the problem. This method is a miracle and has never been passed on to the public (*Qiān Yì*《千翼》). Do not treat flesh tumors; treating them will kill the patient. (*Zhóu Hòu Fāng*《肘後方》says: Do not apply acupuncture and moxibustion).

# 7.13
# *Luǒ Lì*
# 瘰歷
## Scrofula

大迎、五里、臂臑主寒熱，頸瘰歷歷（《千》）。大迎治寒熱，頸痛瘰歷歷（《銅》）。缺盆治寒熱，瘰歷，缺盆中腫，外潰，則生胸中熱滿，腹大，水氣，缺盆中痛，汗出（《明》同）。

Dà Yíng 大迎 (ST 5), Wǔ Lǐ 五里 (LI 13), and Bì Nào 臂臑 (LI 14) govern [sensations of] cold and heat and scrofula of the neck (*Qiān*《千》).

Dà Yíng (ST 5) treats [sensations of] cold and heat and neck pain with scrofula (*Tóng*《銅》).

Quē Pén 缺盆 (ST 12) treats [sensations of] cold and heat, scrofula, and swelling of the empty basin [superclavicular fossa]. When it ulcerates externally, it generates heat and fullness of the chest, enlarged abdomen, water qì, pain of the empty basin, and sweating (*Míng*《明》agrees).

五里治寒熱，瘰歷，咳嗽。臂臑治寒熱，頸項急，瘰歷，肩背痛不得舉。少海療腋下瘰歷，臂疼屈伸不得，風痹疼，疰病（《明》）。天牖療瘰歷寒熱，頸有積氣，暴聾肩痛（《下》）。

Wǔ Lǐ (LI 13) treats [sensations of] cold and heat, scrofula, and cough.

Bì Nào (LI 14) treats [sensations of] cold and heat, neck and nape tension, scrofula, and pain of the shoulders and back with inability to raise them.

Shào Hǎi 少海 (HT 3) cures scrofula under the axilla, arm pain with inability to flex and stretch, pain due to wind *bì*-impediment, and infixation diseases (*Míng*).

Tiān Yǒu 天牖 (SJ 16) cures scrofula with [sensations of] cold and heat, qì accumulations of the neck, sudden deafness, and shoulder pain (*Xià*《下》).

灸一切瘰歷在項上，及觸處但有肉結凝，似作瘻及癰癤者：以獨頭蒜截兩頭留心，大作艾炷如蒜大小，貼歷子上灸之。勿令上破肉，但取熱而已，七壯一易蒜，日日灸之，取消止。一切瘰歷，灸兩胯裡患歷處宛宛中，日一壯止，神驗。又五里、人迎各三十壯。又患人背兩邊腋下後文上，隨年壯。又耳後髮際直脈七壯。

To apply moxibustion for all kinds of scrofula on the nape as well as anywhere there is bound up flesh appearing like a fistula or welling-abscesses: Cut the two ends off a single-clove garlic leaving the core; make cones of moxibustion the size of the garlic, put the garlic on the scrofula, then burn the moxa cones. Do not break the skin; just warm it. Change the garlic every seven cones. Apply this moxibustion every day until the scrofula disappears.

For all scrofula, apply moxibustion in the depression at the affected area and on the inner aspect of the thighs. Burn one cone of moxibustion every day. This is divinely effective. Or apply thirty cones of moxibustion on Wǔ Lǐ 五里 (LI 13) and Rén Yíng 人迎 (ST 9); or burn the same number of the cones as the patient's age above the posterior axillary fold on the side of the back; or apply seven cones of moxibustion on the vertical vessel within the hairline behind the ear.

有同舍項上患歷，人教用忍冬草研細，酒與水煎服，以滓敷而愈（詳見《良方》）。次年復生，用前藥不效，以艾灸之而除根。有小兒耳後生歷，用藥敷不效，亦灸之而愈云。

My co-worker suffered scrofula on the nape; someone told him to grind *rěn dōng cǎo* 忍冬草 into a fine powder, cook it with liquor and water, drink it, then apply the dregs [externally to the site]. The disease was cured (for the details, see *Liáng Fāng*《良方》). The scrofula came back the next year, and the previous herbs did not work. He applied moxibustion and removed the root.

A child suffered scrofula behind the ear. Herbs were applied but did not work. It was cured after moxibustion.

瘰歷初生如梅李，切忌以毒藥點蝕，及針刀鐮割。勞歷為甚，既經蝕取之，後無有不死者，蓋外醫既少慈悲，又利於積日，特宜戒之（《必》）。歷瘍著頸及胸前，灸乳間（見白駁）。

For scrofula that looks like a plum in the beginning, do not apply toxic herbs to erode it, or needle or cut it with the knife.

Taxation scrofula is severe, if it has eroded the channel and you treat it, the patient will die later. External doctors are not so benevolent and are also greedy. Avoid this kind of treatment (*Bì*《必》).

For scrofula and sores on the neck and chest, apply moxibustion on Rǔ Jiān 乳間 ('between the breasts,' possibly Rèn 17) (see the section on white patch [psoriasis]).

腋下瘰歷漏，臂疼屈伸不得，風痹漏瘙，針少海三分，留七呼，瀉五吸。針瘰歷：先拄針皮上三十六息，推針入。納之，追核大小，勿出核，三上三下乃出針。頸漏：天池百壯。又心鳩尾下宛宛中七十。又章門、臨泣、支溝、陽輔（百壯），又肩井隨年，乂以艾炷繞四畔周匝，七壯即止。諸惡漏中冷息肉出，灸足內踝上各三壯（二年者六壯，《千翼》）

Scrofula with fistula under the axilla, arm pain with inability to flex and stretch, wind *bì*-impediment, and fistula with itching: Needle Shào Hǎi 少海 (HT 3) three fēn deep; retain the needle for seven respirations; drain for five respirations.

To needle scrofula: lean the needle against the skin for thirty-six breaths, then push the needle in. After the needle is in, determine the size of the node and do not let the needle go through it. Manipulate the needle up and down three times, then remove the needle.

Neck fistula: Apply a hundred cones of moxibustion on Tiān Chí 天池 (PC 1), or seventy cones of moxibustion in the depression below the xiphoid process; or a hundred cones of moxibustion on Zhāng Mén 章門 (LV 13), Lín Qì 臨泣 (GB 41), Zhī Gōu 支溝 (SJ 6), and Yáng Fǔ 陽輔 (GB 38); or burn the same number of cones as the patient's age on Jiān Jǐng 肩井 (GB 21); or place moxa cones around [the fistula], burn seven cones of moxibustion, and stop.

Malign fistula with coldness and polyps: Apply three cones of moxibustion on the medial malleolus (burn six cones for people have suffered the disease for two years, *Qiān Yì*《千翼》).

# 7.14
## *Fēng Zhěn (Yǐn Zhěn)*
## 風疹（癮疹）

膝 536
偏風 396
風勞 371

### Wind papules
**(Dormant papules)**

曲澤治風疹，臂肘腕善動搖（《銅》）。肩髃治熱風癮疹（《明》云：刺風風虛）。曲池刺風癮疹。涌泉（《明》同）、環跳（見膝）治風疹。下崑崙療刺風，疹風，熱風，冷痹（《明》）。曲池療刺風疹疼痛（見偏風）。伏兔（見風勞）療癮疹。合谷、曲池療大小人遍身風疹（《下》）。

Qū Zé 曲澤 (PC 3) treats wind papules and frequent shaking of the arms, elbows and wrists (*Tóng*《銅》).

Jiān Yú 肩髃 (LI 15) treats hot wind and wind papules (*Míng*《明》says: It treats prickly wind[23] and wind [due to] vacuity).

Qū Chí 曲池 (LI 11) treats prickly wind and wind papules.

Yǒng Quán 涌泉 (KI 1) (*Míng* agrees) and Huán Tiào 環跳 (GB 30) (see the discussion of the knees) treat wind papules.

Xià Kūn Lún 下崑崙 cures prickly wind, papule wind, and hot, wind, or cold *bì*-impediment (*Míng*).

Qū Chí (LI 11) cures prickly wind and rashes with pain (see the section on hemilateral wind).

Fú Tù 伏兔 (ST 32) (see the section on wind taxation) cures dormant papules.

Hé Gǔ 合谷 (LI 4) and Qū Chí (LI 11) cure wind papules all over the body in adults and children (*Xià*《下》).

《千金方》云：人有風疹多必眼暗，先攻其風，其暗自瘥。然則人之目暗，亦有因風疹多而得者，風疹可不先治乎。

23. Prickly wind is caused by wind-cold attacking the skin then transforming to wind heat. The symptoms include a prickly feeling all over the body.

*Qiān Jīn Fāng*《 千金方 》says: People with wind papules usually suffer from dim vision. Dim vision will recover after attacking the wind. So if dim vision is caused by wind papules, we have to treat the wind papules first.

《 千金翼 》灸風熱赤瘮癢，搔之逐手作瘡法：以一條艾蒿長者，以兩手極意尋之著壁，立兩手並蒿竿拓著壁伸十指，當中指頭，以大艾炷灸蒿竿上，令蒿竿斷，即止灸，十十瘥 。瘥後重發，更依法灸，永瘥 。

There is a moxibustion method in *Qiān Jīn Yì*《 千金翼 》to treat wind heat, red and itchy rashes and sores aroused after scratching: Take a long stem of mugwort; fully extend both hands touching a wall. Stand with the two hands and the mugwort stem aligned and press against the wall, extending all ten fingers. Right at the end of the middle finger, burn big mugwort cones on the mugwort stem until the mugwort stem is severed, and then stop the moxibustion. Ten out of ten cases will recover. If there is a relapse after recovery, apply moxibustion again using the same method, and there will be permanent recovery.

癮瘮，曲池灸隨年壯 。頭痛癮瘮，天窗七壯 。

Dormant papules: Apply the same number of cones as the patient's age on Qū Chí 曲池 (LI 11).

Headaches and dormant papules: Apply seven cones of moxibustion on Tiān Chuāng 天窗 (SI 16).

# 7.15
## *Lì Jié Fēng*
## 歷節風
## Joint-running wind

飛揚、涌泉、頷厭、後頂主歷節汗出(《千》見頸項)。飛揚治歷節風，足指不得屈伸，頭目眩逆氣(《銅》)。

Fēi Yáng 飛揚 (UB 58), Yǒng Quán 涌泉 (KI 1), Hàn Yàn 頷厭 (GB 4), and Hòu Dǐng 後頂 (Dū 19) govern joint-running and sweating (see the section on the neck and nape in *Qiān*《千》).

Fēi Yáng (UB 58) treats joint-running wind, inability to flex and stretch the toes, dizzy head and vision, and qì counterflow (*Tóng*《銅》).

麝香丸尤治白虎歷節，諸風疼痛，游走無定，狀如蟲行，晝靜夜劇。許叔微在歙川，有家婦人遍身走注疼痛，至夜則發，如蟲嚙其肌，多作鬼邪治。予曰：此正歷節病也，三服愈（見《本事方》）。

*Shè Xiāng Wán* 麝香丸 (Musk Pill) treats white tiger joint-running and various wind-type wandering pain that feels like insects crawling and is calm in the daytime but worse at night.

Xǔ Shūwēi[24] was in Xī Chuān where a lady suffered influx pain all over her body. The pain occured at night and felt like the insects were biting her skin. She was often given treatment for ghost evils. Xǔ said: This is joint-running disease. It was cured after she took three doses (see [*Pǔ Jì*] *Běn Shì Fāng*《本事方》).

舉體痛癢如蟲嚙，搔之皮便脫作瘡：灸曲池(見疔瘡)。《良方》服治癩藥半月，兩膝眼灸二七壯。丞相長安公醫人無數。

24. Xǔ Shūwēi 許叔微 was the compiler of *Pǔ Jì Běn Shì Fāng*《普濟本事方》(Skillful Formulas for Universal Salvation). See the book appendix.

Generalized pain and itching that feels like the insect are biting, the skin falls off after scratching and sores arise: Apply moxibustion on Qū Chí 曲池 (LI 11) (see the section on clove sores). *Liáng Fāng*《良方》says to take leprosy herbs for half month, then apply two times seven cones of moxibustion on the two Xī Yǎn 膝眼 points. Prime Minister Chángān treated numerous patients this way.

麻風惡疾，《千金》諸方藥甚多，或效或不效。惟兼絲葉細末，地暴米糊丸梧子大，日二三服，每服四五十丸，茶湯下。調藥末服，效尤速，只難服爾。病去後，亦宜服。屢施與人，神效。若更灸曲池、合谷、三里、絕骨等穴尤佳。予與人按此等穴皆酸疼故也。

Leprosy is a malign disease. *Qiān Jīn*《千金》has lots of formulas and herbs for it; some of them work but some do not. Make a fine powder with *jiān sī yè* 兼絲葉 and mix it with rice paste to make pills the size of *wú zǐ* 梧子 (Firmianae Semen). Take forty or fifty pills each time with tea, two or three times a day. It would be quicker just to take the powder, but it is difficult to take. It is appropriate to take it even after the disease is gone. I frequently use it on people, and have had divine effects. It is especially good to apply moxibustion on Qū Chí (LI 11), Hé Gǔ 合谷 (LI 4), Sān Lǐ 三里 (ST 36), Jué Gǔ 絕骨 (GB 39) and so forth. I press these points on people; they are all sore.

# 7.16
## *Dīng Chuāng (Yáng, Yú Qí Chuāng, Wō Chuāng, Gān Chuāng)*
# 疔瘡（瘍　魚臍瘡　窩瘡　疳瘡）

## Clove sores
**(Sores, fish umbilical sores,[25] fossa sores, *gān* sores)**

疔腫，灸掌後橫文後五指，男左女右，七壯即瘥，已用得效。疔腫灸法雖多，然此法甚驗，出於意表（《千》）。刮竹箭上取茹作炷，灸疔腫上二七壯，即消。

Swollen clove sores: Apply moxibustion on the site that is five finger-widths behind the transverse crease proximal to the palms; apply moxibustion on the left side for males and on the right for females. Burning seven cones of moxibustion will cure the disease. The effect has been proven. There are a lot of moxibustion methods for treating swollen clove sores; this is the most effective one, so I put it here (*Qiān*《千》).

Scrape bamboo and make cones with the bamboo shavings; swollen clove sores will disappear immediately when two times seven of these cones are burned on them.

疔瘡灸法《千金》以為神驗。亦有先以針刺魚臍瘡上四畔作孔，擣白苣汁滴瘡孔者；有刺瘡頭及四畔令汁出，擣生栗黃敷（以面圍之，勿令黃出），從旦至午，根拔出者；有用蒼耳根莖苗，但取一色燒灰，醋泔澱和如泥塗，乾即易之，不過十度，拔根出者（疔腫方有千首皆不及此）；有用皂莢子取仁作末敷，五日內瘥者；有用水獺屎敷大良者，可考而知也。

*Qiān Jīn*《千金》took this moxibustion method for clove sores as divinely effective. Or needle around the fish umbilical sore to make holes, then pound white lettuce to make juice and apply it in the holes. Or needle the head of the sores and the area around it, then pound raw yellow chestnuts and apply it on the sores from dawn until noon (surround the sore with flour dough; do not let the yellow paste flow out), this will remove the root. Or burn into the ash the newly grown roots of *cāng ěr gēn* 蒼耳根 (Xanthium Root) that are all the same color, mix it with vinegar to make a

25. Fish umbilical sores: The shape of the sore appears like a fish umbilicus because of the depression in the center.

mud-like paste, then apply it on the sores; change it when it becomes dry. This can remove the root within ten applications (there are a thousand formulas for swollen clove sores, but none is better than this). Or grind *zào jiá zǐ* 皂莢子 (Gleditsiae Semen) into powder, then apply it on the sores. This will cure the disease in five days. Or apply otter feces on the sores. These can all be verified.

有道人傳瓦盤覆蜣螂，安濃米泔小盞，以火逼之，蟲熱吃泔，及困死，取腦中白肉（乃米泔也），新瓦上瞨乾為末，熱酒調二錢服，仍以少傅瘡即愈。胡簽母患此，疼如鐵丁丁然。依此治之效。

There was a Daoist who said to cover dung beetles with a tile plate, place a small bowl of thick rice soup on top, heat the plate to force the insects to drink water from rinsing rice. Once they have died, take the white flesh in their brains (this is the water from rinsing rice), dry it on a new tile, and powder it. Mix two *qián* with warm liquor and drink it; also apply a little on the sores. This will cure the sores. The mother of Hú Qiān suffered this; her pain felt like iron nails. It was effective after this treatment.

小海治瘍腫振寒，太衝、臨泣（見腋腫）治馬刀瘍瘻（《銅》）。一切痼瘡：灸足大指奇間二七壯，灸大指頭亦佳（《千》）。

Xiǎo Hǎi 小海 (SI 8) treats swollen sores and quivering with cold.

Tài Chōng 太衝 (LV 3) and Lín Qì 臨泣 (GB 41) (see the section on swelling of the axilla) treat saber lumps, sores, and fistulas (*Tóng*《銅》).

All fossa sores: Apply two times seven cones of moxibustion in the space next to the big toe. It is also good to apply moxibustion on the tip of the big toe (*Qiān*《千》).

予年少生一瘡，在足內外踝之中，深而疼，陰證瘡也。偶閱古陰陽書，有用青桑漿治袴口瘡者，用之即愈。後在武林，內踝上生一瘡，逾月又生一瘡，令仆往江下取得少黃桑漿，僅可一抹，翌朝愈矣。自是常教人用，皆驗。舍侄腿生瘡不可行，舍弟取桑根搗成膏敷，亦愈。

I had a sore when I was young; it was between the medial and lateral malleolus, deep and painful. It was a yīn pattern sore. I happened to read an ancient *Yīn Yáng Shū* 陰陽書, which said to apply green mulberry liquid to treat sores on the lower legs. The sore was cured after I used this method. Later on in Wǔlín, I had a sore on the medial malleolus [again], then another one came a month later. I asked the servant to get a little yellow mulberry liquid from the lower part of the river, then applied it once. The sores were cured by the next morning. Since then, I always teach other people to use it, and it is always effective. My cousin had sores on his legs and could not walk; my younger brother pounded mulberry root into a paste, applied it on him, and the sores were cured.

舉體痛癢如蟲嚙，癢而搔之，皮便脫落作瘡：灸曲池二穴，隨年壯 。發即灸之，神良（《千》）。凡疔腫 、頭瘡 、魚臍等瘡，一切無名者，皆治（見發背 ）。凡瘡毒久不合：灸合谷各七壯，至七七壯，極驗（仍服內托散 ）。

Generalized body pain and itching that feels like insects biting, the skin falls off after scratching, then sores are formed: Apply moxibustion on Qū Chí 曲池 (LI 11), burning the same number of cones as the patient's age. Applying moxibustion right after the sores flare up has divine effects (*Qiān*《千》). It also treats sores such as swollen clove sores, head sores, fish umbilicus [sores], and so forth, as well as those sores without a name (see the section on sores on the back).

Unhealed enduring toxic sores: Apply seven up to seven times seven cones of moxibustion on Hé Gǔ 合谷 (LI 4); it is extremely effective (in addition take *Nèi Tuō Sǎn* 内托散 (Internal Expulsion Powder)).

小兒疳濕瘡：灸第十五椎俠脊兩傍七壯，未瘥，加七壯（《千》）。疔腫在左，灸左臂曲肘紋前，取病患三指外於臂上處中灸之兩筋間，從不痛至痛，腫在右從右灸，不過三日即瘥（《千》）。

*Gān* damp sores in children: Apply seven cones of moxibustion on the site alongside the fifteenth vertebrae; add another seven cones if it is not cured (*Qiān*).

If swollen clove sores are on the left, apply moxibustion on the depression between two sinews on the upper part of the arm, three finger-widths distal to the elbow crease when the left arm is flexed; if there was no pain at the beginning, burn moxa until the patient feels pain; apply the moxibustion on the right when swelling is on the right. It will cure the disease in three days (*Qiān*).

# 7.17
# Xuǎn Jiè Chuāng (Bái Diàn Fēng, Yóu Mù)
# 癬疥瘡（白癜風　疣目）

## Lichens and scab sores
**(Vitiligo; warts)**

日中時灸病處影上三壯。咒曰：癬中蟲，毛戎戎，若欲治，待日中（《千》）。又法：八月八日日出時，令病患正當東向戶長跪，平舉兩手，持戶兩邊，取肩頭小垂際骨解宛宛中灸，兩火俱下，各三壯，若七壯，十日愈。

Apply three cones of moxibustion on the shadow of the affected area at noon. The incantation [to be chanted during treatment] says: Insects in the lichen, hairy and furry, if you want a treatment, wait until noon (*Qiān*《千》). Another method: At sunrise on the eighth day of the eighth lunar month, ask the patient to kneel toward the east and face the door. Have him lift his arms horizontally against the door frame and apply moxibustion on the depression slightly below the tip of the shoulder joint. Burn the fire on both sides at the same time; apply three or seven cones of moxibustion. This will cure the disease in ten days.

《千金翼》曰：瘡瘑疥癬，皆有諸蟲，三年不瘥，便為惡疾云云。治久癬不瘥方：細研水銀霜如粉，和臘月豬膏。先以泔清洗瘡，拭乾一塗即瘥，再塗永瘥。大陵、支溝、陽谷、後溪主痂疥（《千》）。陽溪治痂疥（《銅》）。合谷、曲池療皮膚痂疥（《明下》）。

*Qiān Jīn Yì*《千金翼》says: Sores, scabs and lichens are all caused by insects. If not cured within three years, malign diseases will arise. The formula to treat enduring lichens: Grind calomelas, mix with lard from the twelfth lunar month. First clean and rinse the sores with the water used to rinse rice and dry them. Applying the ointment once will cure the disease; repeating once will cure the disease forever.

Dà Líng 大陵 (PC 7), Zhī Gōu 支溝 (SJ 6), Yáng Gǔ 陽谷 (SI 5), and Hòu Xī 後溪 (SI 3) govern scabies (*Qiān*).

Yáng Xī 陽溪 (LI 5) treats scabies (*Tóng*《銅》).

Hé Gǔ 合谷 (LI 4) and Qū Chí 曲池 (LI 11) cure scabies of the skin (*Míng Xià*《明下》).

予少患疥，凡十五年，遇冬則為瘡。人教用羊蹄菜根（蛇床子根）片切如錢，米泔浸三二宿，漉出；生薑、礬同研細，裹以生布，遇浴擦洗良久，以水洗，三四次用即除根。後數年再生，用前法愈，神效如此。何以灸為也。

I suffered scabies when I was young; it had been there for 15 years and changed to sores during the winter. Someone told me to slice the root of *yáng tí cài* 羊蹄菜 (*shé chuáng zǐ* 蛇床子(Cnidii Fructus)) into pieces the size of a coin. Soak it in water from rinsing rice for two or three nights and drain it. Then grind it into a fine powder with ginger and alum and wrap it with raw sackcloth. When taking a bath, rub and wash the affected site for a while, then rinse with water. Repeating this three or four times will remove the root [of the disease]. If it comes back years later, use the previous method again; it will be divinely effective. So why apply moxibustion?

白癜風：灸左右手中指節去延外宛中三壯。未瘥，報之。

Vitiligo: Apply three cones of moxibustion in the depression on the lateral side of joints of left and right middle fingers. Repeat moxibustion if the disease is not cured.

《至道單方》治紫癜風：用舶上硫黃細研，綿帛裹，生薑自然汁半盞浸和，綿子塗所患處，稍乾再易。此患多從夏發。但請驗之，予雖未試，想必奇方也。

*Zhì Dào Dān Fāng*《至道單方》(Single-Herb Formulas to Reach the Dào) treatment for purple patch wind (Lichen Planus): Grind *líu huáng* 硫黃 (Sulfur) from a ship into fine powder, wrap it in cotton or silk cloth, and let it sit in half a bowl of fresh ginger juice. Wipe the affected area with a cotton ball of the liquid and repeat when it dries. This disease usually occurs in summer. I request that someone verifies this; I have never tried it, but I thought it was a miracle formula.

《千金翼》灸白癜、白駁等：重午日午時，灸膝外屈腳當文頭隨年壯，一時下火，不得動。又白癜、白駁、浸淫、歷瘍著頭頸胸前：灸兩乳間隨年壯，立瘥。疣目：著艾炷疣目上灸之，三壯即除。支正治生疣目(《銅》)。

Moxibustion for vitiligo and psoriais from *Qiān Jīn Yì*《千金翼》: At noon time on a *Chóng Wǔ* 重午 day (*Duān Wǔ* or the fifth day of the fifth lunar month; the dragon boat festival), apply moxibustion at the end of the crease on the lateral aspect of the knees when the legs are bent. Burn the same number of cones as the patient's age. Once the fire is buring, do not move the legs.

Vitiligo, white patch [psoriasis], wet spreading sores, or tinea versicolor on the head, neck, and chest: Apply the same number of cones as the patient's age on the site between the two nipples. It will cure the disease immediately.

Warts: Apply moxibustion on the warts; burn three cones of moxibustion to remove the warts. Zhī Zhèng 支正 (SI 7) treats warts (*Tóng*《銅》).

疣目雖可灸，《千金方》亦有用杏仁燒令黑，研膏塗上者；有用松柏脂合和塗之，一宿失去者；有用牛口中涎數涂自落者；有用苦酒漬石灰六七日，滴取汁點疣上，小作疣即落者；有以豬脂揩癢處，令少許血出即瘥。神驗無以加者，不必專拘灸也。

Though we can apply moxibustion on warts, *Qiān Jīn Fāng*《千金方》says to fry *xìng rén* 杏仁 (Armeniacae Semen) until black, grind it into a paste, and apply it on the warts; or mix [the *xìng rén*] with pine resin and apply it on the warts, the warts will disappear in one night; or frequently wipe them with drool from an ox's mouth, the warts will fall off automatically; or soak limestone with bitter liquor for six or seven days, then apply drops of the liquid on the warts, small warts will fall off immediately; or wipe the itchy area with pork lard and let a little blood to cure the warts. These all are divinely effective; we do not have to limit ourselves to moxibustion.

# 7.18
## *Gǔ Dú*
# 蠱毒
## **Gǔ-toxins**[26]

巨闕治蠱毒（《銅》見心痛）。俗亦有灸法：初中蠱，於心下捺便大炷灸百壯。並主貓鬼，亦灸得愈。又當足下小指尖上灸三壯，當有物出：酒上得者，有酒出；飯上得者，有飯出；肉菜上得者，有肉菜出。即愈，神驗。皆於灸瘡上出（《千》）。

Jù Quē 巨闕 (Rèn 14) treats *gǔ*-toxins (see the section on heart pain in *Tóng*《銅》). There are moxibustion methods, too: In the initial attacked by *gǔ*, press the area below the heart, then apply a hundred cones on it. This is also effect for cat *gǔ* 蠱.[27] Or apply three cones of moxibustion on the tip of the little toe; something should come out: if [the *gǔ*] came from drinking, liquor will come out; if it came from eating, rice will come out; if it came from meat and vegetables, vegetables and meat will come out. The disease will be cured immediately. Its effects are divine. The *gǔ*-toxins come out from the moxa sores (*Qiān*《千》).

梅師治卒中蠱，下血如雞肝，臟腑敗壞。桔梗搗汁服七分合佳。《錄驗方》亦云：卒中蠱，血如雞肝，晝夜出血，桔梗搗屑，酒服方寸匕，日三。藥不下，校開口灌。又有用馬藺根末水服方寸匕，隨吐則出，極神者。《肘後方》云：凡中蠱令人心腹切痛，如有物咬，或吐下血，不即治，蝕人五臟盡即死。蓖麻一枚去皮，朴硝一錢同研，新水作一服，連進二三服效。此雖未試，亦奇方也。

Master Méi's treatment of sudden *gǔ* attack, with blood in the stool that looks like chicken livers and damage to the organs: It is best to pound *jié gěng* 桔梗 (Platycodonis Radix) and drink seven tenths of a *gě* of juice.

*Lù Yàn Fāng*《錄驗方》(Records of Effective Formulas) also says: for sudden *gǔ* attack with blood that looks like chicken liver, bleeding day and night, pound *jié gěng* (Platycodonis Radix) into

26. *Gǔ* 蠱 is a type of poison from insects or reptiles.

27. *Māo Guǐ Gǔ* 貓鬼蠱 (cat *gǔ*): This is the most poisonous *gǔ* 蠱 from an animal.

bits, take a square-cùn spoonful with liquor three times a day. If someone is unable to get the herbs down, open his mouth forcefully and pour the herbs in. Or drink a square-cùn spoon of powder of *mǎ lìn gēn* 馬藺根 (Iridis Radix) with water. The patient will vomit [the *gǔ*] out. This is extremely miraculous.

*Zhóu Hòu Fāng*《肘後方》(Prescriptions for Emergencies) says: When *gǔ* attacks, the victim has cutting pain of the chest and abdomen that feels like something is biting him, as well as vomiting blood, or bloody diarrhea. If he cannot get treatment in time, the *gǔ* erodes his five viscera and he will die. Grind together one piece of peeled *bì má* 蓖麻 (Ricini Semen) and one *qián* of *pǔ xiāo* 朴硝 (Natrii Sulfas Non-purus) and cook it in enough newly-drawn water to make one dose. Drinking two or three doses will be effective. Though I have never tried this, it is a miraculous formula.

## 7.19
## *Quǎn Shāng (Shé Shāng)*
# 犬傷（蛇傷）
### Dog bite
**(Snake bite)**

外丘治猘犬所傷，毒不出，發寒熱，速以三壯艾可灸嚙處，立愈(《銅》)。春末夏初，狂犬咬人，即令人狂，過百日乃得免。當終身禁食犬肉、蠶蛹，食此則發，不可救也。先去卻惡血，灸瘡中十壯。明日以後，日灸一壯，百日乃止，忌酒。每七日搗韭汁飲一二盞。

Wài Qiū 外丘 (GB 36) treats damage from rabid dog bites, with inability to get toxin out and onset of [sensations of] cold and heat: Apply three cones of moxibustion on the site of bite to cure the disease immediately (*Tóng*《銅》).

At the end of spring and beginning of summer, people suffer mania after rabid dog bites.[28] When a hundred days have passed the danger is over. People should avoid eating dog meat and silkworm chrysalis for the rest of their life. The disease will relapse after eating these things and is not treatable. First remove the malign blood and then apply ten cones of moxibustion on the wound. Apply one cone of moxibustion every day on the second day and after, stopping at a hundred days. Liquor is contraindicated. Pound leeks to make juice and drink one or two cups every seven days.

28. Note that *kuáng* 狂 means rabid for dogs, but mania for people. In fact, this means people get rabies from dogs and then act as if manic.

睡中蛇入七竅，以艾灸蛇尾即出。又法：刀破蛇尾些子，入椒七粒，蛇自出。出後急以雄黄朱砂細研，煎人參湯調灌，取蛇毒(《單》)。

If a snake enters into the seven orifices during sleep, apply moxibustion on the snake's tail and it will come out. Another method: Cut the snake's tail a little bit and apply seven pieces of pepper; the snake will automatically come out. As soon as the snake comes out, grind *xióng huáng* 雄黄 (Realgar) and *zhū shā* 朱砂 (Cinnabaris) into fine powder, cook *Rén Shēn Tāng* 人參湯 (Ginseng Decoction), mix it with the powder and pour it in. It will remove the snake poison (*Dān*《單》).

山居人或被蛇傷，即以溺溺之，拭乾，以艾灸之效。《朝野僉載》記艾炷當毒蛇嚙處灸，引出毒氣瘥。薄切獨頭蒜貼蛇咬處灸，熱徹即止（灸蛇毒上三七壯，無艾，以火頭稱瘡孔大小蒸之。《千翼》）。狂犬咬人，令人吮去惡血盡，灸百壯後（日日灸，百日止。若血不出，一生忌酒豬。《千翼》）。

When people who live in a mountainous area are bitten by a snakes, they urinate on the wound, wipe it dry, then apply moxibustion. This is effective. *Cháo Yě Qiān Zǎi*《朝野僉載》(Combined Chronicle of the Government and the Public) recorded that moxa cones should be applied on the site of a poison snake bite to pull out the poison qì and cure the disease. Or cut single-clove garlic into thin slices and place one on the site of the bite; apply moxibustion on it and stop when the heat penetrates through. [Apply three times seven cones of moxibustion on the site of poison snake bite. If mugwort is not available, use a flame to match the size of the sores to steam it. *Qiān Yì*《千翼》).

For a rabid dog bite, have someone suck all the malign blood out, then apply a hundred cones of moxibustion. (Apply moxibustion daily for a hundred days. If no blood comes out, the victim should avoid liquor and pork for the rest of his life (*Qiān Yì*).

月事
735

# 7.20
## *Rŭ Yōng*
## 乳癰
## Mammary welling-abscess

膺窗治乳癰寒熱，臥不安（《銅》）。臨泣治乳癰（見月事）。神封治乳癰，灑淅惡寒（《明》同）。乳根治乳癰淒慘寒（《千》有熱字）痛，不可按。三里主乳癰（《銅》同）有熱（《千》）。下廉主乳癰，驚，痹，脛重（《銅》作喉痹胻腫），足跗不收，跟痛。

Yīng Chuāng 膺窗 (ST 16) treats mammary welling-abscess with [sensations of] cold and heat and unquiet sleep (*Tóng*《銅》).

Lín Qì 臨泣 (GB 41) treats mammary welling-abscess (see the section on menstruation).

Shén Fēng 神封 (KI 23) treats mammary welling-abscess and aversion to cold as if after soaking in the rain (*Míng*《明》agrees).

Rŭ Gēn 乳根 (ST 18) treats mammary welling-abscess, aversion to cold (*Qiān*《千》has heat) and pain that cannot be pressed.

Sān Lĭ 三里 (ST 36) governs mammary welling-abscess (*Tóng* agrees) with heat (*Qiān*).

Xià Lián 下廉 (ST 39) governs mammary welling-abscess, fright, *bì*-impediment, heaviness of the lower legs (*Tóng* says: throat *bì*-impediment and swollen lower legs), loss of use of the legs, and heel pain.

神封、膺窗主乳癰寒熱短氣，臥不安。天溪、俠溪主乳腫癰潰。論曰：產後宜勤擠乳，不宜令汁蓄積。蓄積不去，便結不復出，惡汁於內引熱，溫壯結堅，牽掣痛，大渴引飲，乳急痛，手不得近，成妬乳，非癰也。急灸兩手魚際二七壯，斷癰脈也。不復惡手近，乳汁亦自出，便可手助迮捋之，則乳汁大出，皆如膿狀。內服連翹湯，外以小豆薄塗之，便瘥。又以繩橫度口，以度從乳上行，灸度頭二七壯（《千翼》）。

Shén Fēng (KI 23) and Yīng Chuāng (ST 16) govern mammary welling-abscess, [sensations of] cold and heat, shortness of breath, and unquiet sleep.

Tiān Xī 天溪 (SP 18) and Xiá Xī 俠溪 (GB 43) govern breast swelling and ulcerated welling-abscesses. The discussion says: It is appropriate to squeeze the breasts after giving birth; do not let the milk accumulate. Accumulations do not go away; they will bind up and never come out. Malign fluids remaining inside will lead to heat and cause warmth, hardness, pulling pain, severe thirst with desire to drink, and acute pain of the breasts that cannot be touched. This will become begrudging milk[29] and is not a welling-abscess. Quickly apply two times seven cones of moxibustion on Yú Jì 魚際 (LU 10) bilaterally to sever the welling-abscess vessels. Then the patient will not be averse to a hand nearing [touching] the breast, and milk will naturally come out. Then when the breasts are manually pressed and stroked, a lot of milk that all looks like pus will come out. Take *Lián Qiào Tāng* 連翹湯 (Forsythia Decoction) internally, and apply a thin layer of red bean [paste] externally. This will cure the disease. Or measure the width of the mouth with a string, then use this length to measure up from the nipples. Apply two times seven cones of moxibustion at the end of the string (*Qiān Yì*《千翼》).

《千金論》曰：女人患乳癰，四十以下，治之多瘥；四十以上，治之多死；不治，自終天年。予有親年七十，生乳癰，不信此論，令外科用刀仗開，時暫雖快，未歲而殂。方知《千金》猶信也。有搗地榆汁敷，有搗蔓菁葉或根敷，熱即易之。有用白芷末溫湯調敷效。

*Qiān Jīn Lun*《千金論》says: Females who suffer mammary welling-abscess can be cured if they are less then forty years old. They will die after treatment if they are over forty years old, but if they do not get any treatment, they will complete their natural life span. I had a seventy-year-old relative who had breast welling-abscess, but she did not believe this theory, and asked an external doctor to lance it open. She was pleased temporally, but died before long. So [what was said in] *Qiān Jīn*《千金》is reliable.

There is also the method of pounding *dì yú* 地榆 (Sanguisorbae Radix) and applying the juice externally. Or pound the roots or the leaves of *màn jīng* 蔓菁 (Brassicae Rapae Tuber et. Folium), then apply it externally, changing it when it feels warm. Or external application of a warm decoction of *bái zhǐ* 白芷 (Angelicae Dahuricae Radix) powder. These are all effective.

29. *Dù rǔ* 妒乳 (begrudging milk): Retention and stagnation of milk in the breast, an early stage of breast abscess.

月事
735
脾疼
309
胸痛
469
驚
323

# 7.21

## *Rǔ Zhǒng Tòng (Rǔ Shǎo, Tǔ Nǎi)*

## 乳腫痛（乳少　吐奶）

## Painful swelling of the breasts

**(Insufficient lactation; vomiting of milk)**

乳根療乳痛（《明》）。肓門（《明》同）治婦人乳有餘疾（《銅》）。《千》云：中極主乳餘疾。氣衝治難乳，子上搶心（見月事）。府舍，厥氣兩乳（見脾疼）。太泉主妒乳膺胸痛（《千》）。天溪治乳腫賁膺（見胸痛）。

Rǔ Gēn 乳根 (ST 18) cures breast pain (*Míng*《明》).

Huāng Mén (UB 51) (*Míng* agrees) treats various breast diseases in women (*Tóng*《銅》). *Qiān*《千》says: Zhōng Jí 中極 (Rèn 3) governs various breast diseases.

Qì Chōng 氣衝 (ST 30) treats difficult lactation and fetal [qì] surging up into the heart (see the section on menstruation).

Fǔ Shě 府舍 (SP 13) treats reversal qì of the two breasts (see the section on spleen pain).

Tài Quán 太泉 (LU 9) governs begrudging milk and pain of the anterior chest (*Qiān*).

Tiān Xī 天溪 (SP 18) treats swelling of the breasts and a sensation of fullness in the chest (see the section on chest pain).

梁丘（見驚）、地五會治乳腫。天牖主乳腫，缺盆中腫（《千》）。足臨泣主乳腫（見月事）。膻中治乳汁少（《銅》）。《明下》云：奶脈滯無汁，下火立愈。小兒吐奶：灸中庭一壯（《明下》）。小兒喉中鳴，咽乳不利：璇璣三壯。

Liáng Qiū 梁丘 (ST 34) (see the section on fright) and Dì Wǔ Huì 地五會 (GB 42) treat swelling of the breasts.

Tiān Yǒu 天牖 (SJ 16) governs swelling of the breasts and swelling of the empty basin (*Qiān*《千》).

月事
735

Zú Lín Qì 足臨泣 (GB 41) governs swelling of the breasts (see the section on menstruation).

Dàn Zhōng 膻中 (Rèn 17) treats insufficient lactation (*Tóng*《銅》). *Míng Xià*《明下》says: It treats blockage in the vessels of the breasts and absence of lactation. It will be cured as soon as moxibustion is applied.

Vomiting of milk in children: Apply one cone of moxibustion on Zhōng Tíng 中庭 (Rèn 16) (*Míng Xià*).

Throat rales in children and inhibited swallowing of milk: Apply three cones of moxibustion on Xuán Jī 璇璣 (Rèn 21).

## 7.22
## *Fù Rén Wú Zǐ*
# 婦人無子
## Infertility

陰廉治婦人絕產。若未經產者，灸三壯即有子（《銅》）。中髎治絕子帶下，月事不調。次髎、涌泉、商丘治絕子。中極治婦人斷緒（見月事，《明》同）。《明下》云：療失精絕子。石關治絕子，臟有惡血上衝，腹痛不可忍。《明下》云：腹厥痛絞刺。

Yīn Lián 陰廉 (LV 11) treats infertility in women. Those who have never been pregnant will conceive after applying three cones of moxibustion (*Tóng*).

Zhōng Liáo 中髎 (UB 33) treats infertility, abnormal vaginal discharge, and irregular menstruation.

Cì Liáo 次髎 (UB 32), Yǒng Quán 涌泉 (KI 1), and Shāng Qiū 商丘 (SP 5) treat infertility.

Zhōng Jí 中極 (Rèn 3) treats infertility (see the section on menstruation; *Míng*《明》agrees). *Míng Xià* says: It cures loss of essence and infertility.

Shí Guān 石關 (KI 18) treats infertility with malign blood rushing upward in the viscera and unbearable abdominal pain (*Míng Xià* says: Reversal pain of the abdomen that feels like twisting a knife).

曲泉主女子疝瘕，按之如以湯沃兩股中，小腹腫，陰挺出痛，經水來下，陰腫或癢，漉青汁如葵羹，血閉無子，不嗜食(《千》)。水原、陰蹻主女不字，陰暴出淋漏，月水不來，多悶心痛。

Qū Quán 曲泉 (LV 8) governs *shàn*-mounting and conglomerations, when pressed it feels like the thighs are being washed with hot water, swelling of the smaller abdomen, pain due to vaginal protrusion (prolapse of the uterus), genital swelling or itching during menstruation, with seepage of greenish vaginal discharge that looks like black nightshade soup, blood blockage, infertility, and no desire to eat (*Qiān*《千》).

Shuǐ Yuán 水原 (KI 5) and Yīn Qiāo 陰蹻 (KI 6 or KI 8) govern infertility in women, sudden prolapse of the uterus, vaginal spotting and leakage, absence of menstruation, and frequent oppressive heart pain.

然谷主不字(《銅》作不孕)，陰暴出，經漏(《千》)。上窌主絕子，瘧寒熱，陰挺出，不禁白瀝，痙，脊反折。陰交主拘攣腹滿疝，月水不下，乳餘疾，絕子，陰癢，賁豚上膜，腹堅痛，下引陰中，不得小便。

Rán Gǔ 然谷 (KI 2) governs infertility (*Tóng*《銅》says: cannot conceive), sudden prolapse of the uterus, and leakage of menstruation (*Qiān*).

Shàng Liáo 上窌 (UB 31) governs infertility, malaria with [sensations of] cold and heat, vaginal protrusion (prolapse of the uterus), incontinence of white vaginal discharge, tetany, and arched-back spine.

Yīn Jiāo 陰交 (Rèn 7) governs hypertonicity, abdominal fullness, *shàn*-mounting, amenorrhea, various breast diseases, infertility, genital itching, running-piglet disease with fullness, hardness and pain of the abdomen that radiates to the genitals, and inability to urinate.

石門主腹滿疝積，乳餘疾，絕子，陰癢，賁豚上膜，小腹堅痛，下引陰中，不得小便，忌灸，絕孕。關元主絕子，血在內不下，胞轉不得尿，小腹滿，石水痛。又主引脅下脹，頭痛身背熱，賁豚，寒，小便數，泄不止.

Shí Mén 石門 (Rèn 5) governs abdominal fullness, *shàn*-mounting, accumulations, various breast diseases, infertility, genital itching, running-piglet disease with fullness, hardness and pain in the smaller abdomen radiating to the genitals, and inability to urinate. Moxibustion on this point is contraindicated; it causes infertility.

Guān Yuán 關元 (Rèn 4) governs infertility with the blood remaining inside and unable to descend, shifted bladder with inability to urinate, fullness of the smaller abdomen, and pain due to stone water. It also governs radiating distention of the rib-sides, headaches, hot body and back, running-piglet disease, coldness, frequent urination, and incessant diarrhea.

中極主子門不端，小腹苦寒，陰癢及痛，賁豚搶心，飢不能食，腹脹，經閉不通，小便不利，乳餘疾，絕子。又主拘攣腹疝，陰癢。築賓主大疝絕子。涌泉主女子無子，咳而短氣。氣衝主無子，小腹痛。陰廉主絕產，若未曾產。

Zhōng Jí 中極 (Rèn 3) governs malposition of the mouth of the uterus, coldness in the abdomen, itching painful genitals, running-piglet prodding the heart, hunger with inability to eat, abdominal distention, amenorrhea, inhibited urination, various breast diseases, and infertility. It also governs hypertonicity of the abdomen with *shàn*-mounting, and genital itching.

Zhù Bīn 築賓 (KI 9) governs great *shàn*-mounting and infertility.

Yǒng Quán 涌泉 (KI 1) governs infertility in women, cough, and shortness of breath.

Qì Chōng 氣衝 (ST 30) governs infertility and pain of the smaller abdomen.

Yīn Lián 陰廉 (LV 11) governs infertility.

婦人絕子：灸然谷五十壯。婦人絕嗣不生，胞門閉塞：關元三十壯，報之。婦人妊子不成，若墮落腹痛，漏見赤：胞門五十壯，在關元左邊二寸是。婦人絕嗣不生：灸氣門，在關元旁三寸，百壯。婦人子臟閉塞，不受精，疼：胞門五十壯。

Infertility in women: Apply fifty cones of moxibustion on Rán Gǔ 然谷 (KI 2).

Infertility in women with blockage of uterus: Apply thirty cones of moxibustion on Guān Yuán 關元 (Rèn 4) and repeat in sessions.

Inability to become pregnant, abdominal pain after miscarriage, and spotting of blood: Apply fifty cones of moxibustion on Bāo Mén 胞門. It is located 2 cùn lateral to Guān Yuán (Rèn 4), on the left side.

Infertility in women: Apply a hundred cones of moxibustion on Qì Mén 氣門. It is located 3 cùn lateral to Guān Yuán (Rèn 4).

Blockage of the uterus, inability to conceive, and pain: Apply fifty cones of moxibustion on Bāo Mén.

婦人絕嗣不生，漏赤白：泉門十壯，三報。月水不利，賁豚上下，並無子：四滿三十壯。婦人胞落頹：臍中三百壯；又身交五十壯，三報，在臍下橫文中；又背脊當臍五十壯；又玉泉五十壯，三報。

Infertility in women, spotting with red and white [discharge]: Apply ten cones of moxibustion on Quán Mén 泉門 (non-channel);[30] repeat for three sessions.

Inhibited menstruation, running-piglet that moves up and down, and infertility: Apply thirty cones of moxibustion on Sì Mǎn 四滿 (KI 14).

Prolapse of the uterus: Apply three hundred cones of moxibustion on Qí Zhōng 臍中 (Rèn 8). Or burn fifty cones of moxibustion on Shēn Jiāo 身交 (non-channel); repeat for three sessions. It is located in the transverse crease below the umbilicus. Or burn fifty cones of moxibustion on the site on the back that is level with the umbilicus. Or apply fifty cones of moxibustion on Yù Quán 玉泉 (Rèn 3); repeat for three sessions.

婦人胞下垂注，陰下脫：灸俠玉泉三寸隨年壯，三報。婦人陰冷腫痛：歸來三十壯，三報。中極，婦人斷緒最要穴（帶下）。關元主斷緒產道冷，針八分，留三呼，瀉五吸，灸亦佳，灸不及針，日灸百壯止。

Prolapse of the uterus in women: Apply moxibustion on the site 3 cùn lateral to Yù Quán 玉泉 (Rèn 3); burn the same number of cones as the patient's age, and repeat for three sessions.

Coldness, swelling, and pain of the genitals in women: Apply thirty cones of moxibustion on Guī Lái 歸來 (ST 29); repeat for three sessions.

Zhōng Jí 中極 (Rèn 3) is the most important point for infertility in women (see the section on [red and white] vaginal discharge).

Guān Yuán 關元 (Rèn 4) governs infertility and coldness of the vagina; needle 8 fēn deep, retain the needle for three respirations, and drain for five breaths. Moxibustion also is good, but not as good as needling. Apply up to a hundred cones of moxibustion.

妊不成，數墮落：玉泉（即中極）五十，三報；又龍門二十壯。婦人無子：針關元（《千翼》，甄權）。涌泉治婦人無子（見虛損）。婦人欲斷產，灸右踝上一寸三壯，即斷（《千》）。石門忌灸，絕孕。《銅》云：針之絕子。《明》云：懷胎必不針關元，若針而落胎。

Inability to become pregnant with frequent miscarriage: Apply fifty cones of moxibustion on Yù Quán (meaning Zhōng Jí (Rèn 3)); repeat for three sessions. Or burn twenty cones of moxibustion on Lóng Mén 龍門.[31]

30. Quán Mén 泉門 is located on the anterior midline below the lower border of symphysis pubis and right above the anterior commisure of the labia majora.

31. Lóng Mén 龍門 is the external opening of the vagina in married women who have never given birth.

Infertility in women: Needle Guān Yuán 關元 (Rèn 4) (*Qiān Yì*《 千翼 》and Zhēn Quán).

Yǒng Quán 涌泉 (KI 1) treats infertility in women (see the section on vacuity detriment).

Women who desire to stop childbirth[32]: Apply three cones of moxibustion on the site 1 cùn above the right ankle. It will stop (*Qiān*《 千 》).

Shí Mén 石門 (Rèn 5) is contraindicated for moxibustion; this will cause infertility. *Tóng*《 銅 》says: Acupuncture on it causes infertility. *Míng*《 明 》says: Acupuncture is contraindicated during pregnancy; the fetus will fall [miscarry] after needling.

胎多不出，針外崑崙立出。陰交灸多，絕孕（《千翼》）。又云：石門、關元相去一寸，針關元治婦人無子；針石門則終身絕嗣。其道幽隱，豈可輕侮哉。

The fetus cannot come out: Needling Wài Kūn Lún 外崑崙 will immediately induce labor.

Applying a lot of moxibustion on Yīn Jiāo 陰交 (Rèn 7) causes infertility (*Qiān Yì*). It also says: There is a difference of one cùn between Shí Mén (Rèn 5) and Guān Yuán (Rèn 4). Needle Guān Yuán (Rèn 4) to treat infertility in women but needling Shí Mén (Rèn 5) causes infertility for the rest of the life. The theory has been secret, but we cannot ignore it.

32. This means to prevent conception.

血崩 728
虛損 174
月事 735

# 7.23
## *Fù Rén Xuè Qì Tòng*
## 婦人血氣痛
### Pain due to blood and qì in women

四滿（又主胞中有血）、石門主子臟有惡血內逆，滿痛（《千》）。四滿治婦人血积冷。陽蹻療婦人血氣（《明》）。陰交治產後惡露不止，繞臍冷痛（見血崩）。涌泉治心痛不嗜食，婦人無子，女子如妊娠，五指端盡痛（見虛損）。婦女本臟氣血癖走刺痛（灸法見腎虛）。陰交治血塊腹痛（餘見月事）。

Sì Mǎn 四滿 (KI 14) (It also governs blood in the uterus) and Shí Mén 石門 (Rèn 5) govern malign blood counterflowing inside in the uterus with fullness and pain (*Qiān*《千》).

Sì Mǎn (KI 14) treats accumulations of cold in the blood.

Yáng Qiāo 陽蹻 (UB 62) cures blood and qì in women (*Míng*《明》).

Yīn Jiāo 陰交 (Rèn 7) treats persistent flow of lochia after childbirth and cold pain around the umbilicus (see the section on flooding of blood).

Yǒng Quán 涌泉 (KI 1) treats heart pain, no desire to eat, infertility in women, and pain of the tips of the fingers during pregnancy (see the section on vacuity detriment).

Qì and blood aggregations, migrating prickly pain of the root organ [unknown term] of women (see the method of moxibustion under kidney vacuity).

Yīn Jiāo 陰交 (Rèn 7) treats blood clots with abdominal pain (for further discussion, see the section on menstruation).

# 7.24
# *Xuè Kuài (Yū Xuè)*
# 血塊（瘀血）

## Blood clots
**(Blood stasis)**

月事 735
淋 222
尸厥 531

石門治婦人因產惡露不止，遂結成塊，崩中(《明》同)漏下(《銅》)。天樞、中極治成塊(並見月事)。下極療因產惡露不止，遂成疝瘕，或因月事不調，血結成塊(《明》)。

Shí Mén 石門 (Rèn 5) treats incessant flow of postpartum lochia that then forms clots, and flooding of blood (*Míng*《明》agrees) or spotting (*Tóng*《銅》).

Tiān Shū 天樞 (ST 25) and Zhōng Jí 中極 (Rèn 3) treat blood clots (for all, see the section on menstruation).

Xià Jí 下極 (KI 11) cures incessant flow of postpartum lochia that becomes *shàn*-mounting and conglomerations or blood clots due to irregular menstruation (*Míng*).

漏谷、曲泉治血瘕(《銅》見痃癖)。曲骨主血癃(《千》)。復溜主血淋。血淋灸丹田等(並見淋)。三里治胸中瘀血(《銅》)。九曲中府主內有瘀血(見尸厥)。

Lòu Gǔ 漏谷 (SP 7) and Qū Quán 曲泉 (LV 8) treat blood conglomerations (see the section on strings and aggregations in *Tóng*).

Qū Gǔ 曲骨 (Rèn 2) governs blood blockage (*Qiān*《千》).

Fù Liū 復溜 (KI 7) governs blood *lín*-strangury.

Apply moxibustion on Dān Tián 丹田 (cinnabar field) and so forth for blood *lín*-strangury (for all, see the section on dribbling).

Sān Lǐ 三里 (ST 36) treats blood stasis in the chest (*Tóng*).

Jiǔ Qū Zhōng Fǔ 九曲中府 governs internal blood stasis (see the section on deathlike reversal).

月事
735
血塊
727
疝
213
無子
721

# 7.25

## *Xuè Bēng (Bēng Zhōng Lòu Xià, È Lù Bù Zhǐ)*

# 血崩（崩中漏下　惡露不止）

## Flooding of blood

**(Flooding and spotting of blood, incessant lochia)**

大敦治血崩不止（《銅》）。合陽治崩中。氣海（見月事）、石門治崩中漏下（見血塊）。中都治崩中，因產惡露不絕。交信、陰谷、太衝、三陰交治女漏血不止。石門治崩中漏下（見血塊）。血海治漏下惡血，月事不調，逆氣腹脹。

Dà Dūn 大敦 (LV 1) treats incessant flooding of blood (*Tóng*《銅》).

Hé Yáng 合陽 (UB 55) treats flooding of blood.

Qì Hǎi 氣海 (Rèn 6) (see the section on menstruation) and Shí Mén 石門 (Rèn 5) treat flooding and spotting of blood (see the section on blood clots).

Zhōng Dū 中都 (LV 6) treats flooding of blood and incessant flow of postpartum lochia.

Jiāo Xìn 交信 (KI 8), Yīn Gǔ 陰谷 (KI 10), Tài Chōng 太衝 (LV 3), and Sān Yīn Jiāo 三陰交 (SP 6) treat incessant spotting of blood in women.

Shí Mén (Rèn 5) treats flooding and spotting of blood (see the section on blood clots).

Xuè Hǎi 血海 (SP 10) treats spotting of malign blood, irregular menstruation, qì counterflow, and abdominal distention.

血海主漏下，若血閉不通，逆氣脹（《千》）。陰谷主漏血，小腹脹，體寒熱，腹偏腫。太衝（見疝）、然谷主經漏（見無子）。陰蹻主陰挺下血，陰腫或癢，漉清汁若葵汁。

Xuè Hǎi (SP 10) governs spotting, blood blockage, qì counterflow, and distention (*Qiān*《千》).

Yīn Gǔ 陰谷 (KI 10) governs spotting of blood, distention of the smaller abdomen, generalized [sensations of] cold and heat, and hemilateral swelling of the abdomen.

Tài Chōng 太衝 (LV 3) (see the section on prominent *shàn*-mounting) and Rán Gǔ 然谷 (KI 2) govern menstrual spotting (see the section on infertility).

Yīn Qiāo 陰蹻 (KI 6 or KI 8) governs prolapsed uterus, bleeding, swelling or itching of the genitals, and seeping of vaginal discharge that looks like black nightshade juice.

白崩：灸小腹横文當臍孔直下百壯，又内踝上三寸，左右各百壯 。陰交 、石門療崩中（ 《 明 》 ）。天樞療漏下赤白（ 交儀 、復溜並同 ），及腹大堅，食不化，面色蒼蒼（ 《 下 》 ）。

White flooding [abnormal vaginal discharge][33]: Apply a hundred cones of moxibustion on the transverse crease of the smaller abdomen, right below the umbilicus. Or bilaterally 3 cùn above the medial malleolus.

Yīn Jiāo 陰交 (Rèn 7) and Shí Mén 石門 (Rèn 5) cure flooding (*Míng* 《 明 》).

Tiān Shū 天樞 (ST 25) cures red and white spotting (same for Jiāo Yí 交儀 (LV 5) and Fù Liū 復溜 (KI 7)), enlarged and hard abdomen, inability to digest food, and greenish facial complexion (*Xià* 《 下 》).

若經候過多，其色瘀黑，甚者崩下，吸吸少氣，臍腹冷極，則汗出如雨，尺脈微小，由衝任虛衰，為風冷客乘胞中，氣不能固：可灸關元百壯，宜鹿茸丸（ 《 指 》 ）。

Profuse menstruation with black color, or flooding, insufficient qì when breathing, extreme cold of the umbilicus and abdomen, sweating like rain, and fragile thin pulse in the *chǐ* position. This is caused by vacuity of the chōng and rèn vessels and wind-cold attacking the uterus, so qì is insecure: Apply a hundred cones of moxibustion on Guān Yuán 關元 (Rèn 4); it is appropriate to take *Lù Róng Wán* 鹿茸丸 (Velvet Deerhorn Pill) (*Zhǐ* 《 指 》).

有皮匠妻患血崩兩月，飲食不進，與鎮靈丹服，少減而未斷，因檢得《耆域方》如聖散：用烏梅、乾薑各一兩，並燒存五分性為末，每服二錢，食前烏梅湯調下（患甚者不過三服），合一劑與服而疾平。又有巡捕之妻，年逾五十，因傷寒而血崩，與加膠艾四物湯，一服漸愈。後因勞復大作，與鎮靈丹十五丸而止。或無此丹，燒鹿角存性為末，酒調服亦佳。以其屢驗，故附於此。

33. White flooding indicates incessant white vaginal discharge.

月事 735 The wife of a leather worker suffered flooding of blood for over two months with inability to eat. After taking *Zhèn Líng Dān* 鎮靈丹 (Settle Spirit Elixir), the bleeding decreased but did not stop. So
血崩 728 I checked and found *Rú Shèng Sǎn* 如聖散 (Sagacious Powder) in the *Qí Yù Fāng*《耆域方》:
赤白帶 739 one *liǎng* each of *wū méi* 烏梅 (Mume Fructus) and *gān jiāng* 乾薑 (Zingiberis Rhizoma). Fry them together until fifty percent of their properties are preserved and then grind them into powder. Before meals, take two *qián* each dose mixed with *Wū Méi Tāng* 烏梅湯 (Mume Decoction) (no more than three doses are needed, even for severe cases). One dose cured the disease.

The wife of a patrol officer was over fifty years old. She suffered flooding of blood due to cold damage. After taking one dose of [*Rú Shèng Sǎn* (Sagacious Powder)] plus *Jiāo Ài Sì Wù Tāng* 膠艾四物湯 (Ass Hide Glue and Mugwort Four Agents Decoction), the disease improved. Later on, because she worked too hard, she relapsed severely, but it stopped after taking 15 pills of *Zhèn Líng Dān* (Settle Spirit Elixir). If this pill is unavailable, fry deer antler to preserve its properties and grind it into powder. Mix it with liquor and drink it. This also will do good. These methods are always effective, so I put them here.

陰交治女子月事不絕，帶下，產後惡露不止，繞臍冷痛（《銅》《明》同）。氣海（見月事）、中都治惡露不止（見血崩）。關元治惡露不止（見赤白帶）。中極（《明》見血塊）、石門（《下》與《銅》同）療惡露不止。

Yīn Jiāo 陰交 (Rèn 7) treats incessant menstruation, abnormal vaginal discharge, incessant flow of postpartum lochia, and cold pain around the umbilicus (*Tóng*《銅》and *Míng*《明》agree).

Qì Hǎi 氣海 (Rèn 6) (see the section on menstruation) and Zhōng Dū 中都 (LV 6) treat incessant lochia (see the section on flooding of blood).

Guān Yuán 關元 (Rèn 4) treats incessant lochia (see the section on red and white vaginal discharge).

Zhōng Jí 中極 (Rèn 3) (see blood clots in *Míng*) and Shí Mén 石門 (Rèn 5) (Xià《下》and *Tóng* agree) cure incessant lochia.

漏胞下血不禁：灸關元兩旁三寸百壯。產難，月水不禁，橫生，胎動：針三陰交。胎動，崩中，下痢，賁氣上逆：針石門寸四分。漏胞見赤，胞門五十，又氣門五十。崩中，帶下：針灸中極（帶下）。

Incessant spotting during pregnancy: Apply a hundred cones of moxibustion on the sites 3 cùn lateral to Guān Yuán (Rèn 4).

Difficult childbirth, incessant menstruation, transverse presentation, and stirring fetus: Needle Sān Yīn Jiāo 三陰交 (SP 6).

Stirring fetus, flooding of blood, dysentery, rushing qì counterflowing upward: Needle Shí Mén 石門 (Rèn 5) 1.4 cùn deep.

Spotting with redness [blood] during pregnancy: Apply fifty cones of moxibustion on Bāo Mén 胞門 (ST 28) and Qì Mén 氣門 [non-channel, three cùn lateral to Guān Yuán 關元 (Rèn 4)].

Flooding of blood and abnormal vaginal discharge: Apply acupuncture and moxibustion on Zhōng Jí 中極 (Rèn 3) (see the section on [red and white] vaginal discharge).

## 7.26
## *Chǎn Hòu Yú Jí (Chǎn Qián)*
# 產後餘疾（產前）
## Postpartum diseases
**(Before childbirth)**

期門治產後餘疾（《銅》見心痛）。《千》云：主產餘疾，食不下，賁豚上下，傷食腹滿。伏兔療婦人八部諸疾（《明》）。婦人產後渾身疼：針百勞穴。遇痛處即針，避筋骨及禁穴（《許》）。《明下》云：產後未滿百日，不宜灸。

Qī Mén 期門 (LV 14) treats postpartum diseases (see the section on heart pain in *Tóng* 《銅》). *Qiān* 《千》 says: It governs diseases related to childbirth, difficulty getting food down, running-piglet [moving] up and down, and food damage with abdominal fullness.

Fú Tù 伏兔 (ST 32) cures the various diseases of the eight sections in women[34] (*Míng* 《明》).

Postpartum pain all over the body: Needle Bǎi Láo Xué 百勞穴 (non-channel). Needle the painful area, but avoid hurting the sinews and bones and contraindicated points (*Xǔ* 《許》).[35] *Míng Xià* 《明下》 says: Moxibustion is contraindicated within one hundred days after giving birth.

34. *Fù rén bā bù* 婦人八部 the eight sections in women: Menstruation, pregnancy, post-partum, abdominal masses, breasts, external genitals, bleeding disorders, and vaginal discharge. This comes from *Tài Píng Shèng Huì Fāng* 《太平聖惠方》 (*Sòng* (宋), 987).

35. See footnote 24 above on page 707.

產後血暈，寒熱往來，或血搶心，惡疾也。予閱《食療本草》，見有用鹿角燒為末，酒調服，日夜數服驗者。偶家有婦人患此，令服此神效。因教他人婦服皆驗，但以產後未可飲酒，以童子小便調服爾，最忌服利藥。

Postpartum blood dizziness, alternating [sensations of] cold and heat, and blood rushing into the heart: this is a malign disease. I read *Shí Liáo Běn Cǎo*《食療本草》(Herbal Foundation of Diet Therapy) and found that people fry deer antler, grind it into powder, mix it with liquor, and then drink several doses day and night. It is effective. A woman in my family suffered this disease, so I asked her to drink this; it is divinely effective. I have asked other women to drink it; it was effective for all of them. Since women cannot drink liquor after giving birth, they can mix it with the urine of young boys and drink it. Harsh herbs are contraindicated.

《明下》云：凡懷孕、不論月數，不宜灸。《銅》云：昔宋太子善醫術，出苑遇一妊婦。太子診曰女。令徐文伯診，曰：一男一女。針之，瀉三陰交，補合谷，應針而落。果如文伯言，故妊娠不可刺。

*Míng Xià*《明下》says: It is inappropriate to apply moxibustion during pregnancy no matter which month. *Tóng*《銅》said: In the past, a prince of *Sòng* was good at medicine. He encountered a pregnant woman on his way while hunting. He examined her and predicted she would have a girl. He asked Xú Wénbó to confirm his diagnosis. Xú said she would have a girl and a boy [twins]. They needled the woman, draining Sān Yīn Jiāo 三陰交 (SP 6) and supplementing Hé Gǔ 合谷 (LI 4). [The fetuses] responded to the needle and she gave birth. It was just as Xú Wénbó said.

# 7.27

## *Nán Chǎn (Bāo Yī Bù Chū, Zǐ Qiǎng Xīn, Luò Tāi)*

月事
735

# 難產（胞衣不出　子搶心　落胎）

## Difficult childbirth

**(Retention of the placenta, fetus surging up into the heart, miscarriage)**

衝門治難產，子上衝心，不得息（《銅》）。張仲文療橫產先出手，諸符藥不捷，灸右腳小指尖頭三壯，炷如小麥，下火立產。中封主小腹大，字難，嗌乾嗜飲，夾臍疝（《千》）。上崑崙主字難，若胞衣不出，泄風從頭至足。

Chōng Mén 衝門 (SP 12) treats difficult childbirth, fetal [qì] rushing upward into the heart, and inability to breathe (*Tóng*《銅》).

Zhāng Zhòngwén treated a case of transverse presentation [in childbirth] with the hands [of the baby] emerging first, but the various incantations and herbs did not work. He applied three cones of moxibustion on the tip of little toe of the right foot [of the mother], burning cones the size of a grain of wheat; it brought on delivery right away.

Zhōng Fēng 中封 (LV 4) governs enlargement of the smaller abdomen, difficult childbirth, dry throat with desire to drink, and *shàn*-mounting along the umbilicus (*Qiān*《千》).

Shàng Kūn Lún 上崑崙 (UB 60) governs difficult childbirth. If there is retention of the placenta, [Shàng Kūn Lún] drains wind from head to toe.

氣衝主胞不出（見月事）。氣衝治子上搶心（《銅》見月事，《千》同）。衝門主乳難，子上衝心，陰疝（《千》、《海上方》治難產及胞衣、死胎不下：蓖麻七粒，去皮研如泥，塗足心，才下急洗去。《本事方》云極驗）。

Qì Chōng 氣衝 (ST 30) governs retention of the placenta (see the section on menstruation).

Qì Chōng (ST 30) treats fetal [qì] surging up into the heart (see the section on menstruation in *Tóng*; *Qiān* agrees).

Chōng Mén 衝門 (SP 12) governs difficult lactation, fetal [qì] rushing upward into the heart, and genital *shàn*-mounting.

(Treatment in *Qiān*《千》and *Hǎi Shàng Fāng*《海上方》for difficult childbirth, retention of placenta, and stillbirth: Peel seven piece of *bì má* 蓖麻 (Ricini Semen), grind it into paste, and apply it on the soles. Wash it off immediately after [the placenta or baby] comes out. [*Pǔ Jì*] *Běn Shì Fāng*《本事方》says this is extremely effective.)

昔胡陽公主每產累不能，終南山道士進枳殼散，神效（枳殼麸炒去穰四兩，甘草炙三兩為細末，每服一大錢匕，空腹沸湯點服，五六月後便可服日一服，八月日三服。始產瘦小，數月後平服）。橫生逆生，宜服黑散（百草霜釜下黑煤是，香白芷等分研匀，每服二錢匕。醋、童子小便各一茶腳調勻，更入少沸湯溫熱服，良久便正生。未知再作，頃刻活二人命）。予教人服屢驗，故附此。

In the past, Princess Hú Yáng always suffered difficult delivery. A Daoist from Zhōng Nán mountain suggested *Zhì Ké Sǎn* 枳殼散 (Bitter Orange Powder); it worked divinely (four *liǎng* of *zhì ké* 枳殼 (Aurantii Fructus) fried with wheat bran and the pulp removed plus three *liǎng* of honey-fried *gān cǎo* 甘草 (licorice); mix them and grind it into fine powder. Each dose is one large *qián*-spoonful, taken with a little boiled water on an empty stomach. After five or six months [of pregnancy], take one dose every day; after eight months, take three doses a day. The baby was a little thin when delivered, but was normal within several months).

For transverse or breech presentation, it is appropriate to take *Hēi Sǎn* 黑散 (equal portions of black coal taken from below a pot used in making *bǎi cǎo shuāng* 百草霜 (Herbarum Ustarum Fuligo), and *xiāng bái zhǐ* 香白芷 (Angelicae Dahuricae Radix), grind them into powder and mix evenly. Each dose is two *qián*-spoonfuls. Mix it with one small tea cup each of vinegar and the urine of young boys, add a little boiled water, and drink it while warm. After a while, the patient will have a normal delivery. Drink it again if there is no response; it can save two people's lives right away). I taught people to drink this and it always works, so I put it here.

婦人墮胎後手足厥逆：針肩井立愈，灸更勝針，可七壯（《銅》）。

Reverse counterflow of the limbs after miscarriage: Needling Jiān Jǐng 肩井 (GB 21) will cure the disease immediately. Moxibustion is better than acupuncture. Apply seven cones of moxibustion (*Tóng*《銅》).

# 7.28
## *Yuè Shì*
# 月事

帶下
739

## Menstruation

氣衝治月水不利，身熱腹痛，潰疝陰腫，難乳，子上搶心，痛不得息，氣衝腰痛不得俯仰（《銅》）。會陰治女子經不通（《千》同）。關元治月脈斷絕（見帶下）。足臨泣治月事不利，季脅支滿，乳癰心痛，周痹痛無常處，逆氣，喘不能行。

Qì Chōng 氣衝 (ST 30) treats inhibited menstruation, body heat, abdominal pain, *shàn*-mounting, genital swelling, difficult lactation, fetal [qì] surging up into the heart, pain with inability to breathe, qì surging into the lower back with pain, and inability to bend forward and backward (*Tóng* 《銅》).

Huì Yīn 會陰 (Rèn 1) treats absence of menstruation (*Qiān* 《千》 agrees).

Guān Yuán 關元 (Rèn 4) treats cessation of menstruation (see the section on [red and white] vaginal discharge).

Zú Lín Qì 足臨泣 (GB 41) treats inhibited menstruation, propping fullness of the rib-sides, mammary welling-abscess, heart pain, generalized *bì*-impediment with migrating pain, qì counterflow, panting, and inability to walk.

中極治婦人斷緒，又因惡露不止，月事不調，血結成塊。天樞治月事不時，血結成塊，腸鳴腹痛，不嗜食。水泉治月事不來，來即多，心下悶痛，目𥆨𥆨不能遠視，陰挺出，小便淋瀝腹痛。

Zhōng Jí 中極 (Rèn 3) treats infertility in women, incessant lochia, irregular menstruation, and clotting of blood.

Tiān Shū 天樞 (ST 25) treats irregular menstruation, clotting of blood, intestinal rumbling, abdominal pain, and no desire to eat.

Shuǐ Quán 水泉 (KI 5) treats amenorrhea, profuse bleeding when menstruation comes, oppression and pain below the heart, blurred vision, inability to see distant objects, vaginal protrusion (prolapsed uterus), and urination with *lín*-strangury and abdominal pain.

無子 721

陰蹻療不月水，驚悲不樂，如墮墜，汗出（《千》作不出），面黑，病飢不欲食，婦人淋瀝，陰挺出，四肢淫濼，心悶（《明》）。《下》云：療月水不調，嗜臥怠惰，善悲不樂，手足偏枯，不能行。

Yīn Qiāo 陰蹻 (KI 6 or KI 8) cures amenorrhea, fright, sorrow and unhappiness, a feeling as if falling down, sweating (*Qiān*《千》says: absence of sweating), dark facial complexion, hunger but with no desire to eat, dribbling in women, vaginal protrusion (prolapsed uterus), and pain and weakness of the four limbs, as well as oppression of the heart (*Míng*《明》). *Xià*《下》says: It cures irregular menstruation, somnolence with fatigue, frequent sorrow and unhappiness, hemilateral withering of the hands and feet, and inability to walk.

太衝療月水不通（《下》）。陰包、交儀療月水不調。陰蹻主經逆，四肢淫濼，陰暴跳，小腹偏痛，又主女子淋，陰挺出，月水不來。行間主月事不利，見赤白而有身反敗，陰寒。足臨泣主月水不利，見血而有身則敗，乳腫。

Tài Chōng 太衝 (LV 3) cures amenorrhea (*Xià*).

Yīn Bāo 陰包 (LV 9) and Jiāo Yí 交儀 (LV 5) cure irregular menstruation.

Yīn Qiāo (KI 6 or KI 8) governs menstrual counterflow, pain and weakness of the four limbs, a sudden pulsating feeling in the genitals, and unilateral pain in smaller abdomen; it also governs *lín*-strangury in women, prolapse of the uterus, and absence of menstruation.

Xíng Jiān 行間 (LV 2) governs inhibited menstruation, appearance of red and white [bleeding and discharge] and miscarriage if pregnant, or yīn [genital] coldness.

Zú Lín Qì 足臨泣 (GB 41) governs inhibited menstruation, appearance of blood and miscarriage if pregnant, or breast swelling.

腰俞主月閉溺赤，脊強互引反折，汗不出。中樞主經閉不通（見無子）。治女人從小至大，月經未嘗來，服黃芩牡丹湯兩劑後，灸乳下一寸黑員際各五十壯。氣穴主月水不通，奔泄氣上下，引腰脊痛。

Yāo Shù 腰俞 (Dū 2) governs amenorrhea, reddish urine, stiffness of the spine that induces arched-back rigidity, and absence of sweating.

Zhōng Shū 中樞 (Dū 7) governs amenorrhea (see the section on infertility).

Primary amenorrhea: take two doses of *Huáng Qín Mǔ Dān Tāng* 黃芩牡丹湯 (Scutellaria and Moutan Decoction), then apply fifty cones of moxibustion on the border of dark circle 1 cùn below the nipple.

Qì Xué 氣穴 (KI 13) governs amenorrhea and qì pouring up and down with pain radiating to the lower back and spine.

天樞主胞中痛，惡血，月水不以時休止，腹脹腸鳴，氣上衝胸。氣衝主月水不利，或暴閉塞，腹脹滿，癃，淫濼，身熱乳難，子上搶心。若胞不出，眾氣盡亂，腹中絞痛不得反息：正仰臥，屈一膝伸一膝。月經不斷：灸內踝下白肉際青脈上，隨年壯。

Tiān Shū 天樞 (ST 25) governs pain of the uterus with malign blood, menses that do not stop on time, abdominal distention, intestinal rumbling, and qì surging up into the chest.

Qì Chōng 氣衝 (ST 30) governs inhibited menstruation or sudden blockage, abdominal distention and fullness, dribbling urinary blockage, weakness and pain, body heat, difficult lactation, and fetal [qì] surging up into the heart. If there is retention of the placenta, derangement of all qì, colicky pain of the abdomen, and inability to breathe: Lie supine, bending one knee and stretching out the other one.

Incessant menstruation: Apply moxibustion on the green vessel at the border of the white flesh below the medial malleolus; burn the same number of cones as the patient's age.

帶脈、俠溪主小腹堅痛，月水不通。水道主小腹脹滿，痛引陰中，月水至則腰背痛，胞中瘕，子門寒，大小便不通。下窌治女子下蒼汁不禁，中痛引小腹疼，大便不利，寒濕內傷（《銅》）。

Dài Mài 帶脈 (Dū 26) and Xiá Xī 俠溪 (GB 43) govern hardness and pain in the smaller abdomen and amenorrhea.

Shuǐ Dào 水道 (ST 28) governs distention and fullness of the smaller abdomen, pain radiating to the genitals, lower and upper back pain when menstruation comes, conglomerations in the uterus, coldness of the vagina, and blockage of stool and urine.

Xià Liáo 下窌 (UB 34) treats incontinence of greenish vaginal discharge with pain [of the vagina] radiating to the smaller abdomen, inhibited defecation, and cold-damp internal damage (*Tóng*《銅》).

漏下 728
小腹痛 209
血崩 728
無子 721
疝瘕 220

隱白治月事過時不止，刺之立愈。陰交治月事不絕。氣海治月事不調，帶下崩中，因產惡露不止，繞臍病痛。氣穴治月事不調，泄利不止，賁氣上下，引腰脊痛。血海（見漏下）、帶脈治月脈不調（見小腹痛）。

Yǐn Bái 隱白 (SP 1) treats prolonged periods; this will be cured immediately after needling.

Yīn Jiāo 陰交 (Rèn 7) treats incessant menstruation.

Qì Hǎi 氣海 (Rèn 6) treats irregular menstruation, abnormal vaginal discharge, flooding of blood, incessant flow of postpartum lochia, and pain around the umbilicus.

Qì Xué 氣穴 (KI 13) treats irregular menstruation, incessant diarrhea, rushing qì that moves up and down, and pain radiating to the lower back and spine.

Xuè Hǎi 血海 (SP 10) (see the section on [flooding and] spotting of blood) and Dài Mài 帶脈 (GB 26) treat irregular menstruation (see the section on pain of the smaller abdomen).

陰交（見血崩）治月事不絕（《千》云不下）。月水不利：灸四滿（並見無子）。月水不調，血結成塊：針間使（見疝瘕）。產後月水不禁，橫生胎動：皆針三陰交（《千翼》）。月水不利，賁血上下，無子，四滿三十。

Yīn Jiāo (Rèn 7) (see the section on flooding of blood) treats incessant menstruation (*Qiān*《千》says: amenorrhea).

Inhibited menstruation: Apply moxibustion on Sì Mǎn 四滿 (KI 14) (for all, see the section on infertility).

Irregular menstruation with clotting of blood: Needle Jiān Shǐ 間使 (PC 5) (see the section on *shàn*-mounting and conglomerations).

Incessant menstruation after giving birth or transverse presentation and stirring fetus: For all, needle Sān Yīn Jiāo 三陰交 (SP 6) (*Qiān Yì*《千翼》).

Inhibited menstruation, rushing blood that moves up and down, and infertility: Apply thirty cones of moxibustion on Sì Mǎn (KI 14).

# 7.29
## *Chì Bái Dài*
## 赤白帶
## Red and white vaginal discharge

月事 735
絕子 721
小腹痛 209
惡露 728

關元治帶下瘕聚，因產惡露不止，月脈斷絕，下經冷（《銅》與《明》同）。氣海（見月事）、小腸俞治帶（《千》、《明》並同）。中髎治帶下，月事不調（見絕子）。帶脈治帶下赤白（見小腹痛）。《明下》又云：脅下氣轉連背，痛不可忍。

Guān Yuán 關元 (Rèn 4) treats vaginal discharge, conglomerations and gatherings, incessant flow of postpartum lochia, cessation of menstruation, and cold menstruation (*Tóng*《銅》and *Míng*《明》agree).

Qì Hǎi 氣海 (Rèn 6) (see the section on menstruation) and Xiǎo Cháng Shù 小腸俞 (UB 27) treat vaginal discharge (*Qiān*《千》and *Míng* agree).

Zhōng Liáo 中髎 (UB 33) treats vaginal discharge and irregular menstruation (see the section on infertility).

Dài Mài 帶脈 (GB 26) treats red and white vaginal discharge (see the section on pain of the smaller abdomen). *Míng Xià*《明下》also says: It treats qì shifting below the rib-sides and radiating to the back with unbearable pain.

陰交（見惡露）療帶下（《明》）。曲骨療帶下赤白，惡合陰陽（《銅》同），小便閉澀不通，但是虛乏冷極，皆宜灸。上窌主白瀝（《千》見絕子）。次髎主赤白瀝，心積脹腰痛。中窌主赤淫時白，氣癃，月事少。

Yīn Jiāo 陰交 (Rèn 7) (see the section on [incessant] lochia) cures vaginal discharge (*Míng*).

Qū Gǔ 曲骨 (Rèn 2) cures red and white vaginal discharge, dislike for sexual activity (*Tóng* agrees), inhibited urination and urinary blockage, and vacuity with extreme cold. It is appropriate to apply moxibustion.

Shàng Liáo 上窌 (UB 31) governs white vaginal discharge (see the section on infertility in *Qiān*).

Cì Liáo 次髎 (UB 32) governs red and white vaginal discharge, distention of the heart, and lower back pain.

Zhōng Liáo 中窌 (UB 33) governs red vaginal discharge that is sometimes white, dribbling qì block, and scant menstruation.

腰尻交主下蒼汁不禁，赤瀝，陰癢痛引小腹控眇不可俯仰 。曲骨主赤白沃，陰中乾痛，惡合陰陽，小腹堅，小便閉 。大赫主赤沃 。

Yāo Kāo Jiāo 腰尻交 (UB 34) governs incontinence of greenish vaginal discharge, red vaginal discharge, itching and pain of the genitals that radiates to the smaller abdomen and pulls on the rib-sides, and inability to bend forward and backward.

Qū Gǔ 曲骨 (Rèn 2) governs red and white vaginal discharge, dry painful genitals, dislike for sexual activity, hardness of the smaller abdomen, and retention of urine.

Dà Hè 大赫 (KI 12) governs red vaginal discharge.

有來覓赤白帶藥者，予並以鎮靈丹與之，鎮靈丹能活血溫中故也。以其神效，故書於此。但有孕不可服爾。若灸帶脈穴，尤奇于此丹也。有婦人患赤白帶，林親得予《針灸經》，初為灸氣海穴未效。次日，為灸帶脈穴。有鬼附患身云：昨日灸亦好，只灸我未着，今灸着我，我今去矣，可為酒食祭我。其家如其言祭之，其病如失，此實事也。

When someone comes for the herbs to treat red and white vaginal discharge, I give them *Zhèn Líng Dān* 鎮靈丹 (Settle Spirit Elixir) because it can move blood and warm the center. It is divinely effective so I put it here. But it is contraindicated during pregnancy; applying moxibustion on Dài Mài 帶脈 (GB 26) would be better than this pill.

A woman suffered red and white vaginal discharge; Lín Qīn 林親 got the *Zhēn Jīu Jīng*《針灸經》from me, and at first applied moxibustion on Qì Hǎi 氣海 (Rèn 6), but it was not effective. The next day he applied moxibustion on Dài Mài 帶脈 (GB 26). There was a ghost attached to her body and it said: Yesterday's moxibustion was good, but it did not catch me; today, it caught me and I am leaving; you can offer liquor and food as a sacrifice to me. The family followed what it said and the disease was gone. This is a true story.

予初怪其事，因思晉景公膏肓之病，蓋有二鬼焉。以其虛勞甚矣，鬼得乘虛而居之。今此婦人之疾，亦有鬼者，豈其用心而虛損，故有此疾，鬼亦乘虛居之。灸既著穴，其鬼不得不去，雖不祭之可也。自此有來覓灸者，每為之按此穴，莫不應手酸疼，予知是正穴也。令歸灸之，無有不愈。其穴在兩脅季肋之下一寸八分。有此疾者，即速炙之。婦人患此疾而喪生者甚多，切不可忽。若更炙百會尤佳，此疾多因用心使然故也。

I had doubts about this in the beginning, but I thought about the Duke Jǐng of Jìn's disease of the *gāo* 膏 [the fatty area below the tip the heart] and the *huāng* 肓 [the space below the heart and above the diaphragm], which may have been due to two ghosts. He [Duke Jǐng of Jìn] had severe vacuity taxation, so the ghosts attacked and remained [inside].

Now the woman's disease was also due to a ghost. She used her heart-mind too much [excessive mental work], causing vacuity taxation, so she suffered this disease but it was also due to a ghost attack. When he applied moxibustion to this point, the ghost had to leave even if he did not offer a sacrifice. So afterwards, when people come for moxibustion, I always press this point on them. If they feel soreness upon pressure, then I know it is the right point. I asked them to apply moxibustion when they go home. Everyone has been cured. The point is located 1.8 cùn below the free ribs on the rib-sides. Apply moxibustion on it immediately when someone suffers this disease. Lots of women have died from this, so we cannot ignore it. It is even better to [also] apply moxibustion on Bǎi Huì 百會 (Dū 20) because this disease is caused by using the heart-mind too much.

帶下：炙間使三十壯（ 見疝瘕 ）。絕嗣不生，漏下赤白：泉門十壯（ 三報 ）。下血，泄白，漏血：足太陰五十壯，在內踝上三寸 。腹中五寒百壯 。漏下赤白，月水不利，灸交儀 。下血漏赤白，營池四穴二十壯，在內踝前後兩邊池上脈，一名陰陽 。

Vaginal discharge: Apply thirty cones of moxibustion on Jiān Shǐ 間使 (PC 5) (see the section on *shàn*-mounting and conglomerations).

Infertility or red and white spotting: Apply ten cones of moxibustion on Quán Mén 泉門 (non-channel, see above) (repeat for three sessions).

Precipitation of blood, white [vaginal discharge], and spotting of blood: Apply fifty cones of moxibustion on Zú Tài Yīn 足太陰 (SP 6), it is located 3 cùn above the medial malleolus. Apply a hundred cones of moxibustion for the five abdominal coldnesses.

Red and white spotting and inhibited menstruation: Apply moxibustion on Jiāo Yí 交儀 (LV 5).

Precipitation of blood with red and white spotting: Apply twenty cones of moxibustion on Yíng Chí 營池. It is located on the vessels in the depression anterior and posterior to the medial malleous. It also named as Yīn Yáng 陰陽.

寒熱 675

漏下赤白，四肢酸削，漏陰三十壯，在內踝下五分微動脈上。赤白漏泄注，灸陰陽穴隨年壯，三報之，在足拇指下屈裡表頭白肉際。崩中帶下，因產惡露不止，婦人斷緒最要穴，針中極四度即有子。若未有，更針，入八分，留十呼，得氣即瀉。灸亦佳，不及針。日灸三十至三百止。帶下，小腸俞五十（見寒熱，《千翼》）。

Red and white spotting and aching pain of the limbs: Apply thirty cones of moxibustion on Lòu Yīn 漏陰. It is located on the pulsating vessel five fēn below the medial malleolus.

Red and white spotting and outpour diarrhea: Apply moxibustion on the Yīn Yáng Xué point 陰陽穴, burning the same number of cones as the patient's age; give it three sessions. It is located on the border of the white flesh, at the end of the crease beneath the big toe.

Flooding of blood, abnormal vaginal discharge, incessant flow of postpartum lochia, and infertility: Needling the most important point, Zhōng Jí 中極 (Rèn 3), four times will result in pregnancy. Needle it again if this does not work. Needle 8 fēn deep, retain the needle for ten respirations, and drain after qì arrives. Moxibustion also is good, but not as good as needling. Apply thirty cones of moxibustion per day and stop at three hundred cones.

Abnormal vaginal discharge: Apply fifty cones of moxibustion on Xiǎo Cháng Shù 小腸俞 (UB 27) (see the section on [sensations of] cold and heat, *Qiān Yì*《千翼》).

# Appendix

# References cited in
# *Zhēn Jīu Zī Shēng Jīng* 《針灸資生經》

*Zhēn Jīu Zī Shēng Jīng* 《針灸資生經》 Life-Promoting Classic of Acupuncture frequently quotes the following literature:

| Title | English | Author | Dynasty and/or Date |
|---|---|---|---|
| *Běn Cǎo Yǎn Yì* 《本草衍義》 | | | *Sòng* (宋) 1116 |
| | Amplification of the Materia Medica | | |
| | | Compiled by Kòu Zōngshì 寇宗奭 | |
| *Běn Shì Fāng* 《本事方》 | | | |
| See *Pǔ Jì Běn Shì Fāng* 《普濟本事方》 | | | |
| *Bì Yòng Fāng* 《必用方》 | | | *Sòng* (宋) 1078-1085 |
| | Formulas of Necessity | | |
| | | Possibly by Chū Yúshì 初虞世 | |
| *Bì Yòng* 《必用》 | | | |
| | Parts of *Bì Yòng Fāng* were cited in *Pǔ Jì Běn Shì Fāng* 《普濟本事方》 (Skillful Formulas for Universal Salvation). | | |
| *Chǎn Lùn* 《產論》 | | | *Sòng* (宋) 1078-1085 |
| | Discussion on Childbirth | | |
| | | Possibly Yáng Zǐjiàn 杨子建 | |
| *Chuán Yán Fāng* 《傳言方》 | | | *Táng* (唐) |
| | Commonly Passed Down Formulas | | |
| | | Liú Yǔxī 劉禹錫 | |
| *Cháo Yě Qiān Zǎi* 《朝野僉載》 | | | *Táng* (唐) |
| | Combined Chronicle of the Government and the Public | | |
| | | By Zháng Zhuó 張鷟 | |
| | A series of novels. | | |
| *Dān Fāng Gē* 《單方歌》 | | | unknown |
| | Single Formula Rhymes | | |
| | | unknown | |
| *Dān Fāng* 《單方》 | | | |
| *Dōng Yī Bǎo Jiàn* 《東醫寶鑒》 (*Dongui Bogam* 동의보감 in Korean) | | | 1613 |
| | Precious Mirror of Korean Medicine | | |
| | | Xǔ Jùn 許浚 (Heo Jun 허준) | |

*Fù Rén Fāng*《 婦人方 》 *Táng*(唐)

Formulas for Women (Volume 2 of *Qīan Jīn Yào Fāng*《 千金要方 》)

By Sūn Sīmĭao 孫思邈

*Gŭ Zhēng Bìng Jiu Fāng*《 骨蒸病灸方 》 *Táng*(唐)

Moxibustion Formulas For Steaming Bone Disease

By Cuī Zhītì 崔知悌

*Hăi Shàng Xiān Míng Fāng*《 海上仙名方 》 *Sòng*(宋)

Famous Formulas from Immortals who Live at the Sea

By Qián Yú 錢竽, using Sūn Sīmiǎo's 孫思邈 name

*Hăi Shàng Fāng*《 海上方 》

Discusses treatment of over 120 different diseases

*Huáng Dì Míng Táng Jiŭ Jīng*《 黃帝明堂灸經 》 *Táng*(唐)

The Yellow Emperor's Moxibustion Classic of the Bright Hall

unknown

*Jiŭ Jīng*《 灸經 》

The Classic of Moxibustion

*Huáng Dì Nèi Jīng*《 黃帝內經 》 Spring and Autumn Period through the Warring States Period (春秋戰國) 1st century BCE.

The Yellow Emperor's Inner Classic

unknown

*Nèi Jīng*《 內經 》 has two parts: See also *Sù Wèn*《 素問 》 (Plain Questions) and *Líng Shū*《 靈樞 》 (Magic Pivot)

*Nèi Jīng*《 內經 》

*Jí Xiào Fāng*《 集效方 》 unknown

Collections of Effective Formulas

unknown

*Jí*《 集 》

Two volumes. The first is a collection of simple empirical folk formulas; the second is a collection of formulas for several diseases. The total number of formulas is around 400.

*Jì Xiao Fāng*《 既效方 》 *Yuán* (元)

Already Effective Formulas

By Wáng Zhízhōng 王執中 (the author of this book)

Wáng collected the formulas from other people. After trying them on himself, he put the effective ones together into this book. It has been lost since the *Yuán* (元) Dynasty.

*Jiă*《 甲 》

*Jiă Yĭ*《 甲乙 》

*Jiă Yĭ Jīng*《 甲乙經 》

See *Zhēn Jiŭ Jiă Yĭ Jīng*《 針灸甲乙經 》

*Jīn Guì Yào Luè*《 金匱要略 》 Eastern *Hàn* (東漢)

Essential Prescriptions of the Golden Cabinet

By Zhāng Zhòngjĭng 張仲景

*Jīn Guì*《 金匱 》

| | |
|---|---|
| *Jīng Fāng Xiǎo Pǐn* 《 經方小品 》 | Between 454-473, the *Nán běi cháo* (南北朝) (Southern and Northern Dynasties, 420-589) |

Short Sketches of Classical Formulas

By Chén Yánzhī 陳延之

*Xiǎo Pǐn Fāng* 《 小品方 》

*Xiǎo Pǐn* 《 小品 》

Short Sketches of Formulas

| | |
|---|---|
| *Jīu Gāo Huāng* 《 灸膏肓 》 | *Sòng* (宋) |

Apply Moxibustion to Gāo Huāng (UB 43)

By Zhuāng Chuò 莊綽

*Jīu Jīng* 《 灸經 》

The Classic of Moxibustion

See *Huáng Dì Míng Táng Jiū Jīng* 《 黃帝明堂灸經 》

| | |
|---|---|
| *Jīu Yōng Jū Fāng* 《 灸癰疽方 》 | unknown |

Applying Moxibustion for Welling- and Flat-Abscesses

By Líu Héshū 劉和叔

The dates are unknown, but Wáng wrote a preface for it so it was probably written in his lifetime.

*Jú Fāng* 局方

See *Tài Píng Huì Mín Hé Jì Jú Fāng* 《 太平惠民和劑局方 》

*Liáng Fāng* 《 良方 》

See *Sū Shěn Liáng Fāng* 《 蘇沈良方 》

| | |
|---|---|
| *Liè Zǐ* 《 列子 》 (Master Liè) | Western scholars believe it was compiled around the 4th century CE. |

Honorifically entitled the *Chōng Xū Zhēn Jīng* 《 衝虛真經 》

True Classic of Simplicity and Vacuity, also known as the Classic of the Perfect Emptiness.

A Dàoist book of philosophy.

| | |
|---|---|
| *Líng Shū* 《 靈樞 》 | Spring and Autumn Period through the Warring States Period (春秋戰國) 1st century BCE. |

Magic Pivot

unknown

*Zhēn Jīng* 《 針經 》

Acupuncture Classic

Part of *Huáng Dì Nèi Jīng* 《 黃帝內經 》 (The Yellow Emperor's Inner Classic)

*Líng Shū·Gǔ Dù* 《 靈樞·骨度 》

Magic Pivot• Bone Measurement Standards, Chapter 14

unknown

*Líng Shū · Yù Bǎn* 《 靈樞·玉版 》

Magic Pivot• The Jade Slip, Chapter 60

unknown

| | |
|---|---|
| *Shuǐ Rè Xué* 《 水熱穴 》 | unknown |

Treatise on points of Water and Heat, Chapter 61.

*Lù Shì Xù Jí Yàn Fāng*《陸氏續集驗方》 Southern *Sòng*(南宋) 1180

Sequel to the Collection of Proven Formulas from Master Lù

By Lù Yóu 陸游

It was written after *Lù Shì Xù Jí Yàn Fāng*《陸氏集驗方》 by Lù Zhí 陸贄 during the *Táng*(唐) Dynasty.

*Lù Yàn Fāng*《錄驗方》 *Táng*(唐)

Records of Effective Formulas

By Zhēn Lìyán 甄立言

This book has been lost.

*Mài Jué*《脈訣》 *Sòng*(宋)

Rhymed Songs of Pulse

By Cuī Jiāyán 崔嘉言

*Mèng Zǐ*《孟子》 *Warring States*

Mencius

Attributed to Mencius

*Míng Yī Lù*《名醫錄》 *Táng*(唐)

Records of Famous Doctors

By Gān Bózōng 甘伯宗

*Míng Táng*《明堂》 Edited during the Western and Eastern *Hàn*(西東漢) (between 138 B.C.E.-106 C.E.)

Bright Hall

unknown

The first book to systematically discuss acupuncture points. The original book has been lost, but its material was include in *Tài Píng Shèng Huì Fāng* (See also that entry).

*Míng Táng Jīng*《明堂經》

Bright Hall Classic

*Míng Táng Shàng Jīng*《明堂上經》

Upper Canon of the Bright Hall Classic

*Míng Shàng*《明上》

*Shàng*《上》

Volume 99 of *Tài Píng Shèng Huì Fāng*《太平聖惠方》(Sage-like Prescriptions of *Tài Píng* Era). (See also *Míng Táng*《明堂》.)

*Míng Táng Xìa Jīng*《明堂下經》

Lower Canon of the Bright Hall

*Míng Xià*《明下》

*Xià*《下》

Volume 100 of *Tài Píng Shèng Huì Fāng*《太平聖惠方》(Sage-like Prescriptions of Tài Píng Era) (See also *Míng Táng*《明堂》.)

*Míng Shàng*《明上》

See *Míng Táng Shàng Jīng*《明堂上經》

*Míng Xià*《明下》

See *Míng Táng Xìa Jīng*《明堂下經》

*Nàn Jīng* 《 難經 》 Late *Hàn* (漢)

Classic of Difficulties

unknown

*Nàn* 《 難 》

*Nàn Jīng Shū* 《 難經疏 》 *Sòng* (宋)

Explanation of the Classic of Difficulties

By Hóu Zìrán 候自然

*Nàn Shū* 《 難疏 》

It had 13 volumes, but the book has been lost.

*Nèi Jīng* 《 內經 》

See *Huáng Dì Nèi Jīng* 《 黃帝內經 》

*Pǔ Jì Běn Shì Fāng* 《 普濟本事方 》 *Sòng* (宋) 1132

Skillful Formulas for Universal Salvation

Compiled By Xǔ Shūwēi 許叔微, also known as Xǔ Zhīkě 許知可

*Běn Shì Fāng* 《 本事方 》

*Pǔ Jì Fāng* 《 普濟方 》

*Qí Yù Fāng* 《 耆域方 》 unknown

Formulas from Qí Yù

unknown

*Qīan* 《 千 》

*Qīan Jīn* 《 千金 》

See *Qīan Jīn Yào Fāng* 《 千金要方 》 or *Qīan Jīn Yì Fāng* 《 千金翼方 》; these could refer to either one.

*Qīan Jīn Yào Fāng* 《 千金要方 》 *Táng* (唐)

Prescriptions Worth a Thousand Pieces of Gold

By Sūn Sīmǐao 孫思邈

*Qiān·Shèn Zàng* 《 千 · 腎藏 》 *Táng* (唐)

Prescriptions Worth a Thousand Pieces of Gold • Kidney (Volume 19)

*Qīan Jīn Yì Fāng* 《 千金翼方 》 *Táng* (唐)

Appendix to Prescriptions Worth a Thousand Pieces of Gold

By Sūn Sīmǐao 孫思邈

*Qīan Jīn* 《 千金 》

*Qīan* 《 千 》

*Shàng* 《 上 》

See *Míng Táng Shàng Jīng* 《 明堂上經 》

*Quán Shēng Zhǐ Mí Fāng* 《 全生指迷方 》 *Sòng* (宋), 1119-1125

Formulas of Comments on Confusion to Rescue Life

By Wáng Kuàng 王貺

*Zhǐ* 《 指 》

*Zhǐ Mí* 《 指迷 》

*Shān Tiào Jīng* 《 山眺經 》 unknown

Mountain View Classic

*Shàng Jīng*《 上經 》 unknown

Upper Canon of the Bright Hall Classic

*Shén Yìng Jīng*《 神應經 》 *Míng* (明)

Divinely Responding Classic

By Chén Huì 陳會, edited by Liú Jǐn 劉瑾

*Shén Yìng Zhēn Jīng Yào Jué*《 神應針經要訣 》 Northern *Sòng* (北宋)

The Acupuncture Classic of Essential Rhymed Songs of Wondrous Response

By Xǔ Xī 許希

*Zhēn Jīng*《 針經 》

The Acupuncture Classic

*Shèng Jì Zǒng Lù*《 聖濟總錄 》 *Sòng* (宋)

Sage's Salvation Records

A Government Publication

*Shǐ Jì*《 史記 》 *Hàn* (漢) 91 B.C.E.

The Records of the Grand Historian

By Sīmǎ Qiān 司馬遷

An important history book. It recounts Chinese history from the time of the Yellow Emperor to King Wǔ 武 of the *Hàn* Dynasty, covering about 3000 years.

*Shí Liáo Běn Cǎo*《 食療本草 》 *Táng* (唐)

Herbal Foundation of Dietary Therapy

By Mèng Shēn 孟詵

*Shì Zhāi Bǎi Yī Xuǎn Fāng*《 是齋百一選方 》 *Sòng* (宋)

One in a Hundred Formulas Selected by Shì Zhāi

By Wáng Qíu 王璆

*Shuō Wén Jiě Zì*《 說文解字 》 Eastern *Hàn* (漢) (early 2nd century CE)

Explaining and Analyzing Characters

By Xǔ Shèn 許慎

*Shuō Wén*《 說文 》

A dictionary of Chinese characters.

*Sù*《 素 》

See *Sù Wèn*《 素問 》

*Sù Nǚ Lùn*《 素女論 》 unknown

Statements of the *Sù Nǚ*

unknown

*Sù Nǚ*《 素女 》

An ancient sexology book. It was lost after the *Táng* Dynasty. But it was partially recorded in the *Yī Xīn Fāng*《 醫心方 》, Volume 28, by Dān Bō Kāng Lài 丹波康賴 in 982. This is a famous Japanese book called Ishimpo in Japanese. *Sù Nǚ* was a goddess of ancient China. She was skilled in music and lived in the same era as Huáng Dì (the Yellow Emperor).

*Sū Shěn Liáng Fāng*《 蘇沈良方 》 *Sòng* (宋)

Good Formulas from Masters Sū and Shěn

unknown

*Liáng Fāng*《 良方 》

This book is a combination of *Shěn Shì Liáng Fāng* 《沈氏良方》( Good Formulas from Master Shěn) by Shěn Kuò 沈括 and *Sū Xué Shì Fāng* 《蘇學士方》(Good Formulas from Master Sū) by Sū Shì 蘇軾. It discusses pulse diagnoses, internal organs, moxibustion, herbology and the treatment of different diseases.

*Sù Wèn* 《素問》 Spring and Autumn Period through the Warring States Period (春秋戰國) 1st century BCE.

Plain Questions

unknown

*Sù* 《素》

Part of *Huáng Dì Nèi Jīng* 《黃帝內經》(The Yellow Emperor's Inner Classic)

*Cì Jìn* 《刺禁》

Treatise on Needling Contraindications, Chapter 52.

*Cì Nüè* 《刺瘧》

Treatise on Needling Malaria, Chapter 36.

*Cì Yāo Tòng Zhù* 《刺腰痛注》

The Annotation to the Treatise on Needling Lower Back Pain, Chapter 41.

*Gǔ Kōng Lùn* 《骨空論》

Treatise on Bone Hollows, Chapter 60.

*Líng Lán Mì Diǎn Lùn* 《靈蘭秘典論》

Treatise of the Arcane Book of the Orchid Chamber of the Spirit Tower, Chapter 8.

*Miù Cì Lùn* 《繆刺論》

Treatise on Cross Needling, Chapter 63.

*Nüè Lùn* 《瘧論》

Treatise on Malaria, Chapter 35.

*Qì Fǔ* 《氣府》

Treatise on the House of Qi, Chapter 49.

*Qì Xué* 《氣穴》

Treatise on Qi Points, Chapter 48.

*Rè Xué Lùn Zhù* 《熱穴論注》

Annotations on the Treatise on Points for Heat, Chapter 61.

*Sù Wèn Zhù* 《素問注》 *Sòng* (宋)

Annotations to Plain Questions

By Wáng Bīng 王冰

*Sù Zhù* 《素注》

These are Wáng Bīng's 王冰 annotations on *Sù Wèn* 《素問》

*Tài Píng Huì Mín Hé Jì Jú Fāng* 《太平惠民和劑局方》

Imperial Grace Pharmacy Formulas

Compiled by the *sòng tài yī jú biān* 宋太醫局編 Sòng Imperial Medical Bureau *Sòng* (宋) (1078-85)

*Jú Fāng* 局方

The official *Sòng* (宋) Dynasty government-published formulary.

*Tài Píng Shèng Huì Fāng*《 太平聖惠方 》 Sòng (宋), 992

Sage-like Prescriptions of Tài Píng Era

By Wáng Huáiyǐn 王懷隱

*Tāng Bù*《 湯簿 》

Book of Decoctions

*Tóng Rén Shū Xuè Zhēn Jīu Tú Jīng*《 銅人腧穴針灸圖經 》 Sòng (宋), 1027

The Bronze Statues Illustrated Classic of Acupuncture Points

By Wáng Wéiyī 王維一

*Tóng*《 銅 》

*Tóng Rén*《 銅人 》

*Wài Tái Mì Yào*《 外臺秘要 》 Táng (唐), 752

Essential Secrets from Outside of the Metropolis

By Wàng Tāo 王燾

*Wài Tái*《 外臺 》

*Míng Táng*《 明堂 》

Bright Hall Classic

*Wǔ Zàng Lùn*《 五臟論 》 Eastern *Hàn* (漢)

Discussion on Five Visceras

By Zhāng Zhòngjǐng 張仲景

*Xià*《 下 》

See *Míng Táng Xia Jīng*《 明堂下經 》

*Xīn Jiào Zhèng*《 新校正 》 Sòng (宋)

New Annotations and Corrections [of *Sù Wèn* (Plain Questions]

Lín Yì 林億 (editor)

A later edited edition of *Sù Wèn*《 素問 》(Plain Questions) with *Sù Wèn Zhù*《 素問注 》(Annotations to Plain Questions) (Also see these)

*Xiǎo Pǐn Fāng*《 小品方 》

See *Jīng Fāng Xiǎo Pǐn*《 經方小品 》

*Yīn Yáng Shū*《 陰陽書 》 Warring States Period (戰國)

Book of Yīn and Yáng

By Zhōu Yán 周衍 and Zhōu Shì 周奭

A book of calendars, divination, and constellations.

*Yù Piān*《 玉篇 》 Liáng 梁 (519-581) circa 543 CE

Jade Chapters

Edited by Gù Yěwáng 顧野王

A Chinese dictionary.

*Zhēn Jīng*《 針經 》

Acupuncture Classic

Unfortunately, this could be one of three things. See also 1. *Líng Shū*《 靈樞 》; 2. *Zhēn Jīng Chāo*《 針經鈔 》; or 3. *Shén Yìng Zhēn Jīng Yào Jué*《 神應針經要訣 》

*Zhēn Jīng Chāo*《 針經鈔 》 Táng (唐)

Copy of the Acupuncture Classic

By Zhēn Quán 甄權

*Zhēn Jīng* 《針經》

Lost.

*Zhēn Jiǔ Jiǎ Yǐ Jīng* 《針灸甲乙經》 282 C.E.

The Systematic Classic of Acupuncture and Moxibustion

By Huángfǔ Mì 皇甫謐

*Jiǎ Yǐ Jīng* 《甲乙經》

*Jiǎ Yǐ* 《甲乙》

*Jiǎ* 《甲》

*Zhēn Jiǔ Míng Zhù Jí Chéng* 《針灸名著集成》 unknown

Grand Compendium of Famous Works on Acupuncture and Moxibustion

Edited by Huáng Lóngxiáng 黃龍祥

*Zhì Dào Dān Fāng* 《至道單方》 unknown

Single-Herb Formulas to Reach the Dào

*Zhǐ Mí* 《指迷》 *Sòng* (宋) 960-1279

[Formulas of] Comments on Confusion

By Wáng Kuàng 王贶

*Zhì Yōng Jū Nóng Dú Fāng* 《治癰疽膿毒方》 unknown

Formulas for treating toxic diseases with pus, welling-abscesses, and flat-abscesses

By Hú Quán 胡權

This book is lost. More information on Hú Quán and when the book was written is not available.

*Zhōng Zàng Jīng* 《中藏經》 Reputed to be Eastern *Hàn* (漢)

Classic of the Central Viscera

Attributed to Huá Tuó 華佗

*Zhóu Hòu Bèi Jí Fāng* 《肘後備急方》 *Jìn* (晉)

Emergency Standby Remedies

By Gě Hóng 葛洪

*Zhóu Hòu Fāng* 《肘後方》

It mainly discusses the treatment of emergency cases.

*Zhū Bìng Yuán Hóu Lùn•Fēng Bìng Zhū Hóu* 《諸病源候論·風病諸候》 *Suí* (隋)

The Origin and Indicators of Disease • Indications of All Wind Disease

By Cháo Yuánfāng 巢元方

*Zuǒ Zhuàn* 《左傳》

Commentary of Mr. Zuǒ

Attributed to Zuǒ Qīumíng 左丘明

*Zhuàn* 《傳》

Among the earliest Chinese works of narrative history, covering the period from 722 to 468 BCE. It is one of the most important sources for understanding the history of the Spring and Autumn Period (*Chūn Qiū* 春秋).

# People

# Texts

# Extra Points

| | | |
|---|---|---|
| Shǒu Tài Yáng 手太陽 | location of this point is unknown. | **670** |
| Shǒu Xīn 手心 | Dà Líng 大陵 (PC 7) | **273**, 402, 404, 507 |
| Shǒu Yángmíng 手陽明 | | **350** |
| Shǒu Wǔ Cè 手五冊 | located on both sides of the transverse crease of the elbow, two points on each arm. | **393** |
| Sì Huā Xué 四花穴 | four flowers point | **187** |
| Xī Yǎn 膝眼 | | **133**, 136, 520, 540, 708 |
| Xià Jiāo Shù 下焦俞 | Lower Burner Transport | **189**, 490 |
| Xié Táng 脅堂 | | **93**, 408, 580 |
| Xiōng Táng 胸膛 | Dàn Zhōng 膻中 (Rèn 17) | **275**, 278, 402, 404, 417, 424, 479, 485, 699–700 |
| Xuán Mìng 懸命 | The point is located on string-like flesh in the center of the inside of the upper lip | **351** |
| Yàn Kǒu 燕口 | swallow mouth (It is located at the corner of the mouth, on the border of dark and light skin, near Dì Cāng 地倉 (ST 4). It has the appearance of the mouth of the swallow, hence its name.) | **329** |
| Yīn Fèng 陰縫 | | **670** |
| Yīn Yáng Xué 陰陽穴 | located on the border of the white flesh, at the end of the crease beneath the big toe. | **742** |
| Yín Mén 寅門 | located on the midline approximately 1.8 cùn posterior to the anterior hairline. | **669** |
| Yíng Chōng 營衝 | located on the vessel in the depression anterior and posterior to the medial malleolus. There are two points on each side. | **237** |
| Zhù Shì 注市 | | **532**, 535 |
| Zú Suǐ Kǒng 足髓空 | located one cùn posterior to the lateral malleolus | **393** |
| Zú Wǔ Cè 足五冊 | located at the end of the transverse crease when the knee is flexed | **393** |

# Regular Points

# A-Z

| | | | |
|---|---|---|---|
| blood rushing into the heart | *xuè qiǎng xīn* | 血搶心 | 732 |
| blood stasis in the chest | *xiōng zhōng yū xuè* | 胸中瘀血 | 132, 403, 484, 727 |
| blood vessels | *xuè mài* | 血脈 | 20, 151, 166, 557 |
| bloody dribbling block | *xuè lóng* | 血癃 | 223, 227 |
| bloody hemorrhoids | *xuè zhì* | 血痔 | 255 |
| bloody *lín*-strangury | *xuè lín* | 血淋 | 222 |
| bloody stool | *biàn xuè* | 便血 | 208, 210, 245, 253–254, 257–258, 260, 369 |
| bloody stool and urine | *dà xiǎo biàn xuè* | 大小便血 | 253 |
| bloody urine | *nì xuè* | 溺血 | 190, 230–233, 466, 693 |
| blue whites of the eyes | *mù zhōng bái jīng qīng* | 目中白睛青 | 589 |
| blurred vision | *mù bù míng* | 目不明 | 22, 132, 190, 303, 322, 388, 418, 553, 569, 572–575, 577–583, 585–587, 590, 592, 638, 640, 649, 656, 667, 735 |
| blurred vision in women | *fù rén mù huāng huāng* | 婦人目䀮䀮 | 580 |
| blurred vision when getting up | *qǐ zé mù huāng huāng* | 起則目䀮䀮 | 418, 580 |
| *Bó Jīng* vessel | *bó jīng mài* | 髆井脈 | 32 |
| body arched backwards | *shēn fǎn zhé* | 身反折 | 179 |
| body feels like it is on fire | *shēn rú huǒ* | 身如火 | 693 |
| body hair | *máo* | 毛 | 151 |
| body heat | *shēn rè* | 身熱 | 189–190, 215, 735, 737 |
| body heat with shivering | *shēn rè zhèn lì* | 身熱振栗 | 190 |
| body pain | *tǐ tòng* | 體痛 | 244, 711 |
| bone *bì*-impediment | *gǔ bì* | 骨痹 | 509, 558, 683 |
| bone flat-abscesses | *gǔ jū* | 骨疽 | 697 |
| bone pain | *gǔ téng* | 骨疼 | 336, 373, 424, 469, 478, 558 |
| bone pain of the anterior chest | *xiōng yīng gǔ téng* | 胸膺骨疼 | 469, 478 |
| bone disease | *gǔ bìng* | 骨病 | 186 |
| bones and marrow | *gǔ suǐ* | 骨髓 | 151–152, 558–559 |
| both testicles retracted upward into the smaller abdominal with pain | *liǎng wán shàng rù xiǎo fù tòng* | 兩丸上入小腹痛 | 215 |
| bowstring tension of the abdomen | *fù xián jí* | 腹弦急 | 442 |
| bowstring tension, fullness, and heat of the smaller abdomen | *xiǎo fù xián jí zhàng rè* | 小腹弦急脹熱 | 212, 442 |
| brain fistulas | *nǎo lòu* | 腦瘻 | 701 |
| brain leakage | *nǎo xiè* | 腦瀉 | 650 |
| brain pain | *nǎo tòng* | 腦痛 | 3, 294, 529, 531, 583, 638, 640, 649–651, 656 |
| brain wind | *nǎo fēng* | 腦風 | 106, 324, 601, 649–650, 656 |
| break the intersecting vessels | *jiāo mài pò jué* | 交脈破決 | 29 |
| breast bone | *yì* | 臆 | 72 |
| breast pain | *rǔ tòng* | 乳痛 | 720 |

| | | | |
|---|---|---|---|
| cold phlegm with qì ascent | *hán tán shàng qì* | 寒痰上氣 | 276 |
| cold qì | *lěng qì* | 冷氣 | 74, 190, 316, 319, 434, 441, 445, 458, 467, 617, 678, 681 |
| cold qì accumulations and gatherings | *lěng qì jī jù* | 冷氣積聚 | 438 |
| cold qì bind | *hán qì jié* | 寒氣結 | 235 |
| cold qì entering the abdomen | *hán qì rù fù* | 寒氣入腹 | 679 |
| cold qì entering the smaller abdomen | *hán qì rù xiǎo fù* | 寒氣入小腹 | 432 |
| cold qì in six bowels | *liù fǔ zhī qì hán* | 六腑之氣寒 | 297, 443 |
| cold qì in six bowels with no desire to eat | *liù fǔ qì hán bù shì shí* | 六腑氣寒不嗜食 | 297 |
| cold qì in the abdomen | *fù zhōng lěng qì* | 腹中冷氣 | 244 |
| cold qì in the flesh with pain | *hán qì zài fēn ròu jiān tòng* | 寒氣在分肉間痛 | 683 |
| cold qì rushing upward to the heart | *lěng qì shàng chōng xīn* | 冷氣上衝心 | 680 |
| cold qì in the stomach with inability to eat | *hán qì bù néng shí* | 寒氣不能食 | 295 |
| cold qì settling between the divisions of the flesh | *hán qì kè yú fēn ròu jiān* | 寒氣客於分肉間 | 269 |
| cold qì settling in the intestines | *hán qì kè yú cháng jiān* | 寒氣客於腸間 | 245 |
| cold reversal | *hán jué* | 寒厥 | 348, 490, 625, 661, 680, 691, 694 |
| cold reversal with hot feet | *hán jué zú rè* | 寒厥足熱 | 306 |
| cold semen | *jīng hán* | 精寒 | 206 |
| cold *shàn* | *hán shàn* | 寒疝 | 213, 217–219, 233, 419 |
| cold *shàn*-mounting in the greater abdomen | *dà fù hán shàn* | 大腹寒疝 | 443 |
| cold shivering in the chest and back | *xiōng bèi hán lì* | 胸背寒栗 | 485 |
| cold shivering of the interstices on the back | *bèi còu hán lì* | 背腠寒栗 | 557 |
| cold shivering of the shoulders | *jiān hán lì* | 肩寒栗 | 490 |
| cold shivering of the shoulders and back | *jiān bèi hán lì* | 肩背寒栗 | 490 |
| cold sinews | *jīn hán* | 筋寒 | 270, 373 |
| cold strike | *hán zhòng* | 寒中 | 227, 244, 253, 292–293, 347, 443, 449 |
| cold sweats | *lěng hàn* | 冷汗 | 662 |
| cold tears | *lěng lèi* | 冷淚 | 574, 585, 590, 592 |
| cold teeth | *chǐ hán* | 齒寒 | 106, 601–602 |
| cold things that can stir up wind | *dòng fēng lěng wù* | 動風冷物 | 169 |
| cold-damp internal damage | *hán shī nèi shāng* | 寒濕內傷 | 683, 737 |
| cold-heat malaria | *hán rè jīe nüè* | 寒熱痎瘧 | 302–305 |
| cold-heat tetany with pain radiating to the bones | *hán rè jìng yǐn gǔ tòng* | 寒熱痙引骨痛 | 355 |
| coldness and numbness | *hán bù rén* | 寒不仁 | 509, 538, 683 |
| coldness and numbness of the legs | *lěng jiǎo bù rén* | 冷腳不仁 | 540 |
| coldness and pain below the heart | *xīn xià yǒu hán tòng* | 心下有寒痛 | 314, 446 |
| coldness down the lower back and legs that feels like [the back was soaked in] cold water | *xià zhì yāo jiǎo rú lěng shuǐ* | 下至腰腳如冷水 | 217 |

| | | | |
|---|---|---|---|
| foxy *shàn*-mounting moving up and down | *hú shàn zǒu shàng xià* | 狐疝走上下 | 214 |
| fragile thin pulse in the *chǐ* position | *chǐ mài wēi xiǎo* | 尺脈微小 | 729 |
| free and diffuse the blood vessels | *xuè mài tōng xuān* | 血脈通宣 | 20 |
| free rib region | *jì xié* | 季脅 | 91–92, 418 |
| frenetic anger | *wàng nù* | 妄怒 | 369 |
| frenetic laughing | *wàng xiào* | 妄笑 | 179 |
| frenetic walking | *kuáng zǒu* | 狂走 | 181, 537 |
| frequent belching | *shàn yī* | 善噫 | 218, 277, 281, 318, 325, 335, 418, 462 |
| frequent belching after childbirth | *chǎn hòu shàn yī* | 產後善噫 | 282 |
| frequent belching of sour fluids | *xǐ yī suān* | 喜噫酸 | 314 |
| frequent biting of one's own cheeks | *xǐ niè jiá* | 喜嚙頰 | 632 |
| frequent bouts of [sensations of] cold and heat with sweating | *duō hán rè hàn chū* | 多寒熱汗出 | 334, 662 |
| frequent coldness | *shí hán* | 時寒 | 478 |
| frequent cough | *shù ké* | 數咳 | 418, 422, 478 |
| frequent coughing | *shàn ké* | 善咳 | 281 |
| frequent defecation | *shí shí yù xià* | 時時欲下 | 299 |
| frequent diarrhea | *dà biàn xiè shù* | 大便泄數 | 241, 250, 252 |
| frequent dysphagia | *shàn yē* | 善噎 | 413, 483, 552 |
| frequent feeling of sleepiness | *shí yàn yàn shì wò* | 時厭厭嗜臥 | 684 |
| frequent fright | *duō jīng* | 多驚 | 321, 325–326, 362, 369, 373, 646, 666 |
| frequent fright and fear | *xǐ jīng kǒng* | 喜驚恐 | 324 |
| frequent generalized dampness | *shēn cháng shī* | 身常濕 | 665, 682 |
| frequent hiccups | *shàn yuě* | 善噦 | 282, 305, 313, 478, 644, 667 |
| frequent incessant laughter | *shàn xiào bù xiū* | 善笑不休 | 693 |
| frequent laughter | *xǐ xiào* | 喜笑 | 503, 529, 532 |
| frequent mild heat | *shí yǒu wéi rè* | 時有微熱 | 668 |
| frequent miscarriage | *shù duò luò* | 數墮落 | 23, 724 |
| frequent needling | *pín cì* | 頻刺 | 44 |
| frequent oppressive heart pain | *duō mèn xīn tòng* | 多悶心痛 | 722 |
| frequent retching | *xǐ ǒu* | 喜嘔 | 271, 274, 280, 283, 334, 432, 445–446, 641, 662, 666–667, 690–691 |
| frequent retching of blood | *shí shí ǒu xuè* | 時時嘔血 | 403 |
| frequent retching when eating | *shí yǐn shàn ǒu* | 食飲善嘔 | 593 |
| frequent rumbling in the intestines | *cháng zhōng cháng míng* | 腸中常鳴 | 263 |
| frequent runny nose with clear snivel in children | *xiǎo ér bí duō qīng tì* | 小兒鼻多清涕 | 616 |
| frequent shaking of the arms, elbows and wrists | *bì zhǒu wàn shàn dòng yáo* | 臂肘腕善動搖 | 705 |
| frequent shaking of the head | *shàn yáo tóu* | 善搖頭 | 673 |

| | | | |
|---|---|---|---|
| hot qì in the sānjiāo, urinary bladder and kidneys | *sānjiāo* 、*páng guāng* 、*shèn zhōng rè qì* | 三焦、膀胱、腎中熱氣 | 185, 205 |
| hot red face | *miàn chì ér rè* | 面赤而熱 | 418, 665 |
| hot red urine | *xiǎo biàn chì rè* | 小便赤熱 | 203, 207 |
| hot water washing from the medial aspect of the genitals to the low back | *tāng wò gǔ nèi zhì yāo* | 湯沃股內至腰 | 220 |
| hot wind | *rè fēng* | 熱風 | 130, 367, 384, 397, 684, 705 |
| hot yáng wind | *rè yáng fēng* | 熱陽風 | 329 |
| human body | *rén shēn* | 人身 | 4, 170, 176, 178 |
| hunchback that looks like a turtle's back | *bèi lóu rú guī bèi* | 背僂如龜背 | 485 |
| hundred diseases of wind taxation | *fēng láo bǎi bìng* | 風勞百病 | 423 |
| hunger | *dà jī* | 大飢 | 152, 169, 736 |
| hunger but no desire to eat | *jī bù yù shí* | 飢不欲食 | 297 |
| hunger with inability to eat | *jī bù néng shí* | 飢不能食 | 294, 438, 723 |
| hyperactive tongue | *nòng shé* | 弄舌 | 369 |
| hypertonicity and pain of the knees | *liǎng xī luán tòng* | 兩膝攣痛 | 537 |
| hypertonicity and pain of the low back and spine | *yāo jí luán tòng* | 腰脊攣痛 | 550, 552, 554 |
| hypertonicity and pain of the sinews and bones | *jīn gǔ luán tòng* | 筋骨攣痛 | 424 |
| hypertonicity and pain of the smaller abdomen | *xiǎo fù jū jí tòng* | 小腹拘急痛 | 209 |
| hypertonicity between the shoulders and chest | *jiān yǐn xiōng bì luán jí* | 肩引胸臂攣急 | 493 |
| hypertonicity of the arms | *shǒu bì luán jí* | 手臂攣急 | 397, 494, 693 |
| hypertonicity of the arms and elbows | *shǒu bì zhǒu luán* | 手臂肘攣 | 500–501 |
| hypertonicity of the arms and wrists | *bì wàn jí* | 臂腕急 | 495 |
| hypertonicity of the arms with inability to stretch | *shǒu luán bù shēn* | 手攣不伸 | 666 |
| hypertonicity of the axilla | *yè jū luán* | 腋拘攣 | 496, 499 |
| hypertonicity of the back | *bèi jū jí* | 背拘急 | 218, 484 |
| hypertonicity of the back and arms | *bèi bó jū jí* | 背膊拘急 | 484 |
| hypertonicity of the chest and back | *xiōng bèi jū jí* | 胸背拘急 | 305, 484 |
| hypertonicity of the elbows | *zhǒu luán* | 肘攣 | 317, 347, 377, 383, 495, 497, 501, 673 |
| hypertonicity of the elbows and propping fullness | *zhǒu luán zhī mǎn* | 肘攣支滿 | 500 |
| hypertonicity of the elbows with stiffness and distention | *zhǒu luán zhù mǎn* | 肘攣柱滿 | 499 |
| hypertonicity of the eyes | *mù nèi luán* | 目內攣 | 569 |
| hypertonicity of the finger joints | *shǒu jié luán suō* | 手節攣縮 | 372 |
| hypertonicity of the fists | *quán luán* | 拳攣 | 368 |
| hypertonicity of the hands | *shǒu luán* | 手攣 | 267, 305, 498, 505 |

| | | | |
|---|---|---|---|
| inability to breathe | *bù dé xī* | 不得息 | 214–215, 267, 272, 284, 307, 312–313, 319, 364, 407–410, 418–419, 421, 427, 430–432, 445, 450, 453, 457, 462, 470, 472–473, 478–480, 490, 534, 546, 600, 612–613, 620–621, 643, 675–676, 733, 735, 737 |
| inability to breathe when sitting up or laying down | *zuò fú bù dé xī* | 坐伏不得息 | 425 |
| inability to chew | *bù kě jué* | 不可嚼 | 591, 606, 609 |
| inability to chew food | *chǐ yá bù jué wù* | 齒牙不嚼物 | 16 |
| inability to chew with pain and swelling from tooth decay | *chǐ yá bù jué wù, qǔ tòng zhǒng* | 齒牙不嚼物，齲痛腫 | 601 |
| inability to close the eyes | *mù bù hé* | 目不合 | 326, 570, 572, 592, 656 |
| inability to contract the lips | *chún wěn bù shōu* | 唇吻不收 | 599, 608, 632, 656 |
| inability to cough | *bù kě ké* | 不可咳 | 403, 548 |
| inability to defecate | *bù dé dà biàn* | 不得大便 | 235, 249, 446 |
| inability to digest food | *shí yǐn bù xiāo* | 食飲不消 | 552, 729 |
| inability to drink water | *bù dé yǐn shuǐ* | 不得飲水 | 593 |
| inability to eat | *bù shí* | 不食 | 251, 259, 278, 288–289, 292, 294–295, 298–299, 313–314, 318, 337, 367, 382, 390, 407, 424, 427, 432–433, 438, 442, 445, 448, 454–456, 464, 526, 535, 624–625, 631, 665, 668, 681, 723, 730 |
| inability to eat and drink | *bù néng yǐn shí* | 不能飲食 | 399 |
| inability to eat or drink | *yǐn shí quán bù jìn* | 飲食全不進 | 41, 74 |
| inability to engender flesh and skin | *bù zuò jī fū* | 不作肌膚 | 252 |
| inability to feel pain | *bù zhī suǒ tòng* | 不知所痛 | 331 |
| inability to feel warm | *bù néng wēn* | 不能溫 | 533 |
| inability to feel where it hurts | *bù zhī suǒ tòng* | 不知所痛 | 384 |
| inability to flex and stretch | *bù dé qū shēn* | 不得屈伸 | 230, 271, 377, 484, 488, 491, 494, 501, 505–506, 516–517, 536, 539, 541, 543, 554, 683, 697, 702, 704 |
| inability to flex and stretch the knees | *xī bù néng qū shēn* | 膝不能屈伸 | 540, 553 |
| inability to flex and stretch the shoulders and arms | *jiān bì bù dé qū shēn* | 肩臂不得屈伸 | 489 |
| inability to flex and stretch the toes | *zhǐ bù dé qū shēn* | 指不得屈伸 | 515, 707 |
| inability to flex the knees | *xī bù dé qū shēn* | 膝不得屈伸 | 146, 536 |
| inability to flex the knees after stretching | *xī shēn bù dé qū* | 膝伸不得屈 | 540 |
| inability to get drinks down | *yǐn yǐn bù xià* | 引飲不下 | 305 |
| inability to get food down | *bù dé xià shí* | 不得下食 | 63, 275–276, 290, 348, 412, 443, 482–483, 668, 698 |
| inability to get up when sitting | *zuò bù néng qǐ* | 坐不能起 | 496, 512, 536, 538 |
| inability to get warm even when wearing thick clothing | *zhòng yì bù dé wen* | 重衣不得溫 | 557 |

| | | | |
|---|---|---|---|
| oppression and derangement in the heart | *xīn zhōng kuì luàn* | 心中憒亂 | 181, 380 |
| oppression and derangement in the heart and chest | *xīn xiōng mèn luàn* | 心胸悶亂 | 181 |
| oppression and heat | *mèn rè* | 悶熱 | 295, 337, 522–523 |
| oppression due to phlegm | *tán mèn* | 痰悶 | 400, 429 |
| oppression due to wind | *fēng mèn* | 風悶 | 640 |
| oppression of the back and scapulae | *bèi jiǎ mèn* | 背胛悶 | 484 |
| oppression of the chest | *xīn zhōng mèn* | 心中悶 | 319, 330, 422, 471, 475, 481, 634 |
| oppression of the chest and diaphragm | *xiōng gé mèn* | 胸膈悶 | 481, 634 |
| oppression of the heart | *xīn mèn* | 心悶 | 225, 330, 336–337, 363, 366, 666, 672, 686, 736 |
| oppressive ghost dreams [nightmares] | *mèng yǎn* | 夢魘 | 342 |
| orange | *jú* | 橘 | 166, 734 |
| original qì is the root | *yuán qì wéi běn* | 元氣為本 | 176 |
| original yáng | *yuán yáng* | 元陽 | 177 |
| other day | *tā rì* | 他日 | 3, 301, 316, 381 |
| other diseases in the abdomen | *fù zhōng yú jí* | 腹中餘疾 | 206 |
| ouch point | *ā shì* | 阿是 | 164 |
| outer | *wài jiān* | 外間 | 27, 143, 158, 389, 391, 537, 540–541, 568–569, 577, 587, 589, 595, 625, 647–648, 655, 671, 683 |
| outpour diarrhea | *xiè zhù* | 泄注 | 241, 244–245, 249–250, 252, 260, 264, 271, 364, 424, 451, 742 |
| outpour diarrhea with precipitation of blood | *lì zhù xià xuè* | 痢注下血 | 250 |
| outside the sinews | *wài jīn* | 外筋 | 64 |
| over-eating | *shí duō* | 食多 | 79, 300 |
| oversized patients | *féi rén* | 肥人 | 72 |
| ox epilepsy | *niú xián* | 牛癇 | 358 |
| ox epilepsy in children | *xiǎo ér niú xián* | 小兒牛癇 | 368 |
| **P** | | | |
| pain along the eyebrows | *xún méi tòng* | 循眉痛 | 575 |
| pain along the spine | *jiā jǐ tòng* | 夾脊痛 | 667 |
| pain and fullness of the abdomen and rib-sides | *fù xié tòng mǎn* | 腹脅痛滿 | 480 |
| pain and fullness under the heart | *xīn xià tòng mǎn* | 心下痛滿 | 430 |
| pain and hardness under the rib-sides | *xié xià jiān tòng* | 脅下堅痛 | 479 |
| pain and itching of the pupils | *mù tóng zǐ tòng yǎng* | 目瞳子痛癢 | 568 |
| pain and swelling due to tooth decay | *qǔ tòng zhǒng* | 齲痛腫 | 16 |
| pain and swelling with inability to cough | *zhǒng tòng bù kě ké* | 腫痛不可咳 | 548 |
| pain and weakness in the anterior aspect of the medial malleolus | *nèi huái qián tòng yín luò* | 內踝前痛淫濼 | 218 |
| pain and weakness of the four limbs | *sì zhī yín luò* | 四肢淫濼 | 219, 225, 736 |

| | | | |
|---|---|---|---|
| posterior hairline | *hòu fà jì* | 後髮際 | 156, 622 |
| posterior to the ear | *ěr hòu* | 耳後 | 15, 17–18 |
| posterior to the root of the ear | *ěr běn hòu* | 耳本後 | 17 |
| postpartum blood dizziness | *chǎn hòu xuè yùn* | 產後血暈 | 732 |
| postpartum diseases | *chǎn hòu yú jí* | 產後餘疾 | 430, 446, 731 |
| postpartum pain all over the body | *fù rén chǎn hòu hún shēn téng* | 婦人產後渾身疼 | 731 |
| pounds up into the throat | *shàng zhú yàn hóu* | 上築咽喉 | 284 |
| pregnancy | *rèn shēn* | 妊娠 | 78, 99, 127, 201, 461, 725–726, 730–732, 734, 740, 742 |
| pregnant woman | *rèn fù* | 妊婦 | 127, 732 |
| preoccupation | *lǜ* | 慮 | 182, 530 |
| prickly wind | *cì fēng* | 刺風 | 522, 705 |
| profuse discharge from the eyes | *duō chī miè* | 多眵瞜 | 584 |
| profuse nasal mucus | *duō bí tì* | 多鼻涕 | 5 |
| profuse sweating | *duō hàn* | 多汗 | 252, 306, 322, 569, 578, 645, 662, 678, 685, 687–688 |
| profuse tearing | *duō lèi* | 多淚 | 573, 584 |
| prognosis | *sǐ shēng* | 死生 | 117 |
| progressively worsening dizzy vision | *mù xuàn yín yín* | 目眩淫淫 | 577 |
| prolapse of the rectum in adults and children | *dà rén 、xiǎo ér tuō gāng* | 大人 、小兒脫肛 | 266 |
| prolapsed rectum | *tuō gāng* | 脫肛 | 40 |
| prolapsed rectum and bloody diarrhea in children | *xiǎo ér tuō gāng xiè xuè* | 小兒脫肛瀉血 | 258 |
| prolapsed rectum in the late fall | *qiū mò tuō gāng* | 秋末脫肛 | 251 |
| prolonged periods | *yuè shì guò shí bù zhǐ* | 月事過時不止 | 738 |
| prominent *shàn*-mounting | *tuí shàn* | 癪疝 | 198–199, 202–203, 205–211, 214, 216, 223–224, 227–228, 239, 243, 259, 268, 276, 281, 323, 468, 537, 540, 542, 544, 546, 554, 557, 628, 689, 729 |
| prominent *shàn*-mounting in men | *zhàng fū tuí shàn* | 丈夫癪疝 | 215 |
| promote stomach qì | *zī wèi qì* | 資胃氣 | 181 |
| prone position | *miǎn* | 俛 | 39–41, 56–57, 146, 160 |
| pronounced cold | *duō hán* | 多寒 | 306, 331 |
| proportional measurement same-body cùn | *tóng shēn cùn* | 同身寸 | 42, 60, 157 |
| propping fullness | *zhī mǎn* | 支滿 | 296, 382, 403, 425, 500–501, 587, 674, 735 |
| propping fullness and pain of the rib-sides | *jì xié zhī mǎn tòng* | 季脅支滿痛 | 661 |
| propping fullness of the abdomen and rib-sides | *fù xié zhī mǎn* | 腹脅支滿 | 215 |

## R

## S

| | | | |
|---|---|---|---|
| stuffy chest | *xiōng mǎn sāi* | 胸滿塞 | 630 |
| sudden and violent epilepsy and dizziness | *cù bào xián xuàn* | 卒暴癇眩 | 357 |
| sudden blockage | *bào bì sāi* | 暴閉塞 | 737 |
| sudden bouts of cold and heat | *zhà hán zhà rè* | 乍寒乍熱 | 269, 666, 676, 679 |
| sudden bouts of crying | *zhà kū* | 乍哭 | 333 |
| sudden collapse after getting up | *zú qǐ jiāng pū* | 卒起僵仆 | 531 |
| sudden collapse with inability to stand for long | *jiāng pū bù néng jiǔ lì* | 僵仆不能久立 | 531 |
| sudden coughing | *zú ké nì* | 卒咳逆 | 421 |
| sudden counterflow in the chest | *xiōng zhōng bào nì* | 胸中暴逆 | 471 |
| sudden counterflow in the rib-sides | *xié zhōng bào nì* | 脅中暴逆 | 629 |
| sudden deafness | *bào dé ěr lóng* | 暴得耳聾 | 303, 564–566, 702 |
| sudden deafness in the ears | *ěr bào lóng* | 耳暴聾 | 564–565 |
| sudden death | *zú sǐ* | 卒死 | 381, 389, 531, 535 |
| sudden death due to ghost strike | *guǐ jī zú sǐ* | 鬼擊卒死 | 530 |
| sudden deathlike reversal | *zú shī jué* | 卒尸厥 | 531, 533 |
| sudden dizziness | *hū tóu xuán* | 忽頭旋 | 569, 579 |
| sudden dry vomiting | *zú yuě* | 卒噦 | 280 |
| sudden facial swelling | *zú miàn zhǒng* | 卒面腫 | 349, 657 |
| sudden fright | *bào jīng* | 暴驚 | 323 |
| sudden green color and pricking pain of the feet | *zú zú qīng tòng rú cì* | 足卒青痛如刺 | 532 |
| sudden heart pain | *zú xīn tòng* | 卒心痛 | 312, 319, 321 |
| sudden infixation attacking the heart and chest | *zú zhù wǔ gōng xīn xiōng* | 卒疰忤攻心胸 | 535 |
| sudden loss of consciousness | *zú bù shí rén* | 卒不識人 | 13, 375, 383–384 |
| sudden loss of speech | *bào yǎ bù néng yán* | 暴啞不能言 | 593, 608 |
| sudden loss of voice | *bào yīn* | 暴喑 | 595 |
| sudden loss of voice and inability to speak | *bào yīn bù néng yán* | 暴喑不能言 | 317, 594, 596 |
| sudden lower back pain | *yāo zú tòng* | 腰卒痛 | 549 |
| sudden malignity strike | *cù zhòng è* | 卒中惡 | 532, 534 |
| sudden mania | *cù kuáng* | 卒狂 | 347, 351, 693 |
| sudden manic raving | *cù kuáng yán* | 卒狂言 | 351 |
| sudden onset of abdominal distention | *bào fù zhàng* | 暴腹脹 | 450 |
| sudden onset of abdominal fullness | *fù bào mǎn* | 腹暴滿 | 447 |
| sudden onset of flesh *bì*-impediment | *cù bìng ròu bì* | 卒病肉痹 | 378 |
| sudden onset of screens in the eyes | *mù cù shēng yì* | 目卒生翳 | 586 |
| sudden onset of wind stroke | *cù zhòng fēng* | 卒中風 | 383, 395 |
| sudden pain | *cù tòng* | 卒痛 | 313, 320, 545, 547 |
| sudden pain of the heart and abdomen | *xīn fù zhōng cù tòng* | 心腹中卒痛 | 320 |
| sudden pain of the lower and upper back | *yāo bèi cù tòng* | 腰背卒痛 | 545, 547 |
| sudden prolapse of the uterus | *yīn bào chū* | 陰暴出 | 722 |

| | | | |
|---|---|---|---|
| tetany | *jìng* | 痓 | 250, 270, 283, 307, 324, 355–356, 360–361, 373–374, 555, 594, 608, 610, 633, 675, 687, 722 |
| tetany with qì ascent | *jìng shàng qì* | 痓上氣 | 596 |
| the arm is unable to reach up to the head | *bù de shàng tóu* | 不得上頭 | 96 |
| the big toe | *zú dà zhǐ* | 足大指 | 117–118, 126, 137, 187, 219, 242, 252, 319, 342, 351, 353, 388, 532, 534, 623, 662, 687, 710, 742 |
| the corner of the nail | *qù zhuǎ jiǎ jiǎo* | 去爪甲角 | 93, 98, 104, 107, 113, 117, 121, 126, 129, 141, 158, 326 |
| the cross-like crease at the seam on the back of the scrotum | *náng hòu fèng shí zì wén* | 囊後縫十字紋 | 216 |
| the disease was acquired internally | *bìng dé zhī nèi* | 病得之內 | 298 |
| the dorsum of wrist | *shǒu biǎo wàn* | 手表腕 | 114 |
| the feet cannot step on the ground | *zú bù dé jiàn dì* | 足不得踐地 | 180, 461 |
| the fetus usually will not come out | *tāi duō bù chū* | 胎多不出 | 78 |
| the five dysphagias | *wǔ yē* | 五噎 | 481 |
| the food enters the abdomen then comes back out | *rù fù huán chū* | 入腹還出 | 289 |
| the four limbs | *sì zhī* | 四肢 | 164–165, 179, 211, 215, 219, 225, 243, 252, 269, 298, 339, 345, 372, 377, 415, 497, 512, 529, 688, 736 |
| the fourth toe | *zú xiǎo zhǐ cì zhǐ* | 足小指次指 | 121–122 |
| the ghost is busy singing and crying | *guǐ máng gē kū* | 鬼忙歌哭 | 344 |
| the hundred diseases | *bǎi bìng* | 百病 | 195, 384, 404, 409, 423, 535, 552, 670 |
| the hundred diseases also arise out of the kidneys | *bǎi bìng jiē shēng yú shèn* | 百病皆生於腎 | 194 |
| the hundred diseases are all governed | *bǎi bìng jiē zhǔ* | 百病皆主 | 4 |
| the hundred diseases arise out of the heart | *bǎi bìng jiē shēng yú xīn* | 百病皆生於心 | 194 |
| the hundred diseases with edema | *bǎi bìng shuǐ zhǒng* | 百病水腫 | 464 |
| the hundred types of wind | *bǎi zhǒng fēng* | 百種風 | 390 |
| the lower legs tend to be thin | *zú jìng piān xì* | 足脛偏細 | 517 |
| the middle finger | *shǒu zhōng zhǐ* | 手中指 | 32, 44, 109–110, 125, 133, 156–158, 187, 332, 372, 504, 570, 586, 609–610, 706 |
| the nail | *zhuǎ jiǎ* | 爪甲 | 93, 98, 104, 107, 109, 113, 117, 121, 126, 129, 141, 158, 219, 242, 326, 332, 343, 351, 353, 522, 532, 534, 635 |
| the palm | *zhǎng* | 掌 | 95, 97, 104–106, 109–111, 302, 344 |
| the qì meets in the sānjiāo | *qì huì sān jiāo* | 氣會三焦 | 64 |
| the qì spreads the yīn and yáng | *qì bù yīn yáng* | 氣布陰陽 | 63 |
| the qì surges upward into the eyes | *qì shàng chōng mù* | 氣上衝目 | 133 |

## U

# W

## X



## Y

# Formulas

# Medicinals

| | | |
|---|---|---|
| *nì fěn* 膩粉 | calomel | 381 |
| *péng é mào* 蓬莪茂 | Curcumae Rhizome | 309 |
| *pò gù zhǐ* 破故紙 | Psoralea Fructus | 299 |
| *pǔ xiāo* 朴硝 | Natrii Sulfas Non-purus | 716 |
| *qīng nèn liǔ pí* 青嫩柳皮 | green tender willow bark | 168 |
| *quán xiē* 全蝎 | scorpions | 194 |
| *rén shēn* 人参 | Ginseng | 391 |
| *rěn dōng cǎo* 忍冬草 | | 703 |
| *ròu dòu kòu* 肉豆蔻 | nutmeg, Myristicae Semen | 299 |
| *sháo yào* 芍藥 | Paeoniae Radix | 583 |
| *shé chuáng zǐ* 蛇床子 | Cnidii Fructus | 713 |
| *shén qū* 神曲 | Medicated Leaven | 247 |
| *shēng dì huáng* 生地黃 | Fresh Rehmanniae | 370 |
| *shēng jiāng* 生薑 | Ginger | 17, 370 |
| *shí gāo* 石膏 | Gypsum Crudum | 17, 370 |
| *sū zǐ* 蘇子 | Perillae Fructus | 238 |
| *suān zǎo rén* 酸棗仁 | Spiny Jujube Semen | 341 |
| *suō shā rén* 縮砂仁 | Amomi Villosi Semen seu Fructus | 194 |
| *táo zhī* 桃枝 | peach twig | 168 |
| *tiān nán xīng* 天南星 | Arisaematis Rhizoma | 701 |
| *tiě jiāng* 鐵漿 | Ferri Aqua | 696 |
| *tíng lì zǐ* 葶藶子 | Lipidii Semen | 256 |
| *tù fù shàng bái xì máo* 兔腹上白細毛 | fine white fur from a rabbit's abdomen in the winter | 168 |
| *wáng bù líu xíng zǐ* 王不留行子 | Vaccariae Semen | 225 |
| *wū méi* 烏梅 | Mume Fructus | 250, 730 |
| *wú zhū yú* 吳茱萸 | Evodiae Fructus | 248 |
| *wǔ bèi zǐ* 五倍子 | Galla Chinensis Galla | 225 |
| *wǔ líng zhǐ* 五靈脂 | Trogopteri Faeces Frictum | 310 |
| *wǔ wèi zǐ* 五味子 | Schisandrae Fructus | 191, 196, 248 |
| *xiāng bái zhǐ* 香白芷 | Angelicae Dahuricae Radix | 734 |
| *xīn mián* 新棉 | new cotton | 168 |
| *xìng rén* 杏仁 | Armeniacae Semen | 247 |
| *xiōng qióng* 芎窮 | Chuān Xiōng Root | 247 |
| *xióng huáng* 雄黃 | Realgar | 717 |
| *yán hú suǒ* 延胡索 | Corydalis Rhizome | 310 |
| *yáng tí cài* 羊蹄菜 | Cnidii Fructus | 713 |
| *yīn chén* 茵陳 | Artemisiae Scopariae Herba | 671 |
| *yīng sù ké* 罌粟殼 | Papaveris Pericarpium | 250 |
| *yú yú liáng* 禹餘糧 | Limonite | 463 |
| *zào jiá zǐ* 皂莢子 | Gleditsiae Semen | 710 |
| *zào jiǎo* 皂角 | Gleditsia | 168 |

# The Chinese Medicine Database

## www.cm-db.com

The Chinese Medicine Database has been organized around one central principle -- translation of Classical Asian texts, and dissemination of that information.

There are thousands of Asian medicine texts that have never been translated. We have compiled a small list on our website of the ones that we have found, but we believe that there are tens of thousands of documents that span from the *Hàn* Dynasty to pre-Republican times. Most of these documents will never be read by people in the West, simply because of lack of translation.

We have created a vehicle, that allows interested practitioners, students, institutions, and scholars to help support and fund the translation of these documents, and then mine and synthesize the data that is gained from these texts.

### The Database contains:

**Monographs on:**

690 Single Herbs
1510 Formulas
Mayway's Patents
ITM's Formulations
Golden Flowers Formulations
Classical Pearls Formulations by Heiner Fruehauf
OBGYN Modifications to Formulas
Single Points: the 361 Regular Points
Time Line of the History of Chinese Medicine

**Beer Hall Lecture Series**

Watch videos from our monthly Beer Hall lecture series with guest speakers such as: Arnaud Versluys, Subhuti Dharmananda, Jason Robertson, Craig Mitchell, Michael Max, Lorraine Wilcox, and Ed Neal.

**Play STORT**

Play our free online game STORT where you can learn Chinese while having a bit of fun (www.cm-db.com/stort).

**15,000 Western Diagnoses with ICD-9 Codes**

**A Chinese-English dictionary:**

Containing over 102,943 terms, including the Eastland and the WHO term sets.

**A Western Book search containing:**

Fenner's Complete Formulary
by B. Fenner

The 1918 Dispensatory of the United States of America
Edited by Joseph P. Remington, Horatio C. Woods and others
The Eclectic Materia Medica, Pharmacology and Therapeutics
by Harvey Wickes Felter, M.D.

**A Personal Dashboard, which allows users to:**

Blog
Take notes on any monograph.
Search for other users by city, state, country and name.
Make friends all around the world.
Share and compare notes with friends.
Personalize your dashboard by adding photos, and information about your practice.

**Translations:**

| | | |
|---|---|---|
| Shāng Hán Lái Sū Jí | 傷寒來蘇集 | Renewal of Treatise on Cold Damage |
| Qí Jīng Bā Mài Kǎo | 奇經八脈考 | Explanation of the Eight Vessels of the Marvellous Meridians |
| Shāng Hán Míng Lǐ Lùn | 傷寒明理論 | Treatise on Enlightening the Principles of Cold Damage |
| Wú Jū Tōng Yī Àn | 吴鞠通医案 | Case Studies of Wú Jūtōng |
| The Nàn Jīng | 難經 | The Classic of Difficulties |
| The Zàng Fǔ Biāo Běn Hán Rè Xū Shí Yòng Yào Shì | 臓腑標本寒熱虛實用藥式 | Viscera and Bowels, Tip and Root, Cold and Heat, Vacuity and Repletion Model for Using Medicinals |
| Wēn Rè Lún | 温熱論 | Treatise on Warm Heat Disease |
| Shāng Hán Shé Jiàn | 傷寒舌鑒 | Tongue Mirror of Cold Damage |
| Xǔ Shì Yī Àn | 許氏醫案 | Case Histories of Master Xǔ |
| Fǔ Xìng Jué Zāng Fǔ Yòng Yào Fǎ Yào | 輔行決臟腑用藥法要 | Secret Instructions for Assisting the Body: Essential Methods for the Application of Drugs to the Viscera & Bowels |
| Biāo Yōu Fù | 標幽賦 | Indicating the Obscure |
| Liú Juān Zǐ Guǐ Yí Fāng | 劉涓子鬼遺方 | Liu Juanzi's Formulas Inherited from Ghosts |
| Shèn Jí Chú Yán | 慎疾芻言 | Precautions in Illness: My Humble Thoughts |
| Yào Zhèng Jì Yí | 藥症忌宜 | Medicinals & Patterns Contraindications & Appropriate [Choices] |
| Fù Kē Wèn Dá | 婦科問答 | Questions and Answers in Gynecology |
| Nèi Jīng Zhī Yào | 內經知要 | Essential Knowledge from the Nèijīng |
| Běn Cǎo Bèi Yào | 本草備要 | The Essential Completion of Traditional Materia Medica |
| Bǎi Zhèng Fù (Jù Yīng) | 百症賦《聚英》 | Ode of the Hundred Diseases from The Great Compendium of Acupuncture-Moxibustion |

**Benefits:**

Subscribers to the Database receive a 10% discount on our published books when they are in pre-release.

We translate texts as often, and in quantities that reflect our user base. The larger amount of subscribers that we have, the more translation that we can accomplish.

## Published Books:

2008 Bèi Jí Qiān Jīn Yào Fāng 備急千金要方: Essential Prescriptions Worth a Thousand Gold Pieces For Emergencies. vol. 2-4 by Sūn Sīmiǎo 孫思邈
Translated by Sabine Wilms.
ISBN 978-0-9799552-0-4
Out of Print

2010 Zhēn Jiǔ Dà Chéng 針灸大成: The Great Compendium of Acupuncture & Moxibustion vol. I by Yáng Jìzhōu 楊繼洲
Translated by Sabine Wilms.
ISBN 978-0-9799552-2-8

2010 Zhēn Jiǔ Dà Chéng 針灸大成: The Great Compendium of Acupuncture & Moxibustion vol. V by Yáng Jìzhōu 楊繼洲
Translated by Lorraine Wilcox.
ISBN 978-0-9799552-4-2

2010 Jīn Guì Fāng Gē Kuò 金匱方歌括: Formulas from the Golden Cabinet with Songs vol. I - III by Chén Xiūyuán 陳修園
Translated by Sabine Wilms.
ISBN 978-0-9799552-5-9

2011 Zhēn Jiǔ Dà Chéng 針灸大成: The Great Compendium of Acupuncture & Moxibustion vol. VIII by Yáng Jìzhōu 楊繼洲
Translated by Yue Lu.
ISBN 978-0-9799552-7-3

2011 Zhēn Jiǔ Dà Chéng 針灸大成: The Great Compendium of Acupuncture & Moxibustion vol. IX by Yáng Jìzhōu 楊繼洲
Translated by Lorraine Wilcox.
ISBN 978-0-9799552-6-6

2012 Raising the Dead and Returning Life: Emergency Medicine of the Qīng Dynasty by Bào Xiāng'áo 鮑相璈
Translated by Lorraine Wilcox.
ISBN 978-0-9799552-3-5

2014 Zhēn Jiǔ Zī Shēng Jīng 針灸資生經: The Classic of Supporting Life with Acupuncture and Moxibustion Vol. I-III by Wáng Zhízhōng 王執中
Translated by Yue Lu.
ISBN 978-0-9799552-1-1

2014 Jīn Guì Fāng Gē Kuò 金匱方歌括: Formulas from the Golden Cabinet with Songs vol. IV - VI by Chén Xiūyuán 陳修園
Translated by Eran Even.
ISBN 978-0-9799552-8-0

www.ingramcontent.com/pod-product-compliance
Lightning Source LLC
LaVergne TN
LVHW082013200926
848481LV00010B/2847
*9780979955297*